FETAL PHYSIOLOGY AND MEDICINE

FETAL PHYSIOLOGY AND MEDICINE

The Basis of Perinatology

EDITED BY

RICHARD W. BEARD, MD, FRCOG

Professor of Obstetrics and Gynaecology, St Mary's Hospital Medical School, London

AND

PETER W. NATHANIELSZ, PhD, MB, BChir

University Lecturer, Physiological Laboratory Cambridge

1976

W. B. Saunders Company Ltd   London · Philadelphia · Toronto

W. B. Saunders Company Ltd: 1 St. Anne's Road
Eastbourne, East Sussex BN21 3UN

West Washington Square
Philadelphia, Pa. 19105

833 Oxford Street
Toronto, Ontario M8Z 5T9

Fetal Physiology and Medicine   ISBN 0–7216–1600–3

Library of Congress Catalog Card Number 76–20126

Text set in 11 pt Photon Times, printed by photolithography, and bound in Great Britain at The Pitman Press, Bath

Last digit is print no: 9 8 7 6 5 4 3 2 1

PREFACE

It was said that Isaac Newton was so premature at birth he could have been fitted into a quart pot. He was born probably in the total absence of any obstetric care, far less the aid of fetal monitors, so why is it that modern obstetrics is so obsessed with care of the fetus? The reason is that, for every Newton, there are a multitude of normal babies who later fail to develop their potential simply because Nature is capricious and cannot be relied upon to protect the fetus from permanent injury.

Modern perinatal medicine has evolved from the convergence of two disciplines—fetal physiology and clinical obstetrics. It was the genius of Barcroft working in Cambridge who recognised that all physiology has its origin in the development that follows the union of sperm and ovum. He and his disciples laid the basis of our present day understanding of intra-uterine life by mapping out the development, function, maternal–fetal inter-relationships, defence mechanisms and finally the adaptive processes occurring at birth. This development has coincided with the growing recognition that the first priority of a mother in particular and of society in general is the delivery of a baby capable of achieving his or her full potential in adult life.

The practice of perinatal medicine started when obstetricians, having resolved most of the problems of the mother, turned their attention to the fetus. Recording of the fetal heart rate has for many years been the only window available to the obstetrician through which to observe the condition of the fetus—a cloudy view of a world full of activity. It was therefore natural that efforts should be made to improve the technology of observation, with the result that systems such as continuous recording of the instantaneous fetal heart rate evolved. At the same time the function of the placenta and indirectly the condition of the fetus were investigated by measuring the many hormones and enzymes produced by that organ. The logic of this approach has often been questioned because so little is known of the physiological purpose of many of the substances manufactured by the placenta. Although a degree of clinical success has been achieved by using the absolute and relative changes in concentration of these substances to predict fetal death, how much more insight into the condition of the fetus would we have if we knew the role of these hormones relative to intra-uterine life?

To many physiologists and obstetricians it seems quite incomprehensible that our two disciplines have taken so long to recognise the need for each other. Clinicians know that the development of techniques for assessing the condition of the fetus cannot progress without knowledge of fetal life which is unobtainable from the human fetus. This basic information is vital in the ultimate establishment of successful intra-uterine therapy. Equally many physiologists acknowledge that fetal physiology, so dependent on the animal model, has limited purpose if it is not ultimately used for the benefit of the human. There are few who

v

would dispute that we should come together, but what is now required is an understanding of each other's needs and, with it, a language that is common to us all.

In this book we have attempted to bring together much of the knowledge of fetal life that is the product of physiological and clinical research. We recognise that the book is not entirely comprehensive, but this is largely a reflection of the almost day-to-day advances that are being made in the subject. The design of the book and the selection of subjects has the objective of stimulating those who have the interest of the fetus at heart, whether as obstetricians taking postgraduate examinations or as research workers seeking information on some aspect of fetal life. It is hoped that it will prove possible to keep the content up to date by frequent revision and reissue of the book.

We, as editors, are grateful to all who have made this book a reality—to the contributors, who so willingly agreed to join the venture, to the publishers, W. B. Saunders, for their faith in us and to our long-suffering assistant Miss Cynthia Knight.

London, 1976   Richard W. Beard
Cambridge, 1976   Peter W. Nathanielsz

CONTRIBUTORS

M. C. ADINOLFI, MD, PhD, Senior Lecturer, Paediatric Research Unit, Guy's Hospital Medical School, London.

EVA ALBERMAN, MD, MFCM, Reader in Child Health, London School of Hygiene and Tropical Medicine; Research Epidemiologist, Paediatric Research Unit, Guy's Hospital Medical School, London.

PETER BAILLIE, MD, FCOG(SA), MRCOG, part-time Lecturer, Department of Obstetrics, University of Cape Town; part-time specialist, Groote Schuur Hospital and Mowbray Maternity Hospital, Cape Town, South Africa.

R. J. BARNES, MA, MB, Demonstrator in Physiology, University of Cambridge.

JOHN M. BASSETT, PhD, Senior Research Officer, Nuffield Institute for Medical Research, University of Oxford.

R. W. BEARD, MD, FRCOG, Professor of Obstetrics and Gynaecology, St Mary's Hospital Medical School, London.

W. D. BILLINGTON, MA, BSc, PhD, Senior Lecturer, Department of Pathology, The Medical School, University of Bristol.

K. BODDY, MB, BS, MRCOG, Senior Lecturer, Department of Obstetrics and Gynaecology, University of Edinburgh; Consultant, Simpson Memorial Maternity Pavilion, Edinburgh.

STUART CAMPBELL, MRCOG, Professor of Obstetrics and Gynaecology, King's College Hospital Medical School, London.

JOHN R. G. CHALLIS, PhD, Junior Research Fellow, Wolfson College, Oxford; Research Scientist, John Radcliffe Hospital and the Nuffield Department of Obstetrics and Gynaecology, University of Oxford.

T. CHARD, MD, FRCOG, Professor of Reproductive Physiology, St Bartholomew's Hospital Medical College, London.

LAWRENCE CHIK, PhD, Assistant Professor of Biomedical Engineering, Department of Reproductive Biology, Case Western Reserve University; Co-director, Biomedical Engineering, Perinatal Clinical Research Center, Cleveland Metropolitan General Hospital, Cleveland, Ohio.

PAMELA DAVIES, MD, FRCP, Senior Lecturer, Institute of Child Health, University of London; Honorary Consultant Paediatrician, Hammersmith Hospital, London.

P. F. FAIRBROTHER, BA, BM, MRCOG, Senior Lecturer, University of Natal; Principal Specialist, King Edward VIII Hospital, Durban, Natal, South Africa.

J. J. HOET, MD, Professor of Medicine, University of Louvain; Chief of Clinic, Endocrinology and Nutrition Service, Hôpital St Pierre, Louvain, and Hôpital St Luc, Louvain La Woluwe, Brussels.

D. HULL, BSc, MB, ChB, FRCP, Professor, Department of Child Health, The Medical School, University of Nottingham; Consultant Paediatrician, North and South Nottingham Health Districts.

M. G. R. HULL, MB, BS, MRCOG, Senior Lecturer in Obstetrics and Gynaecology, The Medical School, University of Bristol; Consultant, Bristol Maternity Hospital, Royal Infirmary and General Hospital, Bristol.

P. M. B. JACK, BSc, MA(Cantab.), PhD, Senior Lecturer in Biology, I. M. Marsh College, Liverpool.

COLIN T. JONES, PhD, Research Officer, Nuffield Institute for Medical Research, University of Oxford.

ALFRED JOST, MD, PhD, Professor of Developmental Physiology, Collège de France, Paris.

G. C. LIGGINS, MB, ChB, PhD, FRCOG, FRCS(Ed.), Professor of Obstetrics and Gynaecological Endocrinology, Postgraduate School of Obstetrics and Gynaecology, University of Auckland; Obstetrical and Gynaecological Consultant, National Women's Hospital, Auckland, New Zealand.

B. S. LINDBLAD, MD, Assistant Professor of Paediatrics, Karolinska Institute, Stockholm; Consultant, Department of Obstetrics, St Erik's Hospital, and Paediatric Department, St Goran's Hospital, Stockholm, Sweden.

PETER W. NATHANIELSZ, PhD, MB, BChir, University Lecturer, Physiological Laboratory, Cambridge.

N. W. OAKLEY, MD, MRCP, Senior Lecturer in Human Metabolism, St Mary's Hospital Medical School; Honorary Consultant Physician, St Mary's Hospital, London.

JAMES F. PEARSON, MD, MRCOG, Senior Lecturer, Welsh National School of Medicine; Consultant Obstetrician and Gynaecologist, University Hospital of Wales, Cardiff.

R. H. PHILPOTT, MD, FRCOG, Professor of Obstetrics and Gynaecology, University of Natal; Head of the Department of Obstetrics and Gynaecology, King Edward VIII Hospital, Durban, Natal, South Africa.

P. RENOU, MB, BS, MRCOG, FAGO, Senior Lecturer, Monash University; Director, Fetal Intensive Care Unit, and Honorary Assistant Obstetrician and Gynaecologist, Queen Victoria Memorial Hospital, Melbourne, Australia.

MORTIMER G. ROSEN, MD, Professor of Reproductive Biology, Case Western Reserve University; Director, Department of Obstetrics and Gynecology, Cleveland Metropolitan General Hospital, Cleveland, Ohio.

D. M. SERR, MD, Professor and Head of the Department of Obstetrics and Gynaecology, University of Tel Aviv Medical School; Director, Department of Obstetrics and Gynaecology, Sheba Medical Centre, Tel Hashomer, Israel.

MARIAN SILVER, MA, PhD, Assistant Director of Research, Physiological Laboratory, Cambridge.

ROBERT J. SOKOL, MD, Assistant Professor of Obstetrics and Gynecology, Department of Reproductive Physiology, Case Western Reserve University; Assistant Program Director, Perinatal Clinical Research Center, Cleveland Metropolitan General Hospital, Cleveland, Ohio.

FRANK M. SULLIVAN, BSc, Senior Lecturer, Department of Pharmacology, Guy's Hospital Medical School, London.

GEOFFREY D. THORBURN, MD, BS, BSc(Med.), MRACP, Member of the External Scientific Staff, Medical Research Council; Honorary Consultant Obstetrician and Gynaecologist, John Radcliffe Hospital and the Nuffield Department of Obstetrics and Gynaecology, University of Oxford.

F. A. VAN ASSCHE, MD, PhD, Professor, University of Louvain; Consultant, Department of Obstetrics and Gynaecology, Academische Ziekenhuis St Raphaël, Louvain, Belgium.

C. R. WHITFIELD, MD, FRCOG, Professor of Midwifery, University of Glasgow; Consultant, Queen Mother's Hospital, Glasgow.

C. WOOD, MB, BS, FRCOG, FAGO, Professor, Monash University; Honorary Obstetrician and Gynaecologist, Queen Victoria Memorial Hospital, Melbourne, Australia.

MAUREEN YOUNG, PhD, Reader in Reproductive Physiology, Department of Obstetrics and Gynaecology, St Thomas' Hospital Medical School, London.

CONTENTS

1

SEXUAL DIFFERENTIATION

Alfred Jost

The fulfilment of reproductive function necessitates the cooperation of males and females. In essence reproduction depends upon four physiological processes, namely: (1) the production of the female and male germ cells, which takes place in the gonads; (2) the realisation of conditions which permit these cells to come into contact, to fuse and to produce the fertilised egg cells—this can be achieved only if the male and the female genital apparatuses are properly formed and functional; (3) the male and female must exhibit proper sex drive and sex behaviour; (4) finally, in mammals, the egg should be provided with a favourable uterine environment in which to develop into a newborn animal, and the young should be given postnatal care and education.

The anatomical, physiological, psychological and behavioural differences between males and females, which become more evident during successive developmental stages, stem from the initial chromosomal dissimilarity established at fertilisation (genetic sex). The future sexual structure of the gonadal primordia (gonadal sex) becomes recognisable before the sexual orientation of the genital tract or other sex characters of the body (body sex). Sexual differentiation therefore involves a long series of events and the sex of an individual is determined by a wide range of factors which, under normal circumstances, develop in harmony, but in the case of genetic or environmental anomalies may not conform to this normal pattern.

In this chapter emphasis will be laid on the development of the genital apparatus, not only because a normal genital tract is the indispensable basis of sexual life and of reproduction, but also because the experimental results obtained from studies of sexual development have shed light on the mechanisms underlying differentiation of other systems in the body, e.g. the nervous system and behaviour.

The male and female sex apparatuses do not differentiate synchronously; in mammals the morphological and endocrinological differentiation of the genital tract occurs earlier in males than in females. This chronological difference, as well as some unsolved problems, will be considered first*. The role of hormones and of genetic factors in sexual differentiation of the genital tract and germ cells will then be discussed. Finally a brief section will be devoted to the development of other sex characteristics, for example sex behaviour.

DIFFERENTIATION AND DEVELOPMENT OF THE GENITAL APPARATUS

During an early and brief *presexual phase* of organogenesis in very young fetuses, there is no indication of a genital apparatus. At this stage (less than 5 mm full length) the fetal kidneys (mesonephros) are developing on the dorsal aspect of the abdominal cavity. These nephric

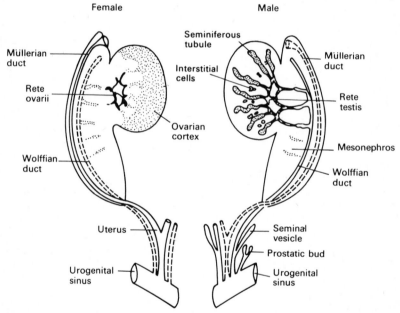

Figure 1.1. Composite scheme showing some homologies in the development of male and female organs from the undifferentiated condition characterised by the presence on the mesonephros of a double set of ducts (wolffian and müllerian ducts) and of a gonadal primordium. In females the wolffian duct and in males the müllerian ducts disappear (interrupted lines). In the presumptive ovaries no ovarian structure has been indicated. From Jost (1970b) with kind permission of the publisher (Berlin: Springer-Verlag).

* In discussing human developmental problems the difficulty of dating young fetuses is met all the time. Age in days is sometimes reckoned from the day of the last missed menses or calculated after subtracting arbitrarily 14 days ('fertilisation age'). The size of the fetus is also a valuable indication because in theory it can be measured with certainty. However, the full length of the fetus or its crown–rump length are difficult to measure in very young fetuses. Moreover, the size and weight of the fetus may be modified by fixative fluids, depending on their concentration. Determinations made on fresh and on fixed fetuses therefore give very different results.

organs will later be intimately related with the development of sex glands and sex ducts (Figures 1.1 and 1.2).

During the presexual period, the mesonephric system comprises bilateral masses made up of undifferentiated cells or developing urinary tubules and an epithelial duct (mesonephric or wolffian duct) extending down to the presumptive urethra. The mesonephros is covered by coelomic epithelium and bulges into the abdominal cavity, the size of the bulge depending on the degree of differentiation.

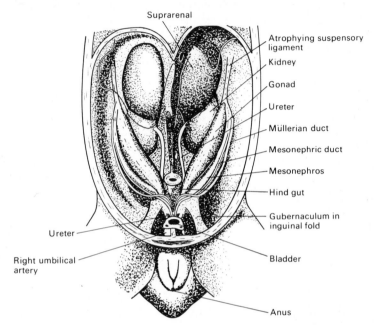

Figure 1.2. A dissection of the posterior abdominal wall in a 26-mm human fetus to show the relationships of the genitourinary apparatus and its associated ducts. The lines of peritoneal reflexion are shown. From Hamilton, Boyd and Mossman (1945) with kind permission of the publisher (London: Macmillan).

The nephric function of the mesonephros is probably unnecessary to the mammalian fetus, and its structure may remain vestigial (for instance, in the rat no true glomeruli are formed). However, the genital system forms in close relation with the mesonephros and in the mammalian fetus the sexual potential of the mesonephros may have transcended its urinary function.

The sexual primordia

The germ cells, i.e. the cells which in the mature individual differentiate into spermatozoa or oocytes, constitute a special line of cells which segregate early in embryonic development. They can first be recognised in varying extragonadal sites, depending on the class of vertebrate (e.g. extra-embryonic germinal crescent of chick embryos, primordial germ cells in the gut of mammalian embryos). In one way or another the primordial germ cells reach the inside of the mesonephros and congregate among or beneath the cells of the coelomic epithelium in the area which becomes the 'genital ridge' or the gonadal primordium. The chemotaxis responsible for the 'attraction' of germ cells into the gonadal primordium has recently been studied in chick embryos (Dubois and Croisille, 1970). In the human fetus, the migration of the primordial germ cells is practically complete by the end of the fifth week postfertilisation (Witschi, 1948).

The gonadal primordium increases in thickness in a way that has not yet been clearly established. Proliferation of cells or proliferation of 'sex cords' from the epithelium have often been invoked. However, no experimental study of the number of mitoses, for instance, has been reported. The word 'cord' itself should be more strictly defined, making clear the distinction between a cord and a haphazard line of nuclei seen in histological section. The gonadal primordium contains large primordial germ cells, usually easily recognisable by histological or histochemical criteria, among a mass of undifferentiated cells. Connecting fibres may be present and a 'basement membrane' may even underlie the superficial cell layer in some places. However, on the whole the somatic cells of the undifferentiated gonadal primordium have an undifferentiated appearance. In many species, especially in the human, this gonadal blastema overlies the Bowman's capsules of the mesonephros.

The primordium is usually referred to as a 'sexually undifferentiated gonad'. However, there are reports in the literature of primordial germ cell counts in the gonadal anlage of bird embryos or of rat fetuses whose genetic sex had been established with the 'sex chromatin' test. These counts displayed differences between male and female embryos before any morphological differentiation of the gonad had occurred. If substantiated or, even better, if complemented by other biochemical differences, these data would suggest that the concept of a sexually indifferent stage in gonadal organogenesis may be questioned. Moreover, it is obvious that an analysis of the sex chromosomes or of the 'sex chromatin' permits an early diagnosis of 'genetic sex' (at least in normal fetuses).

Two other important parts of the presumptive genital tract become recognisable before the stage of about 10 to 15 mm crown–rump (CR) length (sixth week) when the indifferent gonad is formed. These are (1) the genital tubercle (future penis or clitoris), with two lateral genital swellings which later will fuse into a scrotum in males and form the labia majora in females; (2) the primordium of the müllerian ducts, which appears as a bilateral invagination of the coelomic epithelium of the mesonephros at the upper part of the genital ridge. The blind end of this funnel grows along the wolffian duct towards the urogenital sinus, which it reaches much later when the fetus measures 30 mm CR (Figure 1.2). (The müllerian duct which runs alongside the wolffian or mesonephric duct is sometimes called the paramesonephric duct.)

Differentiation of the male genital apparatus

The two sexes can be distinguished morphologically in histological section when in males the gonadal primordium acquires its first testicular characteristics. In the human fetus this occurs when the fetus is around 17 mm CR length, i.e. at approximately the end of the sixth week postfertilisation. In females the gonads remain undifferentiated until much later (Figure 1.3).

Testicular differentiation

The differentiation of the testis from the undifferentiated gonadal anlage involves successive steps:

Differentiation of the seminiferous tubules or seminiferous cords. The first sign of testicular differentiation is the appearance of the future seminiferous tubules or cords, which in their

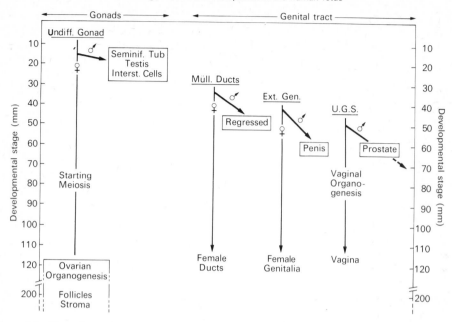

Figure 1.3. Chronology of sexual development indicated according to CR development stage. U.G.S. = urogenital sinus. Adapted from Jost (1972a) with kind permission of the editor of the *Johns Hopkins Medical Journal*.

embryonic condition are solid cellular structures containing the germ cells. The formation of the albuginea testis begins soon afterwards and seems to result from a transformation of the superficial cells into mesenchyme and connective tissue. The mode of differentiation and the origin of the seminiferous tubules have been a subject of controversy for a century. They were reported to arise from a mesonephric proliferation or an ingrowth of 'sex cords' from the superficial epithelium, or from a localised differentiation of the gonadal blastema ('autodifferentiation' of Prenant, 1889). The theory of sex cords is the one most frequently adopted in textbooks. Local differentiation of sex cords in the gonadal blastema has been described by many authors (Felix, 1912 for the human; Brambell, 1927 for the mouse), the usually accepted view being that the blastema is divided into seminiferous tubules by the proliferation and movement of mesenchymal cells. However, by itself this explanation is not sufficient, for the major issue is not the spatial separation of cells but their functional differentiation into testicular cells.

In the rat, the first events that can be recognised in sections are changes occurring at the level of some cells of the blastema (Jost, 1972c). The cells swell, acquire a clear cytoplasm and come into contact either by a large surface or by processes which are extended around germ cells. More and more cells differentiate in this way and make contact with each other. In a 13.5 or 14-day-old rat fetus the seminiferous cord is a structure made up of cells similar to those just described, the early Sertoli cells which encompass the germ cells. Although a definite basement membrane does not appear before day 14.5, the cells of the early seminiferous cord form an entity. This can be demonstrated by placing the testis in a concentrated fixative fluid—the cells constituting the seminiferous tubule shrink together, thus isolating the whole seminiferous cord.

The seminiferous tubules of the rat fetus are especially large but their number is low in comparison with the fetal testis of other species. The details of the formation of the seminiferous tubules may present species differences, but in one way or another the future Sertoli cells differentiate early and encompass the germ cells. It is noteworthy that these germ cells continue to multiply but as a rule they do not enter meiosis until prepuberty.

Differentiation of interstitial cells (Leydig cells). The interstitial cells or Leydig cells, with their cytoplasmic attributes, differentiate during the second developmental phase. They appear among the undifferentiated intertubular mesenchymal cells (in the human fetus this is after the eighth week, in 29 mm CR fetuses, according to Pelliniemi and Niemi, 1969) (Figure 1.3). At that stage their cytoplasm enlarges and acquires a functional aspect, for instance the abundant tubular agranular endoplasmic reticulum of the steroid-secreting cells.

The development (in both number and size) of the interstitial cells reaches a maximum when the fetus is around 10 to 12 cm CR. After that, many interstitial cells degenerate.

Differentiation of the rete tubules and urogenital connections. The rete cords acquire a lumen and form true tubules communicating with the tubuli recti, but only after many other parts of the genital tract, to be mentioned now, have been masculinised.

Masculinisation of the genital tract

The differentiation of the male genital tract involves three mechanisms (Figure 1.4): (1) the disappearance of the müllerian ducts, the ducts which in females differentiate into the fallopian tubes and uterus; (2) the incorporation of part of the mesonephros and of the mesonephric duct into the male genital sphere at the level of the epididymides and of the vasa deferentia and seminal vesicles respectively; (3) the masculinisation of the common structures, e.g. urogenital sinus and external genitalia.

The order in which these mechanisms take place differs between species. Thus in human and rabbit, for example, the müllerian ducts disappear first, and the earliest prostatic buds differentiate on the urogenital sinus before the external genitalia are masculinised. In the calf fetus, on the other hand, masculinisation of the external genitalia becomes discernible on day 47, i.e. before regression of the müllerian ducts (which starts only after day 52) and before the appearance of prostatic buds on days 56 to 58.

In all cases, the differentiation of male characteristics proceeds very rapidly (Figure 1.3). In the human fetus most of the male sexual organs are established when the fetus is 60 mm CR length (see Jirasek, 1967).

Differentiation of the female genital apparatus

Differentiation of the genital apparatus begins later in the female and, with the exception of development of the ovary, is simpler than that in the male.

Ovarian organogenesis

At first, the sex glands destined to become ovaries can be recognised only because they do not become testes. The superficial epithelium is retained and for a long time no structure comparable to that of an adult ovary differentiates in the internal blastema. However, the

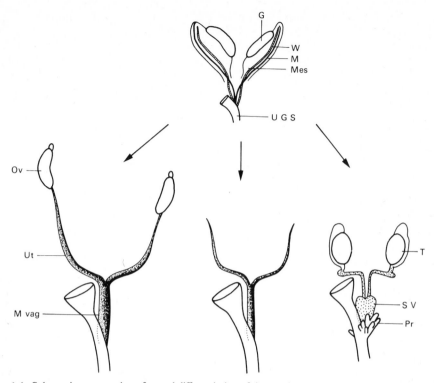

Figure 1.4. Schematic presentation of sexual differentiation of the sex ducts in the rabbit embryo. From the undifferentiated condition (top) may arise either the female structure (bottom left), or the male structure (bottom right), or the gonad-less female structure in castrated embryos of either sex (bottom centre). G = gonad; M = müllerian duct; Mes = mesonephros; M vag = müllerian vagina; Ov = ovary; Pr = prostate; SV = seminal vesicle; T = testis; UGS = urogenital sinus; Ut = uterine horn; W = wolffian duct (stippled). From Jost (1960) with kind permission of the editor of *Memoirs of the Society for Endocrinology*.

glands grow and their germ cells multiply, although they remain less numerous than those in the testes. Whereas in the testes the germ cells multiply throughout the seminiferous cords (and, for a while, in the rete testis), in the developing ovary many of the germ cells are located beneath the superficial epithelium and tend to remain grouped in clusters. During the process of cellular division they are often incompletely separated and communicate by cellular bridges; they therefore have a synchronous evolution. However, as seen in squashed preparations of the developing ovaries of mice (Blandau, White and Rumery, 1963), the germ cells retain a considerable degree of independent locomotive activity; this activity is lost at an early stage in the testis.

The multiplication of the germ cells produces considerable masses of daughter germ cells, more or less regularly separated by small undifferentiated mesenchymal cells or by connective tissue and fibres. These masses, which may eventually contact the inner side of the surface epithelium, are interpreted in many textbooks as 'secondary sex cords' ingrown from the surface epithelium. However, this view has long been criticised (Felix, 1912; Fischel, 1930, etc.). The number of germ cells reaches a peak (fifth month in the human fetus) and after that declines quite quickly as a result of germ cell degeneration. This is a period of critical importance in ovarian organogenesis when several interrelated events are occurring:

1. In the deepest region of the ovigerous nests of the 75 mm CR fetus, a few oogonia enter

the prophase of meiosis. The number of cells entering meiosis increases progressively from the deeper aspect towards the surface of the ovary.

2. Somewhat later (Figure 1.3), the first ovarian follicles are formed in the most central part of the ovigerous nests. A regular layer of small follicular cells surrounds one germ cell ('polyovular' follicles do exist but are exceptional). As soon as the follicle has differentiated the meiotic chromosomes vanish, meiosis stops at the diplotene phase and the nucleus becomes clear again. Many germ cells never become surrounded by follicular cells; they undergo pyknosis and degenerate. In a short time there is a drastic reduction in the number of germ cells. The reason why so many germ cells degenerate is not clear. According to Ohno and Smith (1964) one condition for a germ cell to survive is that it becomes enclosed in a follicle and meiosis ceases.

3. In several species, for instance in the human and in the calf fetus, at the time when the follicles differentiate strands of chromophilic cells extend between the hilus (region of the rete ovarii) and the periphery where follicles are formed. In the past, these strands were described by German authors as 'Markstränge' and have since often been named 'medullary' or 'primary sex cords' (despite their late appearance). In the female calf, for instance, these cellular strands are especially clear at the time when, in the male, the urogenital connections between the seminiferous tubules and the rete testis become clearly established. The role of these cords is not known with certainty. It has been suggested that in the calf fetus they act as channels along which follicular cells pass (Gropp and Ohno, 1966). Byskov (1974) recently gave some evidence that in the rat, a species in which the developing ovary is small and the structures close together, the rete ovarii is an inductor for the differentiation of follicles.

In summary, it should be noted how late true ovaries, provided with follicles, theca and stroma and capable of steroidogenesis, differentiate. By this stage, males have long acquired their male organs; even in the female the genital tract has clearly differentiated before the ovaries are defined.

Feminisation of the genital tract

In females the wolffian or mesonephric ducts are not incorporated into the genital structures (Figure 1.4). Regression occurs at different times in different species. In human females, the diameter of the ducts has already decreased at the 30 mm CR stage, when the müllerian ducts start retrogressing in males. They have almost completely disappeared after the 50 to 55 mm CR stage. This means that henceforth no possibility exists for redifferentiating vasa deferentia, whatever the experimental or pathological conditions.

The müllerian ducts persist and differentiate into fallopian tubes and uterine horns (one uterus in humans, resulting from the fusion of the two ducts). The organogenesis of the vagina, which progressively detaches itself from the urogenital sinus, and the origin of its inner epithelium are by no means simple (Forsberg, 1972). In contrast, the external genitalia diverge little from the undifferentiated condition.

THE ROLE OF HORMONES IN THE DIFFERENTIATION OF THE GENITAL APPARATUS

The view that hormones play a role in the differentiation of the genital organs has a long historical background. It is necessary to consider observations on the effect of exogenous hormones on fetal development as well as the role of the fetus' own hormones.

Action of extraneous hormones

An effect of extraneous hormones on sexual differentiation was first suggested by the study of freemartins in cattle. A freemartin is a genetic female (XX chromosomes in non-circulating cells) that developed as a twin to a male calf fetus, and whose internal sex organs are abnormal. The müllerian derivatives are more or less completely absent but seminal vesicles and epididymides are present; the small gonads may contain a large number of sterile seminiferous tubules and secrete testosterone in the adult (Short et al, 1969). However, the external genitalia are feminine in shape. Lillie (1916, 1917) and Keller and Tandler (1916) explained the condition by the transfer of a fetal testicular hormone from male to female.

The freemartin condition can be reproduced in amphibians by uniting in parabiosis two early larvae of newts (Witschi, 1950; Burns, 1961). With a modification of the technique (orthotopic grafting), Humphrey (1945) observed a long series of changes imposed upon the developing ovaries by a testis grafted in the same animal. In some individuals these alterations finally resulted in a complete morphological and functional sex reversal (genetic female → phenotypic male).

It should be noted that in these observations and experiments the testicular hormones modified the genetically female embryo; the reverse did not occur.

When, in the early 1930s, chemically defined sex hormones (first oestrogens, then androgens) became available, many experiments were performed in all classes of vertebrates to attempt to influence sexual differentiation of the embryos. The results were very variable; no simple law or rule was discernible. Some cases of complete and functional sex reversal, i.e. adult fertile animals functioning phenotypically in the sex opposite to their genotype, were obtained in a few amphibian species, for instance (i) feminisation of genetically male newts (*Pleurodeles waltlii*) (Gallien, 1954) or African clawed toads (*Xenopus laevis*) (Gallien, 1955; Chang and Witschi, 1955) by oestrogens; and (ii) masculinisation of a genetically female Japanese frog by testosterone. It must be emphasised that in those species in which successful sex reversal was possible, it could be produced only in one direction; usually sex was altered in embryos of the homogametic sex (females in frogs, males in newts) by the hormone of the heterogametic sex. In the cyprinodont fish, *Oryzias latipes*, genetic males could be feminised by androgens and females masculinised by androgens, but this is an exception.

In some species of amphibians steroid hormones do not affect gonadal differentiation at all. The same is true in placental mammals in which sex hormones (usually administered to the mother) do not reverse gonadal differentiation even if they influence the genital tract. For instance, in genetic females androgens provoke the persistence and development of wolffian derivatives and masculine shape of the urogenital sinus and external genitalia, but they do not affect ovarian development.

Action of hormones produced by the fetus itself

The role of gonadal hormones in sexual differentiation

The mechanisms controlling the differentiation of the genital tract are quite dissimilar in males and females, as was established a long time ago when rabbit fetuses were surgically castrated in utero before or during sexual differentiation (Figure 1.4) (Jost, 1947, 1953). Experiments in vivo on mice (Raynaud and Frilley, 1947) or in vitro on isolated pieces of the genital tract of rat fetuses (Jost and Bergerard, 1949; Picon, 1969) afforded complementary observations.

The early differentiation of the female condition does not depend on gonadal hormones;

female organs develop in castrated female or male fetuses (Figure 1.4) or in isolated pieces of the genital tract cultivated in vitro in the absence of hormones. In other words, the retrogression of the wolffian ducts (which do not become sexual structures), the persistence of the müllerian ducts and their differentiation into tubal and uterine regions, and the female development of the urogenital sinus and external genitalia do not require gonadal hormones.

On the contrary, the realisation of each part of the male genital apparatus depends on the testicular hormones which impose masculinity on the body. The testes induce the retrogression of the müllerian ducts and the development of the male organs against an inherently feminine developmental trend, a trend that must be suppressed by the testicular hormones.

In comparing males and females it should be recalled that testes differentiate very early, before any sexual orientation of the genital primordia, whereas ovaries form only after the specialisation of the female genital tract has already proceeded. The differentiation of the ovaries appears to complete the basic female programme, when it has not been impaired by early masculinisation. The capacity for steroidogenesis, as judged from the conversion of precursors into hormones in vitro or histochemically detectable enzymatic activities, e.g. 3β hydroxysteroid dehydrogenase, appears in testes when interstitial cells form, but becomes conspicuous in ovaries only after follicles and stroma have differentiated.

The testicular hormones

Experiments done on castrated rabbit fetuses showed that androgens like testosterone or methyltestosterone were no substitute for the intact fetal testis. Androgens provoke the development of all male structures, but they do not induce the retrogression of the müllerian ducts (Figure 1.5). Subsequently many animal experiments or clinical observations supported the view that the fetal testis produces two kinds of hormones, a hormone responsible for the disappearance of the müllerian ducts and androgens responsible for the development of the male organs. Thus, the anti-androgen cyproterone acetate acting in male rabbit or dog fetuses opposes the masculinising effect of the fetal testis, but it does not impair its anti-müllerian activity (Figure 1.5). When treated with cyproterone acetate these genetic males,

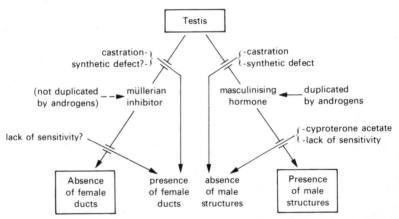

Figure 1.5. Scheme summarising the testicular control of the differentiation of the sex ducts and sex characters. Some conditions capable of interfering with the normal testicular activity are indicated (crossing arrows). The data concerning cyproterone acetate refer to experiments made on rabbit fetuses (in rats the effect is not the same). From Jost (1970b) with kind permission of the publisher (Berlin: Springer-Verlag).

although they possess testes, have no sex ducts but they do have a vagina and female external genitalia (see Neumann, Elger and Steinbeck, 1970; Jost, 1972b). The condition of the genital tract parallels the condition known in humans as 'testicular feminisation', that results from tissue insensitivity to androgens, but not to the anti-müllerian hormone.

The capacity of the fetal testis to produce androgens at an age when the male sex organs differentiate has been studied largely in animal or human tissue in vitro. The nature and concentration of the circulating hormone(s) still needs elucidation. It is not certain whether the major hormone directing the formation of the male organs is exactly the same at different developmental phases or in different animal species. Recent observations on the fetal calf testis suggest that the anti-müllerian hormone is a large protein molecule, and that it is produced by the Sertoli cells. Seminiferous cords dissected out from fetal calf testes showed the anti-müllerian activity which was absent in the intertubular material (Josso, 1973).

These experimental data provide a biological interpretation of many abnormalities of the genital tract. For normal male differentiation two testicular factors must act in the fetus. Developmental defects occur if one or both of these: (1) are not produced, or (2) do not act on the target organs, if the latter are unresponsive. Examples of the first possibility are given by cases of absent gonads (Turner's syndrome) or by enzymatic defects impairing the synthesis of androgens (e.g. 17α-steroid-hydroxylase deficiency); in both cases feminine features of the body sex are evident. Testicular feminisation is an example of the second possibility. The persistence of a uterus in otherwise normal males might result either from defective production of, or lack of sensitivity to, the anti-müllerian hormone.

Mode of action of gonadal hormones

Only a few aspects of the mode of action of hormones during sexual organogenesis have been investigated. Three lines of investigation are now described:

1. The early sex primordia can be influenced by testicular hormones only during a limited period of time—the period of sensitivity. For example, (1) the retrogression of the müllerian ducts of the rat fetus under the influence of a fetal testis is obtained in vitro only if the ducts are taken from 14.5 to 15-day-old fetuses; if taken from older female fetuses the ducts can no longer be inhibited (Picon, 1969). (2) Androgens given to pregnant mammals masculinise the genital tract of the female fetuses only if given during a definite period of time: e.g. the external genitalia of female calf fetuses can be completely masculinised (penis opening under the umbilicus, presence of a scrotum) if androgens are given from days 40 to 60; if androgens are given between days 60 and 80 they fail to masculinise the genitalia (Jost et al, 1973). These observations explain the freemartin phenomenon described earlier; in the first phase of development the genital organs are influenced exclusively by an anti-müllerian and anti-ovarian factor, and androgenisation begins only after day 60, too late to masculinise the external genitalia (Jost et al, 1975).

In cases of the human adrenogenital syndrome the clitoris is usually enlarged but not transformed into a male organ. In some cases, complete masculinisation does occur, and these probably result from an early onset of androgenisation.

2. Studies of androgen action in the prostate of the adult rat have indicated that the mechanism of testosterone action may be mediated by its metabolite, dihydrotestosterone. Dihydrotestosterone is formed in the cytoplasm of the prostatic cells and transferred to the nucleus by a specific cytosol 'receptor' protein.

Some sexual structures (urogenital sinus, genital tubercle) taken from young rabbit or rat fetuses before their masculinisation is complete convert testosterone into dihydrotestosterone in vitro and concentrate dihydrotestosterone from the medium. On the other hand, the lateral parts of the mesonephros containing the müllerian and wolffian ducts have no such capacity before the wolffian ducts have become the male sex ducts (Wilson and Lasnitzki, 1971; Wilson, 1973). These data suggest that the actual steroids working on different parts of the genital tract are not the same.

3. Androgen-insensitive male mice and rats (X-linked Tfm gene for testicular feminisation) are animals with inherited tissue insensitivity to androgens; in these males the müllerian ducts have disappeared normally but all male organs are missing and the external genitalia are feminine. Since adult Tfm 'males' lack sex organs such as a prostate, other tissues present in both sexes and sensitive to androgens were studied, e.g. the kidneys and the preputial glands. In androgen-insensitive 'males' these organs convert testosterone into dihydrotestosterone, but the cells do not concentrate dihydrotestosterone because of the lack of the cytosol androgen 'receptor' protein. The defect in masculinisation might result from the absence of this protein (Gehring, Tomkins and Ohno, 1971; Bullock and Bardin, 1974).

Action of hormones on gonadal differentiation

Several observations, e.g. the nearly testicular structure of the freemartin gonad in cattle or the sex reversal obtained in newts under the influence of a developing testis or, in some other instances, of sex hormones, led many biologists to accept the idea that during normal development the formation of either a testis or an ovary from undifferentiated cells is governed by hormones or diffusible inductors. Witschi (1950, 1967) suggested a possible explanation. The indifferent gonad is considered to be developed from two regions, the cortex and the medulla, which produce antagonistic inductors (distinct from the sex hormones). The medullary inductor(s) oppose(s) ovarian and impose(s) testicular differentiation; the antagonistic cortical inductor(s) compete(s) with the medullary inductor(s) and favour(s) ovarian differentiation. Both cortex and medulla are assumed to participate together in the formation of either type of gonad but to retain the possibility of producing a specific inductor, thus permitting late sex reversal. This rather complex scheme still lacks cytological, histochemical or biochemical evidence. It implies that in the early development of genetic females, inductors are necessary to keep the undifferentiated gonad undifferentiated, and it hardly fits the chronological difference in testicular and ovarian organogenesis.

Other biologists subscribe to the view that sex hormones themselves, produced in the gonadal primordium under genetic control, direct gonadal differentiation. They accept the concept that a testis becomes a testis because it produces testosterone and not that it produces testosterone because it has become a testis. However, humans or animals insensitive to androgens still have histologically nearly normal testes, at least before puberty; similarly patients suffering from enzymatic defects preventing testosterone synthesis and masculinisation of the genital tract nevertheless have testes.

There is no definite evidence that the initial differentiation of the gonads is governed by hormones. It is certainly an oversimplification to admit that one hormone or inductor is responsible for the morphological and physiological differentiation of many different cell types from similar undifferentiated cells.

The development of the abnormal gonads in freemartin fetuses has recently been shown to be a complex and prolonged process (Jost et al, 1973, 1975). In male calves the first seminiferous cords appear around day 40 and the interstitial cells are seen a few days later. In presumptive freemartins and in females the still undifferentiated gonads remain similar for a further week; thereafter the gonads of the freemartins cease growing more or less completely and become stunted. The number of germ cells does not increase any more and the superficial epithelium progressively disappears. After day 75, the germ cells do not enter meiosis as they do in normal females. After day 90 the freemartin gonads resume growing at a reduced rate, and in approximately one-half of the fetuses examined between days 90 and 250, cellular cords closely resembling seminiferous cords appear in the blastema, around the rete. These cords contain germ cells which degenerate before birth. Clusters of cells similar to interstitial cells are seen in a smaller number of freemartins. This testicular-like organogenesis occurs in the freemartin gonad at the time when ovarian follicles develop in females, but the series of intimate mechanisms involved is still not clear. It should be recalled that androgens given to female calf fetuses extensively masculinise the genital tract but do not duplicate the freemartin effect on the gonads.

Another important problem in gonadal development is the almost complete absence of meiosis in the germ cells in the testes (and in the freemartin gonad), whereas early stages of meiosis are characteristic of presumptive ovaries (they are perhaps a prerequisite for folliculogenesis). It remains unknown whether meiosis is triggered by some cellular or hormonal influence in female fetuses, whether it is prevented from occurring in the testes or whether it is directly controlled by the genetic constitution of the germ cells. Recent in vitro experiments indicate that fetal hypophyseal gonado-stimulating hormones are not necessary for the occurrence of premeiotic changes in cultivated presumptive ovaries. Solving this problem would be of great interest for the physiology of the adult gonad.

GENETIC CONTROL OF SEXUAL DIFFERENTIATION

It has long been known that in mammals one pair of chromosomes differs in males and in females: this pair consists of two X chromosomes in females and one X plus one smaller and distinct Y chromosome in males. In 1959 observations made on human patients who had a 44 XXY karyotype, and on XO or XXY mice, led to the demonstration that the Y chromosome is the bearer of the male-determining factor(s). In principle, the mere absence of a Y chromosome results in female determination (no testes, no male sex characters) and the presence of a Y chromosome, whatever the number of X chromosomes (for instance multi-X Klinefelter's syndrome), results in male determination (at least the presence of testes) (see Cattanach, 1974). However, exceptional autosomal genes are known which mimic the presence of a Y chromosome in XX individuals: masculine XX mice bearing the autosomal sex reversal gene Sxr; XX goats homozygous for the gene for polledness (or hornlessness); masculine XX humans. In most of these cases XX germ cells degenerate sooner or later in the testicular surrounding and the individual becomes sterile.

In the normal situation, the Y chromosome is necessary for the successive differentiation of seminiferous cords and of interstitial cells. The early functions of these two components are probably production of anti-müllerian hormone and testicular influence on germ cells for the former component, and secretion of androgen for the second. How these functions are controlled is still not clear. However, it is clear that androgen synthesis requires the formation of an enzymatic chain, depending on a series of genes. If one of these genes is deficient, hormonal synthesis and masculinisation are impaired.

On the other hand, sensitivity of embryonic cells of the reproductive tract to androgens is not a sexual character insofar as it exists in both sexes (females can be masculinised by androgens). In Tfm mice or rats the 'receptor' protein for androgens is absent or very scarce in the various target organs whatever the type of response to hormones expected in normal animals (e.g. formation of a prostate or of male external genitalia). The detailed mechanisms of hormonal intervention in morphogenetic processes and their genetic control are yet to be studied.

Finally, even if it is conceivable that one particular gene located on the Y chromosome triggers a long series of events, including derepression of many other genes, normal sexual differentiation should not be considered to obey a 'one gene, one sex' rule.

OTHER SEX CHARACTERISTICS

Most of the male or female sex characters depend on hormones secreted by the gonad for their expression in adulthood. They become more or less indistinct if the adult animal is castrated, but they can be restored by appropriate hormonal treatment. Eventually they may be sex-reversed if male hormone is given to castrated females or vice versa (e.g. distribution of hair). Other sex characteristics cannot be sex-reversed in adulthood because they have been permanently and irreversibly established during an early critical stage. In such cases the developmental scheme is similar to that governing the differentiation of the genital tract, insofar as the basic programme is feminine and the testicular hormone must repress femaleness and impose the male pattern during a 'critical' phase.

The existence of a permanent 'sexualisation' at the level of nervous structures involved in reproductive physiology has been described in several animal species. In the rat the hypothalamus imposes a continuous gonado-stimulating activity on the hypophysis of the male and a cyclical activity in the female. The male pattern of hypothalamic function is imprinted as a result of the influence of testicular hormones on the hypothalamus at a definite developmental stage (5th postnatal day). The male pattern does not appear in males castrated before that stage; in these early castrated males a cyclical hypothalamic function will prevail in adulthood. The male pattern can be impressed on the hypothalamus of young females by an injection of testosterone at the critical stage. When they reach puberty neonatally androgenised females do not ovulate and are therefore sterile. In 1959 Phoenix et al opened a fascinating chapter when they discovered that in guinea-pigs prenatal androgenisation could influence and 'sexualise' for life the neural structures mediating sex behaviour. Adult female guinea-pigs whose mothers received testosterone during pregnancy could hardly be induced to display female sexual behaviour, while male behaviour was readily elicited by testosterone.

In rats the period of sensitivity to androgens is postnatal (day 4 or 5); for male behaviour to be easily elicited in adulthood, androgenisation of the nervous system must occur during this restricted initial period.

It is not certain that these permanent effects of early testicular or androgenic hormones seen in animals apply to human physiology, but the animal models give valuable indications for further studies on humans.

REFERENCES

Blandau, R. J., White, B. J. & Rumery, R. E. (1963) Observations on the movements of the living primordial germ cells in the mouse. *Fertility and Sterility,* **14,** 482–489.

Brambell, F. W. R. (1927) The development and morphology of the gonads of the mouse. I. The morphogenesis of the indifferent gonad and of the ovary. *Proceedings of the Royal Society of London,* **101B,** 391–409.

Bullock, L. P. & Bardin, C. W. (1974) Androgen receptors in the mouse kidney: a study of male, female and androgen-insensitive (tfm/y) mice. *Endocrinology*, **94**, 746–756.

Burns, R. K. (1961) Role of hormones in the differentiation of sex. In *Sex and Internal Secretions* (Ed.) Young, W.C. Ch.2. Baltimore: Williams and Wilkins.

Byskov, A. G. S. (1974) Does the rete ovarii act as a trigger for the onset of meiosis? *Nature*, **252**, 396–397.

Cattanach, B. M. (1974) Genetic disorders of sex determination in mice and other mammals. In *Birth Defects. Excerpta Medica International Congress Series*, **310**, 129–141.

Chang, C. Y. & Witschi, E. (1955) Breeding of sex-reversed males of Xenopus laevis Daudin. *Proceedings of the Society for Experimental Biology and Medicine*, **89**, 150–152.

Dubois, R. & Croisille, Y. (1970) Germ-cell line and sexual differentiation in birds. *Philosophical Transactions of the Royal Society of London*, **259B**, 73–89.

Felix, W. (1912) The development of the urogenital organs. In *Manual of Human Embryology* (Ed.) Keibel, F. & Mall, F. P. Vol. 2, Ch. 19, pp. 752–979. Philadelphia: J. B. Lippincott.

Fischel, A. (1930) Ueber die Entwicklung der Keimdrüsen der Menschen. *Zeitschrift für Anatomie und Entwicklungsgeschichte*, **92**, 34–72.

Forsberg, G.-J. (1972) Estrogen, vaginal cancer, and vaginal development. *American Journal of Obstetrics and Gynecology*, **113**, 83–87.

Gallien, L. (1954) Inversion expérimentale du sexe sous l'action des hormones sexuelles chez le triton Pleurodeles waltlii Michah. Analyse des conséquences génétiques. *Bulletin de Biologie de France et Belgique*, **88**, 1–51.

Gallien, L. (1955) Descendance unisexuée d'une femelle de Xenopus laevis Daud. ayant subi pendant sa phase larvaire, l'action gynogène du benzoate d'oestradiol. *Compte Rendu de l'Académie des Sciences*, **240**, 913–915.

Gallien, L. (1965) Genetic control of sexual differentiation in vertebrates. In *Organogenesis* (Ed.) De Haan, R. L. & Ursprung, H. pp. 583–610. New York: Holt, Rinehart and Winston.

Gehring, U., Tompkins, G. M. & Ohno, S. (1971) Effect of the androgen insensitivity mutation on a cytoplasmic receptor for dihydrotestosterone. *Nature, New Biology*, **232**, 106–107.

Gropp, A. & Ohno, S. (1966) The presence of a common embryonic blastema for ovarian and testicular parenchymal (follicular, interstitial and tubular) cells in cattle, Bos taurus. *Zeitschrift für Zellforschung*, **74**, 505–528.

Humphrey, R. R. (1945) Sex determination in ambystomid salamanders: a study of the progeny of females experimentally converted into males. *American Journal of Anatomy*, **76**, 33–66.

Jirasek, J. E. (1967) The relationship between the structure of the testis and differentiation of the external genitalia and phenotype in Man. *Ciba Foundation Colloquia in Endocrinology*, **16**, 3–27.

Josso, N. (1973) *In vitro* synthesis of müllerian-inhibiting hormone by seminiferous tubules isolated from the calf fetal testis. *Endocrinology*, **93**, 829–834.

Jost, A. (1947) Recherches sur la différenciation sexuelle de l'embryon de lapin. III. Rôle des gonades foetales dans la différenciation sexuelle somatique. *Archives d'Anatomie Microscopique et de Morphologie Expérimentale*, **36**, 271–315.

Jost, A. (1953) Problems of fetal endocrinology: the gonadal and hypophyseal hormones. *Recent Progress in Hormone Research*, **8**, 379–418.

Jost, A. (1970a) Hormonal factors in the sex differentiation of the mammalian foetus. (In Discussion on Determination of Sex. *Philosophical Transactions of the Royal Society of London*, **259B**, 119–130.

Jost, A. (1970b) General outline about reproductive physiology and its developmental background. In *Mammalian Reproduction, 21; Colloquium der Gesellschaft für biologische Chemie, Mosbach* (Ed.) Gibian, H. & Plotz, E. J. pp. 1–32, Berlin: Springer-Verlag.

Jost, A. (1971) Embryonic sexual differentiation (morphology, physiology, abnormalities). In *Hermaphroditism, Anomalies and Related Endocrine Disorders* (Ed.) Jones, H. W. & Scott, W. W. pp. 16–64, 2nd revised edition. Baltimore: Williams and Wilkins.

Jost, A. (1972a) A new look at the mechanisms controlling sex differentiation in mammals. *Johns Hopkins Medical Journal*, **130**, 38–53.

Jost, A. (1972b) Use of androgen antagonists and antiandrogens in studies on sex differentiation. *Gynecological Investigation*, **2**, 180–201.

Jost, A. (1972c) Données préliminaires sur les stades initiaux de la différenciation du testicule chez le rat. *Archives d'Anatomie Microscopique et de Morphologie Expérimentale*, **61**, 415–438.

Jost, A. & Bergerard, Y. (1949) Culture in vitro d'ébauches du tractus génital du foetus de rat. *Compte Rendu de la Société de Biologie*, **143**, 608–609.

Jost, A., Perchellet, J. P., Prepin, J. & Vigier, B. (1975) The prenatal development of bovine freemartins. In *Intersexuality in the Animal Kingdom* (Ed.) Reinboth, R. pp. 392–406. Berlin, Heidelberg, New York: Springer-Verlag.

Jost, A., Vigier, B., Prepin, J. & Perchellet, J. P. (1973) Studies on sex differentiation in mammals. *Recent Progress in Hormone Research*, **29**, 1–41.

Keller, K. & Tandler, J. (1916) Uber das Verhalten der Eihäute bei der Zwillingsträchtikeit des Rindes. Untersuchungen über die Entstehungsursache der Geschlechtlichen Unterentwicklung von weiblichen Zwillingskälbern welche neben einem männlichen Kalbe zur Entwicklung gelangen. *Wiener Tierarztliche Wochenschrift*, **3**, 513–526.

Lillie, F. (1916) The theory of the freemartin. *Science*, **43**, 611–613.

Lillie, F. (1917) The freemartin, a study of the action of sex hormones in fetal life of cattle. *Journal of Experimental Zoology*, **23**, 371–451.

Mittwoch, U. (1973). *Genetics of Sex Differentiation*. New York, London: Academic Press.

Neumann, F., Elger, W. & Steinbeck, H. (1970) Antiandrogens and reproductive development. *Philosophical Transactions of the Royal Society of London*, **259B**, 179–184.

Ohno, S. & Smith, J. B. (1964) Role of fetal follicular cells in meiosis of mammalian oöcytes. *Cytogenetics*, **3**, 324–333.

Pelliniemi, L. J. & Niemi, M. (1969) Fine structure of the human foetal testis. I. The interstitial tissue. *Zeitschrift für Zellforschung*, **99**, 507–522.

Phoenix, C. H., Goy, R. W., Gerall, A. A. & Young, W. C. (1959) Organizing action of prenatally administered testosterone propionate on the tissues mediating mating behaviour in the female guinea-pig. *Endocrinology*, **65**, 369–382.

Picon, R. (1969) Action du testicule foetal sur le développement *in vitro* des canaux de Müller chez le rat. *Archives d'Anatomie Microscopique et de Morphologie Expérimentale*, **58**, 1–19.

Prenant, A. (1889) Contribution à l'histogenèse du tube séminifère. *Internationale Monatsschrift für Anatomie und Physiologie*, **6**, 1–30.

Raynaud, A. & Frilley, M. (1947) Destruction des glandes génitales de l'embryon de souris, par irradiation au moyen de rayons X, à l'âge de treize jours. *Annales d'Endocrinologie*, **8**, 400–419.

Short, R. V., Smith, J., Mann, T., Evans, E. P., Hallett, J., Fryer, A. & Hamerton, J. L. (1969) Cytogenetic and endocrine studies of a freemartin heifer and its bull co-twin. *Cytogenetics*, **8**, 369–388.

Wilson, J. D. (1973) Testosterone uptake by the urogenital tract of the rabbit embryo. *Endocrinology*, **92**, 1192–1199.

Wilson, J. D. & Lasnitzki, I. (1971) Dihydrotestosterone formation in fetal tissues of the rabbit and rat. *Endocrinology*, **89**, 659–668.

Witschi, E. (1948) Migration of the germ cells of human embryos from the yolk sac to the primitive gonadal folds. *Contributions in Embryology*, **32**, 69–80. (Carnegie Institute, Washington, Publication No. 575.)

Witschi, E. (1950) Génétique et physiologie de la differenciation du sexe. *Archives d'Anatomie Microscopique et de Morphologie Expérimentale*, **39**, 215–240.

Witschi, E. (1967) Biochemistry of sex differentiation in vertebrate embryos. In *The Biochemistry of Animal Development* (Ed.) Weber, R. Vol. 2, pp. 193–225. New York: Academic Press.

2

ONTOGENY OF ACQUIRED IMMUNITY AND FETO-MATERNAL IMMUNOLOGICAL INTERACTIONS

M. C. Adinolfi and W. D. Billington

As an essential factor in the ability of the individual to preserve the integrity of the body the immune system must be highly functional from the moment of birth. This is achieved during fetal life not only by the development of specialised organs and the differentiation of immunologically active cells but also by the temporary acquisition of maternally derived immunity. The intimate association of the fetus with maternal tissues in the sheltered intra-uterine environment also brings with it a serious problem. The fetus inherits from the father genetic characteristics that are foreign to the mother and hence presents her with an antigenic challenge that should be capable of eliciting immunological rejection reactions. This chapter analyses the complex and changing immunological interrelationships that are involved in the maintenance of the fetus as an intra-uterine allograft and in the establishment of the immune defence mechanisms of the newborn. Although the evidence presented relates as far as possible to studies in man, it is frequently necessary to draw upon observations from experimental animals.

DEVELOPMENT OF THE IMMUNE RESPONSE

For many years it was claimed that the human fetus was not capable of producing specific antibodies and that the immunological defences of the newborn were based exclusively upon the presence of maternal antibodies which had crossed the human placenta. However, studies carried out during the last decade have demonstrated that, although maternal antibodies play a very important role in protecting the human newborn against bacterial and viral infections, the maturation of both humoral (antibody-mediated) and cellular (cell-mediated) immune responses starts at an early stage of development in the human fetus and in the fetuses of other mammals (Sterzl and Silverstein, 1967; Adinolfi and Wood, 1969; Lawton and Cooper, 1973).

It has also been shown that other plasma proteins involved in the immunological mechanisms of protection against bacterial and viral infections, such as the components of complement (C), lysozyme (LZM) and interferon, start to be produced at an early stage of fetal development (Adinolfi, 1972).

Organisation of the lymphoid system

It is now evident that in most vertebrates the entire haemopoietic system develops from stem cells which appear first in the yolk sac and then migrate to the fetal liver, thymus and bone marrow (Metcalf and Moore, 1971; Owen, 1973). The differentiation of the stem cells into specific cell types depends upon interaction with the inductive tissues in which these cells are proliferating. Release and relocation of cells permit new interactions between emerging, diversified cell types and result in the production of stable cell lines capable of clonal proliferation (Figure 2.1). Depending upon the inducing influence of the environmental tissues, the stem cells may differentiate along one or another of the haemopoietic lines, into red cells, granulocytes, monocytes, megakaryocytes or lymphoid cells (Yoffey and Courtice, 1970; Metcalf and Moore, 1971; Owen, 1973). Current evidence suggests that in humans migration of stem cells from the yolk sac occurs at about the sixth week of fetal life.

The maturation of T-lymphocytes

Migration of stem cells into the thymus will lead to the proliferation of several types of thymocytes (T-cells) with characteristic immunological properties and expressing specific surface antigens. Thymocytes are capable of prolonged recirculation, are endowed with immunological memory and are mainly involved in the cell mediated types of immune response. These cells are characterised by the presence of specific membrane antigens (theta, θ), have a high degree of radio-resistance and respond in vitro to phytohaemagglutinin (PHA) stimulation and to mitomycin-treated or irradiated allogeneic cells (Miller and Osoba, 1967; Talmage, 1969; Mitchison, 1971; Katz and Benacerraf, 1972).

Although T-lymphocytes in peripheral organs are derived from the thymus there are substantial differences between thymus and peripheral T-cells in terms of their functions and cell surface antigens. Thus only a minority of thymus lymphocytes have been shown to be immunologically responsive and this population, like the peripheral T-cells, is less sensitive to the cytolytic effects of corticosteroids than the majority of the T-cells.

These and other studies reviewed by Owen (1973) have established the fact that there are two categories of T-cells, one immunologically inert (immature) and a minority, probably located in the thymus medulla, immunologically responsive. The expression of histocompatibility antigens (H) and thymus-specific antigens (TL and theta) is different in the two populations (Figure 2.1).

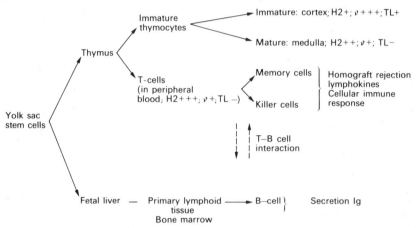

Figure 2.1. Migration of yolk sac cells and production of T and B-cells.

In human fetuses, the thymus is an active lymphoid organ after six weeks of gestation. Lymphopoiesis is intense and is independent of antigenic stimulation (Metcalf, 1966; Adinolfi and Wood, 1969). Recent studies have shown that the thymus of human fetuses of more than 14 weeks contains antigen-binding cells (Dwyer and MacKay, 1970). The number of thymocytes binding specific antigens may be greater in the fetal thymus than in the postnatal or adult thymus.

The maturation of B-lymphocytes

Counterpoint to the T-cells stands the system of the antibody-producing cells, or bone marrow-derived B-cells. In fully differentiated form, these are cells capable of producing and secreting immunoglobulin molecules (Katz and Benacerraf, 1972; Warner, 1974).

Studies of human myeloma proteins derived from single clones of cells, together with the analysis of isolated antibodies and immunofluorescence techniques, have shown that each antibody-producing cell synthesises only one class or subclass of immunoglobulin (Pernis, 1967; Natvig and Kunkel, 1968, 1973). This restriction is extended to the products of allelic genes; in fact B-cells produce only one genetic type of immunoglobulin molecule in heterozygous individuals. The exception to this rule is represented by the expression on the cell surface of both IgM and IgD molecules with the same type of light chain (Rowe et al, 1973).

Small lymph nodes showing active lymphopoiesis have been observed in the connective tissue of the neck of fetuses 25 to 28 mm long (Gilmour, 1941). At this stage of gestation a few lymphocytes are present in the peripheral blood. Definite lymph nodes can be seen in fetuses more than 48 mm long, when lymphocytes can be detected inside lymph vessels and in bone marrow. Lymphocyte counts near 1000 cells/mm³ have been observed in fetuses 12 weeks old. The number of these cells reaches values between 5000 and 10 000 cells/mm³ in fetuses 24 weeks old (Playfair, Wolfendale and Kay, 1963).

Other tissues appear to have lymphopoietic potentialities during life in utero. The presence of potentially immunocompetent cells in fetal liver has been repeatedly demonstrated in man and other mammals; their maturation is dependent upon an intact thymic function (Tyan, Cole and Herzenberg, 1967). The placenta is another tissue which has been considered as potentially immunocompetent (Dancis, Braverman and Lind, 1957).

The functional duality of the immune system is reflected in certain immunological disorders (Davis, 1973; Hitzig, 1973; Stiehm, 1973). In Di George's syndrome, for example, children born without a thymus have a deficiency of lymphocytes and of cell-mediated immune responses. Plasma cells and immunoglobulins are present, suggesting an independent development of B-cells. On the other hand, the Bruton type of immunological deficiency is characterised by a lack of plasma cells and consequently the inability to produce antibodies; cell-mediated functions are present, enabling the young patients to resist most viral and fungal infections. There is, however, a considerable body of evidence, in man and in experimental animals, suggesting that most immunological responses are the result of cooperation between T and B-cells, including the genetic mechanisms controlling immune responses (McDevitt and Benacerraf, 1969; Green, 1974).

Classes of immunoglobulins

Five different classes of immunoglobulins have been identified in man on the basis of the discrete physicochemical properties and antigenic specificities associated with the polypeptide chains forming these molecules (Cohen, 1971; Natvig and Kunkel, 1973; Porter, 1973). In order of relative concentration in serum, these five classes are IgG, IgA, IgM, IgD and IgE globulins (Table 2.1). By virtue of subtle antigenic differences, four subclasses of IgG (IgG1, IgG2, IgG3 and IgG4) and two subclasses of IgA have been recognised to date.

IgG. The largest part of the circulating antibodies is formed by IgG molecules with a molecular weight near 150 000 and a coefficient of sedimentation between 6.6 and 7S.

Table 2.1. *Human immunoglobulins.*

Classes	Subclasses	Heavy chains	Light chain	Other chains [a]	Some physiological properties
IgG	IgG1, 2, 3, 4	γ	κ or λ	–	Placental transfer
IgA	IgA1, IgA2	α	κ or λ	J and SC	In external secretion
IgM		μ	κ or λ	J	Early immune response
IgD		δ	κ or λ	–	Unknown
IgE		ε	κ or λ	–	Reaginic activity; mast cell fixation

[a] J = 'joining' chain in IgA and IgM; SC = secretory piece in IgA only.

IgA. IgA constitute about 20 per cent of the total Ig in serum; colostrum, milk, parotid and bronchial secretions are rich in IgA molecules.

IgM. About eight to ten per cent of total Ig in serums are IgM; these molecules have a coefficient of sedimentation of 19S and a molecular weight near 900 000. Several specific antibodies such as cold agglutinins, anti-I, anti-D isoagglutinins and antibodies against O antigen of *Salmonella* are almost entirely confined to IgM.

IgD. The function of IgD remains to be established; this class of Ig is present in normal sera in concentration between 2.3 and 40 mg/100 ml.

IgE. Studies of the nature of skin-sensitising antibodies and myeloma proteins have led to the discovery of IgE. The blood levels of IgE are increased in about 50 per cent of patients with allergic diseases.

Gm, Am and Inv markers. A genetic polymorphism has been observed for the IgG and IgA molecules; the two genetic systems are referred to as the Gm and Am groups. Genetic variants (Inv system) of one of the light chains(x-chain) of Ig have also been demonstrated (Grubb, 1970). Gm, Am and Inv markers are controlled by autosomal dominant genes; this means that no offspring 'positive' for one of the markers has been observed in families where both parents were of the 'minus' type; for example Gm (a+) children cannot be born to parents who are both Gm (a−).

Transfer of immunoglobulins across the placenta

The route and the degree to which the various classes of immunoglobulins are transferred to the offspring vary in different species of mammals (Table 2.2) (Brambell, 1970; Wild, 1973; Hemmings, 1974).

Not all types of maternal Ig are transferred into the fetal circulation. There is evidence that maternal–fetal transfer is not related to the number or thickness of the placental membranes, but it depends upon the capacity of the cells forming such membranes to allow a percentage of endocytosed proteins to be transferred across without being degraded (Brambell, 1970; Wild, 1973).

Table 2.2. *Time and route of transmission of passive immunity in different species.*

Species	Transmission		Route	
	Prenatal	Postnatal	Prenatal	Postnatal
Man	+++	0	Placenta	−
Monkey	+++	0	Placenta	−
Rabbit	+++	0	Yolk sac (+placenta?)	−
Guinea-pig	+++	0	Yolk sac	−
Rat, mouse	+	++	Yolk sac	Gut
Dog, cat	+	++	Unknown	Gut
Horse, pig	0	+++	−	Gut
Ruminants	0	+++	−	Gut

From Brambell (1970) with kind permission of the publisher (Amsterdam: North Holland).

Studies on the transfer of plasma proteins, reviewed by Gitlin (1974), have shown that diffusion is most likely the process whereby albumin reaches the fetal circulation from the maternal plasma, whereas an active transport is involved in the process of transfer of IgG molecules.

The concentration of a maternal plasma protein in the fetal blood is not a simple expression of its transfer rate; it depends upon several factors, such as the concentration of the protein in the maternal blood, the rate of its degradation in the fetus, the diffusion of the protein from the plasma into the fetal interstitial fluids, and eventually the transfer of the same protein once again in the maternal circulation. If the rates of degradation of two proteins are different in the mother, or the fetus, or both, their concentration in maternal and fetal blood will be different even if their transfer is identical.

In man, transmission of immunoglobulins occurs exclusively by way of the chorio-allantoic placenta (Brambell, 1970). Selection is perhaps one of the most remarkable features of this transfer; in fact, only IgG molecules readily cross the placental barrier, whilst other classes of maternal immunoglobulins are either not transferred or only cross the placenta in small quantities (Wiener and Berlin, 1947; Vahlquist, 1958; Hitzig, 1959; Freda, 1962).

Maternal IgG molecules are first detectable in the fetal blood after 10 weeks gestation; at this stage of development maternal anti-Rh antibodies have been found in human Rh negative fetuses (Mollison, 1967). At the end of normal gestation, the mean level of IgG in newborn sera is slightly higher than that in the corresponding maternal blood. Variations in the total levels of IgG in the mother are usually reflected in the concentration of this class of proteins in cord blood. The levels of IgG2 are slightly lower in cord sera than in the corresponding maternal samples. However, this subclass of IgG has been detected in fetal blood at 11 weeks together with IgG1 and IgG3. On the other hand, IgG4 molecules have been detected occasionally after 14 weeks and constantly after 19 weeks (Schur, Alpert and Alper, 1973).

Table 2.3. *Gm(a) at birth and at one year of age.*

Mother	Infant	
	at birth	at 1 year
Gm(a+)	Gm(a+)	Gm(a+)
Gm(a+)	Gm(a+)	Gm(a−)
Gm(a−)	Gm(a−)	Gm(a−)
Gm(a−)	Gm(a−)	Gm(a+)

Gm (a) type in pairs of maternal and newborn sera; at birth the phenotype of the child resembles that of the mother; the maternal IgG molecules are slowly replaced by the infant IgG and at about 1 year of age the serum contains the product of the child's Gm genes.

Evidence that the major part of IgG present in fetal and newborn circulation is derived from the maternal blood has been confirmed by studies of the genetic markers of these proteins in pairs of maternal and cord samples. In fact, the IgG molecules present in the newborn carry Gm factors similar to those present in the corresponding maternal serum, irrespective of the genotype of the infants (Table 2.3). During the first months of life the maternal IgG molecules are replaced gradually by similar immunoglobulins produced by the infants; at about one year of age, the IgG molecules will express exclusively the infants own Gm markers.

The mechanisms involved in the active transfer of IgG across the human placenta are not yet known. The complexity of the problem is exemplified by the contradictory results of studies of the transfer of two fragments (Fab and Fc) obtained by enzymatic digestion of IgG molecules. Brambell et al (1960) have studied the transfer of labelled Fab and Fc fragments of rabbit IgG by measuring the amount of radioactive fragments in the fetuses 24 hours after inoculation into the uterine lumen of pregnant rabbits. They observed that whilst the concentration of the Fc fragment in the fetal serum was one-quarter of that attained using intact IgG molecules, the levels of the Fab fragments were only from one-sixth to one-tenth those of the Fc fragments. These results suggested that the transport of IgG molecules across the placenta was mediated through a receptor on the Fc fragment. However, these findings could not be confirmed by Gitlin and collaborators (Gitlin et al, 1964; Gitlin, 1974), who injected labelled IgG fragments into pregnant women. In fact, the half-lives of the two fragments proved to be different from each other; the half-life of the Fc fragment being about four days whilst that of the Fab was only 0.3 days. When the transfer of the fragments was re-evaluated taking into consideration their degradation, it became apparent that they were transferred with identical rates. However, further studies are needed to clarify the role of Fc as a placenta receptor site of IgG. The presence of the receptor has recently been demonstrated on the surface of the trophoblast at ten weeks and at term (Jenkinson, Billington and Elson, 1975).

According to Gitlin (1974), the rate of active transport of human IgG varies in the course of normal gestation. Between 6 and 16 weeks of pregnancy the concentrations of IgG range between 100 and 200 mg/100 ml. After 22 weeks of gestation, however, the transfer of maternal IgG increases and concentrations similar to those detectable in maternal sera are reached at 26 weeks. This increase in permeability seems selective for IgG, since there is no concomitant increase in the passage of other maternal plasma proteins. The observed increased transfer of AFP from fetal into the maternal circulation towards the end of gestation appears to confirm that the permeability of the placenta varies during pregnancy.

In sera from normal infants born at term, specific maternal antibodies associated with IgM and IgA cannot be detected and IgD molecules are either absent or present at low levels. Specific maternal IgE reaginic antibodies are not detectable in the corresponding cord blood. There is in fact good evidence that the IgM, IgA and IgE present in newborn blood are produced by the fetus during life in utero.

Synthesis of immunoglobulins by the fetus

The concentration of IgG estimated in infants bled at intervals soon after birth appears to decrease during the first three months of life. For many years this phenomenon was interpreted as evidence for the slow catabolism of the maternal IgG molecules, which were not replaced by similar proteins produced by the infants. However, as early as 1959, Trevorrow showed that if the dilution of serum proteins was taken into account, the amount of immunoglobulins during the first months of life was relatively constant. On the basis of these observations Trevorrow suggested that immunoglobulins are synthesised during life in utero in the course of normal pregnancy.

The low number of plasma cells in normal human fetuses, even during the last months of gestation, seems to be the effect of the absence of environmental stimulation rather than the cause of an inefficient antibody response. In fact, following intra-uterine infections, the human fetuses may respond to antigenic stimulation by the proliferation of plasma cells after the sixth month of gestation. Both congenital syphilis and toxoplasmosis have been found to be associated with infiltration of plasma cells into various fetal tissues (Pund and Von Haam,

1957; Silverstein and Lukes, 1962). Very young fetuses may, however, have positive staining for *Treponema* in the absence of an inflammatory response.

Early infection may not cause sufficient damage to result in the death of the fetus. The immunological immaturity of the fetus may allow the infective agent to persist in the tissues; however, this does not necessarily imply that the fetus becomes tolerant to the invading organism (Silverstein, 1972).

Following intra-uterine infections, specific antibodies and high levels of IgM have been detected in cord sera. Abnormal levels of IgM have been observed in sera from infants with congenital rubella, with a cytomegalic inclusion disease, or with infections of *Toxoplasma gondii* (Alford, 1965; McCraken and Shinefield, 1965; Remington and Miller, 1966; Alford et al, 1967; Adinolfi, 1974). The correlation between intra-uterine infection and high levels of IgM has been repeatedly observed and long-sustained antigenic stimulation during fetal life has been found to affect the synthesis of IgG during infancy (Soothill, Hayes and Dudgeon, 1966). For instance, low levels of IgG have been detected during the first 12 months in infants with congenital rubella and high levels of IgM at birth. Some of these infants showed a high susceptibility to infection. Antibodies associated with IgM globulins have also been detected in normal newborns; these antibodies are directed against red cell and, occasionally, bacterial antigens (Adinolfi, 1974). It is of interest that immunoglobulin molecules which behave as 7S proteins, as judged by gel filtration, but are antigenically related to IgM, have been detected in human cord blood (Perchalski, Clem and Small, 1968); 7S IgM have also been detected in lower vertebrates (Clem and Leslie, 1969).

In vitro cultures of fetal tissues in the presence of labelled amino acids and the analysis of the culture fluids by immunoelectrophoresis and autoradiography have confirmed that the human fetus is capable of producing IgG and IgM after the 12th week of gestation (Figure 2.2). Spleen and lymph nodes are the main sites of synthesis (van Furth, Schuit and Hijmans,

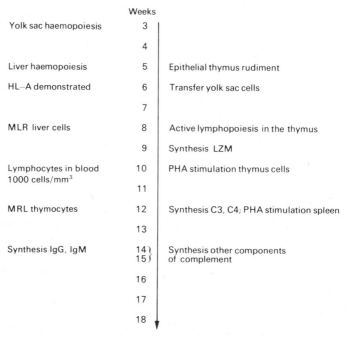

	Weeks	
Yolk sac haemopoiesis	3	
	4	
Liver haemopoiesis	5	Epithelial thymus rudiment
HL–A demonstrated	6	Transfer yolk sac cells
	7	
MLR liver cells	8	Active lymphopoiesis in the thymus
	9	Synthesis LZM
Lymphocytes in blood 1000 cells/mm³	10	PHA stimulation thymus cells
	11	
MRL thymocytes	12	Synthesis C3, C4; PHA stimulation spleen
	13	
Synthesis IgG, IgM	14 } 15 }	Synthesis other components of complement
	16	
	17	
	18	

Figure 2.2. Maturation of acquired immunity.

1965; Gitlin and Biasucci, 1969). Immunofluorescent staining of fetal spleen tissue has demonstrated that medium-size and large lymphoid cells, as well as plasma cells, secrete IgM and IgG molecules.

The number of B-cells in cord blood bearing surface Ig has been investigated by Fröland and Natvig (1971); the mean value for cells containing IgM was 9·7 per cent, that for IgG was 7.9 per cent. It is of interest that the dominant subclass of IgG expressed on cord lymphocytes was IgG2. No cells positive for IgA were detected in peripheral newborn blood. In fact only low levels of IgA have been detected in serum of normal neonates. However, high values of IgA have been detected in infants with congenital infections and in infants previously transfused during life in utero (Stiehm and Fudenberg, 1966; Hobbs, Hughes and Walker, 1968).

IgD immunoglobulins are usually absent or are present only in low concentrations in sera of normal human newborns. However, these molecules present on the surface of 3.5 per cent of B cells in normal adults have been detected in as many as 18 per cent of the lymphocytes from cord blood, usually in association with IgM molecules (Rowe et al, 1973). During the fetal stages of development, IgD molecules appear to behave more as cell 'receptors' than as humoral immunoglobulins.

IgE globulins are present in sera from normal newborns. The concentrations in paired cord and maternal blood samples are not correlated and specific maternal reaginic antibodies are not present in the newborn blood. In vitro cultures of fetal tissues have confirmed that IgE is synthesised during life in utero.

The evidence that the human fetus is capable of producing antibodies at an early stage of development is in agreement with studies on the ontogeny of acquired immunity in other species. Synthesis of antibodies during life in utero has been observed in the monkey, lamb, cow and guinea-pig (Solomon, 1971). In the lamb there is evidence that immunological competence to various antigens does not arise simultaneously but as a step-wise maturation of the ability to respond to different antigens at different stages of development (Silverstein, 1972).

These data lend support to the hypothesis that the specific events of immunological maturation in the fetus are finely timed. It should be noted, however, that in other species, notably the mouse and the rabbit, immunological maturity is attained only after birth. An important point which has emerged from studies on the ontogeny of acquired immunity in experimental animals is that the rate at which the antibody response to certain antigens develops in the immediate postnatal period is under genetic control (Playfair, 1968a, b).

Ontogeny of cellular immune response

The response of lymphocytes to phytohaemagglutinin (PHA) or to allogeneic stimuli has been used by various investigators to detect the onset of the functional development of T-cells in the human fetus. Thymocytes have been found to respond to PHA after 10 weeks of gestation (Pegrum, Ready and Thompson, 1968; Papiernik, 1970a, b; August et al, 1971; Ceppellini et al, 1971; Pegrum, 1971; Prindull, 1974; Stites, Carr and Fudenberg, 1974). At this stage of development a well-demarked thymic cortex and medulla are present. PHA-responsiveness of spleen and peripheral lymphocytes follows that in the thymus in time; this is consistent with the supposed thymic origin of these cells (Figure 2.2).

The formation of 'rosettes' between human lymphocytes and sheep red cells has been recognised as a property of the thymus-derived cells. In a study of 13 fetuses, a maximum of 65 per cent rosette-forming cells (RFC) were found in the thymus, with a poor correlation between incidence and fetal age. Only a small proportion of RFC was found in fetal bone marrow and spleen (Stites, Carr and Fudenberg, 1974). The results of these studies are consistent with the notion that RFC originate from the thymus and gradually migrate to peripheral blood during embryogenesis. Recent studies have also shown that 95 to 100 per cent of fetal thymocytes from fetuses between 12 and 20 weeks react specifically by immunofluorescence with an immune serum containing antibodies against fetal thymocyte antigens (Stites, Carr and Fudenberg, 1974).

Of great interest is the observation that the ability to respond to allogeneic lymphocytes by the mixed lymphocyte reaction (MLR) is first detectable at 7.5 weeks using hepatic cells; similar reactivity has been first observed in the thymus at 12.5 weeks (Figure 2.2) (Stites et al, 1972; Stites, Carr and Fudenberg, 1974).

Using in vitro tests of thymocytes, spleen cells and peripheral lymphocytes, a tendency for PHA-dependent DNA synthesis to increase with age has been noted. The highest reaction occurs near 19 weeks and thereafter the responsiveness declines.

It is worth stressing that peripheral lymphocytes from normal newborns, cultured without PHA, incorporate approximately six to ten times more radioactive thymidine into DNA than adult cells. Therefore, allowance should be made for such increased synthesis in studies of allogeneic stimulation of cord lymphocytes with maternal or paternal cells and unrelated mitomycin-treated adult lymphocytes. In the one-way mixed lymphocyte reaction, recognition of histocompatibility differences triggers proliferative response of the responding lymphocytes; the kinetics of this response have been found to be predictably altered by previous exposures to the appropriate antigens, producing either tolerance or sensitisation.

The MLR, therefore, appears particularly suitable to investigate whether specific modifications of cellular immunity are produced in the mother against the alien fetal histocompatibility antigens or in the fetus against the maternal or paternal antigens (Ceppellini et al, 1971; Bonnard and Lemos, 1972; Carr, Stites and Fudenberg, 1974).

There is good agreement that after calculation of the stimulation ratios, in many instances cord lymphocytes are less reactive against allogeneic stimuli from unrelated adult cells. According to Ceppellini and his collaborators (1971) maternal lymphocytes are a poorer stimulus than unrelated cells. However, Carr, Stites and Fudenberg (1974) have observed that when the temporal kinetics of the stimulation of maternal and adult unrelated cells are compared, the results do not suggest any specific tolerance or sensitisation of the fetal lymphocytes towards the maternal histocompatibility antigens.

It has also been suggested by Ceppellini et al (1971) that maternal lymphocytes, collected at time of delivery, are often less responsive to the corresponding newborn lymphocytes than to cell histocompatibility antigens from unrelated adults. However, according to Carr, Stites and Fudenberg (1974) the kinetic reactions of maternal lymphocytes in the MLR have the appearance of the usual allogeneic responses and the results do not suggest specific tolerance or specific sensitisation toward fetal histocompatibility antigens. Although stimulation with related mitomycin-treated cord lymphocytes is usually poorer than against unrelated cells, this is not unexpected since at least one-half of the histocompatibility antigens is similar in related mothers and newborns.

Although the results of the studies so far published show some discrepancies, they clearly suggest that an immunological depression of the maternal lymphocytes with respect to the related fetal histocompatibility antigens is not essential to the fetal survival, at least in human pregnancies.

During the last few years, evidence has also been produced that specific plasma proteins present in fetal serum and crossing the human placenta—such as alpha-fetoprotein (AFP)—or produced during pregnancy—such as the pregnancy zone protein (PZ)—may be responsible for an impaired immune reaction of lymphocytes in vitro and in vivo (Beckman, Beckman and Von Schoultz, 1974; Von Schoultz, Stigbrand and Tärnivik, 1974; Murgita and

Tomasi, 1975a, b). At the present time of research the roles that these proteins play in reducing the maternal cellular immunity and in the protection of the fetus are not yet clear. It is worth emphasising, however, that whatever their role, about ten per cent of pregnant women seem to be unable to produce PZ in detectable levels and that the fetus is capable of immune response in the presence of high levels of AFP in serum.

The evidence that transplantation immunity in man develops at an early stage of gestation is in good agreement with the observed early maturation of cell-mediated immunity in fetal lamb and monkey (Silverstein and Prendergast, 1970; Silverstein, 1972). This is not so in all species, since for example transplantation of allogeneic tissues in mice is successfully achieved when performed during perinatal life. Unfortunately, the early maturation of cell-mediated immunity in man makes it difficult to transplant normal tissues into human new-borns with inherited disorders; the only successful transplants so far achieved are those attempted in children with thymus-dependent immunological deficiencies (Van Bekkum and Dicke, 1972; Thomas, 1974).

Ontogeny of complement and lysozyme

It has long been recognised that even in the absence of deliberate immunisation and subsequent synthesis of antibodies, vertebrates possess an innate or natural resistance to infection. It is now generally accepted that endocytic cells, components of complement (C) and lysozyme (LZM) greatly influence the course and outcome of host defences. Deficiencies of components of C (Rosen and Alper, 1973) or the natural defence mechanisms associated with leucocyte functions (Miller, 1973) can be responsible for severe disorders.

Studies on the ontogeny of human C have shown that the mean level of total C activity in newborn sera is about half that detected in maternal blood (Adinolfi, 1972; Rosen, 1974). The introduction of the radial diffusion technique and of sensitive haemolytic tests for the estimation of single components of C have made it possible to evaluate the levels of these proteins in fetal and newborn sera. C3 and C4 have been detected in sera from human fetuses after 14 weeks and occasionally in nine to ten-week-old fetuses (Figure 2.2). C1, C3 activator, C5, C7 and C9 have also been detected at an early stage of fetal development (Adinolfi, 1972; Adinolfi and Beck, 1975).

The estimation of the levels of C3, C4, C6 and C7, and C3 activator in paired maternal and cord blood samples has shown that the mean concentration of these proteins in newborn samples is about half the values detected in maternal or adult sera. The only exceptions are for C8 and C9, which are present in cord blood in concentrations of 10 to 25 per cent of the mean in samples from normal adult subjects (Adinolfi, 1972, 1974; Adinolfi and Beck, 1975).

Direct evidence that C1, C3, C4 and C5 are produced during fetal life has been obtained by incubating fetal tissues in media containing labelled amino acids (Adinolfi, Gardiner and Wood, 1968; Gitlin and Biasucci, 1969; Adinolfi, 1972; Köhler, 1973). Analysis of the culture fluids for the presence of specific newly synthesised components of C, either using haemolytic tests or by autoradiography of the immunoelectrophoretic plates, has shown that C3 was produced in the liver cultures from fetuses more than 14 weeks old; in addition, haemolytically active de novo synthesised C3 has been isolated from the supernatants of fetal liver cultures. Similarly, synthesis of C4 has been demonstrated in liver tissue cultures obtained from fetuses more than eight weeks old.

Human peritoneal and alveolar cells from fetuses more than 14 weeks old have been shown to produce C3 and C4 in vitro. These findings are in agreement with evidence that these components of C are produced by liver, lung and peritoneal cells from adult monkeys, rats, rabbits and guinea-pigs. In man and experimental animals, macrophages collected from adult tissues seem to be capable of in vitro synthesis of C4 and C2. When human fetal liver macrophages were separated from other hepatic cells on a discontinuous albumin gradient, C4 was found to be produced in a fraction rich in macrophages (Colten, 1974).

The type of cells involved in the synthesis of C5 during fetal life is not yet known. In vitro cultures suggest that human C5 is produced mainly in fetal liver and spleen, but there is some evidence of C5 biosynthesis by fetal colon, lung, thymus, placenta, and peritoneal and bone marrow cells in culture (Köhler, 1973; Colten, 1974).

In a single experiment, in vitro synthesis of the first component of C1 was observed by Colten et al (1968) using tissues obtained from a 19-week-old fetus. Isolated fragments of the small intestine and colon were found to be capable of in vitro production of haemolytically active C1. No significant synthesis was observed in the culture fluids of fetal liver, lung, kidney, thymus, spleen and stomach.

Gitlin and Biasucci (1969) have also investigated the synthesis of C1-inhibitor by the autoradiographic techniques. Newly produced C1-inhibitor was detected in the culture fluid of liver tissue from four-week-old human fetuses. Early production of C1-inhibitor in fetal liver has been confirmed by Colten (1972), who noticed that the rate of synthesis of C1-inhibitor in an 11-week-old fetus appeared to be similar to that observed in normal adult subjects.

Lysozyme (LZM) is also produced at an early stage of fetal development; the enzyme has been detected in sera from fetuses more than nine weeks old and all cord samples tested; levels similar to those detected in normal adults are reached at about 18 weeks of gestation (Glynn, Martin and Adinolfi, 1970; Adinolfi, 1972). Using an immunoperoxidase technique, LZM has been detected in the alveolar macrophages of lung in human fetuses as well as in fetuses of experimental animals (Klockars, Adinolfi and Ossermann, 1974).

FETO-MATERNAL IMMUNOLOGICAL INTERACTIONS

The development of a fetus within the uterine environment is now known to have a profound effect on the immunological status of the mother. In man and in experimental animals there is evidence for both humoral and cell-mediated immune responses elicited by antigens of fetal origin. Whilst much of the data, and this chapter, concern reactivity largely to histocompatibility and blood group antigens, it is also clear that many other fetal antigens can be involved, particularly those of a tissue-specific, phase-specific and fetal serum protein nature. The influence is not solely in one direction. There is a certain amount of evidence for maternal modification of the fetal immune system, such as impaired responsiveness to maternal antigen, allotype suppression and inhibition of paternal histocompatibility antigen expression.

Maternal response to pregnancy

The existence of antibodies in the maternal serum directed against paternally inherited histocompatibility antigens (human leucocyte antigen or HL-A) of the human fetus is well-established. Lymphocytotoxic and leucoagglutinating antibodies are detectable at significant levels in women of different parity. Although estimates vary, it appears that up to 20 per cent of women in their first pregnancy may possess lymphocytotoxins, and that this may rise to 50 per cent or more in some multiparous groups. Leucoagglutinin response is lower, with positive findings in about 5 and 20 per cent of cases respectively (Jones, 1971). These figures may to some extent simply reflect the sensitivity of the techniques employed as well as the type of antibody identified, and the use of newer assays such as antibody-dependent cell-mediated lympholysis (Perlmann, Perlmann and Wigzell, 1972) may reveal the frequencies to be higher. The reason why only a proportion of women show detectable responses is not known. Since it is estimated that 99 per cent of women have histoincompatible pregnancies, it must presumably relate to quantitative variation in fetal stimulus or genetically determined variation (HL-A linked?) in the ability of the female to respond. It is also possible that some of the non-responsiveness could be explained by cross-reactivity of the HL-A antigens of the fetus with the mother. The findings on maternal antibody production parallel closely those of extensive investigations on pregnancy in the mouse.

There has been considerable debate as to whether or not certain pathological conditions of pregnancy, particularly pre-eclampsia, are associated, either as cause or effect, with changes in the maternal antibody response. Most investigators appear to have been unable to detect significant variation from that seen in normal pregnancies, but the matter is still in dispute (see section on pregnancy disorders). Claims have also been made for elevated HL-A sensitisation in female sterility, but the data are not yet convincing.

Maternal sensitisation against the fetal blood cell antigens may also occur under particular circumstances, the most well-known being rhesus and platelet isoimmunisation. Fetal A and B blood group antigens cannot induce a primary immunisation since 'naturally occurring' antibodies are already present in ABO incompatible mothers.

Evidence for the induction of a specific cell-mediated response to fetal antigen is less extensive, with most of the compelling data obtained from studies on inbred strains of mice and rats. In allogeneic pregnancy there is a significant and specific hypertrophy of the lymph nodes draining the uterus. In addition, lymphoid cells removed from females multiparous by allogeneic males have been shown to have specific immune reactivity to the antigens of the male strain, as assessed by their ability to induce splenomegaly, fibroblast colony inhibition, popliteal lymph node enlargement and erythrocyte rosette formation in appropriate test situations. It has so far proved much more difficult to demonstrate a significant response during the course of a first pregnancy, although recent unpublished studies in our laboratory (G. F. Eldred and W. D. Billington) using a mouse macrophage migration inhibition (MIF) test, indicate that this can occur.

Attempts to detect the presence of cell-mediated immunity by classical skin-grafting techniques have led to the unexpected and apparently paradoxical finding of a *prolonged* survival of grafts following allogeneic pregnancy. This phenomenon, referred to as 'tolerance' by its discoverers and 'unresponsiveness' by later investigators, may well be explicable in terms of current knowledge on the mechanism of immunological enhancement. The coexistence of cellular and humoral immunity can lead to the blocking of cell-mediated tissue rejection by the attachment of the antibody or, more likely, antigen–antibody complexes to the target and/or effector cell surface. This blocking system may well play a role in the protection of the fetal allograft as well as the test skin graft (see section on mechanisms for fetal protection).

Evidence for the induction of cellular immunity in human pregnancy is not yet so well documented. There have been no reports of a uterine lymph node hypertrophy comparable to that observed in the laboratory animals. Since many of the experimental approaches are not possible in man, in vitro assays of lymphocyte reactivity have been extensively employed. One of these, the MIF test, has recently indicated that a cell-mediated immunity is present and persists for some months into the postpartum period (Dossetor et al, 1974). Many findings have in fact demonstrated that lymphocytes from pregnant women are *hyporeactive* towards those from paternal or cord blood as compared to those from an unrelated donor. However, it has also been shown that various factors present in maternal serum can be responsible for this diminished response, since their removal from the cultures allows full lymphocyte reactivity to return. It seems reasonable to conclude that specific cellular immunity to fetal antigen is present in the pregnant woman, but that the immunity is suppressed in vivo by one or many of the factors reported to reduce lymphocyte reactivity in vitro. These factors may be specific, such as IgG (or antigen–antibody complexes), or non-specific, such as the placental protein hormones human chorionic gonadotrophin (hCG) and human placental lactogen (hPL), steroid hormones, the so-called 'pregnancy zone' proteins and serum seromucoid glycoproteins.

Antigen expression during fetal development

The specific humoral and cell-mediated responses in the pregnant female must be stimulated by appropriate fetal antigens. Although in the case of Rh sensitisation and platelet isoimmunisation the source of the antigenic stimulus is quite clear, this is not so for the responses to paternally inherited histocompatibility antigen of the fetus, and a number of alternatives must be considered.

The first antigenic challenge to the female comes from a massive 'inoculation' of spermatozoa and seminal fluid. It has been suggested that this is responsible for the induction of anti-HL-A antibody in normal pregnancy and also in some cases of infertility. Although this could possibly be a contributory factor, it is unlikely to be the main method of sensitisation for a number of reasons: the extent of expression of histocompatibility antigens on the human spermatozoon has not been fully established, the levels of maternal immunity encountered are unlikely to be reached by this means on those occasions when pregnancy follows a single sexual experience and, in experimental animals, it has proved exceedingly difficult to induce a response against histocompatibility antigens by injection of spermatozoa. The crucial experiment would be to investigate antibody production in animals in which pregnancy had been accomplished by the transfer of fertilised eggs to virgin females.

Whether or not spermatozoa are excluded, it is pertinent to consider the expression of antigens on the embryo. Studies on the mouse have demonstrated that the strong histocompatibility antigen complex (H-2) is expressed very early, at the blastocyst stage of development, whilst the weaker antigens (non-H-2) are present even on the cleaving egg. The time of paternal antigen expression probably relates quite closely to this. In the human there is direct evidence, from a mixed agglutination technique, for the presence of HL-A antigens on the six-week conceptus, the earliest stage so far examined. The liver and fetal membranes were detectably antigenic at this time, whereas many other tissues did not react positively until a few weeks later (Seigler and Metzgar, 1970).

The evidence from studies on mouse and man thus indicates the presence of histocompatibility antigens from the earliest embryonic stages. How do these antigens stimulate the maternal immune system? It is widely believed that the leucoagglutinating and lymphocytotoxic antibodies in pregnant women are indicative of stimulation by transplacentally transferred fetal leucocytes. In fact, evidence for any such cell transfer is far from convincing, and the few reports claiming to have detected fetal leucocytes in maternal blood can be seriously questioned. Attempts have been based on identification of male 46XY cells by karyotype analysis or Y-chromosome fluorescence using quinacrine mustard. Since both these techniques can give false-positive results in non-pregnant controls and in women with a subsequently delivered female offspring, the issue is by no means fully resolved. On grounds such as these, some authors have extended their studies and retracted conclusions based on earlier data. On the other hand, it should be noted that evidence for fetal red cell transfer to the maternal circulation in normal pregnancy, and of course in cases of rhesus incompatibility, is fairly substantial. Although it would seem reasonable to expect that the transfer of leucocytes would at least parallel, if not on the basis of their motility actually exceed that of red cells, this need not inevitably be so. Some form of specific trapping mechanism might operate.

It has been suggested that cytotoxic antibody can appear in a primigravida prior to significant leucocyte development in the fetus, and that this would argue against these cells being responsible for the immunity. However, it would seem on present evidence that the antibody cannot be detected much before the seventh week of pregnancy, whilst lymphoid cell proliferation is already extensive in the sixth week.

There are two other possible sources of stimulatory histocompatibility antigen: on placental trophoblast tissue and in a transferred soluble form. Trophoblast is the only fetal material in direct and continuous contact with the maternal tissues and would seem to be ideally situated to present a prolonged immunogenic challenge. In addition, at least in man and one or two other species, the trophoblastic elements are shed from the placenta into the maternal circulation throughout much of pregnancy, and could contribute significantly to this challenge. Unfortunately for this theory, there is as yet no satisfactory proof of the expression of histocompatibility antigens on the trophoblast. This has profound importance for many aspects of reproductive immunology and is considered in detail below. As far as the second possibility is concerned, little is known about the release and in vivo solubility of fetal histocompatibility antigen. Experimental procedures do, however, indicate that this is likely to occur to a much greater extent than with adult tissues. Techniques are now available for the detection of free antigen in body fluids and it would be interesting to see these applied to the pregnancy situation.

Mechanisms for fetal protection

The presence of an antigenically active fetus capable of inducing specific humoral and cellular immunity in its maternal host raises the question of why the fetus does not undergo rejection in the face of this immunity. This has been considered as "one of the major unsolved problems of transplantation immunology" (Billingham, 1964) and has been the subject of intense investigation and speculation. Answers to this problem are likely to be of interest not only for an understanding of normal and abnormal pregnancy but also for new approaches to tumour immunotherapy and organ transplantation.

The following six sections give brief consideration to the major hypotheses that have been advanced for fetal survival (for more detailed reviews see Beer and Billingham, 1971; Edidin, 1972).

Vascular isolation

The conceptus is not vascularised in the manner of a surgically constructed graft, and the circulatory systems of the mother and fetus, although coming into close contact within the placenta, remain entirely independent. This is believed to be an important factor in restricting the exchange of immunological information that would under other transplantation circumstances lead to tissue rejection.

Fetal antigenic immaturity

An absence, or relatively low level, of histocompatibility antigens on fetal tissues could prevent either the induction of a significant immune response or the destruction of the tissues by any pre-existing immunity. However, it is now known, as indicated above, that these antigens are detectable from the earliest stages of development, and are responsible for the state of maternal immunity directed specifically against them. There is, nevertheless, much to be learned about their precise nature, location and immunogenicity, and this may give further clues to the insusceptibility of the fetus to immune attack. It should also be acknowledged that the relevance of the antigenic status of the fetus in this respect has still to be fully defined, since it is the placenta that has direct contact with maternal tissues and has to face the major part of the immunity, particularly in the form of immunocompetent lymphocytes.

Maternal immunological unresponsiveness

Despite the existence of a specific immune reactivity in the mother, it is possible that there may be modifying forces able to render it ineffective in fetal rejection. These could be of a nonspecific or a specific nature. A slight overall nonspecific effect could be mediated by the high levels of corticosteroids during pregnancy, which are known to produce a transient lymphocytopenia and have a weak immunosuppressive action. Studies on the suppression of lymphocyte transformation in vitro by the variety of pregnancy serum factors mentioned previously also point to a likely system operating in vivo. It has recently been suggested that extremely high levels of hCG may have a local immunosuppressive effect at the trophoblast cell surface. Whilst this may offer an attractive explanation for the presence of this hormone in human pregnancy, it should be stressed that techniques are not yet available for the quantitative assay of localised hormone, and that hCG is not known to have a counterpart in all mammalian species.

Specific maternal unresponsiveness was at one time considered in terms of the induction of a state of classical immunological tolerance. There is now little support for this, and current views largely favour the concept of enhancement, with blocking antibody or immune complexes operating in a manner similar to that described for tumour survival in immune hosts (see Hellström and Hellström, 1974). Blocking systems tend to be promoted by a prolonged release of low doses of weak antigen, conditions which the fetus or, more likely, the placenta could well provide.

It is now clear that although there is no gross maternal inertia—in most situations the pregnant female shows little or no alteration of reactivity to allogeneic skin grafts, injected antigen or pathogenic organisms—there are rather more subtle regulations of the immune response occurring at this time. It seems possible that both specific and nonspecific factors are in operation, perhaps at different stages of pregnancy and at various levels of suppression.

Immunological privilege of the uterine environment

It is possible that the uterus may have features in common with such sites as the anterior chamber of the eye and the brain, and allow the extended survival of tissue allografts. However, unlike these sites, the uterus is not overtly deficient in either its vascular supply or lymphatic drainage and has now in fact been shown in experimental animals to express a normal state of transplantation immunity, at least to non-fetal grafts. Although this hypothesis is frequently discarded, it should be noted that the experiments designed to test it have been carried out almost entirely on the non-pregnant uterus and have not always taken into account the existence in pregnancy of the uterine decidual tissue, which is known under certain conditions to possess immunological quarantining properties.

Anatomical barrier

Allograft rejection reactions could in theory be frustrated by the presence of a partial or total barrier to either the afferent or efferent arm of the immunological response. It would seem from the evidence on the induction of maternal immunity that in the pregnancy situation any barrier must be largely efferent. If this were in an anatomical form, it would have to involve a structure providing a continuous interface between intimately apposed maternal and fetal tissues. The only material that answers this description at the important placental level is the trophoblast, although the outermost fetal membrane, which has direct contact with the uterine wall, must also be taken into account. In humans this membrane is the chorion, which is trophoblastic in nature, but in other species it may be of quite different embryological origin. Very little is known of the fetal membranes in this respect, with the exception of the mouse yolk sac (see Jenkinson and Billington, 1974).

An anatomical barrier of this type must not only be effective against any maternal immune response directed against the fetus but must itself be insusceptible to immune attack. It is therefore important to establish whether or not trophoblast possesses transplantation antigens. This has proved an exceedingly difficult task that has given rise to a considerable amount of confusing and controversial evidence. To a large extent, the problems relate to the fact that many investigators have apparently been unaware of the variety of biological forms of the trophoblast, not only in different species but during particular phases of development and in the mature placenta. In addition, in most cases it has not yet been possible to extract the tissue in a pure form suitable for immunological analysis. The issue has been fully discussed in a recent review (Billington, 1975), and is considered in the section on trophoblast as an immunological barrier.

Immunological competence of the placenta

Although not normally included in a list of possible reasons for the survival of the fetal allograft, it is perhaps worth considering that an ability on the part of the placenta to participate in immune reactivity could have certain advantages for the fetus. As pointed out by Douglas (1965), the main one might be the provision of a line of defence against the entry of potentially injurious antigens. His other suggestions, that the placenta might by this means limit the passage of maternal cells and even mount a local graft-versus-host reaction against maternal tissue, are much less acceptable in view of the antigenic relationship between the mother and her F_1 placenta.

Experimental evidence for immunological competence of the placenta is in fact limited and as yet unconvincing. The report of an agammaglobulinaemic woman who raised antibodies to injected typhoid bacilli during pregnancy, but was non-responsive after delivery, with no antibody in the baby (Good and Zak, 1956), provides one of the few positive clinical indications. The nature of the fetal cell type in the placenta responsible for such activity is unknown.

The trophoblast as an immunological barrier

A lack of effective antigenicity would appear to be an important feature for a tissue believed to be involved in a barrier role. That the trophoblast fulfils this condition is clear from the wide variety of transplantation and in vitro studies that have documented its insusceptibility to specific immune destruction. This was originally suggested to be due to either an absence or severe intrinsic deficit of histocompatibility antigens (Simmons and Russell, 1962), but there is the alternative possibility that such antigens may be present yet prevented from being recognised to any detectable degree (Kirby et al, 1964; Currie and Bagshawe, 1967). From studies on the mouse placenta, Kirby and his colleagues initially proposed that a fibrinoid-like material coating the trophoblast could provide a mechanism for the lack of recognition of underlying antigens. Subsequent examination of both normal and pathological human trophoblast, using more refined techniques of electron-histochemistry, demonstrated that the coating material was actually a membrane-bound mucoprotein, and quite distinct from the gross fibrinoid deposits in other regions of the placenta (Bradbury et al, 1970). The immunological implications of the trophoblast cell surface mucoprotein have recently been considered in detail (Billington, 1975).

Experiments have been designed to test the theory of antigen masking by mucoprotein. A number of these have involved human mixed lymphocyte–trophoblast cultures following trypsinisation of placental tissue, but have generally been unsatisfactory because of the difficulty of establishing the identity of the trophoblast and of setting up adequate specificity controls. The first apparently convincing evidence came from Currie, van Doorninck and Bagshawe (1968) who reported that the injection of neuraminidase-treated early mouse trophoblast into allogeneic recipients induced sensitisation to subsequent skin grafts. By analogy with similar experiments on certain tumour cells, this was interpreted as indicating the unmasking of antigens by enzymatic removal of neuraminic acid from cell-surface sialomucins. Unfortunately, two independent investigations have failed to confirm these findings and this, together with other evidence (see Searle, Jenkinson and Johnson, 1975), seems to rule out the mucoprotein masking hypothesis, at least as far as the early differentiating mouse trophoblast is concerned. However, it must be stressed that this does *not* necessarily mean that other antigen-masking systems do not operate (see Billington, 1976), nor even that mucoprotein cannot be the effective agent on later stages of trophoblast, particularly in the placenta, in which the electron-microscopical and histochemical identification of the material has been fully confirmed (Wynn, 1971). It has not yet proved possible to pursue a satisfactory experimental approach with such a mature trophoblast, since a method has not been found for obtaining pure trophoblast from the placenta. There are in fact considerable difficulties in assessing the specific involvement of trophoblastic elements in nearly all immunological analyses of placental tissues, and especially using in vitro techniques.

Discussions on masking phenomena and other possible mechanisms for the apparent insusceptibility of gestational trophoblast to in vivo maternal immunological attack are of relevance only if this fetal tissue actually possesses appropriate antigenic determinants. Despite intense research effort, there is still no conclusive proof that this is so, although most investigators believe that the weight of evidence is in this direction (see Billington, 1976).

The so-called 'placental barrier', of which the trophoblast has been identified as the important component, relates mainly to the prevention of access of deleterious agents to the immunologically immature fetus, particularly immunocompetent maternal cells and pathogenic microorganisms. The trophoblast of course also allows the transfer of many substances, although often exhibiting great selectivity, particularly with respect to the passage of protein molecules (see the first part of this chapter). Although it is not therefore a complete barrier—there is an increasing tendency to refer to it as a 'filter'—the placenta clearly plays an important role in fetal protection. From the few exceedingly rare cases of severe graft-versus-host disease in human neonates that are believed to be due to transplacentally transmitted maternal leucocytes, it is apparent that the placenta must provide an effective barrier to these cells in normal pregnancy. Studies on experimental animals, using chromosomal and radioactive tracers, and examination of the peripheral blood of human male neonates for cells of 46XX karyotype, have shown that little or no traffic occurs. Those few cells that have been detected are likely to have crossed near to the end of pregnancy, when the structural integrity of the placenta is breaking down, and there can be little immunological significance in their presence. This is supported by the findings that only by exposure of pregnant female rodents to agents that are known to cause placental damage (e.g. x-irradiation and hyaluronidase) can significant modification of fetal immune responses and maternal cell transfer be demonstrated.

Recent studies using in vitro techniques have also shown suppression of mitosis of maternal lymphocytes when mixed with neonatal cells in the presence of mitotic agents or in a two-way mixed lymphocyte culture (Olding et al, 1974; Lawler et al, 1975).

The final consideration concerns the question of the selective transmission of antibody across the placenta. Not all of the maternal immunoglobulins will be of the beneficial type that endow the fetus with its passive immunity. As will be clear from the preceding discussion on maternal immune responses in pregnancy, some will be directed specifically against the antigens of the fetus and hence constitute a potential danger. Although it has been suggested that under certain experimental conditions cytotoxic 7S antibody may be able to cross the placenta and localise without demonstrable harm on the fetal tissues (Lanman and Herod, 1965), this is by no means fully established. It may in fact be important in normal pregnancy for the trophoblast to prevent the transfer of most, if not all, of the anti-fetal antibody. One mechanism for this could be the possession of an array of antigenic determinants able to 'trap' such antibody by specific attachment, whilst being in a form insusceptible to immune lytic reaction. Another recent suggestion is that some of the antibody in the form of immune complexes, such as that believed to be involved in 'blocking' systems, may be bound to trophoblast by means of cell-surface Fc receptors (Elson, Jenkinson and Billington, 1975).

Immunological factors in pregnancy disorders

The information on normal pregnancy indicates that the successful maintenance of the fetal–maternal relationship probably depends upon a complex and dynamic immunological equilibrium involving the constant interplay of many factors. As with any biological control system this is liable to break down and lead to complications for the relationship. Numerous clinical abnormalities of pregnancy have been examined for an immunological causation and although the evidence is often fragmentary, sometimes conflicting and rarely conclusive, several of these abnormalities may have an immunological basis (see Jones and Scott, 1976).

Spontaneous abortion

From skin grafting tests and mixed lymphocyte cultures it is apparent that habitual aborters frequently possess an increased reactivity to their consort's antigens by comparison with those of an unrelated male. Although this might be taken to indicate that histoincompatibility is associated with abortion, it is not yet clear in what way this could operate. It is also possible that a specific sensitisation to paternally derived fetal antigen is induced. If this is the case, it is perhaps surprising that secundigravida who have had a normal first pregnancy appear to have higher HL-A antibody responses than those having had a previous spontaneous abortion (Burke and Johansen, 1974), although this of course does not relate directly to the previously implied state of cellular immunity.

A number of reports provide data showing an increase in the incidence of abortion in ABO blood group incompatible matings, and it has been suggested that two per cent of all zygotes may die as a result of such incompatibility (Chung and Morton, 1961).

Toxaemia

An immunological basis for pregnancy toxaemia was first proposed at the beginning of the century, and although evidence has slowly accumulated from several directions this is still not conclusive. There are hallmarks of immune conflict in the placenta and kidneys during toxaemia, with extensive infarction and fibrinoid necrosis showing deposition of immunoglobulins, complement, fibrinogen and fibrin. Injection of placental extracts produces similar effects in the kidneys of experimental animals.

More recently, attempts have been made to correlate the disorder with the HL-A antigen relationship between husband and wife. Some data suggest a shift towards histoincompatibility whilst other data show no deviation. There appears to be an increase in the serum seromucoid levels in pre-eclampsia/eclampsia, and this may be related to the clinical severity of the condition. This is of interest here since it is known that these glycoproteins are particularly influenced by immune stress. Jenkins (1974) has also presented evidence for an association between maternal–paternal HL-A antigen disparity and the seromucoid levels, supporting histoincompatibility as a related factor. This could also be an implication of the findings of Carretti et al (1974) of an increased frequency of anti-HL-A antibody in toxaemic groups, although here again not all investigators have detected differences from normal pregnancy.

Dysmaturity

Intra-uterine growth retardation, leading to 'small-for-dates' babies, is frequently associated with placental insufficiency. In such cases the placenta may have histological characteristics in common with those described in toxaemia and indicative of an immune reaction. Some overtly dysmature babies exhibit features similar to those found in experimentally induced runt disease in laboratory animals, produced by the injection of immunocompetent allogeneic cells into neonates. As mentioned previously, there are in fact a few very rare instances of human male neonates with severe symptoms of runting (graft-versus-host disease) believed to result from transplacentally transferred maternal lymphocytes. A report that runting can be induced in experimental animals by immunisation of the mother to paternal antigens either before or during pregnancy (Beer and Billingham, 1973) has not been confirmed in our laboratory (G. F. Eldred and W. D. Billington, 1974, unpublished observations).

Rhesus disease

Maternal isoimmunisation to the Rh(D) antigen of the fetal erythrocyte is a well-defined phenomenon. Sensitisation commonly occurs at the time of placental degeneration approaching term, or actually at delivery, although it is now recognised that earlier bleeds can occur, particularly following therapeutic abortion. Fetal distress or death results from the transmission of the maternal antibody across the placenta, usually in the subsequent pregnancy.

In the present context it is of interest to consider the small group (two to four per cent) of

Rh-negative women who have anti-D antibodies during their first pregnancy. This could be explained in terms of a very early fetal bleed or of the exposure of the Rh-negative mother to D antigen stimulation during her own intra-uterine development in an Rh-positive female. In the latter case, re-exposure in the woman's first Rh incompatible pregnancy would produce an extensive secondary response. The finding of small numbers of Rh-negative infants with anti-D antibody supports this hypothesis, and also indicates the desirability of screening newborns for immunoglobulin treatment. Whether or not this would be effective might depend upon the length of time since sensitisation occurred in utero.

Congenital malformation

It has been claimed that the incidence of congenital defects is higher in infants of women with raised HL-A antibody levels in pregnancy (Terasaki et al, 1970), although this could not be confirmed in a later study by these workers. Whilst further data are clearly needed, it may be significant that maternal immunisation against paternal antigens has not so far been shown to have deleterious effect on the fetus in a number of different experimental animal situations. If antibody could ever be proved to have such an effect, a possible mechanism for this might be interference with cellular interaction during morphogenesis. There are claims in the Russian literature of developmental anomalies resulting from disturbances of anti-fetal organ-specific antibody levels in pregnant women (see Volkova and Maysky, 1969).

Choriocarcinoma

A variety of immunological and genetic factors appears to have a role in the development of this trophoblastic tumour. Early data suggested an increased frequency of choriocarcinoma in women from inbreeding communities and also in women with a relative ABO compatibility with their husbands, indicating consanguinity as a predisposing factor. Although choriocarcinoma patients usually accept a graft of their husband's skin for extended periods there is in fact no evidence for HL-A compatibility between such individuals (Bagshawe, 1974). This could be taken to indicate some form of maternal 'tolerance' to the paternal antigens of the tumour, perhaps in the form of blocking antibodies. However, it should perhaps also be noted that, as in normal pregnancy, there are responders and non-responders for anti-HL-A cytotoxic antibody production.

Recent analyses of ABO relationships in choriocarcinoma show a considerably increased risk for group A women with group O husbands compared to those with group A husbands. The basis for this is unknown.

Despite previous assertions to the contrary, it is now clear that there is a host cellular immune response to this tumour. Mononuclear cell invasion occurs to varying degrees and correlates strongly with susceptibility to chemotherapy; the greater the host response the better the prognosis.

As with all the pregnancy disorders described, further understanding of the aetiology of choriocarcinoma, and approaches to its prevention, may depend upon a greater awareness of the immunological mechanisms in normal fetal–maternal relationships.

REFERENCES

Adinolfi, M. (1972) Ontogeny of components of complement and lysozyme. In *Ontogeny of Acquired Immunity*, pp. 65–81, Ciba Foundation Symposium. Amsterdam: Associated Scientific Publishers.

Adinolfi, M. (1974) The development of lymphoid tissues and immunity. In *Scientific Foundation of Paediatrics* (Ed.) Davis, J. A. & Dobbing, J. New York: Heineman.

Adinolfi, M. & Beck, S. (1975) Human complement—C7 and C9—in fetal and newborn sera. *Archives of Disease in Childhood*, **50**, 562–564.

Adinolfi, M. & Wood, C. (1969) Ontogenesis of immunoglobulins and components of complement in man. In *Immunology and Development* (Ed.) Adinolfi, M. pp. 27–61. London: Spastics International Medical Publications.

Adinolfi, M., Gardner, B. & Wood, C. B. S. (1968) Ontogenesis of two components of human complement, βIE and βIC–IA globulins. *Nature*, **219**, 189–191.

Alford, C. A. (1965) Studies on antibody in congenital rubella infection. I. Physico-chemical and immunological investigation of rubella neutralizing antibody. *American Journal of Diseases of Children*, **100**, 455–463.

Alford, C. A., Schaefer, J., Blankenship, W. J., Straumfjord, J. V. & Cassidy, G. (1967) A correlative immunologic, microbiologic and clinical approach to the diagnosis of acute and chronic infections in newborn infants. *New England Journal of Medicine*, **277**, 437–449.

August, C. S., Izzet Berkel, A., Driscoll, S. & Merler, E. (1971) Onset of lymphocyte function in the developing human fetus. *Paediatric Research*, **5**, 539–547.

Bagshawe, K. D. (1974) A review of some immunological relationships in trophoblastic neoplasia. In *Immunology in Obstetrics and Gynaecology* (Ed.) Centaro, A. & Caretti, N. pp. 287–291. Amsterdam: Excerpta Medica.

Beckman, G., Beckman, L. & Von Schoultz, B. (1974) Relationship between serum concentration of the pregnancy zone protein and mother–child incompatibility. *Human Heredity*, **24**, 558–562.

Beer, A. E. & Billingham, R. E. (1971) Immunobiology of mammalian reproduction. *Advances in Immunology*, **14**, 1–84.

Beer, A. E. & Billingham, R. E. (1973) Maternally acquired runt disease. *Science*, **179**, 240–243.

Bekkum, D. W. & Dicke, K. A. (1972) Treatment of immune deficiency with bone marrow stem cell concentrates. In *Ontogeny of Acquired Immunity*, pp. 223–236. Amsterdam: Associated Scientific Publishers.

Billingham, R. E. (1964) Transplantation immunity and the maternal–foetal relation. *New England Journal of Medicine*, **270**, 667–672, 720–725.

Billington, W. D. (1975) Organisation, ultrastructure and histochemistry of the placenta: immunological considerations. In *Immunobiology of Trophoblast* (Ed.) Edwards, R. G., Howe, C. W. S. & Johnson, M. H. pp. 67–85. London: Cambridge University Press.

Billington, W. D. (1976) The immunobiology of trophoblast. In *Immunology of Human Reproduction* (Ed.) Jones, W. R. & Scott, J. S. London: Academic Press. In press.

Bonnard, G. D. & Lemos, L. (1972) The cellular immunity of mother versus child at delivery: sensitisation in unidirectional mixed lymphocyte culture and subsequent ^{51}Cr-release cytoxicity test. *Transplantation Proceedings*, **4**, 177–180.

Bradbury, S., Billington, W. D., Kirby, D. R. S. & Williams, E. A. (1970) Histochemical characterization of the surface mucoprotein of normal and abnormal human trophoblast. *Histochemical Journal*, **2**, 263–274.

Brambell, F. W. R. (1970) *The Transmission of Passive Immunity from the Mother to Young*. Vol. 18. Amsterdam: North-Holland Publishing Company.

Brambell, F. W. R., Hemmings, W. A., Oakley, C. L. & Porter, R. R. (1960) The relative transmission of the fractions of papain hydrolyzed homologous γ-globulin from the uterine cavity to the foetal circulation in the rabbit. *Proceedings of the Royal Society of London*, **151B**, 478–482.

Burke, J. & Johansen, K. (1974) The formation of HL-A antibodies in pregnancy. The antigenicity of aborted and term foetuses. *Journal of Obstetrics and Gynaecology of the British Commonwealth*, **81**, 222–228.

Carr, M. C., Stites, D. P. & Fudenberg, H. H. (1974) Cellular immune aspects of the human fetal–maternal relationship. III. Mixed lymphocyte reactivity between related maternal and cord blood lymphocytes. *Cellular Immunology*, **11**, 332–341.

Carretti, N., Chiaramonte, P., Pasini, C., Zanetti, M. & Fagiolo, U. (1974) Association of anti-HL-A antibodies with toxaemia in pregnancy. In *Immunology in Obstetrics and Gynaecology* (Ed.) Centaro, A. & Carretti, N. pp. 221–225. Amsterdam: Excerpta Medica.

Ceppellini, R., Bonnard, G. D., Coppu, F., Miggiano, V. C., Pospisil, M., Curtoni, E. S. & Pellegrino, M. (1971) Mixed leukocyte cultures and HL-A antigens. I. Reactivity of young foetuses, newborns and mothers at delivery. *Transplantation Proceedings*, **3**, 58–71.

Chung, C. S. & Morton, N. E. (1961) Selection at the ABO locus. *American Journal of Human Genetics*, **13**, 9–27.

Clem, L. W. & Leslie, G. A. (1969) Phylogeny of immunoglobulin structure and function. In *Immunology and Development* (Ed.) Adinolfi, M. pp. 55–88. London: Spastics International Medical Publications.

Cohen, S. (1971) Structure and biological properties of antibodies. In *Immunological Diseases* (Ed.) Samter, M. 2nd edition, pp. 39–65. Boston: Little, Brown.

Colten, H. R. (1972) Ontogeny of human complement system: *in vitro* biosynthesis of individual complement components by fetal tissues. *Journal of Clinical Investigation*, **51**, 725–730.

Colten, H. R. (1974) Synthesis and metabolism of complement proteins. *Transplantation Proceedings*, **6**, 33–38.

Colten, H. R., Gordon, J. M., Borsos, T. & Rapp, H. Y. (1968) Synthesis of the first component of human complement *in vitro*. *Journal of Experimental Medicine*, **128**, 595–604.

Currie, G. A. & Bagshawe, K. D. (1967) The masking of antigens on trophoblast and cancer cells. *Lancet*, **i**, 708–710.

Currie, G. A., van Doorninck, W. & Bagshawe, K. D. (1968) Effect of neuraminidase on the immunogenicity of early mouse trophoblast. *Nature*, **219**, 191–192.

Dancis, J., Braverman, N. & Lind, J. (1957) Plasma protein synthesis in the human fetus and placenta. *Journal of Clinical Investigation*, **36**, 398–404.

Davis, S. D. (1973) Antibody deficiency disorders. In *Immunologic Disorders in Infants and Children* (Ed.) Stiehm, E. R. & Fulginiti, V. A. pp. 184–198. Philadelphia: W. B. Saunders.

Dossetor, J. B., Kovithavongs, T., Boyd, J. J., Lockwood, B., Lao, V., Schlaut, J., Liburd, E. M., Olson, L. & Russell, A. S. (1974) Humoral and cell-mediated immunity in parous women. In *Immunology in Obstetrics and Gynaecology* (Ed.) Centaro, A. & Carretti, N. pp. 192–199. Amsterdam: Excerpta Medica.

Douglas, G. W. (1965) The immunologic role of the placenta. *Obstetrics and Gynaecology Survey*, **20**, 442–451.

Dwyer, J. M. & MacKay, I. R. (1970) Antigen-binding lymphocytes in human fetal thymus. *Lancet*, **i**, 1119–1212.

Edidin, M. (1972) Histocompatibility genes, transplantation antigens and pregnancy. In *Transplantation Antigens: Markers of Biological Individuality* (Ed.) Kahan, B. D. & Reisfeld, R. A. pp. 75–114. New York and London: Academic Press.

Elson, J., Jenkinson, E. J. & Billington, W. D. (1975) Fc receptors on mouse placental and yolk sac cells. *Nature*, **255**, 412–414.

Freda, V. J. (1962) Placental transfer of antibodies in man. *American Journal of Obstetrics and Gynecology*, **84**, 1756–1777.

Fröland, S. & Natvig, I. B. (1971) Surface-bound immunoglobulin as a marker of B lymphocytes in man. *Nature, New Biology*, **234**, 251–252.

Gilmour, J. R. (1941) Normal haemopoiesis in intra-uterine and neonatal life. *Journal of Pathology and Bacteriology*, **52**, 25–55.

Gitlin, D. (1974) Protein transport across the placenta and protein turnover between amniotic fluid, maternal and fetal circulations. In *The Placenta: Biological and Clinical Aspects* (Ed.) Moghissi, K. S. & Hatze, E. S. E. pp. 151–191. Illinois: Charles C. Thomas.

Gitlin, D. & Biasucci, A. (1969) Development of γG, γA, γM, β1C/β1A, C1 esterase inhibitor, ceruloplasmin, transferrin, hemopexin, haptoglobin, fibrinogen, plasminogen, α_1-antitrypsin, orosomucoid, β-lipoprotein, α_2-macroglobulin and prealbumin in the human conceptus. *Journal of Clinical Investigation*, **48**, 1433–1446.

Gitlin, D., Kumate, J., Urrusti, J. & Morlaes, C. (1964) The selectivity of the human placenta in the transfer of plasma proteins from mother to fetus. *Journal of Clinical Investigation*, **43**, 1938–1951.

Glynn, A., Martin, W. & Adinolfi, M. (1970) Levels of lysozyme in human foetuses and newborns. *Nature*, **225**, 77–78.

Good, R. A. & Zak, S. J. (1956) Disturbances in gamma globulin synthesis as 'experiments of nature'. *Pediatrics*, **18**, 109–149.

Green, I. (1974) Genetic control of immune response. *Immunogenetics*, **1**, 4–21.

Grubb, R. (1970) *The Genetic Markers of Human Immunoglobulins*. London: Chapman and Hall.

Hellström, K. E. & Hellström, I. (1974) Lymphocyte-mediated cytotoxicity and blocking serum activity to tumour antigens. *Advances in Immunology*, **18**, 209.

Hemmings, W. A. (1974) Transport of maternal antibodies to the rabbit foetus. In *Immunology in Obstetrics and Gynaecology* (Ed.) Centaro, A. & Carretti, N. pp. 252–264. Amsterdam: Excerpta Medica.

Hitzig, W. H. (1959) Über die transplacentare Übertragung von Antikörper. *Schweizerische medizinische Wochenschrift*, **89**, 1249–1253.

Hitzig, W. H. (1973) Congenital thymic and lymphocytic deficiency disorders. In *Immunologic Disorders in Infants and Children* (Ed.) Stiehm, E. R. & Fulginiti, V. A. pp. 215–235. Philadelphia: W. B. Saunders.

Hobbs, J. R., Hughes, M. I. & Walker, W. (1968) Immunoglobulin levels in infants after intrauterine transfusion. *Lancet*, **i**, 1400–1402.

Jenkins, D. M. (1974) Immunologic aspects of pre-eclampsia/eclampsia. In *Immunology in Obstetrics and Gynaecology* (Ed.) Centaro, A. & Carretti, N. pp. 211–215. Amsterdam: Excerpta Medica.

Jenkinson, E. J. & Billington, W. D. (1974) Studies on the immunobiology of mouse foetal membranes: the effect of cell-mediated immunity on yolk sac cells *in vitro*. *Journal of Reproduction and Fertility*, **41**, 403–412.

Jenkinson, E. J., Billington, W. D. & Elson, J. (1976) Detection of receptors for immunoglobulin on human placenta by EA rosette formation. *Clinical and Experimental Immunology*, **23**, 456–461.

Jones, W. R. (1971) Immunological factors in pregnancy. In *Scientific Basis of Obstetrics and Gynaecology* (Ed.) Macdonald, R. R. pp. 183–208. London: J. & A. Churchill.

Jones, W. R. & Scott, J. S. (1976) *Immunology of Human Reproduction*. London: Academic Press. In press.

Katz, D. H. & Benacerraf, B. (1972) The regulation influence of activated T cells and B cell responses to antigens. *Advances in Immunology*, **15**, 2–94.

Kirby, D. R. S., Billington, W. D., Bradbury, S. & Goldstein, D. J. (1964) Antigen barrier of the mouse placenta. *Nature*, **204**, 548–549.

Klockars, M., Adinolfi, M. & Osserman, E. F. (1974) Ontogeny of lysozyme in the rat. *Proceedings of the Society for Experimental Biology and Medicine*, **145**, 604–609

Köhler, P. E. (1973) Maturation of the human complement system. I onset time and sites of fetal C19, C4, C3 and C5 synthesis. *Journal of Clinical Investigation*, **52**, 671–677.

Lanman, J. T. & Herod, L. (1965) Homograft immunity in pregnancy. The placental transfer of cytotoxic antibody in rabbits. *Journal of Experimental Medicine*, **122**, 579–586.

Lawler, S. D., Ukaejiofo, E. O. & Reeves, B. R. (1975) Interaction of maternal and neonatal cells in mixed-lymphocyte cultures. *Lancet*, **ii**, 1185–1187.

Lawton, A. R. & Cooper, M. D. (1973) Development of immunity: phylogeny and ontogeny. In *Immunological Disorders in Infants and Children* (Ed.) Stiehm, E. R. & Fulginiti, V. A. pp. 28–41. Philadelphia: W. B. Saunders.

McCracken, G. H. & Shinefield, H. R. (1965) Immunoglobulin concentrations in newborn infants with congenital cytomegalic inclusion disease. *Pediatrics*, **36**, 933–937.

McDevitt, H. O. & Benacerraf, B. (1969) Genetic control of specific immune responses. *Advances in Immunology*, **11**, 31–74.

Metcalf, D. (1966) The nature and regulation of lymphopoiesis in the normal and neoplastic thymus. In *The Thymus: Experimental and Clinical Studies* (Ed.) Wolstenholme, G. W. E. & Porter, R. Ciba Foundation Symposium. Boston: Little, Brown.

Metcalf, D. & Moore, M. A. S. (1971) *Haempoietic Cells*. Amsterdam: North Holland Publishing Company.

Miller, J. F. A. & Osoba, D. (1967) Current concepts of the immunological function of the thymus. *Physiological Reviews*, **47**, 437–520.

Miller, M. E. (1973) Natural defense mechanisms: development and characterization of innate immunity. In *Immunological Disorders in Infants and Children* (Ed.) Stiehm, E. R. & Fulginiti, V. A. pp. 127–144. Philadelphia: W. B. Saunders.

Mitchison, N. A. (1971) Cell co-operation in the immune response: the hypothesis of an antigen presentation mechanism. In *Immunopathology, VIth International Symposium, Basle* (Ed.) Miescher, P. A. pp. 52–64. Stuttgart: Schwabe.

Mollison, P. L. (1967) *Blood Transfusion in Clinical Medicine*, 4th edition. Oxford: Blackwell.

Murgita, R. A. & Tomasi, T. B. Jr (1975a) Suppression of the immune response by α-fetoprotein. I. The effect of mouse α-fetoprotein on the primary and secondary antibody response. *Journal of Experimental Medicine*, **141**, 269–286.

Murgita, R. A. & Tomasi, T. B. Jr (1975b) Suppression of the immune response by α-fetoprotein. II. The effect of mouse α-fetoprotein on mixed lymphocyte reactivity and mitogen-induced lymphocyte transformation. *Journal of Experimental Medicine*, **141**, 440–452.

Natvig, J. B. & Kunkel, H. G. (1968) Genetic markers of human immunoglobulins. The Gm and Inv system. In *Serum Groups* (Ed.) Jensen, K. G. & Killman, S. Vol. 1, pp. 66–96. Copenhagen: Munksgaard.

Natvig, J. G. & Kunkel, H. G. (1973) Human immunoglobulins: classes, subclasses, genetic variants and idiotypes. *Advances in Immunology*, **16**, 1–59.

Owen, J. J. T. (1973) Anatomy of the lymphoid system. In *Defence and Recognition, MIT International Review of Science* (Ed.) Porter, R. R. Biochemistry Series I. Vol. 10, pp. 36–64. London: Butterworths.

Olding, L. B., Benirschke, K. & Oldstone, M. B. A. (1974) Inhibition of mitosis of lymphocytes from human adults by lymphocytes from human newborns. *Clinical Immunology and Immunopathology*, **1**, 79–89.

Papiernik, M. (1970a) Lymphocyte transformation test in the fetus, premature baby and child. Micro and macrotechnique. *Pathologie et Biologie*, **18**, 1119–1123.

Papiernik, M. (1970b) Correlation of lymphocyte transformation and morphology in the human fetal thymus. *Blood*, **36**, 470–479.

Pegrum, G. D. (1971) Mixed cultures of human foetal and adult cells. *Immunology*, **21**, 159–167.

Pegrum, G. D., Ready, D. & Thompson, E. (1968) The effect of phytohaemagglutinin on human foetal cells grown in culture. *British Journal of Haematology*, **15**, 371–376.

Perchalski, J. E., Clem, L. W. & Small, P. A. (1968) 7S gamma M immunoglobulins in human cord serum. *American Journal of the Medical Sciences*, **256**, 107–111.

Perlmann, P., Perlmann, H. & Wigzell, H. (1972) Lymphocyte mediated cytotoxicity *in vitro*. Induction and inhibition by humoral antibody and nature of effector cells. *Transplantation Reviews*, **13**, 91–114.

Pernis, B. (1967) Relationships between the heterogeneity of immunoglobulins and the differentiation of plasma cells. In *Antibodies. Cold Spring Harbor Symposia on Quantitative Biology*, pp. 333–341.

Playfair, J. H. L. (1968a) Strain differences in the immune response of mice. I. The neonatal response to sheep red cells. *Immunology*, **15**, 35–50.

Playfair, J. H. L. (1968b) Strain differences in the immune response of mice. II. Responses by neonatal cells in irradiated adult hosts. *Immunology*, **15**, 815–826.

Playfair, J. H., Wolfendale, M. R. & Kay, H. E. M. (1963) The leucocytes of peripheral blood in human foetus. *British Journal of Haematology*, **9**, 336–334.

Porter, R. R. (1973) Immunoglobulin structure. In *Defence and Recognition. MIT International Review of Science* (Ed.) Porter, R. R. Biochemistry Series I, Vol. 10, pp. 159–197. London: Butterworths.

Prindull, G. (1974) Maturation of cellular and humoral immunity during human embryonic development. *Acta Paediatrica Scandinavica*, **63**, 607–615.

Pund, E. R. & Von Haam, E. (1957) Spirochetal and venereal disease. In *Pathology* (Ed.) Anderson, W. A. D. p. 264. St. Louis: C. V. Mosby.

Remington, J. S. & Miller, M. J. (1966) 19S and 7S anti-toxoplasma antibodies in the diagnosis of acute congenital and acquired toxoplasmosis. *Proceedings of the Society for Experimental Biology*, **21**, 357–363.

Rosen, F. S. (1974) Complement: ontogeny and phylogeny. *Transplantation Proceedings*, **6**, 47–50.

Rosen, F. S. & Alper, C. A. (1973) Disorders of the human complement. In *Immunologic Disorders in Infants and Children* (Ed.) Stiehm, E. R. & Fulginiti, V. A. pp. 289–330. Philadelphia: W. B. Saunders.

Rowe, D. S., Hug, K., Forni, L. & Pernis, B. (1973) Immunoglobulin D as a lymphocyte receptor. *Journal of Experimental Medicine*, **138**, 965–977.

Schur, P. H., Alpert, E. & Alper, C. (1973) Gamma G subgroups in human fetal, cord and maternal sera. *Clinical Immunology and Immunopathology*, **2**, 62–66.

Searle, R. F., Jenkinson, E. J. & Johnson, M. H. (1975) Immunogenicity of mouse trophoblast and embryonic sac. *Nature*, **255**, 719–720.

Seigler, H. F. & Metzgar, R. S. (1970) Embryonic development of human transplantation antigens. *Transplantation*, **9**, 478–486.

Silverstein, A. M. (1972) Immunological maturation in the foetus: modulation of the pathogenesis of congenital infectious disease. In *Ontogeny of Acquired Immunity*. Ciba Foundation Symposium, pp. 17–25. Amsterdam: Associated Scientific Publishers.

Silverstein, A. M. & Lukes, R. J. (1962) Fetal response to antigenic stimulus. I. Plasma-cellular and lymphoid reactions in the human fetus to intrauterine infection. *Laboratory Investigation*, **11**, 918–932.

Silverstein, A. M. & Prendergast, R. A. (1970) Lymphogenesis, immunogenesis and the generation of immunologic diversity. In *Developmental Aspects of Antibody Formation and Structure* (Ed.) Sterzl, J. & Riha, I. pp. 69–77. New York and London: Academic Press.

Simmons, R. L. & Russell, P. S. (1962) The antigenicity of mouse trophoblast. *Annals of the New York Academy of Sciences*, **99**, 717–732.

Solomon, J. B. (1971) *Foetal and Neonatal Immunology. Frontiers of Biology* (Ed.) Neuberger, A. & Tatum, E. L. Amsterdam: North Holland Publishing Company.

Soothill, J. F., Hayes, K. & Dudgeon, J. A. (1966) The immunoglobulins in congenital rubella. *Lancet*, **i**, 1385–1388.

Sterzl, J. & Silverstein, A. M. (1967) Developmental aspects of immunity. *Advances in Immunology*, **6**, 337–459.

Stiehm, E. R. (1973) Immunodeficiency disorders: general considerations. In *Immunological Disorders in Infants and Children* (Ed.) Stiehm, E. R. & Fulginiti, V. A. pp. 145–167. Philadelphia: W. B. Saunders.

Stiehm, E. R. & Fudenberg, H. H. (1966) Serum levels of immune globulins in health and disease. A survey. *Pediatrics*, **27**, 715–727.

Stites, D. P., Carr, M. C. & Fudenberg, H. H. (1974) Ontogeny of cellular immunity in the human fetus. Development of responses to phytohaemagglutinin and allogeneic cells. *Cellular Immunology*, **11**, 257–271.

Stites, D. P., Wybran, J., Carr, M. C. & Fudenberg, H. H. (1972) Development of cellular immune competence in man. In *Ontogeny of Acquired Immunity*, Ciba Foundation Symposium, pp. 113–132. Amsterdam: Associated Scientific Publishers.

Talmage, D. W. (1969) The nature of the immunological response. In *Immunology and Development* (Ed.) Adinolfi, M. pp. 1–26. London: Spastics International Medical Publications.

Terasaki, P. I., Mickey, M. R., Yamazaki, J. N. & Vredevoe, D. (1970) Maternal–foetal incompatibility. I. Incidence of HL–A antibodies and possible association with congenital anomalies. *Transplantation*, **9**, 538–543.

Thomas, E. D. (1974) Bone marrow transplantation. In *Clinical Immunobiology* (Ed.) Bach, F. H. & Good, R. A. Vol. 2, pp. 2–32. New York and London: Academic Press.

Trevorrow, V. E. (1959) Concentration of gamma-globulin in the serum of infants during the first 3 months of life. *Paediatrics*, **24**, 746–751.

Tyan, M. L., Cole, L. J. & Herzenberg, L. A. (1967) Fetal liver: a source of immunoglobulin producing cells in the mouse. *Proceedings of the Society for Experimental Biology and Medicine*, **124**, 1161–1163.

Vahlquist, B. (1958) The transfer of antibodies from mother to offspring. *Advances in Pediatrics*, **10**, 305–325.

van Furth, R., Schuit, H. R. E. & Hijmans, W. (1965) The immunological development of the human fetus. *Journal of Experimental Medicine*, **122**, 1173–1188.

Volkova, L. S. & Maysky, I. N. (1969) Immunological interaction between mother and embryo. In *Immunology and Reproduction* (Ed.) Edwards, R. G. pp. 211–230. London: International Planned Parenthood Federation.

von Schoultz, B., Stigbrand, T. & Tärnivik, A. (1974) Inhibition of PHA-induced lymphocyte stimulation by the pregnancy zone protein. *Federation of European Biochemical Societies Letters*, **38**, 23.

Warner, N. L. (1974) Membrane immunoglobulins and antigen receptors on B and T lymphocytes. *Advances in Immunology*, **19**, 67–216.

Wiener, A. S. & Berlin, R. B. (1947) Perméabilité du placenta humain aux iso-anticorps. *Revue Hématologie*, **2**, 260.

Wild, A. E. (1973) Transport of immunoglobulins and other proteins from mother to young. In *Lysosomes in Biology and Pathology* (Ed.) Dingle, J. T. pp. 169–215. Amsterdam: North-Holland Publishing Company.

Wynn, R. M. (1971) Immunological implications of comparative placental ultrastructure. In *The Biology of the Blastocyst* (Ed.) Blandau, R. J. pp. 495–514. Chicago: University of Chicago Press.

Yoffey, J. M. & Courtice, F. C. (1970) *Lymphatics, Lymph and Lymphomyeloid Complex*. London: Academic Press.

3

EFFECTS OF DRUGS ON FETAL DEVELOPMENT

Frank M. Sullivan

It is now generally recognised that drugs taken by pregnant women may produce malformations in the developing child. There is, however, a good deal of misunderstanding about the full extent of the problem, and many physicians and obstetricians are unaware of the nature and diversity of the effects which drugs can exert. Attitudes vary widely—some physicians state categorically that no drugs at all should ever be given to pregnant women. Since the embryo is at risk from the very earliest stages, even before the woman may know she is pregnant, this attitude of therapeutic nihilism would deny drug treatment to all women between 15 and 50 years of age. Others imagine that the risk to the child exists only during the first trimester of pregnancy. This ignores the fact that brain development, for example, proceeds well into the postnatal period and is susceptible to environmental influences for all of that time. Yet others (Roberts and Lowe, 1975) suggest that since the malformation rate is so much higher among aborted fetuses than in live births, 90 per cent or more of defective conceptuses may in fact be aborted. The deformed infant is then seen as one of the few 'failed abortions' in whom genetic influences are of paramount importance and environmental factors of little significance.

Many environmental factors are known to affect reproduction in women—climate, altitude, social class, parity, food, water, minerals, vitamins, infections, stress, smoking, drugs. Because of the diversity and interactions between these factors and the lack of controlled conditions, it is impossible to assess the overall influence that drugs alone may have on the unborn child. However, from studies in animals, it is possible to demonstrate what types of effect drugs can have. A knowledge of such studies can then allow one to suggest what effects drugs may possibly produce in humans and so permit a view which is hopefully neither totally depressive nor unguardedly optimistic.

LEGAL REQUIREMENTS FOR DRUG TESTING

In most countries of the World it is now mandatory that all new drugs should be tested for effects on reproduction. Prior to 1960 such tests were practically never done, although there was clear evidence that drugs could affect fetal development in animals and sometimes even in man (Ciba Foundation Symposium on Congenital Malformations, 1960). After the thalidomide disaster, however, it became clear that tighter control to ensure adequate toxicity testing of new drugs was required, and among other requirements, tests for teratogenicity were included routinely for the first time. In many countries including Great Britain this merely required administration of the new drug to pregnant females of two species during the period of embryogenesis, with examination of the fetuses at term for the presence of structural malformations. It was hoped that this would help to prevent the recurrence of a tragedy like that seen when thalidomide was taken during pregnancy. Other countries, however, recognised that drugs might well produce different effects on pregnancy by an action outside the period of embryogenesis. Workers in the USA led this field and produced excellent guidelines for carrying out tests to cover various stages of reproduction and including effects on the male (Food and Drug Administration, 1966). From 1975 the Committee on Safety of Medicines in Great Britain has widened its requirements from a simple teratology test to include other possible drug effects on reproduction.

SCOPE OF REPRODUCTIVE TOXICITY TESTS

The new British requirements include essentially three phases of testing:

1. A comprehensive fertility test in which animals are treated from before mating until the end of pregnancy. By treating male rats for 60 to 80 days before mating all stages of spermatogenesis can be covered. This first phase gives an indication of drug effects on gametogenesis which may result in sterility, reduced fertility or production of abnormal offspring. By killing some of the mated animals in mid-pregnancy and examining carefully for evidence of early fetal deaths, one can also consider this as a dominant lethal test for drug-induced mutations, since such mutagenic effects will often allow embryogenesis to proceed up to the post-implantation stage before death occurs. Direct toxic effects of the drug on the developing embryo must of course be excluded.

2. At least two species (one a non-rodent) are treated during the period of embryogenesis, and the offspring delivered by caesarian section on the day prior to parturition and examined for structural abnormalities. This can be considered as the classical 'teratological' test. It is necessary to deliver the fetuses by caesarian section since rodents will often cannibalise any abnormal fetuses delivered and these would then escape detection.

3. Animals are treated during the latter part of pregnancy (not covered in 2 above), through parturition and up to weaning. This tests for toxic effects of the drug or its metabolites on fetal and uterine growth, parturition and postnatal development and suckling of the progeny, as well as for effects on lactation.

Some of the offspring from parts 1 and 3 are allowed to grow up so that late effects on behaviour, auditory and visual function and reproductive capacity may be assessed.

The above tests, which are similar to those required in the USA and Canada, would seem to allow a reasonably good chance of detecting potentially toxic drugs and so act as a safeguard for the human. There are, however, many unresolved problems in extrapolating from animal experiments to predict human safety. There are, for example, wide species differences in response to drugs. Cortisone, which will produce 100 per cent cleft palates in the fetuses of some strains of mice, will hardly affect other strains of mice, has no effect at all in the rat and probably not in the human (Wilson, 1973). Thalidomide, which is highly teratogenic in the human, affecting almost every woman who took it at the appropriate stage of pregnancy, is also teratogenic in the subhuman primate but virtually not at all in the rat or mouse, and only in very high doses (about $100 \times$ the human dose) in the rabbit.

Sometimes these differences can be explained by species variation in drug metabolism and sometimes by differences in the physiology of reproduction in the different species. There is always the worrying possibility, however, that drugs which seem completely safe in the animal species tested may nevertheless be highly toxic for man.

MECHANISMS BY WHICH DRUGS MAY AFFECT FETAL DEVELOPMENT

It may seem reasonable that if a drug does not cross the placenta it could not be teratogenic. Unfortunately this assumption is too naive, and it can be demonstrated that drugs can cause a wide range of fetal abnormalities without passing into the fetus at all. Drugs may act on at least one of four possible sites to produce teratogenic effects. These are: directly on the embryo/fetus, on the feto-placental unit, on the mother or on the father, and at each of these sites there are a number of different ways by which drugs can exert their effect. These have been discussed in more detail elsewhere (Sullivan, 1972), but some examples will illustrate the diversity of mechanisms by which drugs can affect the fetus.

Drugs acting directly on the fetus

Drugs may act on the fetus in a number of different ways. The drug itself may be toxic to the developing embryo, or metabolites of the drug produced by the mother or in the fetus may be toxic. The drug may be indirectly toxic by acting, for example, as a vitamin antagonist; it may produce pharmacodynamic effects on the fetus causing abnormalities; or it may interfere with the endocrine balance of the fetus and produce genital or other abnormalities.

Directly toxic drugs or metabolites

Thalidomide is an example of a drug or metabolite acting directly on the fetus. This produced a characteristic pattern of defects of a very rare but immediately obvious type. Undoubtedly it was because of this that the causal relationship was so convincingly established. It is cautionary, however, that it nevertheless took about five years and 8000 deformed babies before the link was established.

The tetracycline group of antibiotics, if taken during pregnancy, produces a characteristic deformity and discolouration of the teeth when these subsequently erupt in the child (Douglas, 1963; Weyman, 1965). Other antibiotics may also be directly toxic to the fetus (Carter and Wilson, 1965), including, for example, deafness in children induced by streptomycin treatment of the mother during pregnancy (Robinson and Cambon, 1964).

The anticonvulsant drugs seem very likely to be teratogenic in man producing at least a doubling of the malformation rate with cleft lip and palate as the most commonly reported defect (Speidel and Meadow, 1972, 1974). Because multiple drug therapy is so common in epilepsy, it is not possible to say with any degree of certainty which drugs are or are not teratogenic, but from the human and animal evidence available it would seem that the three major drugs for grand mal epilepsy—phenobarbitone, phenytoin and primidone—may all be involved, as well as trimethadione used for petit mal epilepsy (German, Kowal and Ehlers, 1970). There is also some doubt about whether these drugs are directly toxic or whether they may be teratogenic by some action involving an interference with folic acid absorption, action or metabolism (Reynolds, 1973).

Drugs acting as vitamin antagonists

Apart from the anti-convulsants mentioned above which may interfere with folic acid, the pure folic acid antagonists like aminopterin which were used in an attempt to produce therapeutic abortion were quickly found to be powerful teratogens in man (Thiersch, 1956; Goetsch, 1962). Of over 40 women reported on by these authors, about one-third failed to abort and three of the surviving fetuses were deformed. Methotrexate, another folic acid antagonist has also been implicated as a teratogen in man (Milunsky, Graef and Gaynor, 1968). No particular individual type of malformation is produced by these compounds but, as in animals, the effect may depend on the time of gestation when the drug is administered. It is very interesting from the drug safety testing point of view that although the human and the rat are both very susceptible to the teratogenic action of folic acid antagonists, attempts to produce such malformations in subhuman primates have so far been unsuccessful (Wilson, 1974).

Drugs producing pharmacodynamic effects in the fetus

Drugs which produce profound pharmacodynamic effects on the mother may be expected to produce similar effects on the fetus if they cross the placenta. In fact, because of the general lack of drug-metabolising enzymes in the fetus, the effects may be even more marked and prolonged in the fetus than in the mother. Vasoconstrictor drugs like catecholamines, and vasopressin have been shown to be teratogenic in the mouse, rat and rabbit (Jost, 1953; Sullivan, 1965), and part of their action is due to transfer to the fetus, where they produce a long-lasting severe vasoconstriction which can result in gangrenous necrosis and loss of limbs. Paralytic ileus and neonatal death of infants following administration of the ganglion-blocking agent hexamethonium to hypertensive mothers is another example of an excessive pharmacodynamic action of a drug on the fetus. Despite the fact that hexamethonium is a charged quaternary ammonium compound which does not readily cross the placenta or other membranes, sufficient drug accumulated in the fetus to cause paralysis of the gastrointestinal tract (Morris, 1953).

It is very important to realise that irrespective of charge, low lipid solubility, high protein binding, etc., the majority of drugs will cross the placenta in significant amounts provided that a therapeutic blood level persists in the mother for an adequate amount of time. A very interesting discussion of the pharmacokinetics of placental transfer has been given by Goldstein, Aronow and Kalman (1969), and other aspects of fetal pharmacology by Van Petten (1975).

Drugs affecting the endocrine balance of the fetus

Proper genital development of the fetus is dependent on the sex hormone environment of the fetus at the appropriate time of fetal development. It is well recognised that administration of oestrogens, androgens or progestogens to mothers may result in virilisation of female fetuses with clitoral enlargement and varying degrees of fusion of the labio-scrotal fold (Wilkins, 1960). These effects may be due to direct actions of the hormones or their metabolites, or may be due to stimulation of the fetal adrenal to produce excess androgens (Bongiovanni, Di George and Grumbach, 1959).

Drugs acting at sites other than the fetus

In this chapter it is not possible to discuss all of the drugs which may act at other sites to affect the fetus indirectly. An indication, however, of other possible actions follows.

Drugs acting on the feto-placental unit

This includes actions on the umbilical cord, amniotic fluid volume, fetal or maternal placental blood flow, and placental function, e.g. transfer of nutrients.

As mentioned above, cortisone will produce 100 per cent of cleft palates in the offspring of some strains of mice but not at all in rats. Harris (1964) has shown that in these susceptible strains, cortisone reduces amniotic fluid volume by 15 to 40 per cent causing a fixed flexion of the fetal head, so that the tongue is kept in the elevated position. Failure of the tongue to descend from a position between the palatal shelves prevents palatal closure and so results in cleft palate at birth. Jost (1969) supported this concept by showing that in susceptible animals, cleft palate could be induced by simple withdrawal of amniotic fluid.

It is well known from animal experiments that reduction in placental blood flow or interference with the active transport or other nutritive functions of the placenta can result in a wide variety of congenital malformations or fetal death if sufficiently severe. All of these effects are presumably produced by depriving the fetus of adequate nutrition or oxygenation at critical stages of development, and the type of defect produced depends usually on the developmental stage of the fetus at the time of exposure. Trypan blue (Beck, Lloyd and Griffiths, 1967), 5-hydroxytryptamine (Davies, Robson and Sullivan, 1969), anoxia (Ingalls and Curley, 1957) and direct uterine blood flow reduction (Brent and Franklin, 1960) are all teratogens which act in this way.

Drugs acting on the mother to affect fetal development

Substances producing marked biochemical changes in the mother, e.g. hyperglycaemia or hyperlipidaemia (Tuchmann-Duplessis, 1969), may produce congenital malformations in the offspring. Psychotropic drugs like the phenothiazines or anti-depressants can produce marked changes in the endocrine balance of mothers both in animals and man, and certainly in animals this can result in congenital malformations in the offspring. Certain amine oxidase inhibitors for example have been shown to inhibit the release of LH from the pituitary and to have various anti-progesterone effects as well as being embryo-toxic in mice (Jaitly et al, 1968). The teratogenic and embryo-lethal effects of these compounds could be prevented by simultaneous administration of excess progesterone (Poulson, Robson and Sullivan, 1965).

Drugs acting on the father to affect fetal development

It is surprising that most people, when considering drug hazards for the fetus, seem to forget that the male is also concerned in the reproductive process. That a drug taken by the father could affect children conceived subsequently may seem at first sight surprising, but there is no doubt that such effects have been repeatedly demonstrated to occur in animal experiments. Furthermore, drugs may affect only specific stages of spermatogenesis so that, for example, offspring conceived soon after drug administration may be completely normal, but those conceived between the 36th to 49th day later may be severely affected. This corresponds to the time at which an effect would be seen if the drug acted only at the spermatocyte stage in the rat (Hemsworth and Jackson, 1965). Many of the effects seen following treatment of the male are the result of drug-induced mutations. Epstein (1972) has reviewed the many diverse effects such as abortion, congenital malformation, genetic disease, lowered resistance to disease, decreased life span, infertility, mental retardation, senility and cancer which may follow such mutations.

MULTIPLE OR COMBINED ACTIONS OF DRUGS

Actions of sex hormones

It would be wrong to assume that drugs may affect fetal development only by actions at one site or by one mechanism. Pharmacological investigation of drugs usually reveals several different actions and this applies to their teratogenic actions as well. An interesting example is the diversity of teratogenic effects which has been described following sex hormone administration. These are among the relatively few drugs for which convincing evidence of teratogenicity in man has been produced. From clinical and animal studies one could consider the teratogenic risks of sex hormones under the four following headings:

Endocrine effects on developing sex organs and brain

As mentioned earlier, virilisation of female fetuses is known to occur following administration of progestogens—especially those related to testosterone like ethisterone and norethisterone—and by testosterone itself (Grumbach and Ducharme, 1960). Oestrogens on the other hand can produce feminisation of male fetuses in various species (Greene, Burrill and Ivy, 1940; Saunders, 1968) as can the anti-androgen cyproterone (Forsberg, Jacobsohn and Norgren, 1968). Administration of oestrogens or androgens to mice or rats in the neonatal period may also produce permanent sterility by an action on the hypothalamus producing a permanent change in the pattern of gonadotrophin release (Brown-Grant, 1973).

Miscellaneous congenital malformations not related to sex organs

A number of non-genital defects have been reported recently following sex hormone administration during pregnancy in humans. Gal, Kirman and Stern (1967) reported an increase in neural tube defects, especially spina bifida, following the use of hormonal pregnancy tests, but this has been disputed by Sever (1973) on the basis of the time of administration since the neural tube closes on day 28 and the test tablets would usually be given after that time. Malformations of the oesophagus have been ascribed to the use of hormonal pregnancy tests (Oakley, Flynt and Falek, 1973), and congenital heart defects and transposition of the great veins have also been reported after the use of hormones in pregnancy (Levy, Cohen and Fraser, 1973). A syndrome of defects known by the acronym VACTERL to denote vertebral, anal, cardiac, tracheal, oesophageal, renal and limb defects has been described by Kaufman (1973) following the inadvertent use of oral contraceptives in early pregnancy when women were not aware they were pregnant, and also following the use of hormonal pregnancy tests. Janerich, Piper and Glebatis (1973, 1974) also reported limb reduction deformities including absence of arms, legs, fingers and toes following the use of oral contraceptives or other hormones for pregnancy tests or supportive therapy. All affected cases were males and they suggest the effect may be sex-linked.

Chromosomal effects

Chromosomal effects of sex steroids are less well documented but the incidence of nuclear sex chromatin bodies has been reported to be depressed following administration of testosterone or progesterone, and to be increased by stilboestrol (Dokumov and Spasov, 1967). Carr (1970) reported a significant increase in triploidy and tetraploidy in the abortuses of women using oral contraceptives compared with a control group, but Rice-Wray, Marquez-Monter and Gorodovsky (1970) did not find any chromosomal abnormalities in the live born from such mothers.

Transplacental carcinogenic effects

Treatment during pregnancy with synthetic oestrogens, especially stilboestrol, has been shown to lead to the development in some of the exposed offspring of a rare type of adenocarcinoma of the vagina (Greenwald et al, 1971; Herbst, Ulfelder and Poskanzer, 1971). This appears in the affected girls 15 to 22 years after exposure of the mother and may be related to the presence of aberrant tissue in the vagina, since vaginal adenosis has been reported to be present in 13 of 34 women examined whose mothers had been exposed to stilboestrol in doses ranging from 10 mg/day upwards before the 12th week of pregnancy (Herbst, Kurman and Scully, 1972). The incidence of vaginal cancer in exposed girls is not known with certainty but has been estimated to be less than four per 1000 (Lanier et al, 1973).

Thus it is clear that one group of drugs, in this case the sex hormones, can have a wide variety of embryo-toxic or teratogenic effects presumably reflecting the different types of molecular interactions in which these compounds can take part. Considering the close relationship between cytotoxicity, teratogenicity, mutagenicity and carcinogenicity, it is probable that many other groups of compounds could exhibit such diverse embryotoxic effects.

Combined actions of drugs

Just as one drug may have many different actions, so several drugs acting together may produce effects which are not simply the sum of various component actions. Potentiation may occur and effects may even be produced which none of the component drugs individually could achieve; this type of interaction is said to be coalitive (Herxheimer, 1973). Drug interactions of various types can occur also in the field of teratology, which is not surprising since most teratologists believe that the majority of spontaneously occurring malformations are the result of a combination of many genetic and environmental factors. Effects of combined treatments are often additive, but Wilson (1964) reviews a surprising number of instances where potentiation has been shown to occur even when similarity of mode of action of the individual components seemed unlikely. An even more worrying situation is when two or more agents which are not teratogenic by themselves may combine and produce unexpected malformations (Gibson and Becker, 1968). Physical factors such as food deprivation or stress may also potentiate the teratogenic effects of drugs (Goldman and Yakovac, 1963). The interaction between various environmental factors in the aetiology of birth defects is discussed in an excellent book by Wilson (1973), which is also a good practical guide to teratological problems.

The types of drug-induced effects are described in the four sections that follow.

MAJOR TYPES OF DRUG INDUCED EFFECT

Structural abnormalities

Because thalidomide produced severe gross structural malformations, legislative requirements in toxicity testing tend to emphasise tests which could detect that type of drug-induced defect. It would be a mistake, however, to think that this is the only, or even the most important, adverse action that drugs could have on the unborn child.

One way of classifying drug effects in the fetus is in terms of when the effect produced will be recognised. This can range from:

1. Immediate effects—such as fetal death and abortion seen within hours of drug administration.

2. Effects recognisable at birth—includes gross effects like the absence of limbs seen with thalidomide and minor anomalies like clitoral enlargement following norethisterone.

3. Effects not recognised for a few years—this may range from internal structural defects like congenital heart disorders to abnormal behavioural effects recognised when the child starts school, as has been demonstrated in the slight backwardness of children whose mothers smoked during pregnancy (Butler and Goldstein, 1973).

4. Effects recognised only after many years—such as the transplacental induction of cancer of the vagina as described above under the actions of sex hormones. It is not known to what extent other cancers developing even later in life may be dependent on prenatal influences.

5. Effects which are not fully recognised until expressed in subsequent generations. It is known from animal experiments that certain drugs, particularly cytotoxic drugs, if given for example to male rats or mice may produce a slight transient reduction in fertility. When the offspring are allowed to grow up, it is found that their fertility is low or absent and subsequent generations may be completely infertile (Hemsworth and Jackson, 1965; Cattanach, Pollard and Isaacson, 1968).

Thus, when considering the embryopathic activity of drugs, one must look over a wide horizon. Obviously, the longer after the event that the action of a drug is manifest, the more difficult it is to associate the drug taken with the effect produced. Even the few months during pregnancy can dim the memory of a woman for drugs taken during the crucial stages of embryogenesis in the early weeks after conception. How much more difficult it will be to establish cause and effect relationships when the events are separated by many years. That it can be done is demonstrated by the detection of the transplacental carcinogenic effect of stilboestrol referred to above, but this involved a physician seeing over a short period of time a surprising number of cases of a hitherto extremely rare type of cancer. Whether one could detect such a relationship in a more common situation remains to be seen. There is reason to suspect that under certain circumstances the sex hormones used in oral contraceptives may affect the genetic material in the ovum. It is obviously extremely important to be sure that girls taking oral contraceptives in the early years of marriage before starting a family should not be exposed to any mutagenic risk which could affect, for example, the fertility of their subsequent offspring. By the late 1970s the first children of the 'pill' era will be reaching their own reproductive period and it is important that adequate prospective and retrospective trials should be carried out to look for any possible adverse mutagenic effects of such widely used drugs.

Behavioural abnormalities

Among the more subtle long-term effects which drugs taken during pregnancy could have on the offspring is the possibility of an effect on the central nervous system. That drugs can produce gross disorganisation of the central nervous system resulting in such effects as anencephaly or spina bifida has been known for a long time. What would happen if one took smaller amounts of such drugs, or took other drugs which produced much milder effects? Would it be possible to produce such slight anatomical or functional changes in the brain that the only result would be a change in behaviour or intelligence? There is indeed much evidence from animal experiments and some evidence from human studies that such changes can be produced. The term 'behavioural teratology' was first used by Werboff and Gottlieb (1963) to describe this newly recognised system susceptible to the teratogenic action of drugs, i.e. 'the behaviour or functional adaptation of the offspring to its environment'. Public interest was first aroused by the observation of Werboff and his colleagues (Werboff, 1962) that administration of the then widely used tranquilliser, meprobamate, to pregnant rats could affect the learning capacity of the offspring.

It has been known for many years that a wide spectrum of adverse effects in children such as cerebral palsy, epilepsy, mental retardation, behavioural, speech and reading disorders are associated with maternal complications of pregnancy such as toxaemia, vaginal bleeding and premature delivery (see the excellent comprehensive review by Joffe, 1969). Individual aetiological features such as low socioeconomic status, poor nutrition, smoking and stress have all been investigated and shown to play a role in mental development. Similarly infections, like cytomegalovirus infection during gestation, are some of the most important known causes of mental retardation in children (Dudgeon, 1973).

Environmental chemicals are known to be important in this regard. The tragedy in Minamata Bay in Japan in which effluent containing methyl mercury was poured into the sea amply confirmed this. The toxic chemical accumulated in fish which were consumed by the local villagers. Six per cent of the children born to mothers who had eaten the contaminated fish had cerebral palsy (Miller, 1974). Food additives (Olney, 1969; Nagasawa, Yanai and Kikuyama, 1974) and damaged food (Poswillo et al, 1973) are also of interest in regard to possible brain toxicity.

The most important groups of drugs studied so far for effects on offspring behaviour in animals are the psychotropic drugs. Tranquillisers such as reserpine and chlorpromazine given to pregnant rats may affect offspring activity, impair maze learning ability, condition avoidance response (Hoffeld, McNew and Webster, 1968; Clarke, Gorman and Vernadakis, 1970) and render the offspring more susceptible to stress (Young, 1965). Other drugs such as bromide (Harned, Hamilton and Cole, 1944), barbiturates (Armitage, 1952) and even salicylate (Butcher, Voorhees and Kimmel, 1972) all impair maze learning ability in rat offspring in the absence of any gross CNS deformity. Various hormones—growth, thyroid, adrenal and sex—have all been shown to affect brain development and behaviour following administration in utero and have been interestingly reviewed by Balázs (1972) and Joffe (1969). In humans, it has been suggested that prenatal exposure to androgens can result in a higher I.Q. and improved school performance (Money, 1971).

It is always difficult to separate prenatal and postnatal influences on behaviour though this can be done in animals by the use of suitable fostering and cross-fostering techniques.

Effects on neurotransmitters

There is an increasing amount of information on the relationships between the activities of certain neurotransmitters and behaviour (Kempf et al, 1974). The catecholamines and 5-hydroxytryptamine are thought to play an important role in behaviour, mood, locomotor activity and hypothalamic functions such as control of sleep rhythms and gonadotrophin release (Essman, 1971). It has been shown that depressants like chlorpromazine and stimulants like amphetamine given to pregnant rats and rabbits can produce permanent changes in brain level of noradrenaline, dopamine, 5-hydroxytryptamine and their metabolites in the offspring (Tonge, 1973a; Engel et al, 1974).

Thus, from behavioural, anatomical and biochemical studies in animals, there is plenty of evidence that drugs given during pregnancy can affect the subsequent brain development, behaviour and intelligence of the offspring. Methodology for drug testing is different in this particular field, but possible testing methods have been reviewed by Barlow and Sullivan (1975). This is certainly potentially a most important field of teratological research. A drop of a few points in the I.Q. of a population or some subtle change in behaviour would be most difficult to detect but would be of overwhelming importance. Some attention to the subsequent growth, function, and behaviour of the offspring of animals used in teratological studies has been a requirement of the Committee on Safety of Medicines in Britain since 1975.

Transplacental carcinogenesis and mutagenesis

As indicated above, it is already known that the synthetic sex hormone stilboestrol, if taken by pregnant women, may lead to the development of vaginal cancer in their offspring many years later. This is probably not an isolated occurrence, since over 30 different chemicals have been shown to be capable of inducing cancer in the offspring of animals if administered during pregnancy. A comprehensive survey of the literature has been given by Tomatis (1974). Although the incidence of cancer is highest in the older age groups, childhood cancer is by no means rare, with a peak in the age group 0 to 4 years and has been observed at birth and even in stillbirths. This certainly suggests a prenatal influence, and an association of childhood cancer and congenital defects has been reported by Miller (1973). There are other similarities between transplacental carcinogenesis and teratogenesis. For example, just as drugs will produce certain types of malformation by an action at specific times during embryogenesis, so the fetus is susceptible to the action of certain carcinogens at specific times during pregnancy (Druckrey, 1973). The fetus, however, is sometimes 100 times more susceptible than the mother to the carcinogenic action of the chemicals involved and so may present a special risk. There may also be a shortening of the latent period before the development of tumours following prenatal exposure (Tomatis, 1974).

Other drugs which have been suspected as transplacental carcinogens in man are the folic acid antagonists aminopterin and methotrexate, phenytoin, chloramphenicol and immunosuppressive drugs (see Tomatis, 1974). There may well be other drugs which act as carcinogens in man since, although a connection has been shown between mothers contracting influenza or chicken pox during pregnancy and an increased incidence of cancer in their offspring (Fedrick and Alberman, 1972; Bithell, Draper and Gorbach, 1973), it is still not known whether it is the actual viruses which act as the carcinogens or the drugs the mother may have taken to treat the diseases which are responsible.

Many experts believe that there is a close connection between mutagenesis and carcinogenesis (Röhrborn, 1973), and both are obviously of great importance as toxicological hazards for man. Although methodology is difficult, time-consuming and expensive, it is important that attention should be given to the possibility of screening new and widely used drugs for these possible toxicological hazards. Methods for conducting such tests have been outlined together with extensive bibliographies by the United States Department of Health, Education and Welfare (1969) and by the Department of Health and Welfare, Canada (Health and Welfare, Canada, 1973).

DETECTION OF HUMAN TERATOGENS

Monitoring systems

In the past 10 years a great deal of information has accumulated about the teratogenic effects of drugs in animals, and a useful catalogue of teratogenic agents has been compiled by Shepard (1973). Extrapolation from animal experiments to man still presents great difficulties, however, and it is to be hoped that the preclinical screening of all new drugs may help to prevent a repetition of the thalidomide disaster without excluding too many potentially useful drugs in the process. Because of doubts about the validity of extrapolating results from animals to man, it is clear that careful monitoring of the incidence of congenital malformations in the population is necessary to allow early detection of any new drug-induced increase. It is very difficult, however, to know which system of monitoring can be used with confidence to detect new teratogenic hazards. One system which has been tried in Britain is to ask doctors to report any suspected adverse drug reactions to the Committee on Safety of Medicines. Inman (1972) has stated the problem of under-reporting is more serious in relation to congenital abnormalities than in any other area. He estimates that about a quarter of a million abnormal babies were born in the United Kingdom in the period under review and many of the mothers of these babies would have been exposed to one or more drugs during the relevant pregnancy. Despite this, a total of only 353 reports of congenital abnormalities were received by the Committee over that seven-year period. He concludes that the voluntary reporting system is not a reliable means of detecting human teratogens.

The opposite approach is to set up registries of all congenital malformations on a national level. It is hoped that this would be able to detect increases in malformation rates very quickly and so act as a safeguard. However, experience has shown that teratogens increase the rates of specific malformations but not of total malformations or malformations grouped according to organ systems. Thus the reduction deformities of the limbs caused by thalidomide were previously so rare that they would have been lost under the catch-all category of 'other anomalies of the musculoskeletal system' (Miller, 1974). The unfortunate truth is that to date no human teratogens have been identified by registries of malformations in hospitals, cities, regions or nations, nor has any registry confirmed the teratogenicity of an agent once it has been recognised or suspected from clinical observations. There is no doubt, however, that registries are useful for providing background information on malformation rates and for provision of individual data and sources for retrospective investigations.

Most important discoveries of adverse reactions to drugs, and all human teratogens to date, have been made by individual bright doctors noticing a coincidence and then following it up. The American Academy of Pediatrics has attempted to exploit this system by setting up an 'Alert Practitioner Reporting System' (Miller, 1974). This makes use of suitably trained medical students to take detailed case histories from the parents and other family members of malformed babies in the hope that some clue as to aetiology may be obtained. Already some hopeful results have been obtained and it is certainly a most interesting approach to this difficult problem.

How teratogenic must a drug be before it is detected?

Another aspect of detection of environmental teratogens is to consider how teratogenic a compound must be before it can be detected. This involves statistical questions on how big a chance one is willing to take of missing an active teratogen and how certain one wishes to be not to accuse an inactive drug falsely. This question has been discussed by Sullivan (1974). It has been shown that in a situation where one wishes to have a 95 per cent chance of detecting an active teratogen, and only a one per cent chance of falsely accusing a harmless drug, no fewer than 23 000 pregnant women exposed to the drug in question would have to be studied, to detect a doubling of the incidence of a defect like anencephaly, which has a spontaneous incidence of about one per 1000. Even with much slacker criteria, several thousands of women who took the drug at the relevant stage of pregnancy would still have to be studied to detect a doubling of incidence of any single malformation. From such statistical studies it is possible to calculate that there is no realistic chance of ever detecting mild teratogens which doubled or trebled the incidence of specific defects. From the history of the thalidomide episode it can be calculated that exposure to this particular agent led to an increase in malformations of a specific type of the order of 50 000 to 500 000 times greater than normal. With these figures in mind it seems unlikely that any of the surveillance systems outlined above would be able to detect any specific increases in malformations unless they were several thousand times greater than normal.

It is important to realise that one should not think of a drug simply in qualitative terms of whether or not it is teratogenic; one should instead consider quantatively how teratogenic a drug may be. Any surveillance system for the detection of teratogenic hazards to humans must take account of how big the effect will have to be before it can be detected.

REFERENCES

Armitage, S. G. (1952) The effects of barbiturate on the behaviour of rat offspring as measured on learning and reasoning situations. *Journal of Comparative and Physiological Psychology*, **45**, 146–152.

Balázs, R. (1972) Hormonal aspects of brain development. In *The Brain in Unclassified Mental Retardation* (Ed.) Cavanagh, J. B. p. 61. Edinburgh, London: Churchill Livingstone.

Barlow, S. M. & Sullivan, F. M. (1975) Behavioural teratology. In *Teratology, Trends and Applications* (Ed.) Berry, C. L. & Poswillo, D. E. Berlin: Springer-Verlag.

Beck, F., Lloyd, J. B. & Griffiths, A. (1967) Lysosomal enzyme inhibition by trypan blue: a theory of teratogenesis. *Science*, **157**, 1180–1182.

Bithell, J. F., Draper, G. J. & Gorbach, P. D. (1973) Association between malignant disease in children and maternal virus infections. *British Medical Journal*, **i**, 706–708.

Bongiovanni, A. M., Di George, A. M. & Grumbach, M. M. (1959) Masculinization of the female infant associated with oestrogenic therapy alone during gestation: four cases. *Journal of Clinical Endocrinology and Metabolism*, **19**, 1004–1011.

Brent, R. L. & Franklin, J. B. (1960) Uterine vascular clamping: new procedures for the study of congenital malformations. *Science*, **132**, 89.

Brown-Grant, K. (1973) Recent studies in the sexual differentiation of the brain. In *Foetal and Neonatal Physiology* (Ed.) Comline, K. S., Cross, K. W., Dawes, G. S. & Nathanielsz, P. W. p. 527. London: Cambridge University Press.

Butcher, R. E., Voorhees, C. V. & Kimmel, C. A. (1972) Learning impairment from maternal salicylate treatment in rats. *Nature, New Biology*, **236**, 211–212.

Butler, N. R. & Goldstein, H. (1973) Smoking in pregnancy and subsequent child development. *British Medical Journal*, **iv**, 573–575.

Carr, D. H. (1970) Chromosome studies in selected spontaneous abortions: 1. Conception after oral contraceptives. *Canadian Medical Association Journal*, **103**, 343–348.

Carter, M. P. & Wilson, F. (1965) Antibiotics in early pregnancy and congenital malformations. *Developmental Medicine and Child Neurology*, **7**, 353–359.

Cattanach, B. M., Pollard, C. E. & Isaacson, J. H. (1968) Ethyl methane-sulphonate induced chromosome breakage in the mouse. *Mutation Research*, **6**, 297–307.

Ciba Foundation Symposium (1960) *Congenital Malformations* (Ed.) Wolstenholme, G. E. W. & O'Conner, C. M. London: J. & A. Churchill.

Clarke, C. V. H., Gorman, D. & Vernadakis, A. (1970) Effects of prenatal administration of psychotropic drugs on behaviour of developing rats. *Developmental Psychobiology*, **3**, 225–235.

Davies, J., Robson, J. M. & Sullivan, F. M. (1969) Effects of drugs on placental function and their relation to congenital abnormalities. *Proceedings of the Royal Society of Medicine*, **62**, 317–318.

Dokumov, S. I. & Spasov, S. A. (1967) Sex chromatin and sex hormones. *American Journal of Obstetrics and Gynecology*, **97**, 714–718.

Douglas, A. C. (1963) The deposition of tetracycline in human nails and teeth: a complication of long term treatment. *British Journal of Diseases of the Chest*, **57**, 44–47.

Druckrey, H. (1973) Chemical structure and action in transplacental carcinogenesis and teratogenesis. In *Transplacental Carcinogenesis* (Ed.) Tomatis, L. & Mohr, U. p. 45, World Health Organisation, International Agency for Research on Cancer. Scientific Publication, No. 4. Lyon: International Agency for Research on Cancer.

Dudgeon, J. A. (1973) Chairman's summary. *Intrauterine Infections, Ciba Foundation Symposium No. 10* (New Series), p. 200. Amsterdam: Excerpta Medica.

Engel, J., Ahlenius, S., Brown, R. & Lundborg, P. (1974) Behavioural effects in offspring of nursing mothers given neuroleptic drugs. In *Experimental Model Systems in Toxicology and their Significance in Man. Proceedings of the European Society, Study of Drug Toxicity*, Vol. XV (Ed.) Duncan, W. A. M. p. 20. Amsterdam: Excerpta Medica.

Epstein, S. S. (1972) Environmental pathology: a review. *American Journal of Pathology*, **66**, 352–373.

Essman, W. B. (1971) Isolation-induced behavioural modification; some neurochemical correlates. In *Brain Development and Behaviour* (Ed.) Sterman, M. B., McGinty, D. J. & Adinolfi, A. M. p. 265. New York, London: Academic Press.

Fedrick, J. & Alberman, E. D. (1972) Reported influenza in pregnancy and subsequent cancer in the child. *British Medical Journal*, ii, 485–488.

Food and Drug Administration (1966) *Guidelines for Reproductive Studies for Safety Evaluation of Drugs for Human Use.* Washington: Food and Drug Administration.

Forsberg, J. G., Jacobsohn, D. & Norgren, A. (1968) Development of the urogenital tract in male offspring of rats injected during pregnancy with a substance with anti-androgenic properties (cyproterone). *Zeitschrift für Anatomie und Entwicklungsgeschichte*, 126, 320–321.

Gal, I., Kirman, B. & Stern, J. (1967) Hormonal pregnancy tests and congenital malformations. *Nature*, 216, 83.

German, J., Kowal, A. & Ehlers, K. H. (1970) Trimethadione and human teratogenesis. *Teratology*, 3, 349–362.

Gibson, J. E. & Becker, B. A. (1968) Effect of phenobarbital and SKF 525-A on the teratogenicity of cyclophosphamide in mice. *Teratology*, 1, 393–398.

Goetsch, C. (1962) An evaluation of aminopterin as an abortifacient. *American Journal of Obstetrics and Gynecology*, 83, 1474–1477.

Goldman, A. S. & Yakovac, W. C. (1963) The enhancement of salicylate teratogenicity by maternal immobilisation in the rat. *Journal of Pharmacology and Experimental Therapeutics*, 142, 351–357.

Goldstein, A., Aronow, L. & Kalman, S. M. (1969) The absorption, distribution and elimination of drugs—passage of drugs across the placenta. In *Principles of Drug Action*, Ch. 2, p. 179. New York: Harper and Row.

Greene, R. R., Burrill, M. W. & Ivy, A. C. (1940) Experimental intersexuality: the effects of estrogens on the antenatal sexual development of the rat. *American Journal of Anatomy*, 67, 305–345.

Greenwald, P., Barlow, J. J., Nasca, P. C. & Burnett, W. S. (1971) Vaginal cancer after maternal treatment with synthetic oestrogen. *New England Journal of Medicine*, 285, 390–392.

Grumbach, M. M. & Ducharme, J. R. (1960) The effects of androgens on foetal sexual development; androgen induced female pseudohermaphroditism. *Fertility and Sterility*, 11, 157–180.

Harned, B. K., Hamilton, H. C. & Cole, B. B. (1974) The effect of administration of sodium bromide to pregnant rats on the learning ability of the offspring. II. Maze test. *Journal of Pharmacology and Experimental Therapeutics*, 82, 215.

Harris, J. W. S. (1964) Oligohydramnios and cortisone induced cleft palate. *Nature*, 203, 533–534.

Health and Welfare, Canada (1973) *The Testing of Chemicals for Carcinogenicity, Mutagenicity, and Teratogenicity.* Canada: Ministry of Health and Welfare.

Hemsworth, B. N. & Jackson, H. (1965) Embryopathies induced by cytotoxic substances. In *Embryopathic Activity of Drugs* (Ed.) Robson, J. M., Sullivan, F. M. & Smith, R. L. p. 116. London: J. & A. Churchill.

Herbst, A. L., Kurman, R. J. & Scully, R. E. (1972) Vaginal and cervical abnormalities after exposure to stilboestrol in utero. *Obstetrics and Gynecology*, 40, 287–298.

Herbst, A. L., Ulfeder, H. & Poskanzer, D. C. (1971) Adenocarcinoma of the vagina: association of maternal stilboestrol therapy with tumour appearance in young women. *New England Journal of Medicine*, 284, 878–881.

Herxheimer, A. (1973) Investigating the effects of drug combinations. In *International Aspects of Drug Evaluation and Usage* (Ed.) Jouhar, A. J. & Grayson, M. F. p. 275. Edinburgh: Churchill Livingstone.

Hoffeld, D. R., McNew, J. & Webster, R. L. (1968) Effect of tranquillising drugs during pregnancy on activity of offspring. *Nature*, 218, 357–358.

Ingalls, T. H. & Curley, F. J. (1957) Principles governing the genesis of congenital malformations induced in mice by anoxia. *New England Journal of Medicine*, 257, 1121–1127.

Inman, W. H. W. (1972) Monitoring by voluntary reporting at national level. In *Adverse Drug Reactions* (Ed.) Richards, D. J. & Rondel, R. K. p. 86. Edinburgh: Churchill Livingstone.

Jaitly, K. D., Robson, J. M., Sullivan, F. M. & Wilson, C. (1968) The effect of amine oxidase inhibitors on ovulation, implantation and pregnancy. *Journal of Reproduction and Fertility*, Supplement, 4, 75–79.

Janerich, D. T., Piper, J. M. & Glebatis, D. M. (1973) Hormones and limb-reduction deformities. *Lancet*, ii, 96–97.

Janerich, D. T., Piper, J. M. & Glebatis, D. M. (1974) Oral contraceptives and congenital limb-reduction defects. *New England Journal of Medicine*, 219, 697–700.

Joffe, J. M. (1969) Pre-natal determinants of behaviour. *International Series of Monographs in Experimental Psychology*, Vol. 7. Oxford: Pergamon Press.

Jost, A. (1953) La dégénerescence des extrémités du foetus de rat sous des actions hormonales (acroblapsie expérimentale) et la théorie des bulles myelencephaliques de Bonnevie. *Archives Francaises de Pediatrie*, 10, 865–870.

Jost, A. (1969) *Discussion in Foetal Autonomy* (Ed.) Wolstenholme, G. E. W. & O'Conner, N. p. 269. London J. & A. Churchill.

Kaufman, R. L. (1973) Birth defects and oral contraceptives. *Lancet*, ii, 1396.

Kempf, E., Greilsamer, J., Mack, G. & Mendel, P. (1974) Correlation of behavioural differences in three strains of mice with differences in brain amines. *Nature*, **247**, 483–485.

Lanier, A. P., Noller, K. L., Decker, D. G., Elveback, L. R. & Kurland, L. T. (1973) Cancer and stilboestrol. *Mayo Clinic Proceedings*, **48**, 793–799.

Levy, E. P., Cohen, A. & Fraser, F. C. (1973) Hormone treatment during pregnancy and congenital heart defects. *Lancet*, **i**, 611.

Miller, R. W. (1973) Prenatal origins of cancer in man: Epidemiological evidence. In *Transplacental Carcinogenesis* (Ed.) Tomatis, L. & Mohr, U. p. 175. World Health Organisation, International Agency for Research on Cancer. Scientific Publication No. 4. Lyon: International Agency for Research on Cancer.

Miller, R. W. (1974) How environmental effects on child health are recognised. *Pediatrics*, **53**, 792–796.

Milunsky, A., Graef, J. W. & Gaynor, M. F. (1968) Methotrexate induced congenital malformations, with a review of the literature. *Journal of Pediatrics*, **72**, 790–795.

Money, J. (1971) Prenatal hormones and intelligence: a possible relationship. *Impact of Science on Society*, **21**, 285–290.

Morris, N. (1953) Hexamethonium compounds in the treatment of pre-eclampsia and essential hypertension during pregnancy. *Lancet*, **i**, 322–324.

Nagasawa, H., Yanai, R. & Kikuyama, S. (1974) Irreversible inhibition of pituitary prolactin and growth hormone secretion and of mammary gland development in mice by monosodium glutamate administered neonatally. *Acta Endocrinologica*, **75**, 249–259.

Oakley, G. P., Flynt, J. W. & Falek, A. (1973) Hormonal pregnancy tests and congenital malformation. *Lancet*, **ii**, 256–257.

Olney, J. W. (1969) Brain lesions, obesity and other disturbances in mice treated with monosodium glutamate. *Science*, **164**, 719–721.

Poswillo, D. E., Sopher, D., Mitchell, S. J., Coxon, D. T., Curtis, R. F. & Price, K. R. (1973) Further investigation into the teratogenic potential of imperfect potatoes. *Nature*, **244**, 367–368.

Poulson, E., Robson, J. M. & Sullivan, F. M. (1965) Embryopathic effects of progesterone deficiency. *Journal of Endocrinology*, **31**, 28.

Reynolds, E. H. (1973) Anticonvulsants, folic acid and epilepsy. *Lancet*, **i**, 1376–1378.

Rice-Wray, E., Marquez-Monter, H. & Gorodovsky, J. (1970) Chromosomal studies in children born to mothers who previously used hormone contraceptives. *Contraception*, **1**, 81–86.

Roberts, C. J. & Lowe, C. R. (1975) Where have all the conceptions gone? *Lancet*, **i**, 498–499.

Robinson, G. C. & Cambon, K. G. (1964) Hearing loss in infants of tuberculous mothers treated with streptomycin during pregnancy. *New England Journal of Medicine*, **271**, 949–951.

Röhrborn, B. (1973) Correlation between mutagenesis and carcinogenesis. In *Transplacental Carcinogenesis* (Ed.) Tomatis, L. & Mohr, U. p. 168. World Health Organisation, International Agency for Research on Cancer. Scientific publications, No. 4. Lyon: International Agency for Research on Cancer.

Saunders, F. J. (1968) Effects of sex steroids and related compounds in pregnancy and on development of the young. *Physiological Review*, **48**, 601–643.

Sever, L. E. (1973) Hormonal pregnancy tests and spina bifida. *Nature*, **242**, 410–411.

Shepard, T. H. (1973) *Catalog of Teratogenic agents*. Baltimore: Johns Hopkins University Press.

Speidel, B. D. & Meadow, S. R. (1972) Maternal epilepsy and abnormalities of the fetus and newborn. *Lancet*, **ii**, 839–843.

Speidel, B. D. & Meadow, S. R. (1974) Epilepsy, anticonvulsants and congenital malformations. *Drugs*, **8**, 354–365.

Sullivan, F. M. (1965) Discussion. In *Embryopathic Activity of Drugs* (Ed.) Robson, J. M., Sullivan, F. M. & Smith, R. L. p. 110. London: J. & A. Churchill.

Sullivan, F. M. (1972) Mechanisms of teratogenesis. In *Adverse Drug Reactions* (Ed.) Richards, D. J. & Rondell, R. K. Ch. 3. Edinburgh: Churchill Livingstone.

Sullivan, F. M. (1974) General discussion. *Pediatrics*, **53**, 798–799.

Thiersch, J. B. (1956) The control of reproduction in rats with the aid of antimetabolites and early experiments with antimetabolites as abortifacient agents in man. *Acta Endocrinologica*, Supplement 28, **23**, 37–45.

Tomatis, L. (1973) Transplacental carcinogenesis. In *Modern Trends in Oncology* (Ed.) Raven, R. p. 99. London: Butterworths.

Tomatis, L. (1974) Role of prenatal events in determining cancer risks. In *Modern Trends in Toxicology*, No. 2 (Ed.) Boyland, E. & Goulding, R. p. 163. London: Butterworths.

Tonge, S. R. (1973a) Permanent alterations in catecholamine concentration in discrete areas of brain in the offspring of rats treated with methylamphetamine and chlorpromazine. *British Journal of Pharmacology*, **47**, 425–427.

Tonge, S. R. (1973b) Permanent alterations in 5-hydroxyindole concentrations in discrete areas of rat brain produced by pre- and neonatal administration of methylamphetamine and chlorpromazine. *Journal of Neurochemistry*, **20**, 625–627.

Tuchmann-Duplessis, H. (1969) In *Foetal Autonomy* (Ed.) Wolstenholme, G. E. W. & O'Conner, N. p. 245. London: J. & A. Churchill.

United States Department of Health, Education and Welfare (1969) *Report of the Secretary's Commission on Pesticides and their Relationship to Environmental Health.* Washington D.C.: United States Government Printing Office.

Van Petten, G. R. (1975) Pharmacology and the fetus. *British Medical Bulletin,* **31,** 75–79.

Werboff, J. (1962) Effects of prenatal administration of tranquillisers on maze learning ability. *American Psychologist,* **17,** 397.

Werboff, J. & Gottlieb, J. S. (1963) Drugs in pregnancy: behavioural teratology. *Obstetrical and Gyecological Survey,* **18,** 420–423.

Weyman, J. (1965) The clinical appearances of tetracycline staining of the teeth. *British Dental Journal,* **118,** 289–291.

Wilkins, L. (1960) Masculinization due to orally given progestins. *Journal of the American Medical Association,* **172,** 1028–1032.

Wilson, J. G. (1964) Teratogenic interaction of chemical agents in the rat. *Journal of Pharmacology and Experimental Therapeutics,* **144,** 429–436.

Wilson, J. G. (1973) *Environment and Birth Defects.* New York: Academic Press.

Wilson, J. G. (1974) Teratological causation in man and its evaluation in non-human primates. In *Birth Defects, Proceedings of the 4th International Conference, Vienna, 1973* (Ed.) Motulsky, A. G. & Lenz, W. p. 191. Amsterdam: Excerpta Medica.

Young, R. D. (1965) Effects of differential early experiences and neonatal tranquillisation on later behaviour. *Psychological Report,* **17,** 675–680.

4

THE ACCUMULATION OF PROTEIN BY THE FETUS

Maureen Young

The transfer of nitrogen from the mammalian mother to her fetus has four important features which are common to all species. First, fetal protein is synthesised in situ from free amino acids transported across the placental membrane from the maternal circulation; small amounts of gammaglobulin are also transferred in some animals. Second, the free amino acid concentrations are higher in the fetal than in the maternal plasma and transport occurs against this concentration. Third, the amino acid composition of fetal carcass protein is very similar to that in the adult and all the amino acids are probably 'essential' for the fetus until its full complement of enzymes is developed. Finally, the net transfer of α-amino nitrogen is quantitatively small and occurs mostly during the last third of gestational life. The rate of protein accumulation, however, differs between and within species due to the interaction of the genetic capacity of the fetus for growth and the opportunity for placental exchange of nutrients between the fetus and mother. The latter is also under both genetic and environmental influences; Widdowson (1969) pointed out that, since the composition of the maternal plasma does not vary markedly from species to species, differences in fetal growth rate will be due to genetic differences in the supply of nutrients by the maternal placental blood flow. Further, the concept of the fetus as a parasite is now modified by the evidence for the influence of the fetal environment on birthweight and quality of the newborn. Using the method of correlation coefficients it has been shown for the human subject in Western Society that genetic factors provide only 40 per cent of birthweight variation in comparison with 60 per cent due to the effect of the fetal environment; much of the latter is due to such factors as maternal health and nutrition, but at least half is due to the intra-uterine environment itself, in which the maternal sociocultural environment is also reflected (Penrose, see Polani, 1974).

Descriptions of the interrelationships of the amino acid pools in the body, and their organisation for protein synthesis, form a very rich literature (see Munro, 1969, 1970) and are discussed in relation to fetal growth and metabolism elsewhere in this volume (Chapter 5). The purpose of the present chapter is to outline the evidence for the nature and control of the processes concerned with the transport of nitrogen-containing molecules across the membrane separating the maternal and fetal blood streams. They are put into context by sketching the net protein requirements of the fetus, and describing the free amino acid pools which determine the characteristics of the transport mechanisms.

PROTEINS OF THE CONCEPTUS

The total protein content of the newborn is characteristically lower than that of the adult; in the human the respective values are 12 and 15 per cent. There is a gradual increase during development (Widdowson and Spray, 1951) which accompanies a decrease in total body water from 95 per cent in the small embryo to 73 per cent in the newborn (Friis-Hansen, 1957).

The amino acid composition of the mixed proteins of the fetus or placenta has been found to be very similar to that of the adult protein in a number of species (Williams et al, 1954; Southgate, 1971).

The placenta

The human placenta contains about 1.3 g DNA, 1.6 g RNA and 60 g protein at term, 40 g of the protein is laid down by 20 weeks gestation and the DNA: protein ratio remains constant throughout gestation (Winick, Brasel and Rosso, 1972; Laga, Driscoll and Munro, 1973). The RNA content, however, is high in the young placenta during the period of maximum growth, the concentration being greater in the microsomes than in the mitochondria. At five months gestation, the position is reversed and mitochondrial RNA content becomes the larger, corresponding with the change from a predominantly protein synthetic function to that of higher energy-requiring processes (Szabo and Grimaldi, 1970). The oxygen utilisation of the sheep placenta, 10 ml/kg/min, is greater than that of the fetus, 6 ml/kg/min (Dawes, 1968; see Chapter 10). This is probably due to the high requirements for steroid biosynthesis because transport processes, as will be seen, have a relatively low energy dependence. The pattern of nucleic acid and protein synthesis has also been studied extensively in the rat placenta (Winick and Noble, 1966); DNA synthesis ceases before term, while RNA synthesis increases to term.

Human placental tissue has been very thoroughly investigated for the presence of a large number of enzymes by histochemical methods and functional studies of metabolic pathways (Hagerman, 1964). As expected, it has been found to have an enzyme structure enabling it to carry out a wide variety of metabolic processes, the most important of which are concerned with the provision of energy for its transport functions, steroid synthesis, and the regulation of storage and release of carbohydrate for the fetus. Many of the placental enzymes have electrophoretically separable isoenzyme forms. The most outstanding difference between the placental and liver enzyme make-up is the absence of the urea cycle enzymes throughout gestation. This might be expected teleologically since the placenta is the source of amino acids for the fetus; a variety of transaminases are, however, present. Finally, it is the most readily available source of fresh human tissue in which to study enzyme activity. Many studies of the development of enzyme activity in rat and guinea-pig placentas have also been made.

The placenta also takes no part in the production of fetal plasma proteins, but synthesises two protein hormones which are released into the maternal blood stream, namely chorionic gonadotrophin (hCG) and human placental lactogen (hPL) (see Chapter 19). hCG is of syncytial origin and production corresponds initially to its growth rate but declines in the second and third trimester. The half-life is relatively long, 20 to 30 hours (Midgley and Jaffe, 1968), in comparison with that for hPL which is 32 min. A production rate of 0.3 to 1.0 g/day is indicated for hPL.

Little is known of the control of protein synthesis by the placenta. It has been shown that uptake of labelled amino acids into protein in human placental tissue slices is stimulated by small amounts of oestrogen and progesterone, but inhibited by larger amounts. The effect of insulin would be of great interest since Posner (1974) has identified membrane binding sites for the hormone in placental cytoplasm.

The fetus

The normal term human infant has acquired about 500 g protein. In the pre-implantation period, isolated embryos require protein or amino acids in the culture medium but not those generally considered essential for growth later in life, suggesting that endogenous stores provide the missing amino acids (Brinster, 1971; New, 1973). Blastocyst formation and expansion need a greater variety of amino acids.

Net protein synthesis rate can be accurately, though laboriously, measured in fetuses by measuring the nitrogen accumulated at various stages of gestation in a given species (Blaxter, 1964). The net maternal to fetal nitrogen transfer rate in man is about 54 mmoles/day (9 m-moles/100 g placenta/day); in the sheep it is 115 mmoles/day (23 mmoles/100 g placenta/day) and in the guinea-pig 3.4 mmoles/day (86 mmoles/100 g placenta/day). The considerable capacity for oxygen transport of the guinea-pig placenta in comparison with that of the ewe and of the human was also calculated by Bartels (1970). Protein turnover rate has only been measured during the last trimester in the fetal lamb, in chronic preparations in utero (Young, unpublished observations, 1976) by determining the rate of incorporation of a labelled amino acid into protein from the specific activity of the protein and extracellular fluid in the steady state (Waterlow and Stephen, 1967). The results are in substantial agreement with those of Soltesz, Joyce and Young (1973) in the newborn lamb: the fractional synthesis rate of proteins in liver is 100 per cent per day, while that for cardiac and skeletal muscle is 35 and 25 per cent respectively. Total leucine flux is 90 μmol/kg/day. Surprisingly both these measurements indicate a protein synthesis rate which is faster than that previously observed for liver and muscle in young rats (Waterlow and Stephen, 1968), yet the growth rate of the neonatal lamb as measured by nitrogen accumulation rate is only half as fast as that of the neonatal rat (Blaxter, 1964).

The rate of weight increase varies for each organ during fetal development; data have been derived from autopsy material in the human (Schulz, Giordano and Schulz, 1962). Contributing to these differences in weight gain will be the rates of cell division and the time at which this ceases, and the rate at which protein is laid down in the cell (Winick, Brasel and

Rosso, 1972); Widdowson (1972) has evaluated this most elegantly in a lecture entitled 'The Harmony of Growth'. All these relative changes must make a complicated contribution to the inter-organ fluxes of amino acids during development and influence the final free amino acid pattern observed in the body fluids.

In the human infant, the brain and skeletal muscle are the largest organs during late intra-uterine life; the liver weighs only 130 g at this time, one-quarter of that of the placenta but, in comparison with the adult, it is twice the size relative to the body weight, forming four per cent. The production of plasma protein fractions is one of the first functions of the fetal liver to develop, but more important to the subject of fetal nutrition is the development of the necessary intermediary pathways for amino acid metabolism. It has already been pointed out that all the amino acids are probably essential to the fetus until a certain degree of enzyme development has taken place. All the amino acids have been shown to be transferred across the placental membrane, but the arteriovenous differences are small and the use of the Fick principle to relate transport rate to fetal requirements would be inaccurate. Particular interest has centred around the dependence of the fetus upon the maternal to fetal transfer of the non-essential amino acids cystine, tyrosine and arginine (Bessman, 1972), the importance of the development of enzyme systems converting two of them from essential amino acids, and the function of the citrulline–arginine cycle.

FREE AMINO ACID COMPOSITION OF THE BODY FLUIDS

Twenty to twenty-five amino acids are usually separated from protein-free filtrates of body fluids, by column gradient elution techniques for ion exchange chromatography, with estimation by the ninhydrin colour reaction. Twenty of these are found in protein. The amino acids are eluted from the column according to a sequence determined by the properties of the third radical on the α-carbon atom namely, acidic, neutral straight-chain, neutral branched-chain and basic. The first two groups are the most labile metabolically; the acidic group is represented by aspartic and glutamic acid, and the straight-chain neutral by glycine, alanine, serine and threonine, which are potentially gluconeogenic. The latter two groups are primarily concerned with protein structure and contain the majority of the essential amino acids: the neutral branched-chain amino acids, represented by isoleucine, leucine and valine, are potentially ketogenic, and the basic amino acids are represented by histidine, ornithine, lysine and arginine. The pyrolidine and sulphur-containing amino acids—proline, cystine and methionine—are eluted amongst the neutral amino acids and those containing a benzene ring—phenylalanine, tyrosine and tryptophan—between the neutral branched-chain and the basic. The transport groups also fall into these main divisions (see page 68) which do, however, oversimplify the very complicated metabolic interrelationships between the amino acids and other metabolic pathways (Scriver and Rosenberg, 1973).

Over 50 years ago, van Slyke observed that the free α-amino nitrogen concentration was higher in the fetal plasma than in the maternal. As the methods became available, paper chromatography and ion exchange chromatography were quickly used to study the individual free amino acids, so that by 1960 the changes in the maternal plasma resulting from pregnancy and the differences between the mother and her fetus were defined. These relationships are shown, for the human, in the aminograms in Figure 4.1. References to the earlier investigators contributing the data in the following descriptions will all be found in three reviews (Young and Prenton, 1969; Young, 1971; Young and McFadyen, 1973).

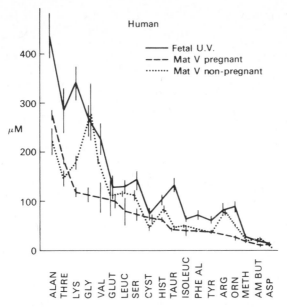

Figure 4.1. Venous plasma free amino acid concentration in the term pregnant woman and umbilical vein at delivery, and in the non-pregnant woman. The aminograms are arranged in order of magnitude of the concentrations occurring in the pregnant woman (± s.e.). The fetal levels are higher than the maternal levels with different concentration ratios for each amino acid. The fetal and non-pregnant levels and pattern are similar except for the higher fetal alanine, lysine and threonine. Redrawn from Young and Prenton (1969) with kind permission of the editor of *Journal of Obstetrics and Gynaecology of the British Commonwealth.*

Maternal plasma

Plasma total α-amino nitrogen is reduced from about 3.0 to 2.3 mmol/l in human pregnancy, a fall in concentration of the majority of the amino acids contributing to this. In Figure 4.1 the aminogram of the pregnant woman at term has been used as the reference, with the amino acids arranged in order of magnitude of the concentrations present. The fall in concentration can be observed within the first month of pregnancy and is a continuation of the reduction occurring in the luteal phase of the menstrual cycle (Croft and Wise, 1969) and is, therefore, not due to the demands of the fetus but to the changing hormone pattern. Similar changes can be induced in the human male and in the non-pregnant ewe by giving oestrogen and progesterone together; nevertheless, the increased renal excretion of amino acids during pregnancy is not observed unless glucocorticoids are also given. The fall in plasma amino acid concentration during pregnancy is in keeping with that observed for glucose and the electrolytes and is part of the resetting of maternal homeostasis by the fetus; it is probable that the free amino acid pool is little changed because of the simultaneous increase in plasma volume.

The relatively greater fall in glycine during pregnancy may be an indication of the catabolic influence of progesterone in the human (Landau and Poulos, 1971). The rise in free alanine levels suggests that gluconeogenesis is not so active during pregnancy; this amino acid has been shown to be the main precursor for this function in the non-pregnant subject (Felig et al, 1970). However, Freinkel et al (1972) provided evidence for protein-sparing mechanisms in the pregnant woman, and suggested a limitation in the supply of this substrate as the cause of the hypoglycaemia which occurs more readily during starvation than in the non-pregnant state. Though the maternal and fetal aminograms in the rabbit (Christensen and Streicher, 1948), the guinea-pig (Hill and Young, 1973) and the sheep (Young and McFadyen, 1973; Schulman et al, 1974) can be compared, the differences between pregnant and non-pregnant animals have not been studied. The majority of the amino acids have very similar levels to those in the human with the exception that glycine is high in both rabbit and sheep maternal plasma.

Fetal plasma

In the human, the total α-amino nitrogen in fetal plasma is 3.8 mmol/l, giving an F: M ratio of 1.7. All the free amino acid concentrations in the umbilical artery and vein are higher than in the maternal antecubital vein, but the F : M ratios are different for each. The pattern of the individual free amino acids in the plasma of the term fetus is similar to that found in the non-pregnant woman (Figure 4.1). The particularly high values for fetal alanine would suggest, again, relatively poor gluconeogenic activity and in the guinea-pig, the uptake by the fetal liver of a model non-metabolisable amino acid, amino-isobutyric acid, which is transported by the same mechanisms as alanine, is not active until after delivery (Christensen and Clifford, 1963). However, in the fetal lamb right auricular plasma contains less alanine and glycine than umbilical vein plasma, demonstrating hepatic uptake of these amino acids (Young et al, 1975). The close relationship between maternal and fetal glucose concentrations suggests that fetal gluconeogenesis would not necessarily be essential to the fetus. The high level of the waste product taurine in fetal plasma suggests that the liver conjugating mechanisms are poor, also that it is transported relatively slowly into the maternal circulation. The high threonine and lysine concentrations are unexplained. It is not possible to investigate with certainty the influence of gestational age on plasma amino acid concentrations because sampling interferes with the circulation in young fetuses and spuriously high values are obtained (Young and Prenton, 1969). Again, the concentrations of the majority of the amino acids in fetal plasma are similar amongst the species; glycine is particularly elevated in both the sheep and guinea-pig, and threonine and serine are high in the sheep.

The reason for the higher levels of free amino acids in the fetal plasma, which exceed those in the non-pregnant woman, is probably the quicker turnover rate of protein in the rapidly growing animal (Waterlow and Stephen, 1968; Soltesz, Joyce and Young, 1973). The part played by fetal metabolism in determining the fetal plasma amino acid pattern was demonstrated simply in the guinea-pig fetal placenta perfused in situ with an intact maternal placental circulation, after removal of the fetus; the pattern of the amino acids transferred into the perfusate was similar to that of the maternal plasma, not that of the fetal plasma (Young and Hill, 1973) An examination of the umbilical vein–artery differences also indicates that the fetal plasma pattern is dominated by its own metabolism; each is small, and difficult to prove significantly different from zero, after vaginal delivery and at caesarean section, in both the human and sheep (Figure 4.2). The arteriovenous differences across the maternal side of the circulation are also small in both these species. It is not yet clear whether the high fetal plasma concentrations ensure faster uptake by the fetal tissues.

Interrelationships between normal maternal and fetal plasma concentrations have been attempted by all workers, but the results, however significant, must be regarded as tenuous because of the sampling procedure from the umbilical vein (Young and Prenton, 1969). The greatest number of significant positive correlations were observed in postmature pregnancies, the slopes of the straight-chain neutral and branched-chain amino acids being less steep than those for the basic. Cockburn et al (1971) found the largest number of significant cor-

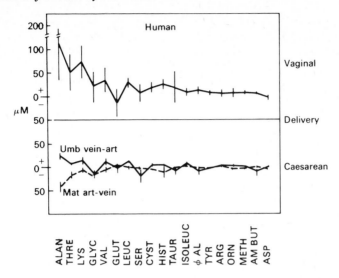

Figure 4.2. Umbilical vein–artery differences in term human vaginal deliveries and at caesarean section, with uterine A–V differences (± s.e.). Each value is small and seldom statistically different from zero. Redrawn from Prenton and Young (1969) with kind permission of the editor of *Journal of Obstetrics and Gynaecology of the British Commonwealth.*

relations between maternal and fetal values in samples from diabetic patients; of the 10 which were significant out of 20, five belonged to the neutral straight-chain and branched-chain groups and none to the basic amino acid group.

Maternal and fetal plasma in toxaemia and diabetes

Investigations of the interrelationships between maternal or fetal plasma composition and fetal size have, on the whole, proved disappointing. It is well established that the plasma amino acids are raised in the mother with pre-eclampsia and Cockburn et al (1971) suggested that this was due to the reduction in circulating hormones resulting from impairment of placental function; the rise in glycine and lysine would be in accord with this theory (Landau and Poulos, 1970). The plasma levels were slightly elevated in the small infants. No significant differences from the normal were observed in the plasma of mothers of small-for-dates infants uncomplicated by toxaemia (Young and Preton, 1969) and the umbilical vein values were also normal.

In diabetic pregnancies, both maternal and fetal plasma concentrations are comparable with normal pregnancies (Cockburn et al, 1971); the close relationship between at least half of the amino acids suggests a greater permeability of the diabetic placental membrane as one cause for the relatively large infant, besides the greater blood flow through the large placenta. It would therefore appear that fetal amino acid homeostasis in utero is maintained in the face of both an increased and a decreased nutrient supply; the withdrawal of nutrients following labour and in the neonatal period unmasks the intra-uterine deficiencies and causes changes in the free amino acid pattern characteristic of malnutrition namely, a rise in alanine and glycine and a fall in the branched chain amino acids (Lindblad, 1971).

Trophoblast

The concentration of free amino acids is particularly high in the intracellular fluid of the fetal liver in comparison with that of the adult and is comparable to that in regenerating liver or malignant growths. Pearse and Sornson (1969) observed that the free amino acids are also higher in human placental tissue than in maternal or fetal plasmas. An accurate measurement is difficult because of the problems associated with accounting for the contamination with maternal and fetal blood and determining the extracellular space. Hill and Young (1974)

Table 4.1. *Concentration ratios of free amino acids.*

| | Plasmas fetal: maternal | Placental levels related to: | |
		Maternal plasma	Fetal plasma
Aspartate	3.9	60.6	21.5
Glutamate	4.0	74.7	22.7
Glycine	6.1	14.7	2.9
Alanine	6.0	12.5	2.4
Valine	2.8	5.5	1.5
Leucine	3.8	9.1	2.7
Lysine	4.2	7.2	2.0
Histidine	3.2	5.8	1.9

published values for the guinea-pig placenta, finding the levels high and variable. Table 4.1 shows the F : M plasma concentration ratios for eight amino acids, and the corresponding relationships between the trophoblast free amino acids and maternal or fetal plasma concentrations. The placental concentrations for the acidic amino acids are very high in the trophoblast in comparison with the maternal plasma, moderately high for the neutral straight-chain amino acids, and smallest for the branched-chain and basic amino acids. With the exception of the acidic amino acids having placental:fetal plasma ratios of about 20, the concentration for all the amino acids in the trophoblast was about twice that in the fetal plasma. Schneider and Dancis (1974) also found high intracellular accumulation rates for the acidic amino acids by human placental slices. The significance of these concentration ratios in relation to transport is discussed later.

Amniotic fluid and fetal urine

The concentration of free amino acids in human amniotic fluid at 15 to 20 weeks gestation, collected from hysterotomies for the termination of pregnancy (Cockburn, Robins and Forfar, 1970) is lower than those in fetal plasma, and similar to those in maternal plasma, but with higher serine, glutamine and citrulline levels. The concentrations in the fetal urine were more closely related to those in the fetal plasma. However, at term the amino acids in both amniotic fluids and fetal urine taken at caesarean section, were lower than the maternal plasma concentrations (Emery et al, 1970; Cockburn et al, 1973). The fall in amniotic fluid amino acid concentration during pregnancy is similar to the decrease in concentration of the other constituents which occurs as a result of the development of the reabsorbtive capacity of the fetal kidney. The contribution of amino acids from other sources such as the skin and lungs is not known.

No significant relationships between the concentrations of amino acids in the amniotic fluid and the maternal or fetal plasma or fetal urine are normally found, with the possible exception of those between the fetal urine and amniotic fluid in early pregnancies. However, with a gross abnormality such as occurs in phenylketonuria, the high maternal levels are reflected in the fetal plasma and urine and in the amniotic fluid (Cockburn et al, 1972). Oral loads or the continuous infusion of phenylalanine, given to patients before termination of pregnancy, also result in high concentrations in the body fluids which confirms observations made in the Rhesus monkey (Kerr et al, 1968). The high fetal plasma levels in phenylketonuria imply that the human placenta does not protect the infant from the maternal imbalance. In fact, the mechanism which is normally so important to ensure a net retention of amino acid by the fetus is detrimental to the fetus in this context, maintaining the F : M ratio above one at all maternal plasma levels. Other congenital abnormalities, such as maple syrup disease, have not been investigated in this way.

Sugawa, Nakamura and Osaki (1963) observed that amino acids can be transferred across the isolated human chorio-amnion and it is of considerable interest that an infusion of amino acids into the human amniotic cavity influences the composition of the maternal but not the fetal aminogram (Reynaud et al, 1972).

Maternal urine

The renal excretion of amino acids is raised during pregnancy more predictably than that of glucose. Hytten and Cheyne (1972) found the neutral straight-chain amino acids, together with histidine, to be lost in the greatest amount; the rise in excretion rate started soon after implantation and continued to term, when it was four-fold the non-pregnant quantity. Excretion of the neutral branched-chain and basic amino acids also increased early but was not maintained. The renal clearance was 30 ml/min for glycine and histidine and some 20 per cent of the filtered load was excreted, amounting to a loss equivalent to 2 g protein/day. This is considerable when compared with the 3 g protein accumulated by the fetus each day during the last trimester over the steep part of the growth curve, and with the 6 g/day stored by the whole conceptus. It would be interesting to know whether this loss of nitrogen is reduced during pregnancy in some of the developing countries when the maternal diet is very restricted. The raised amino acid and glucose concentrations in pregnant urine improve its quality as a culture medium and may account for some of the increased incidence of urinary infection in pregnancy.

PLACENTAL TRANSFER OF FREE AMINO ACIDS

The higher concentration of free amino acids in fetal, in comparison with maternal plasma, suggested to Christensen and Streicher in 1948 that an active transfer mechanism must exist between the two compartments. From studies of the uptake characteristics of ascites tumour cells and absorption by the small intestine, Christensen (1968) divided the amino acids broadly into the three groups summarised in Table 4.2. The correspondence between the metabolic divisions (page 62) of the amino acids and their transfer groups has been included. The 'A'-preferring transport system is so called because the transfer properties of these amino acids are similar to those of alanine, and the 'L'-preferring group has properties similar to those of leucine (Oxender, 1972). The overlap between the groupings is con-

Table 4.2. *Plan of general structure and metabolic characteristics of the three main amino acid transport mediating systems: 'L', leucine-preferring and 'A', alanine-preferring neutral amino acids and basic amino acids.*

Amino acids	Metabolic	Transport	Non-essential
'L' Neutral Branched chain	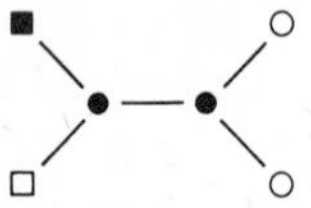 Leucine Isoleucine, etc. Ketogenic	Exchange	5
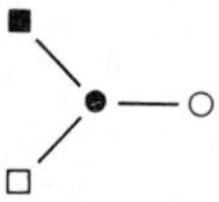 'A' Straight chain	Glycine Alanine, etc. Gluconeogenic	Active-uphill Na^+ and P_{O_2} dependent	1
Basic	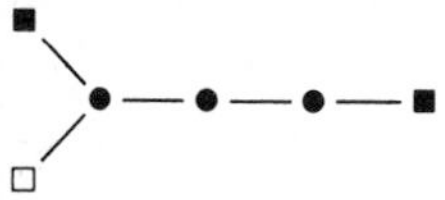 Lysine Arginine, etc.		3

Modified from Christensen (1968).

● carbon atoms
■ amino group
□ carboxyl group
○ third radical

siderable. The following summary shows that the transfer of amino acids from the mother to the fetus has similar characteristics to that across other multicellular membranes.

Active transport

Active transport of amino acids has to satisfy three criteria: (1) stereospecificity, which is never quite complete, (2) competitive inhibition, and (3) uphill transfer, against both concentration and electrochemical gradients. Much of the evidence quoted in this section has been obtained in the pregnant guinea-pig, with the placenta perfused in situ following removal of the fetus to eliminate any influence by its metabolism; the transfer rate in good preparations was about 60 per cent of that expected (Reynolds and Young, 1971).

Selective transport of the L-isomers of amino acids has been observed in the human subject and in the guinea-pig using both labelled and unlabelled isomers (see Reynolds and Young, 1971; Young and McFadyen, 1973). Competition between the mechanisms for glycine and histidine, and methionine and proline, has also been demonstrated, and saturation of the mechanism for histidine transport; the concentrations used to show these effects were much higher than those usually present in physiological fluids. Uphill transfer was shown in the guinea-pig with the fetal placenta infused in situ through the umbilical vessels after removal of the fetus, the maternal circulation being intact (Hill and Young, 1973). With closed circuit perfusion, amino acids accumulated in the perfusion fluid until an equilibrium concentration was reached equivalent to about twice that of the fetal plasma, indicating the reserve capacity of the placenta for amino acid transfer. The concentration of the individual amino acids in the closed circuit at equilibrium was very similar to the levels observed in the placental parenchyma.

Activity of the placental transfer mechanism for amino acids is poorly represented by the F:M plasma concentration ratios. The placental concentrations of free amino acids are much higher than those in the fetal plasma (Table 4.1) and the uphill gradient is better expressed by the placental:maternal plasma ratio. The active uptake may occur in the microvilli on the maternal surface of the syncytiotrophoblast, as at the microvillous surface of the small intestine (Faust, Burns and Misch, 1970), and is followed by diffusion down the concentration gradient from the trophoblast into the fetal plasma, as in other multicellular membranes. It is possible that part of the transfer takes place in the endoplasmic vesicles formed at the microvillous surface, for their number has been observed to increase in small intestine epithelia during amino acid uptake (Bronk and Leese, 1974). These authors also suggest that metabolism of the molecules does not occur during transfer because uptake was not dependent upon concentration. Bidirectional flux measurements across the guinea-pig placenta showed that transfer from mother to fetus was by two routes, a constant secretion from the maternal plasma and diffusion from a metabolic pool (Hill and Young, 1974).

Membrane transport processes have lower energy requirements than protein synthesis and may be conveniently studied separately from the latter by using model non-metabolisable amino acids. Longo, Yuen and Gusseck (1973) investigated the uptake of α-amino-isobutyric acid (AIB) by human placental slices in the presence of various metabolic inhibitors and showed that its accumulation was only slightly decreased when oxygen was replaced by nitrogen in the incubation chamber (Figure 4.3). A 40 per cent reduction in uptake occurred when dinitrophenol was added to the medium and complete inhibition when glycolysis was prevented by arsenate. Depletion of tissue glycogen also inhibited AIB uptake

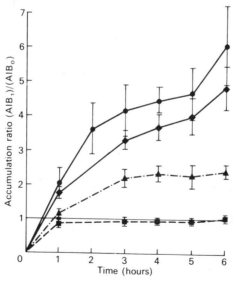

Figure 4.3. Ratio of concentration of α-amino-isobutyric acid (AIB) in free water of placental tissue to its concentration in the media, as a function of time at 25°C following 45 min preincubation. Control (●): 100 per cent N_2 atmosphere; 10^{-4} M dinitrophenol (▲); 10^{-1} M sodium arsenate (■). An accumulation ratio of 1 indicates diffusion equilibrium. Each point is the mean of nine determinations on these animals; bars represent 1 s.d. Redrawn from Longo, Yuen and Gusseck (1973) with kind permission of the authors and the editor of *Nature*.

The y-axis of the figure is labelled: Accumulation ratio $(AIB_1)/(AIB_0)$. The x-axis is labelled: Time (hours).

which was restored when glucose was added to the medium. These observations are in keeping with the anaerobic uptake of amino acids by fetal and newborn rabbit gut and the anaerobic maintenance of sodium, potassium and water gradients by immature and newborn rabbit and kidney slices.

The relation of amino acid transfer to the electrochemical gradient across the placenta has not been investigated. The potential difference measurement is only well established in the sheep; the transplacental potential difference is 36 mV with the fetus negative (Mellor, 1970). The sodium dependence of the transfer of amino acids belonging to the 'A'-preferring and basic groups has also not been studied.

Cahill et al (1972) found that the red cells may play an important role in amino acid transfer to tissues, and Meister (1974) has evidence to support the importance of the γ-glutamyl cycle in mediating the transport of amino acids into tissues together with the function of glutathione in supplying the carrier needed. Neither of these aspects of amino acid transport has been investigated for the placenta.

Influence of maternal–fetal gradients

No controlled studies of the influence of varying concentrations of amino acid in the maternal blood stream on transfer into the fetal compartment are available; the majority of investigators have studied single injections of unphysiological amounts of amino acid (see Young and McFadyen, 1973). However, using single injections of moderate quantities designed to raise the plasma levels five-fold, in the pregnant ewe under spinal anaesthesia, the latter authors observed that an elevation in the neutral branched-chain amino acid concentration had the most influence on the fetal levels; the neutral straight-chain and basic amino acids had little effect. This result was in keeping with the differences in transport rate observed between these groups of amino acids in the isolated gut. Placental transfer does not, therefore, appear to be related to essentiality of the amino acids, and the relative independence of the fetal levels upon the maternal would suggest a secretory process. The data also provided plasma clearance rates: those for the basic amino acids were faster than for both neutral transport groups, and no differences were observed between the mother and fetus. The latter observation is perhaps not surprising since the measurements are crude and depend upon the uptake by a variety of tissues with different relative mass, rate of metabolism and blood flow in mother and fetus.

Net placental transfer of free amino acids against varying concentrations in the fetal placental perfusate has been investigated in the guinea-pig (Hill and Young, 1973). During open-circuit perfusion of the fetal placenta in situ, the transfer of amino N and the individual amino acids was found to be indirectly proportional to the concentration in the medium perfusing the fetal side of the placenta in the steady state and, further, no significant difference between the regressions of transfer on concentration was observed between the three transport groups. This is in accord with the concept of passive transfer down a concentration gradient on the fetal side of the membrane, and would also suggest that the fetal uptake of amino acids would play a part in regulating transfer.

The influence of blood flow

Amino acid transfer rate was found to be independent of blood flow changes on the fetal side of the placenta in the guinea-pig fetal placenta perfused in situ; this would again lend support to the suggestion that they are secreted into the fetal blood by the syncytiotrophoblast.

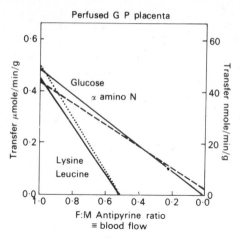

Figure 4.4. The influence of a reduction in materno-placental blood flow on the placental transfer of glucose (—) and total α-amino N (- - - -) expressed as μmol/min/g and leucine (· · · ·) and lysine (—) expressed as nmol/min/g. Redrawn from Young (1974) with kind permission of Ciba Foundation.

Transfer rate was, however, directly related to maternal blood flow in this preparation (Young, 1974). Absolute measurements of blood flow were not made, but changes were monitored continuously by relating the concentration of the freely diffusable antipyrine in the effluent perfusate to the constant level maintained in the maternal circulation. In Figure 4.4 it is seen that a 30 per cent reduction in perfusate : maternal plasma antipyrine concentration ratio is accompanied by an equal fall in total α-amino nitrogen transfer and of glucose; however, the transfer of two essential amino acids belonging to the branched-chain neutral and the basic groups was reduced by about 50 per cent. Similar reductions were observed for other members of these groups, while the transfer of the straight-chain and acidic amino acids was rather variable and usually uninfluenced by the changes in maternal placental blood flow. These results would suggest that an imbalance in the transfer of nutrients, with a relative deficiency of the essential amino acids, might occur when the placental blood flow becomes inappropriately low in utero.

REGULATION OF AMINO ACID TRANSPORT

The secretory, uphill nature of amino acid transport from mother to fetus is quite different from that of the diffusional gradient-dependent transfer of oxygen or glucose. Nevertheless, the influence of maternal blood flow and fetal plasma levels suggests that the quantity transferred is subject to the interaction of the same overall controlling mechanisms as that for other nutrients, namely supply and demand. There is well documented evidence in many species that the supply line is impaired when birthweight is below that expected. But it is difficult to put a quantitative value on the relative importance of each of the factors ensuring its optimum function: the anatomical and metabolic integrity of the membrane, the area for exchange and the blood flow relationships on either side of the placenta. Tighe, Garrod and Curran (1967) found that microvilli were frequently absent from the chorionic villi in some areas of human placentas in toxaemic pregnancies, which provides a microanatomical basis for the impairment of active transport for amino acids and glucose. The grosser anatomical deficiency, a smaller chorionic villous surface area and fetal capillary surface area in these placentas, and those of small-for-dates infants, demonstrates that the exchange of the more freely diffusible substances, such as gases and electrolytes, will also be restricted (Aherne and Dunnill, 1966). The small placenta suggests low blood flows, both maternal and fetal.

These inadequacies of supply over demand affect the final synthesis and storage of protein as well as glycogen deposition, but not, in general, the final homeostatic mechanisms within the fetus as indicated by the plasma free amino acid levels. Because proteins and their associated cellular components form part of the structural basis of the body, measurement of net accumulation over a period of time provides a more accurate determination of the quantity and quality of the transport functions for nitrogen than is possible with many acute animal experiments. The dependence of protein storage on the gestational period in which nutrient transfer is decreased, and upon the severity and duration of intra-uterine malnutrition is well known. The importance of the maternal energy sources available and the capacity of the placenta to adapt, in some measure, to the fetal requirement of nutrients, by hypertrophy or by increasing its transport capacity in the face of deprivation, has also been shown. The evidence comes from investigations into fetal and placental weight relationships in naturally occurring growth retardation in the human (Gruenwald, 1974), rodent (McKeowen, Record and Eckstein, 1965) and sheep (Alexander, 1974), together with experiments designed to impair the appropriate nutrient supply for genetic demand by the fetus. The latter have been varied; the maternal placental blood flow has been reduced by ligating the artery to one uterine horn in rodents (Winick and Noble, 1966; Wigglesworth, 1968), by heat stress in the pregnant ewe (Alexander, 1974), and by embolising the small maternal placental vessels in pregnant sheep (Creasey et al, 1973). Interference with the development of the maternal placental vasculature has been produced by dietary restriction of protein or protein and calories in rodents (Winick, Brasel and Rosso, 1972), and in sheep (Sykes and Field, 1972). Reduction in functioning placental mass has been investigated in the sheep by removal of placental caruncles (Alexander, 1974) and in the Rhesus monkey by tying the vessels between the two placentas (Hill, 1974).

Both placentas and fetuses are lighter than expected for their gestational age following the experiments just described to reduce nutrient supply, but the fetal:placental weight ratio is usually increased, as it is in the clinical conditions, suggesting a metabolic response of the small placenta, and possibly the fetus itself, which enhances its transport capacity. Winick (1968) found high RNA contents in the small placentas resulting from unilateral uterine artery ligation in the rat, and recent observations in pregnant guinea-pigs fed diets low either in calories or in protein during the last half of gestation demonstrated an increase in amino acid uptake on the low protein diet when the calorie supply was adequate (Young and Widdowson, 1975). The fetal:placental weight ratio was the same in the control and restricted calorie group, but doubled in the low protein group. These experiments also provided the interesting information that the capacity of the placenta for amino acid uptake was three-fold that of the maternal liver per unit weight. The relative importance of an adequate maternal intake of calories, in comparison with protein, in determining birthweight has also been observed in humans by Habicht et al (1974) in Guatamala, where undernourished mothers were given various supplements during pregnancy. Mobilisation of maternal protein, the largest reserve of nutrient in the body must, therefore, be very important in pregnancy.

The temporal importance of impaired nutrient supply to the fetus has been of great interest with regard to the quality of the fetus. Winick, Brasel and Rosso (1972) have shown that early deprivation decreases the rate of cell division, resulting in small placentas and fetuses with a relatively small number of cells; while deprivation in the last trimester, during the period of rapid growth, influences fetal weight particularly, through cell size. Because each organ is developed at a specific time and growth should proceed at a definite rate, the period when intra-uterine malnutrition affects a particular physiological function will be critical and will also depend upon the species. The significance of this in relation to the development of various areas of the brain has been reviewed by Dobbing (1974) and Brasel (1974). Brain size is relatively spared by a restriction of nutrient supply in the third trimester, skeletal muscle mass is the most influenced, while the liver, cerebellum and endocrine organs are also particularly vulnerable. Some liver enzymes for bilirubin conjugation, regulation of gluconeogenesis and cystathionase activity are slow to develop in the newborn small-for-dates infant due to a deficiency of substrate transfer in utero. In contrast, there are fetal mechanisms which develop more rapidly under the stress of intra-uterine malnutrition; in the rat fetus, the eyes open and skin develops earlier, while in the human infant, pulmonary development may be enhanced.

Any summary of the factors influencing placental and fetal size and quality, no matter how superficial, begs the questions "What regulates the maternal placental blood flow during a pregnancy?" and "What is the extent of the placental reserve?". The nutritional studies suggest that it would be valuable to study the influence of maternal malnutrition on the metabolic pathways concerned with oestrogen production at various stages of gestation. This information might in turn suggest the mechanisms causing the lower oestrogen production by the placenta observed in the small-for-dates syndrome, when the restricted placental blood flow is due to many other causes (Ounsted, 1968). Recent studies have shown that the plasma prolactin and progesterone levels are low in the pregnant rat fed protein-free diets but that the LH and oestrogen concentrations are normal (Köhler, Wojnorowicz and Borner, 1975). It was also observed that the implantation site contained not only less nitrogen, DNA and RNA, but also an imbalance of free amino acids; the concentrations of the essential amino acids were relatively low in the pool and those of the non-essential relatively higher than in animals fed a normal diet. This change in pattern of free amino acids is similar to that usually found in the plasma in undernourished states, and it is of great interest that it may be reversed in the pregnant rat on a protein-free diet by the administration of a combination of progesterone and oestrogen.

PLACENTAL TRANSFER OF UREA AND AMMONIA

The placental transfer of urea is discussed fully on page 184. The urea concentration in fetal plasma and amniotic fluid is slightly higher than that of the maternal plasma in all the species investigated, and the umbilical artery–uterine artery gradient is about 3 mg per cent in the pregnant ewe in good chronic preparations (Battaglia and Meschia, 1973). Urea clearance across the placenta is approximately 0.54 mg/min/kg fetal weight at term, twice that of the adult and well below the maximum capacity of the membrane for this function. On the basis of these observations, it has been suggested that protein might provide about 25 per cent of the energy source in the fetal lamb.

Freinkel and his group (1972) have suggested that it would be important to conserve maternal nitrogen during pregnancy and that ammonia might be the source of some of the fetal nitrogen, because it would transfer readily across the placental membrane. In support of this hypothesis, an enzyme carbamyl phosphate synthetase II, necessary for the de novo biosynthesis of pyrimidines from ammonia and glutamine, has been found in fetal liver and other tissues; pyrimidines, therefore, need not be transferred across the placental membrane.

TRANSFER OF IMMUNOGLOBULINS, ANTIBODIES AND HORMONES

The time relations of the first appearance of the immunologically competent cells, from the thymus and other lymphoid tissues, varies from species to species (Miller, 1966). In the human, lymphoid tissue is present in the thymus by 12 weeks gestational age, and in the spleen by 20 weeks when the synthesis of gammaglobulins starts. De novo antibody production has been demonstrated by studying the incorporation of labelled isotopes in cultured tissue: IgM, MW 900 000, appears first and is followed by IgA, MW 150 000 to 400 000, and finally IgG, MW 150 000. This latent capacity for antibody production is seldom invoked in utero except during infection of the placenta and fetus by the rubella virus and the syphilis spirochaete.

The passive transfer of specific antibodies from the maternal to the fetal circulation, which starts early in gestation, affords some protection to the fetus but may also interfere with its own antibody development, either by inactivation or by some feedback mechanism. IgG is the only gammaglobulin transferred in utero and at birth the concentrations are 1.0 g per cent in human maternal and fetal plasmas; the amount of fetal globulin contributing to this level is unknown; the half-life in the newborn child is 20 days. The maternal isohaemagglutinins, anti-A and anti-B, MW 1 000 000, are absent from newborn serum and do not develop until three to six months postnatal age; the Rh antibody produced in response to rhesus-positive cells in the mother is a gammaglobulin and is transferred across the placental membrane. Gamma-A-globulin, to which the skin allergens belong, is also absent from newborn plasma.

Table 4.3. *Routes of passive transfer of immunoglobulins from mother to fetus.*

	Route of transfer		
Species	Yolk sac	Placenta	Colostrum or milk
Avian	+		
Rodents	+	−	+
Porcine	−	±	+
Bovine	−	±	+
Ovine	−	−	+
Primates	−	+	−

From Miller (1966) with kind permission of the author and the editor of *British Medical Bulletin*.

+ Transfer occurs.
± Minimum transfer occurs.
− Transfer does not occur.

The differences between the routes through which fetal and newborn animals acquire passive immunity are well known (Brambell, 1970; Solomon, 1971) and are summarised in Table 4.3. The mode of transfer of gamma-G-globulin across membranes such as the primate placenta, the newborn small intestine in ungulates, and the yolk sac splanchnopleure in rodents, is very remarkable. Most of the observations on the transmission of large molecules have been made in the yolk sac of the rabbit, which has an electron-microscopic structure very similar to the other membranes. The free surfaces of the cells are covered with abundant microvilli and, at the bases of the caveoli, the cytoplasm is filled with cisternae and vacuoles. All these structures are covered or lined with glycocalyx. The cytoplasm of the cells is rich in enzymes, including proteolytic enzymes, and lysosomes are plentiful. Pinocytosis of a variety of colloids can be demonstrated, and their ultimate appearance in the basement membrane, en route to vessels, observed, but the manner of their discharge from the cells is much less clear.

Transfer is selective and operates in favour of homologous IgG. Brambell's (1970) working hypothesis suggested that this selectivity could be most readily understood by assuming the presence of specific intracellular receptors for gamma-G-globulins and postulating that the remainder of the proteins taken up by pinocytosis were hydrolysed within the cell. The process is shown diagrammatically in Figure 4.5. The receptors are thought to be on the surface of the microvilli and carry the globulin into the cell as the caveoli are formed; this protein remains protected on the walls of vacuoles as they migrate through the cell and is eventually released to cross the basement membrane. Protein not so attached, albumin and other globulins are thought to be degraded by the lysosomes in the vesicles, and escape from the cell by diffusion. The idea is attractive because the large molecules do not have to traverse the cell membrane and there is nothing new about the concept of pinocytosis

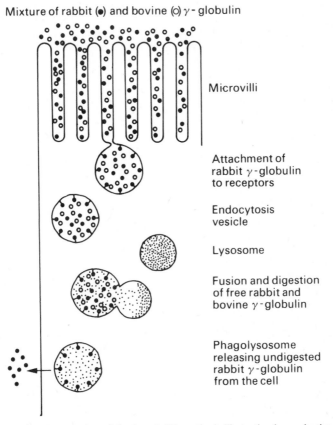

Mixture of rabbit (●) and bovine (○) γ - globulin

Microvilli

Attachment of
rabbit γ-globulin
to receptors

Endocytosis
vesicle

Lysosome

Fusion and digestion
of free rabbit and
bovine γ-globulin

Phagolysosome
releasing undigested
rabbit γ-globulin
from the cell

Figure 4.5 Diagrammatic representation of the Brambell hypothesis illustrating how selective transmission of gammaglobulin according to species of origin may be brought about in the endodermal cell. Redrawn from Brambell (1970) with kind permission of the publisher (Amsterdam: North Holland).

nor of specific receptors for biologically active molecules; studies with gamma-G-globulins treated with pepsin or papain indicate that the C-terminal halves of the molecules determine their transcellular passage. A rate-limiting factor will be the population of available receptors and the kinetics of attachment and release of the globulin. Brambell considered that it would be still more attractive to postulate a variety of receptors so that the much slower transfer of albumin might also be accounted for without interfering with that of globulin. Further, he suggested that the receptors for amino acid transport might also be situated in the glycocalyx, which would fit well with the possibility suggested earlier for active uptake by the placental microvilli. Functional mosaicism has been shown in the plasma membranes of leucocytes (see Allison and Davies, 1974).

Observations designed to reinvestigate Brambell's hypothesis have been reviewed by Wild (1974). His own studies provide elegant evidence for mixed fluid endocytosis by the yolk sac endoderm, using fluorescent labelled molecules, two of which can be detected simultaneously in the vacuoles. The intracellular event is contrasted with the intercellular passage of the same molecules through the paraplacental chorion, which admits albumin and globulins to the excoelomic fluid, and hence into the amniotic fluid in the rabbit. Evidence for receptors is strengthened by the finding of saturation of the transport mechanism by high concentrations and the occasional blocking by heterologous gamma-G-globulins. Fusion of lysosomes with the pinocytotic vesicles has been observed, but in vivo evidence for protein hydrolysis is still lacking in this system; albumin degradation has been shown in sarcoma cells (Ryser, 1968). The basement membrane offers no barrier to protein transmission into the vascular mesenchyme and hence across the vascular endothelium into the vitelline vessels by intercellular routes and, possibly, micropinocytosis. It remains for the mechanism to be investigated in the syncytiotrophoblast of the chorio-allantoic primate placenta.

There is no evidence for maternal to fetal transfer of the growth-promoting hormones with a protein structure (Jost and Picon, 1970; Liggins, 1974), whether the origin is hypophyseal, the thyroid gland or the pancreatic islets; they may be subject to the intracellular hydrolysis just described for the plasma proteins, in the pinocytotic vesicles of the syncytium. The mechanism whereby the protein hormones elaborated by the placenta itself, hCG and hPL, enter the maternal circulation in much greater amounts than into the fetal circulation, remains to be explored. The insulin receptors found in the placenta (Posner, 1974) suggest that there may be a special relationship between this maternal hormone and the conceptus: is the syncytium protecting the fetus against this most active of the growth-promoting hormones? It is also important to remember that the placenta affords little protection of the human fetus against maternal hyperglycaemia, and the consequences are fetal islet hypertrophy and raised plasma insulin levels which probably promote fetal growth by enhancing both glucose and amino acid uptake by the tissues.

Acknowledgements

The author wishes to thank all colleagues for good counsel and hard work, and both the Wellcome Trust and Medical Research Council for financial support.

REFERENCES

Aherne, W. & Dunnill, M. S. (1966) Quantitative aspects of placental structure. *Journal of Pathology and Bacteriology*, **91**, 123–139.

Alexander, G. (1974) Birth weight of lambs: influences and consequences. In *Size at Birth, Ciba Foundation Symposium*, 27 (new series), pp. 215–246. Amsterdam: Associated Scientific Publishers.

Allison, A. C. & Davies, P. (1974) Mechanisms of endocytosis and exocytosis. *Transport at the Cellular Level, Symposia of the Society for Experimental Biology*, **28**, 419–446.

Bartels, H. (1970) *Prenatal Respiration*. Amsterdam: North-Holland.

Battaglia, F. C. & Meschia, G. (1973) Fetal metabolism and substrate utilization. In *Fetal and Neonatal Physiology, Barcroft Centenary Symposium*, pp. 382–397. Cambridge: Cambridge University Press.

Bessman, S. P. (1972) Genetic failure of fetal amino acid 'justification': a common basis for many forms of metabolic nutritional and 'nonspecific' mental retardation. *Journal of Pediatrics*, **81**, 834–842.

Blaxter, K. L. (1964) Protein metabolism and requirements in pregnancy and lactation. In *Mammalian Protein Metabolism* (Ed.) Munro, H. N. & Allison, J. B. Vol. II, pp. 173–223. New York, London: Academic Press.

Brambell, F. W. R. (1970) The transmission of passive immunity from mother to young. In *Frontiers of Biology* (Ed.) Neuberger, A. & Tatum, E. L. Vol. 18. Amsterdam: North-Holland.

Brasel, J. A. (1974) Cellular changes in intrauterine malnutrition. In *Nutrition and Fetal Development. Current Concepts in Nutrition*, Vol. 2 (Ed.) Winick, M. P. pp. 13–26. New York: John Wiley.

Brinster, R. L. (1971) Biochemistry of the early mammalian embryo. In *The Biochemistry of Development. Clinics in Developmental Medicine*, No. 37 (Ed.) Benson, P. E. pp. 161–174. London: Heinemann Medical.

Bronk, J. R. & Leese, H. J. (1974) Accumulation of amino acids and glucose by the mammalian small intestine. In *Transport at the Cellular Level. Symposia of the Society for Experimental Biology*, **28**, 283–304.

Cahill, G. F., Aoki, T. T., Brennan, M. F. & Müller, W. A. (1972) Insulin and muscle amino acid balance. *Proceedings of the Nutrition Society*, **31**, 233–238.

Christensen, H. N. (1968) Relevance of transport across the plasma membrane to the interpretation of the plasma amino acid pattern. In *Protein Nutrition and Free Amino Acid Patterns* (Ed.) Leathem, J. H. pp. 40–52. New Brunswick: Rutgers University Press.

Christensen, H. N. & Clifford, J. B. (1963) Early postnatal intensification of hepatic accumulation of amino acids. *Journal of Biological Chemistry*, **238**, 1743–1745.

Christensen, H. N. & Streicher, J. A. (1948) Association between rapid growth and elevated cell concentrations of amino acids in fetal tissues. *Journal of Biological Chemistry*, **175**, 95–100.

Cockburn, F., Robins, S. P. & Forfar, J. O. (1970) Free amino-acid concentrations in fetal fluids. *British Medical Journal*, **ii**, 747–750.

Cockburn, F., Blagden, A., Michie, E. A. & Forfar, J. O. (1971) The influence of pre-eclampsia and diabetes mellitus on plasma free amino acids in maternal, umbilical vein and infant blood. *Journal of Obstetrics and Gynaecology of the British Commonwealth*, **78**, 215–231.

Cockburn, F., Farquhar, J. W., Forfar, J. O., Giles, M. & Robins, S. P. (1972) Maternal hyperphenylalaninaemia in the normal and phenylketonuric mother and its influence on maternal plasma and fetal fluid amino acid concentrations. *Journal of Obstetrics and Gynaecology of the British Commonwealth*, **79**, 698–707.

Cockburn, F., Giles, M., Robins, S. P. & Forfar, J. O. (1973) Free amino acid composition of human amniotic fluid at term. *Journal of Obstetrics and Gynaecology of the British Commonwealth*, **80**, 10–18.

Craft, I. L. & Wise, I. J. (1969) Changes in amino acid metabolism during the menstrual cycle. *Journal of Obstetrics and Gynaecology of the British Commonwealth*, **76**, 928–933.

Creasey, R. K., de Swiet, M., Kahanpää, K. V., Young, W. P. & Rudolph, A. M. (1973) Pathophysiological changes in the fetal lamb with growth retardation. In *Fetal and Neonatal Physiology, Barcroft Centenary Symposium*, pp. 398–402. Cambridge: Cambridge University Press.

Dawes, G. S. (1968) *Fetal and Neonatal Physiology*. Chicago: Year Book Radical Publishers.

Dobbing, J. (1974) Later development of the brain and its vulnerability. In *Scientific Foundations of Pediatrics* (Ed.) Davies, J. A. & Dobbing, J. pp. 565–576. London: Heinemann Medical.

Emery, A. E. H., Burt, D., Nelson, M. M. & Scrimgeour, J. B. (1970) Antenatal diagnosis and amino acid composition of amniotic fluid. *Lancet*, **i**, 1307–1308.

Faust, R. G., Burns, M. J. & Misch, D. W. (1970) Sodium dependent binding of L-histidine to a fraction of mucosal brush borders from hamster jejunum. *Biochimica et Biophysica Acta*, **219**, 507–511.

Felig, P., Pozefsky, T., Marliss, E. & Cahill, G. F. (1970) Alanine: key role in gluconeogenesis. *Science*, **167**, 1003–1004.

Freinkel, N., Metzger, B. E., Nitzan, M., Hare, J. W., Shambaugh, G. E., Marhsall, R. T., Surmaczuska, B. Z. & Nagel, T. C. (1972) 'Accelerated starvation' and mechanisms for the conservation of maternal nitrogen during pregnancy. *Israel Journal of Medical Sciences*, **8**, 426–439.

Friis-Hansen, B. (1957) Changes in body water compartments during growth. *Acta Pediatrica*, Supplement 110, **46**, 1–68.

Gruenwald, P. (1974) Pathology of the deprived fetus and its supply line. In *Size at Birth, Ciba Symposium 27* (new series) (Ed.) Elliott, K. & Knight, J. pp. 3–26. Amsterdam: Associated Scientific Publishers.

Habicht, J. P., Lechtig, A., Yarborough, C. & Klein, R. E. (1974) Maternal nutrition, birth weight and infant mortality. In *Size at Birth, Ciba Symposium 27* (new series) (Ed.) Elliott, K. & Knight, K. pp. 353–377. Amsterdam: Associated Scientific Publishers.

Hagerman, D. D. (1964) Enzymatic capabilities of the placenta. *Federation Proceedings*, **23**, 785–790.

Hill, D. E. (1974) Experimental growth retardation in Rhesus monkeys. In *Size at Birth, Ciba Symposium 27* (new series) (Ed.) Elliott, K. & Knight, K. pp. 99–126. Amsterdam: Associated Scientific Publishers.

Hill, P. M. M. & Young, M. (1973) Net placental transfer of free amino acids against varying concentrations. *Journal of Physiology*, **235**, 409–422.

Hill, P. M. M. & Young, M. (1974) Bidirectional fluxes of leucine and lysine across the placental membranes. *Proceedings of the International Union of Physiological Sciences*, **XI**, 26.

Hytten, F. E. & Cheyne, G. A. (1972) The aminoaciduria of pregnancy. *Journal of Obstetrics and Gynaecology of the British Commonwealth*, **79**, 424–432.

Jost, A. & Picon, L. (1970) Hormonal control of fetal development and metabolism. In *Advances in Metabolic Disorders* (Ed.) Levine, R. & Luft, R. Vol. 4, pp. 123–184. New York: Academic Press.

Kerr, G. R., Chamove, A. S., Harlow, H. F. & Waisman, H. A. (1968) 'Fetal PKU': The effect of maternal hyperphenylalaninemia during pregnancy in the Rhesus monkey (Macaca Mulatta). *Pediatrics*, **42**, 27–36.

Köhler, E., Wojnorowicz, F. & Borner, K. (1975) Effects of a protein-free diet on amino acids and sex hormones of rats during the early post implantation stages of pregnancy. *Journal of Reproduction and Fertility*, **42**, 9–21.

Laga, E. M., Driscoll, S. G. & Munro, N. (1973) Quantitative studies of human placenta. II. Biochemical characteristics. *Biology of the Neonate*, **23**, 260–283.

Landau, R. L. & Poulos, J. T. (1971) The metabolic influence of progestins. In *Advances in Metabolic Disorders* (Ed.) Levine, R. & Luft, R. Vol. 5, pp. 119–147. New York: Academic Press.

Liggins, G. C. (1974) The influence of the fetal hypothalamus and pituitary on growth. In *Size at Birth, Ciba Foundation Symposium 27* (new series), pp. 165–183. Amsterdam: Associated Scientific Publishers.

Longo, L. D., Yuen, P. & Gusseck, D. J. (1973) Anaerobic, glycogen-dependent transport of amino acids by the placenta. *Nature*, **243**, 531–533.

McKeowen, P., Record, R. G. & Eckstein, P. (1965) Variation in placental weight according to litter size in the guinea pig. *Journal of Endocrinology*, **12**, 108–114.

Mellor, D. J. (1970) Distribution of ions and electrical potential differences between mother and fetus at different gestational ages in goats and sheep. *Journal of Physiology*, **207**, 133–150.

Meister, A. (1973) On the enzymology of amino acid transport. *Science*, **180**, 33–39.

Midgley, A. R. & Jaffe, R. B. (1968) Regulation of human gonadotrophins: II. Disappearance of human chorionic gonadotrophin following delivery. *Journal of Clinical Endocrinology and Metabolism*, **28**, 1712–1718.

Miller, J. F. A. P. (1966) Immunity in the fetus and the new-born. *British Medical Bulltein*, **22**, 21–26.

Munro, H. N. (Ed.) (1969) *Mammalian Protein Metabolism*, Vol. III. New York, London: Academic Press.

Munro, H. N. (Ed.) (1970) *Mammalian Protein Metabolism*, Vol. IV. New York, London: Academic Press.

New, D. A. T. (1973) Studies on mammalian fetuses in vitro during the period of organogenesis. In *The Mammalian Fetus in Vitro* (Ed.) Austin, C. R. pp. 15–65. London: Chapman and Hall.

Ounsted, M. (1968) The regulation of fetal growth. In *Aspects of Prematurity and Dysmaturity. Nutricia Symposium* (Ed.) Jonxis, J. H. P., Visser, H. K. A. & Troelstra, J. A. pp. 167–188. Leiden: Steinfert-Kroese.

Oxender, D. L. (1972) Membrane transport. *Annual Review of Biochemistry*, **41**, 777–814.

Pearse, W. H. & Sornson, H. (1969) Free amino acids of normal and abnormal human placentas. *American Journal of Obstetrics and Gynecology*, **105**, 696–701.

Polani, P. E. (1974) Chromosomal and other genetic influences on birth weight variation. In *Size at Birth, Ciba Foundation Symposium 27* (new series), pp. 127–164. Amsterdam: Associated Scientific Publishers.

Posner, B. I. (1974) Insulin receptors in human and animal placental tissue. *Diabetes*, **23**, 209–217.

Prenton, M. A. & Young, M. (1969) Umbilical vein–artery and uterine arteriovenous plasma amino acid differences. *Journal of Obstetrics and Gynaecology of the British Commonwealth*, **76**, 404–411.

Reynaud, R., Vincedon, G., Boog, G., Brettes, J. P., Schumacher, J. C., Koehl, C., Kirchstetter, L. & Gandar, R. (1972) Injections intra-amniotiques d'acides amines dan les cas de malnutrition foetal. *Journal de Gynecologie Obstetrique et Biologie de la Reproduction*, **1**, 231–244.

Reynolds, M. L. & Young, M. (1971) The transfer of free α-amino nitrogen across the placental membrane in the guinea-pig. *Journal of Physiology*, **214**, 583–597.

Ryser, H. J. P. (1968) Uptake of protein by mammalian cells: an underdeveloped area. *Science*, **159**, 390–396.

Schneider, H. & Dancis, J. (1974) Amino acid transport in human placental slices. *American Journal of Obstetrics and Gynaecology*, **120**, 1092–1098.

Schulman, J. D., Mann, L. I., Doores, L., Duchin, S., Halverstam, J. & Mastrantonio, J. (1974) Amino acid metabolism by the fetal brain during normal and hypoglycaemic conditions. *Biology of the Neonate*, **25**, 57–65.

Schulz, D. M., Giordano, D. A. & Schulz, D. H. (1962) Weights of fetuses and infants. *Archives of Pathology*, **74**, 80–86.

Scriver, C. R. & Rosenberg, L. E. (1973) Amino acid metabolism and its disorders. In *Major Problems in Clinical Pediatrics*, Vol. X. Philadelphia: Saunders.

Solomon, J. B. (1971) Foetal and neonatal immunology. In *Frontiers of Biology* (Ed.) Neuberger, A. & Tatum, E. L. Vol. 20. Amsterdam: North-Holland.

Soltesz, G., Joyce, J. & Young, M. (1973) Protein synthesis rate in the newborn lamb. *Biology of the Neonate*, **23**, 139–148.

Southgate, D. A. T. (1971) The accumulation of amino acids in the products of conception of the rat and in the young animal after birth. *Biology of the Neonate*, **19**, 272–292.

Sugawa, T., Nakamura, K. & Osaki, M. (1963) Studies on the amino acid and protein metabolism in fetal growth: III Dynamics of free amino acids on the amniotic fluid and its nutritive role in the fetus. *Journal of the Japanese Obstetrical and Gynaecological Society*, **10**, 1–7.

Sykes, A. R. & Field, A. C. (1972) Effects of dietary deficiencies of energy, protein and calcium on the pregnant ewe. II Body composition and mineral content of the lamb. *Journal of Agricultural Science*, **78**, 119–125.

Szabo, A. J. & Grimaldi, R. D. (1970) The metabolism of the placenta. In *Advances in Metabolic Disorders* (Ed.) Levine, R. & Luft, R. Vol. 4, pp. 185–228. New York: Academic Press.

Tighe, J. R., Garrod, P. R. & Curran, R. C. (1967) The trophoblast of the human chorionic villus. *Journal of Pathology and Bacteriology*, **93**, 559–567.

Waterlow, J. C. & Stephen, J. M. L. (1967) Measurement of total lysine turnover in the rat by intravenous infusion of L-^{14}C-lysine. *Clinical Science*, **33**, 489–506.

Waterlow, J. C. & Stephen, J. M. L. (1968) The effect of low protein diets on the turnover rates of serum, liver and muscle proteins in the rat, measured by continuous infusion of L-^{14}C-lysine. *Clinical Science*, **35**, 287–305.

Widdowson, E. M. (1969) How the fetus is fed. *Proceedings of the Nutrition Society*, **28**, 17–24.

Widdowson, E. M. (1970) Harmony of growth. *Lancet*, **i**, 901–905.

Widdowson, E. M. & Spray, C. M. (1951) Chemical development 'in utero'. *Archives of Disease in Childhood*, **26**, 205–214.

Wigglesworth, J. S. (1968) Dysmaturity in the experimental animal. In *Aspects of Prematurity and Dysmaturity* (Ed.) Jonxis, J. H. P., Visser, H. K. A. & Troelstra, J. A. pp. 119–126. Leiden: Stenfert Kioese.

Wild, A. E. (1974) Protein transport across the placenta. In *Transport at the Cellular Level. Symposium of the Society for Experimental Biology*, **28**, 521–546.

Williams, H. H., Vurtin, L. V., Abraham, J., Loosli, J. K. & Maynard, L. A. (1954) Estimations of growth requirements for amino acids by assay of the carcass. *Journal of Biological Chemistry*, **208**, 277–285.

Winick, M. (1968) Cellular growth of the placenta as an indicator of abnormal fetal growth. In *Diagnosis and Treatment of Fetal Disorders* (Ed.) Adamsons, K. pp. 83–101. New York: Springer.

Winick, M. & Noble, A. (1966) Cellular response in rats during malnutrition at various ages. *Journal of Nutrition*, **89**, 300–306.

Winick, M., Brasel, J. A. & Rosso, P. (1972) Nutrition and cell growth. In *Nutrition and Development. Current Concepts in Nutrition*, Vol. 1 (Ed.) Winick, M. pp. 49–89. New York: Wiley.

Young, M. (1971) Placental transport of free amino acids. In *Metabolic Processes in the Foetus and Newborn Infant, Nutricia Symposium* (Ed.) Jonxis, J. H. P., Visser, H. K. A. & Troelstra, J. A. pp. 97–110. Leiden: Stenfert Kroese.

Young, M. (1974) In *Size at Birth* (Ed.) Elliott, K. & Knight, J. *Ciba Foundation Symposium 27* (New series), p. 21. Amsterdam: Associated Scientific Publishers.

Young, M. & Hill, P. M. M. (1973) Free amino acid transfer across the placental membrane. In *Foetal and Neonatal Physiology, Barcroft Centenary Symposium*, pp. 329–338. Cambridge: Cambridge University Press.

Young, M. & McFadyen, I. R. (1973) Placental transfer and fetal uptake of amino acids in the pregnant ewe. *Journal of Perinatal Medicine*, **1**, 174–182.

Young, M. & Prenton, M. A. (1969) Maternal and fetal plasma amino acid concentrations during gestation and in retarded fetal growth. *Journal of Obstetrics and Gynaecology of the British Commonwealth*, **76**, 333–344.

Young, M. & Widdowson, E. M. (1975) The influence of diets deficient in energy or in protein on conceptus weight and the placental transfer of a non-metabolisable amino acid in the guinea pig. *Biology of the Neonate*, **27**, 184–191.

Young, M., Soltesz, Gy., Noakes, D., Joyce, J., McFadyen, I. & Lewis, B. V. (1975) The influence of intra-uterine surgery and of fetal intravenous nutritional supplements 'in utero' on plasma free amino acid homeostasis in the pregnant ewe. *Journal of Perinatal Medicine*, **3**, 180–197.

5

PROTEIN AND AMINO ACID METABOLISM DURING FETAL DEVELOPMENT

B. S. Lindblad

The fetus accumulates, in a programmed and regulated manner, body proteins of many types and functions which are essential to its metabolism. In order to achieve this, a balanced input of amino acids is necessary. The respective roles of mother and placenta in fetal amino acid homeostasis have been discussed in Chapter 4. This chapter deals with investigations of the development and extent of fetal autonomy. Studies of the very early embryo or of lower organisms are excluded. Chemical embryology, as based on chicken embryo analyses, was summarised in the opus magnum of Needham (1931). An extensive review of the biochemistry of animal development in relation to functional differentiation has been edited by Weber (1965). Considerable information has accumulated since then concerning protein synthesis during fetal development and the regulation of enzymic activity, with implications for the study of mental retardation, teratological mechanisms, the action of hormones, amino acid transport systems, the development of immunological competence and tumour growth.

The clinical implications of the pattern of enzyme induction are manifold. The intra-uterine detection of inborn errors of metabolism requires detailed knowledge of normal enzymatic development. In obstetrics, an accurate assessment of fetal metabolic maturity is essential prior to premature termination of pregnancy (indicated by such maternal conditions as diabetes or hypertensive disorders) in order to determine if the fetus is better off in utero or in the ward. In neonatology, knowledge about the metabolic situation of the newborn baby is a fundamental prerequisite when attempting to avoid lasting brain damage due to a defective capacity to adapt to the requirements of extra-uterine life. This field has, until quite recently, been dominated by studies of 'fuel', or energy metabolism, neglecting the study of the 'machinery', or the enzymatic set-up.

There are indications in recent literature that in the future it may be possible to interfere with prenatal enzymatic development, and in this way facilitate adaptation of the premature baby to extra-uterine life. It is quite clear that before such intervention is implemented on a broader scale the specificity and nature of the extragenetic mechanisms directing enzyme synthesis must be studied in depth.

METHODS

Estimation of pools of amino acids and metabolites

Carcass analysis (Southgate, 1971) may provide information about the amounts and proportions of fetal amino acid requirements. The free amino acid concentration of fetal liver (Ryan and Carver, 1966) and brain (Marks, Stern and Lajtha, 1975) has been used to relate change in amino acid metabolism to the development of tissue and subcellular fractions (Lajtha and Piccoli, 1971). The appearance of tissue-specific marker proteins (Zuckermann, Herschmann and Levine, 1970; Unsworth, 1975) can be used to demonstrate tissue differentiation. Amniotic fluid analysis (Doran et al, 1974) may develop into a valuable tool for the assessment of fetal maturity.

In vitro conversion of markers in fetal liver slices, homogenates and tissue culture

The cytoheterogenicity of organs makes the investigation of homogenates an approximation. Incubation of fetal tissues with ^{14}C-labelled amino acids, followed by immunoelectrophoresis and radioautography has been used by Gitlin, Pericelli and Gitlin (1972). For a description of the technique and demonstration of the importance of using fresh tissue for liver homogenates, the reader is referred to Cartwright, Connellan and Dawks (1973).

Culture systems of organ explants provide a system for the maintenance of tissue in a chemically defined environment for a prolonged period. Changes provide information as to the competence of the fetal tissue to respond to externally administered agents. Specific prenatal diagnoses may be achieved by assay of cultured amniotic fluid cells (Kaback, Leonard and Parmley, 1971) after careful morphological identification of the cell type (Gerbie et al, 1972). The technique of liver organ culture has been used extensively in the investigation of hormone induction of fetal liver enzymes (Wicks, 1968; Räihä, Schwartz and Lindroos, 1971) and lung epithelial differentiation (Adamson and Bowden, 1975). De novo synthesis of specific proteins has been shown by addition of ^{14}C-leucine to the perfusion medium, followed by electrophoresis on cellulose acetate and immunoelectrophoresis or immunodiffusion of the tissue (Kekomäki, Seppälä and Schwartz, 1971).

Perfused liver systems have been used, particularly in the investigation of hormone induction of fetal liver enzymes (Barnabei and Sereni, 1964).

In vivo incorporation of radioactive substances into protein

The effects on the fetal cerebral cortex of an imbalanced supply of amino acids to the mother has been investigated by in vivo incorporation of radioactive substances into protein (Wong and Justice, 1972).

Fetal RNA synthesis may be studied through ^{3}H-cytidine administration to the pregnant animal (Larkin and Stevens, 1972). In vivo investigation of RNA synthesis in the fetus has been hampered by the inability of the rat fetus to incorporate labelled uridine. The efficiency of protein synthesis in different fetal organs has been studied by Mori and Iso (1965) with the use of ^{35}S-methionine administration to pregnant rabbits. The extent of catabolism in the fetus has been studied by means of catheterisation of whole fetuses (Gresham et al, 1972).

Studies of the immature newborn during the immediate neonatal period

In order to form a true picture of the fetus's capabilities at a specific point in its development, the results of the in vitro studies above have to be correlated with in vivo conversion studies of the whole fetus or the intact animal after premature birth. Such a correlation must be made with caution in view of the unknown factors induced by the birth process itself. The homeostatic response of the newborn infant to a varied amino acid and protein intake, perorally or intravenously, may add valuable information to the prenatal data (Levy et al, 1969). The increase of tyrosine and the less marked fall of phenylalanine immediately after birth in the human (Lindblad, 1971) and hypertyrosinaemic response to total intravenous feeding of newborn babies (Lindblad et al, 1975) (Figure 5.1) are examples of how studies of the plasma amino acid homeostasis in the immediate neonatal period can correlate studies in humans with in vivo studies of fetal protein metabolism during late gestation in animals. Constant or increasing serum protein concentration in the neonate during the immediate neonatal period suggests that the protein has been synthesised by the fetus. Conversely, the fall in serum protein concentration after birth at a rate equal to the half-life of that protein suggests either a cessation or a lack of fetal synthesis (Krasilnikoff, 1967; Gitlin and Biasucci, 1969).

NORMAL FETAL AMINO ACID AND PROTEIN METABOLISM

Amino acid synthesis in the prenatal liver

There seems to be a close relationship between metabolic requirements and the development of enzyme systems. In rat fetuses, the enzymes involved in protein synthesis are especially active, while those catalysing protein metabolism are less well developed (Sereni and Prin-

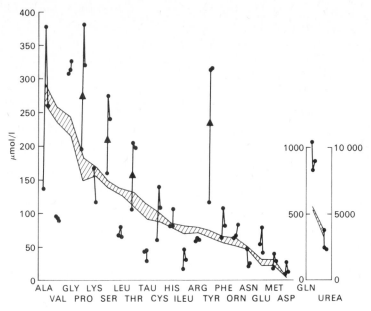

Figure 5.1. Plasma free amino acids before, during and 30 min after cessation of total intravenous feeding of a starving, prematurely born human infant (Lindblad et al, 1975). The striped area represents normal levels of infants, mean ± s.e.m. (Stegink and Baker, 1971). The 'intolerance' to tyrosine is demonstrated. The low alanine, valine, leucine and isoleucine levels and the high glycine levels, characteristic of starvation in adults (Adibi, 1968; Lindblad, 1972), are reflected in newborn infants suffering from food deprivation.

cipi, 1965). As fetal life represents an explosive rate of cellular proliferation and growth not comparable to any other period in life (the human fetus at eight weeks gestation weighs one gram and is 2.5 cm long; at 12 weeks weighs 14 g and is 7.5 cm long; whereas at the end of the second trimester he weighs 1000 g and is 35 cm long) very high enzyme activity is seen in nucleic acid synthesis.

Differentiation of the enzymatic patterns seems to occur in steps, each consisting of the addition of new enzyme clusters (Table 5.1). Two aspects of each step, the chemical mechanisms that regulate the formation of the enzyme and the physiological consequences regulated *by* the enzyme, will now be described and illustrated by the examples below.

The trans-sulphuration pathway

One of the more remarkable findings in the development of amino acid metabolism is that cystathionase is lacking in human fetal liver while in the rat fetus the enzyme is present as early as at 12 days gestation (Gaull, Sturman and Räihä, 1972). The low activity of this enzyme in the conversion of methionine into cysteine is not seen in the other enzymes of the trans-sulphuration pathway, which all show considerable activity. Immunochemical evidence for absence of cystathionase from human fetal liver also exists (Pascal, Gillian and Gaull, 1972). Further evidence for the inactivity of the trans-sulphuration pathway in human fetuses is the high methionine concentration seen in cord blood of prematurely born human babies (Lindblad, 1971), the high methionine levels seen in total intravenous feeding of newborn babies (Stegink and Baker, 1971; Das and Filler, 1973), and the hypermethioninaemia (Levy et

Table 5.1. *Developmental enzyme formations in the metabolism of amino acids.*

Enzyme	Induced in relation to birth
Rat liver	
Tyrosine aminotransferase[a]	+12 hours
p-OH-phenylpyruvate oxidase	+ 1 week
Phenylalanine hydroxylase	+ 1 week
Tryptophan oxygenase[c]	+ 2 weeks
Urea cycle	+ 1 week
Arginase[b,c]	late neonatal
Asparaginase[c]	late neonatal
Histidine decarboxylase	0
Serine dehydratase[a]	0
Ornithine aminotransferase[c]	late neonatal
Alanine aminotransferase[c]	late neonatal
Rat brain	
Glutamate decarboxylase	+12 days
Hydroxytryptophan decarboxylase	− 4 days
Glutamine synthetase	0
Rat kidney	
Hydroxytryptophan decarboxylase	+1 day
Glutaminase	+2 weeks
Arginase	+2 weeks
Ornithine aminotransferase	+3 weeks
Human liver, relatively low activities at birth.[d]	
Tyrosine aminotransferase (low activity)	
p-OH-phenylpyruvate oxidase (inactive form of the protein present)	
Cystathionase (absent, liver and brain)	

For references see Greengaard (1971).

[a]Experimentally enhanced by glucagon.
[b]Experimentally enhanced by thyroxine.
[c]Experimentally enhanced by hydrocortisone.
[d]For references see Räiha and Kekomäki (1975).

al, 1969) and the cystathioninuria (Przyrenbel and Bremer, 1972) in preterm human infants on high protein diets.

Adults metabolise 90 per cent of ingested methionine to cysteine via the trans-sulphuration pathway (Rose and Wixon, 1955). Apparently inorganic sulphate cannot be utilised as a sulphur donor for cysteine synthesis in human fetal liver.

In view of the overwhelming evidence for the absence of cystathionase, the last trans-sulphuration enzyme, in the human fetal liver it seems unlikely that the transfer of sulphur from labelled methionine into cysteine may occur via this route. However, cystathionine-β-synthetase, facilitating cysteine synthesis from serine and sulphide (previously not described in man) has recently been suggested to be identical to human serine dehydratase. This would make possible a transfer of homocystine sulphur (originally derived from methionine) into sulphide and then utilisation of sulphide in a sulphydration reaction of serine with the resultant formation of cysteine. Thus, cystathionine-β-synthetase may be especially important during fetal development by providing a pathway for cysteine synthesis independent of cystathionase. However, high levels of sulphide in relation to homocystine (1.5) seem necessary to trigger the reaction (Porter, Grishaver and Jones, 1974), and whether or not it plays a physiological role is still to be proved.

The human fetus, compared with other mammals, usually shows well-developed enzymatic activities in amino acid metabolism. It is therefore likely that the low activity of cystathionase is an example of a meaningful adaptation to intra-uterine life. Cystathionase deficiency could result in a channelling of the β-carbon of serine into thymidylate (required for DNA synthesis) and in the conservation of the sulphur of methionine for incorporation into protein and for synthesis of polyamines (via-S-adenosyl-methionine) in those tissues which actively synthesise RNA and protein. It would also conserve methionine in the form of S-adenosyl-methionine to facilitate methylation reactions. Evidence favouring this conclusion is the twenty-fold increase in the specific activity of S-adenosyl-methionine decarboxylase in fetal and in adult human liver and a high polyamine concentration in fetal liver (Sturman and Gaull, 1974). The relative activities found in the different methyltransferases are evidence in favour of a turning off of the trans-sulphuration pathway in favour of the folate B_{12} remethylation pathway.

The advantage of an adaptation would be that the β-carbon of serine would be shunted into DNA synthesis at this period of rapid cellular multiplication, rather than having the entire carbon skeleton accept this sulphur from homocysteine to form cysteine. Utilisation of the sulphide into the sulphydration reaction of serine with the formation of cysteine (Porter, Grishaver and Jones, 1974) would not only tentatively provide a protective mechanism for sulphide detoxication, but also mean that there is a mechanism whereby cysteine can be synthesised by the fetus and that cysteine is therefore *not* an essential amino acid for the newborn human baby.

The hydroxylation of phenylalanine to tyrosine

In the complex enzyme system which converts phenylalanine into tyrosine (Kauffman, 1971), the final reaction forming tyrosine requires the enzyme phenylalanine hydroxylase. Phenylalanine hydroxylase activity is present in human fetal liver from the eighth week of gestation, and activities comparable to adult liver are reached after the 13th week (Räihä, 1973). Both phenylalanine hydroxylase, dihydropteridine reductase and the cofactor are present in liver of human fetuses less than 11 weeks (Jakubovic, 1971). ^{14}C-phenylalanine injected postmortem into the umbilical vein of prematurely born human fetuses is readily converted to ^{14}C-tyrosine (Ryan and Orr, 1966). In contrast the fetal rat is not able to metabolise, as rapidly as the mother, a load of phenylalanine delivered by the placenta (Lines and Waisman, 1971).

However, the capacity of the human fetus of eight to ten weeks gestation to metabolise phenylalanine into tyrosine is limited as compared to children of eight weeks to seven years of age (McLean, Harwick and Clayton, 1973), and under certain circumstances the newborn baby seems to be intolerant to a phenylalanine load during total intravenous feeding (Das and Filler, 1973). The relatively slow lowering of the phenylalanine level immediately after birth in the premature human baby is another indication of this (Lindblad, 1971).

In view of the present data, the formerly held view that tyrosine is essential to the newborn human baby is unlikely. However, despite the indications of ability to convert phenylalanine into tyrosine neonatally, this function is limited and tyrosine should be given in the diet to promote optimal growth.

Fetal synthesis of ornithine, arginine, histidine and glycine

Ornithine ketoacid aminotransferase (OKT) is present before the 20th week of gestation in the human fetus. The development pattern of OKT found in human liver is different from that in rat liver (Kekomäki, Räihä and Bickel, 1969). This can be compared with what is known about urea synthesis during fetal life in the two species (Table 5.1). It may be that the main role of the urea cycle during the intensive growth of human fetal life is the synthesis of arginine to supplement a low provision from the mother's blood. These findings are in agreement with the non-essentiality of arginine found in newborn infants (Snyderman, Boyer and Holt, 1959).

The essentiality of histidine during growth of the human infant is well documented (Snyderman, Prose and Holt, 1959). It is therefore highly probable that histidine is also essential for the fetus, but histidine biosynthesis does not seem to have been studied at the biochemical level in fetal tissues. There seems to be competence for glycine synthesis in fetal tissues (Gaull et al, 1973).

Amino acid degradation and urea formation

The combination of intensive growth, low blood flow to the liver and high insulin concentrations (Girard et al, 1973) might explain the low activity of many liver enzymes responsible for the degradation of amino acids found in experimental animals. The high insulin levels of the fetus and the taurinaemia of the newborn (Lindblad, 1971) may reflect a low liver uptake and low biliary acid production. The relatively high lysine concentrations may be secondary to the fact that this amino acid alone takes no part in transamination processes and that the amino acid degrading enzymes might be low in fetal liver.

Taurine metabolism

The homeostasis of taurine in the fetus and newborn seems to be unique. The free taurine level of human fetal liver and brain is increased (Ryan and Carver, 1966; Sturman and Gaull, 1975). The ratio of fetal to maternal plasma concentrations of taurine is very high >4 : 1 (Lindblad, 1971). The plasma levels of taurine fall rapidly to normal during the first days of extra-uterine life, except in the early born where there is a temporary increase (Lindblad, 1971). The high excretion of taurine in the newborn is well known, and was first described as a transient characteristic of the normal full-term neonate's urine by Bickel and Souchon (1955). The taurine level of rabbit and monkey brain is known to decrease during the neonatal period (Agrawal, Davis and Hinwich, 1967; Sturman and Gaull, 1975). Taken together, these facts may suggest that there is an efficient excretion of fetally accumulated taurine during the neonatal period. The synthesis of taurine has been studied mostly in adult animals. The tissues of chicken and calf embryos exhibit certain peculiarities of sulphur metabolism which distinguish them from the tissues of adult animals. Thus, 65 per cent of ^{35}S-sulphate administered to the chicken embryo at 34 hours of age is recovered as taurine at one day of postnatal age (Machlin, Pearson and Denton, 1955). It has also been shown that cysteate in the calf embryo is rapidly decarboxylated to taurine (Chapeville and Fromageot, 1957). Thus it seems that taurine in the chicken and calf embryo could be an end product in metabolism of sulphur-containing amino acids. In contrast, the adult animal excretes 75 per cent of sulphur in the form of sulphate. It seems possible that the high amino acid nitrogen concentrations of cord blood in premature deliveries seen by Lichtenstein (1931) could be due to the occasional exaggeratedly high taurine and lysine concentrations found in cord blood of premature babies (Lindblad, 1971).

Tyrosine metabolism

The further metabolism of tyrosine has been studied extensively in fetal and perinatal liver tissues with special emphasis on the response of the enzyme activity to hormones. The first enzyme in the oxidation of tyrosine, tyrosine aminotransferase (TAT), shows a uniquely slow increase in the fetal liver to a level of approximately 10 per cent of adult values in the liver of premature infants (Räihä, Schwartz and Lindroos, 1971).

The dramatic increase of TAT from low fetal levels to double adult levels 12 hours post-partum in the rat has made it an ideal system for the study of perinatal enzyme induction. Cortisone or adrenalectomy during the initial minutes after birth influence the normal post-natal increase of TAT activity in the rat. Protein synthesis inhibitors nullify the effect, so there is a de novo synthesis of enzyme protein (Sereni, Kenney and Kretchmer, 1959; Kretchmer and Greenberg, 1966). Glucagon, adrenalin and cyclic AMP administered during the last two days of gestation to the rat stimulate enzyme activity in vivo (Greengard and Dewey, 1967). This has also been demonstrated on fetal liver in vitro (Räihä, 1971). In man, as well as in the rat, it has been demonstrated that TAT activity can be induced by corticosteroids in fetal liver explants in culture from about 60 per cent of the duration of gestation (Räihä, 1971).

The spontaneous increase of TAT activity in rat fetal liver cultures has given rise to the hypothesis that there is an intra-uterine inhibition of the enzymatic activity. The fact that hydrocortisone and glucagon are ineffective in fetal liver in vivo, but that both hydrocortisone and glucagon are effective in small fetuses in vitro (Wicks, 1969), is a further indication of fetal in vivo inhibition. Growth hormone represses TAT activity in adult liver and might repress the TAT activity in utero (Rutter, 1969). It has been proposed that the hypoglycaemia developed during the perinatal period leads to glucagon release and an enzyme induction. However, adult activities are not reached at this stage. Premature infants have little or no tyrosine oxidizing activity; it is three to five times higher in term infants and 10 to 30 times higher in adults, according to a study of liver homogenates (Kretchmer et al, 1956).

There are four main principles to be drawn from the studies of tyrosine aminotransferase activity:

1. Mammalian liver responds to hormone-induced enzyme synthesis only after a certain developmental stage is reached and the effects of hydrocortisone and glucagon represent different mechanisms (Räihä, Schartz and Lindroos, 1971). TAT is induced in fetal rat four to three days before term by cyclic AMP only, and at two to one days by cyclic AMP, adrenalin and glucagon (Greengard, 1969). After birth, it is inducible only by hydrocortisone (Sereni and Sereni, 1971).

2. The general phenomenon of interspecies differences of enzymatic development. Thus Räihä, Schwartz and Lindroos (1971) could show no increase in TAT activity in human fetal liver in organ culture at 14 to 24 weeks of gestation, but there was increased enzymatic activity after hydrocortisone, glucagon and insulin treatment from the 18th day to term in rat fetal liver in organ culture.

3. Based on the differences between in vivo and in vitro inducibility of TAT is the hypothesis of intra-uterine enzyme inhibition. However, as yet no convincing evidence for an intracellular repressor in vivo has been presented. The spontaneous TAT and alanine aminotransferase activity increase seen during incubation of liver fragments in organ culture (Sereni and Sereni, 1969) could be due to the release from the ribosomal fraction due to cyclic AMP, FFA, acetyl coenzyme A or other substances accumulating during the early period of culture (Monder and Coufalic, 1975).

4. The final hypothetical generalisation that can be made from the studies of the tyrosine

oxidating system is based on the fact that while the development of TAT activity is slow, the next enzyme in the chain (parahydroxyphenyl-pyruvate oxidase activity) first develops one week later than TAT. This emphasises the importance of substrate activation in the development of enzyme activity (Räihä, 1974).

A human neonatal correlation to the experimental findings is the high plasma tyrosine levels seen at four to six hours of age in the premature human baby (Lindblad, 1971); the tyrosinaemia known to occur later in premature babies, especially if put on a diet providing over 5.0 g protein/kg body weight/day (Mathews and Partington, 1964); and the tyrosinuria and increase of parahydroxyphenylpyruvic acid in the urine of premature infants if given a high protein–low ascorbic acid diet (Gordon and Maples, 1941).

Tryptophan metabolism

The use of tryptophan oxygenase as an experimental model is based on the fact that enzyme activity is absent in the fetal liver of rats, mice, rabbits and guinea-pigs, while adult activity is reached 24 hours postnatally in the rabbit and guinea-pig and 15 days postnatally in the rat and mouse. The developmental increase has been shown to be related to the birth process and not to chronological age. Protein synthesis inhibitors to guinea-pigs have shown that we are dealing with a developmental increase of new enzyme molecules associated with synthesis of RNA (Nemeth, 1963). Further studies have shown that cortisone seems to act by activation of messenger RNA synthesis, while the substrate, tryptophan, acts by stabilising tryptophan oxygenase and possibly making more sites on the ribosomal complex available for protein synthesis. Phenomena similar to these may be seen in regenerating liver of actively growing adult rats.

A close correlation seems to exist between metabolic requirements and the development of enzyme systems. During development, enzymes involved in protein synthesis seem to be active, while those catalysing protein catabolism are less developed. The explanation may lie in the increase of amino acid concentration in the intracellular space prior to active growth causing enhancement of the enzymatic activities of nucleic acid synthesis. An immediate postnatal increase in amino acid influx to the liver occurs in neonates (Christensen and Clifford, 1963). Tryptophan oxygenase can be induced by substrate in adult man, and in the adult rat, rabbit and guinea-pig, but cannot be induced in the fetus or infant (Nemeth, 1963). Following a spontaneous upsurge, tryptophan oxygenase becomes inducible by substrate; thus substrate induction is a *consequence* of differentiation and not a cause of it. The responsiveness to an inducer itself depends on prior differentiation.

The causal factor behind the induction of tryptophan oxygenase is not known; it is certainly not due to the appearance of an isoenzyme (Dawkins, 1966). Transient induction of tryptophan oxygenase can be reached prematurely by hydrocortisone priming followed by trytophan (Greengard, 1971). It seems that tryptophan oxygenase is a rate-limiting step in regulating the brain levels of catecholamines during early development (Eiduson, 1971).

Urea formation

There are indications that nitrogen catabolism with urea formation and energy production from amino acids plays an important role in fetal life, especially during starvation and surgical stress (Gresham et al, 1972). The extent to which this occurs has not been clarified. Newborn infants may produce concentrated urine if fed a high protein diet and it is known that in the human, in sharp contrast to most experimental animals, urea synthesis develops during early gestation (Edelman, Barnett and Troupkan, 1960; Räihä and Suihkonen, 1968). Arginine synthetase shows the lowest relative activity (detectable at eight weeks, considerable activity at birth—40 per cent of adult liver), indicating that it is also a rate-limiting enzyme of the human fetal urea cycle (Räihä and Suihkonen, 1968).

The first human clinical correlations of these findings are the report of urea and uric acid in the bladder of a human embryo in utero by Prout in the early 19th century (cited by Needham, 1931). However, even if the capacity is there, the truth is probably that expressed already by Lindsay (1911) (cited by Needham, 1931) "the picture of fetal metabolism shown by the chemical composition of the earlier amniotic liquid is one of low deaminising power, indicated by the low urea output, the absence of ammonia and the high proportion of amino acids". After the 30th week, creatinine (0.4 to 2.5 mg per cent) and urea (16 to 40 mg per cent) increase steadily in amniotic fluid to levels higher than those of maternal plasma (Lind, 1971). Urea formation as a route for the removal of excess nitrogen is probably small during gestation, as evidenced by alanine perfusion of human fetal liver (Räihä and Kekomäki, 1975; see Chapter 10).

The study of ornithine transcarbamylase (OTC) activity in rat liver is of special interest. There is a peak activity before birth, with a sharp decrease during the first hours of extra-uterine life. During this period, enzymatic activity catalysing the synthesis of carbamylphosphate and production of excretable nitrogen atoms increases more than the metabolism to arginine and ornithine ('amino acid carriers'). This might indicate a rapid rate of protein turnover during the final days of gestation with accumulation of products for enzyme induction. The neonatal drop might be a result of temporarily decreased food intake, as OTC activity has been shown to be proportional to protein intake (Schuit and Dickie, 1973). The synthesis of carbamylphosphate during amino acid catabolism could be a step in the excretion of nitrogen atoms in ureotelic animals. It is not clear if it could be induced by a substrate or if it is due to de novo synthesis as in adult rats (Schimke, 1962).

Protein synthesis

From studies of maternally administered ^{35}S-methionine (Mori and Iso, 1965), it seems that the origin of fetal protein is the free amino acid transferred from mother to fetus. The major direct precursor of fetal protein is not the protein synthesised in the placenta from the amino acids of maternal circulation, or products degraded in the placenta from maternal plasma protein, or the actual transfer of plasma proteins intact through the placenta. It has also been shown that the fetus uses free amino acids transferred from the maternal circulation to an extent sufficient for the synthesis of its own plasma proteins, with the exception of gammaglobulin (Dancis, Braverman and Lind, 1957). During the last trimester of human fetal life there is a very active protein synthesis, ca. 5 g/day (Waisman and Kerr, 1965). This is at first mainly directed towards structural growth, with an active detoxification of the products by the placenta. The developmental behaviour of aspartate carbamyltransferase, an enzyme essential for pyrimidine and therefore for nucleic acid synthesis, may be related to growth. In the guinea-pig, a species which undergoes much of its total body growth during fetal life, the enzyme diminishes to low adult levels by term, whereas in the rat, which continues its rapid growth postnatally, the same enzyme is maintained at a relatively high level for some time after birth (Kretchmer, Hurwitz and Räihä, 1966; Greengard, 1971). Towards the end of pregnancy, there are increasing demands for fetal organ function and the maternally derived amino acids are directed into enzyme and protein hormone synthesis, the synthesis of specific substances like thyroxine and melanin (from tyrosine), serotonin (from tryptophan), histamine (from histidine), steroids (from leucine) and epinephrine and norepinephrine (from phenylalanine). Methyl groups for choline synthesis are derived from methionine, and nucleic acid synthesis requires non-disturbed transfer of glycine and aspartic acid from the mother. The increasing demands for ammonia detoxification by the organs to be met by ammonia excretion in the kidneys and by the placenta means increasing demands for glutamic acid influx. In this way, the fetus develops a high degree of autonomy. Perhaps the maternal system plays no significant role in the regulation of fetal development other than to provide basic nutrients and the appropriate physical environment. In other words, fetal enzyme differentiation may be independent of maternal regulation (Rutter, 1969). The fetus also seems to be less dependent on hormonal regulation of growth, reacting more to localised tissue interactions, than maternal effectors or fetal endocrine control.

There is first a selective differentiation of 'primary' proteins (fundamental metabolic pathways, present in all cells), then of 'secondary' proteins (for example urea cycle enzymes, more than one cell type) and then tertiary proteins (for example hormones, in single cell type). After this, effectors like hormones, nutrients, metabolites and drugs lead to a functional modulation with quantitative changes in protein synthesis.

Very little is yet known about fetal protein breakdown, which is an important prerequisite for remodelling of tissues during morphogenesis (Gan and Jeffay, 1967). More than 50 per cent of the free amino acid pool required as precursors for protein synthesis in adult tissues is contributed by breakdown (Gan and Jeffay, 1967). In adult tissue the re-utilisation of nucleotides is important; the question of whether the placenta acts as a barrier against preformed bases or nucleotides is a question which is yet to be solved (Roux, 1971b). Certainly thymidine seems to cross the placenta freely. The peak activity of pyrimidine nucleotide synthesis correlates with the highest proliferative phase of the organ, but the role of the 'salvage pathway' is unclear. An indication of the very high degree of utilisation of nitrogen for growth during later fetal life is the very strong anabolism during human neonatal life, where four per cent of the calories are derived from protein against 17 per cent in the starving adult (McCance and Strangeways, 1954).

Organ growth and functional differentiation

One main characteristic of tissue development is the relative decrease of water in fat-free tissue and increase of nitrogen. The concentration of total nitrogen at birth in different organs and soft tissues (Dickerson and Widdowson, 1960; Widdowson and Dickerson, 1960; Widdowson, 1964) is given in Table 5.2. From this table it can be seen that heart, liver and kidney are nearer adult levels than skeletal muscle, or skin. Does this reflect different speeds of functional maturation? In the pig, the heart beats before the 21st day when the fetus weighs only 0.2 g. Liver is a haemopoietic organ during intra-uterine life and kidneys produce urine very early during fetal life. The fetal heart does not show the large amount of extracellular material that is found in skeletal muscle (Dickerson and Widdowson, 1960). The free amino acid levels of fetal liver, kidney, subcutaneous muscle and plasma have been determined by Steve and Armstrong (1973). Total free amino acid levels of muscle of rabbit fetuses immediately before birth are four times the adult value, and the levels of ornithine are ten times the adult levels. As compared to the adult, the free amino acid levels of fetal liver are also high, with the exception of valine and cystine (Ryan and Carver, 1966).

The total creatine and protein content of the fetus increases exponentially and in parallel from the 13th to the 19th day of gestation in the rat (Koszalka, Jensh and Brent, 1972). This is also demonstrated by the maximum rate of incorporation of amino acids in the rat at the 20th day of gestation (Southgate, 1971). The placenta does not contain appreciable amounts of either of the two principal enzymes involved in the biosynthesis of creatine (trans-

Table 5.2. *Nitrogen concentration in fetal organs.*

Total N in g/kg BW:

20–25 week fetus	15
premature infant	19
term infant	23
adult	34

Concentration N as percentage adult value at birth:

whole body	67
skin	50
muscle	67
kidney	78
liver	80
heart	86

Concentration N as g/kg fresh organ:

	14th week fetus	20–22 week fetus	newborn	adult
Muscle				
extracell. protein N	0.6	1.8	3.8	1.4
intracell. protein N	10.5	12.0	14.6	28.3
Skin	11.6	11.9	26.5	53.0
Heart		14.0	20.0	23.0
Liver	20.2	22.1	22.6	28.2
Kidney	12.5	14.2	19.2	24.5
Brain	9.6	8.4	9.3	17.1

For references see Dickerson and Widdowson (1960), Widdowson and Dickerson (1960) and Widdowson (1964).

aminase and guanidoacetate-N-methyltransferase). Creatine seems to be derived by synthesis of the fetus and/or transport of creatine across the placenta (Koszalka, Jensch and Brent, 1972).

Variations in the DNA content of a monoploid cell fall mostly within rather narrow limits. Because of this stability, DNA has been used as a reference substance in terms of which the chemical composition of a tissue may be expressed. Thus the RNA:DNA ratio and the protein:DNA ratio may indicate the content of RNA or of protein per cell respectively. Moreover, by estimating the total content of DNA in a particular part of tissue the number of cells in that tissue portion can be ascertained. According to the concentration in human fetal organs (Kapeller-Adler and Hammad, 1972), maximal growth of the liver by cell division seems to occur during the third and fourth month, followed by a progressive organ growth by cell enlargement.

Maturation at birth in respect of cell size, or protein:DNA ratio is 175 in man, 104 in the guinea-pig, 38 in the pig and 15 in the rat (Widdowson, 1971). The heart and brain show maximum growth by cell division at a very early stage of human development (before six to eight weeks); subsequent growth takes place mainly by cell enlargement. The heterogeneity of brain makes this a very broad generalisation. The lungs are comparatively small in early pregnancy and are relatively late to achieve their maximum development. They show a progressive increase in the DNA concentration during the first half of pregnancy. The kidney, like the lung, may be late in achieving its maximum intra-uterine development. Studies on the control of the differentiation of alveolar epithelium suggest that there is a relationship between mitosis and differentiation of epithelial cells. When differentiation is accelerated, division is slowed (Adamson and Bowden, 1975).

The time sequence of increased nucleic acid, pyrimidine and urea synthesis and the increase of the free amino acid pool varies between different organs. However, protein synthetic activity during development follows a certain sequence of events. The first event is an increase of DNA parallel to hyperplastic growth, or increase in cell number. This is followed by an increase in RNA synthesis during hypertrophic growth or increase in cell size. Finally, in combination with an increase in free amino acids in the liver, the tissue protein synthetic activity increases. Hormones may have a significant role in regulating the permeability of cell membranes to amino acids. Glucagon or adrenal activity would distribute amino acids for protein synthesis in the liver, while insulin causes a flow of amino acids to muscles. Interferences in substrate availability could lead to decreased protein synthesis and lack of maturation of the organ.

It is during the periods of hyperplasia that nutritional deficiency may result in permanent and irrevocable changes. The pools of amino acids may be critical, the regulation of protein synthesis by hormones being mostly 'permissive' to cell permeability, and the gene acting as a coarse control, establishing limits but not determining the ultimate extent or state of development (Miller, 1969).

In rats, there is a sharp postnatal increase in liver RNA and protein synthesis (Christensen and Clifford, 1963). The non-metabolisable amino acid analogue (cycloleucine) given to the fetus shows, in less than 24 hours postnatally, an increase of 2.5 in the liver cell water: plasma ratio. This is reflected in the general phenomena of postnatal activation of liver RNA and protein synthesis, e.g. in vitamin K-dependent coagulation factors, and albumin synthesis. The factor(s) behind this could be a complex interaction of corticosteroid, glucagon and thyroxine stimulation.

[14]C-Phenylalanine incorporation into brain protein of newborn pigs falls sharply after birth (Schain et al, 1967). There seems to exist some factor in the uterine environment promoting incorporation of amino acids into brain protein (Johnson, 1968).

Requirement for individual amino acids probably varies during gestation. Different organs grow at different speeds and different organs have a different protein content and different amino acid composition. In the chick and mouse embryo it has been shown that the lysine : leucine : tryptophan ratio changes through gestation (Singer, Hochstrasser and Cerecedi, 1956). Studies of nucleic acid synthesis in various organs of the human fetus from 8 to 15 weeks of gestation by incorporation of radioactive precursors into DNA and RNA of liver, kidney, heart, skin, spleen, lung and brain by autoradiography have shown that the curves for DNA and RNA synthesis are mere images of each other (Mukherjee, Hastings and Cohen, 1973). This indicates a periodicity and unique pattern for nucleic acid synthesis in developing organs at various gestational ages. Physical and chemical factors effecting nucleic acid synthesis may be deleterious during these 'waves' of nucleic acid synthesis. Thus, the kidney seems to have definite peaks of DNA synthesis in the 8th and 15th week of gestation. These waves may be interpreted as division followed by metabolic activity or

Table 5.3. *Comparison of some brain enzyme activity upsurge in relation to birth (days before or after) in different species (the length of gestation in days is given in brackets).*

	Rat (22 days)	Rabbit (32 days)	Guinea-pig (63 days)
Glutamate decarboxylase	+12	+10	−20
NAD nucleosidase	+ 2		−28
Choline acetyltransferase		−10	−32
Carbonic anhydrase	+12		−27
Succinate dehydrogenase	+10		−25
Cytochrome oxidase	+10		−20

For references see Greengard (1971).

differentiation (by which is meant the sum of all processes whereby differential protein synhesis is initiated and regulated in the cells of an embryo).

It has been shown that ^{14}C-phenylalanine incorporation into brain protein falls sharply after birth in the pig. This fall seems to be related to birth rather than to gestational age, although increase in gestational age gives a gradual decrease in brain protein synthesis. It may be that premature delivery, and thus decrease in brain protein synthesis during a critical period of growth of the central nervous system leads to cerebral syndromes later and that this explains the high risk in premature babies of minimal brain dysfunction (Schain et al, 1967). In mouse brain tissue rapid decrease of protein and nucleic acid synthesis has been found during the critical perinatal period (Johnson, 1968). The interspecies difference in cerebral maturation is considerable; Table 5.3 shows six brain enzymes whose developmental formation reflects the marked interspecies difference in cerebral maturation (Greengard, 1971).

Protein digestion and absorption

The extent to which the human fetus digests and/or absorbs protein is not clear. 24 g of amniotic fluid protein/kg/day is cleared, 80 per cent by fetal swallowing (Gitlin et al, 1972). A large fraction of protein-bound activity of amino acid labelled erythrocytes injected into the amniotic fluid appears in maternal urine as protein-free radioactivity. This suggests the occurrence of fetal absorption and metabolism. The low birthweight for gestational age of infants with congenital oesophageal or intestinal atresia (10 per cent deficiency at term) might be explained by the lack of this route of fetal nutrition.

There seems to be a morphological basis for the existence of this intestinal absorption pathway (Lev and Orlic, 1972). Horseradish peroxidase (MW 40 000) was found six hours after infusion into amniotic fluid in the microvillous border of absorptive cells, in the region above the absorptive cells, in the extracellular space between adjacent epithelial cells, and on the luminal surface of the endothelial lining of stromal vessels in the villi. It seems as though the middle and distal segments of the human fetal small intestine are capable of protein uptake from the 14th week of pregnancy to some point before birth. The cessation of uptake of macromolecular substances by the intestine ('closure') occurs in rats simultaneously with the preparation for weaning, whereas in man it may represent a preparation for extra-uterine life (Baintner, 1973). In rabbits and rats (Sugawa, Nakamura and Ozaki, 1963) it has been established how free amino acids of the amniotic fluid are precursors of protein synthesis in the fetus. The role of amniotic fluid in the nutrition of the growing organism is, however, not established, even though the question of whether the embryo is nourished orally by the amniotic liquid, in addition to the umbilical blood, was raised by Harvey as early as 1651 (cited by Needham, 1931).

In the human fetus it has been shown that amino peptidase activities rise significantly in the ileum as compared to the duodenum after the 12th week (Koldovsky et al, 1968). Developmental studies in experimental animals have been made to determine the development of absorption of different amino acids, where an asynchronous development would be direct evidence of individuality in the different transport systems (Wilson, 1966). No conclusive evidence has been found as yet, except the general conclusion that intestinal transport systems for amino acids develop early during fetal life, with the single exception of the imino acid system (proline, hydroxyproline and glycine) (Rubino, 1975). Insulin and glucagon activities appear at the same time as the dramatic increase in the exocrine proteins (15 to 18 days in the rat). Are insulin and glucagon of fetal origin directly involved in the primary transition of the exocrine cells? Digestion and absorption during development is an interesting problem with special implications for the immunology of animals and man through transfer of intact protein molecules across the mucosa. It is not yet known whether some functional properties are lacking, such as the low digestion of protein in the stomach, or whether some unknown mechanisms are present in the small intestine which can facilitate the absorption of intact proteins. Pancreolytic activity increases from the third month of gestational age. Dipeptidase activity is present at two months, increases from the third month and is fully developed at 11 to 23 weeks (Lindberg, 1966). Glycyl-proline uptake in the jejunum of fetal rabbits is more effective than glycine uptake. It increases rapidly from the 25th day and reaches a peak at 10 times the adult level at birth (Rubino, 1975). Trypsinogen and chymotrypsinogen are present in fetuses over 500 g, but are probably still low in premature babies below 2000 g birthweight. Enterokinase activating capacity is present in prematures over and above 1500 g (Koldovsky, 1970). Proteins seemingly enter enterocytes by pinocytosis during the fetal life of mammals, but this capacity is lost in postnatal life. Pinocytosis of *fat* droplets, however, still occurs in the adult, indicating a selective change of pinocytosis through development. Decreased absorption of intact protein can be seen in newborn puppies when hydrocortisone, aldosterone and ACTH are given intravenously to the bitch prior to delivery, while neonatal starvation prolongs protein absorption (Koldovsky, 1970).

Serum protein synthesis

The synthesis of different serum proteins in the human fetus has been studied in tissue cultures using ^{14}C-labelled amino acids, followed by radioimmunoelectrophoresis (Gitlin and Biasucci, 1969).

The best known examples of proteins characteristic of embryonic life are calf fetuin and human α-fetoprotein (Bergstrand and Czar, 1956). Alpha-fetoprotein is synthesised from the sixth week by the fetal hepatocyte, with a repressed synthesis at birth and a half-life of 3.5 days in the circulation of the neonate (Gitlin et al, 1972). (Genetic derepression of α-fetoprotein might explain its presence in hepatoma and certain non-neoplastic diseases during the first years of life. Haemoglobin F is another example of such derepression in some forms of anaemia.) De novo synthesis of specific serum proteins has also been studied in perfusion of isolated human fetal liver, where leucine-^{14}C was added to the perfusion medium followed by plasma protein electrophoresis, immunoelectrophoresis or immunodiffusion. The fetal albumin synthesis rate rises to 1.0 g albumin/kg/day, which is higher than in adults. There is a failure to increase synthesis of α-fetoprotein in proportion to growth (Kekomäki et al, 1971). Alpha-fetoprotein is also lowered in the serum, while albumin increases, and it is clear that there is a more rapid turnover of α-fetoprotein than albumin in vivo. Haptoglobin has been identified in fetal sera, being of a different immunological type than that of the mother (Hirschfeld and Lunell, 1962). It has no haemoglobin-binding capacity; this appears first during the first neonatal weeks to reach adult level at two to four months of postnatal age (Fine et al, 1961).

The first verification of active plasma protein synthesis by the human fetus was found in tissue slices by Dancis, Braverman and Lind (1957). By three to four months of gestation the human fetal liver already actively synthesises all plasma protein fractions except the gammaglobulins. On the other hand, the placenta from pregnancies of three to four months gestation does not synthesise any detectable plasma protein. It was also shown that in guinea-pig fetuses (Dancis and Shafran, 1958), the fetus effectively uses amino acids from the maternal circulation for plasma protein synthesis, whereas the placenta in vitro has no proteolytic powers. Another indication of the active albumin synthesis of the fetus has been given by the study of Krasilnikoff (1967). Albumin synthesis was found to be 0.50 g/kg/day in premature babies weighing 1900 to 2400 g, against 0.32 g in infants and 0.16 g in adults. The fractional catabolic rate of the percentage of intravascularly administered albumin was 20 per cent in premature babies, compared to 8.5 per cent in bigger children and adults. Seventy-two per cent of ^{14}C-leucine perfused into isolated human fetal liver (Kekomäki et al, 1971) was incorporated into albumin and α-fetoprotein, with an increasing proportion of albumin incorporation in relation to gestational age. There is a deficiency of the coagulation factors II, VII, IX and X in the plasma of man at birth, of which factor VII has been shown to depend on a lower rate of synthesis (Sereni and Luppis, 1968). The fibrinogen stabilising factor (factor XIII) has been shown to be 5 ± 3.5 iu/ml at 17 to 24 gestational weeks, against 21 ± 5.6 iu/ml in the adult (Henriksson et al, 1974). It has been suggested that low fibrinogen stabilising factor may afford some safeguard against lasting coagulation damage.

ABNORMAL FETAL PROTEIN METABOLISM

Maternal nutritional deprivation

In the human, maternal undernutrition before the third trimester has no influence on fetal body, organ (brain, thymus, heart, lungs, spleen, liver, adrenals, kidneys) and cellular growth, whereas such effects are pronounced in late gestation. When not too severe, the growth retardation of brain and other organs associated with fetal undernutrition during late gestation is probably reversible with adequate nutrition after birth (Naeye, Blanc and Paul, 1973). It is very difficult to detach effects of maternal undernutrition from the other factors prevailing in the maternal environment that could affect fetal growth and metabolism. It has been suggested that the plasma glycine:valine ratio may serve as an index of subclinical protein malnutrition (low intake of dietary nitrogen) of mother and fetus in the study of the effects of undernutrition on the metabolic situation of the newborn, the adaptation to extra-uterine life and the long-term prognosis for physical and mental development (Lindblad, 1971).

Guinea-pigs born to undernourished mothers show a lower protein content of all organs (Widdowson, 1971). The size of cells and the protein:DNA ratio are less affected than in placental insufficiency, the muscles being more affected than the other tissues. The fetal metabolic response to maternal starvation has been studied in sheep (Simmons et al, 1974). Fetal blood glucose levels stabilise at 15 instead of 25 mg per cent. Urea production seems to double temporarily from the fourth until the seventh day. Transplacental glucose uptake was calculated as 40 per cent of normal during prolonged starvation. All of this indicates a higher rate of amino acid utilisation for energy purposes through the metabolism of amino acids.

The experiments involving temporary starvation during pregnancy of experimental animals have little bearing on the human problem of maternal undernutrition, neither have the studies performed during World War II, which also represent short-term maternal undernutrition. The problem of developing countries is characterised by long-term *prematernal* and maternal undernutrition. An ingenious multigenerational rat model has been used by Stewart, Preece and Sheppard (1975) in order to simulate multigenerational undernutrition and its effect on growth and development.

Knowledge about the effects of more specific nutritional deficiencies on fetal metabolism is limited. At the end of gestation riboflavin deficiency delays the appearance of rapid isoenzymes of alkaline phosphatase in the whole fetus and of LDH in the fetal kidneys, suggesting a similar delay in the course of metabolic differentiation of the skeleton and of kidney tissue. Placental alkaline phosphatase activity is greatly reduced, suggesting the participation of the enzyme in the general hypotrophy of the fetus by a decrease in nutrients carried by the placenta (Potier de Courcy et al, 1974).

Placental insufficiency

A study of runt pigs who show stunted growth in utero because of a bad position and placental insufficiency has shown low protein content partly because they are small and partly because they have a low concentration of protein as compared to normal term pigs (Widdowson, 1971). There is a higher content of protein than in fetuses of a similar weight, indicating that the so-called small-for-gestational-age pig is more mature than the fetus of the same size. Protein concentration was lower, however, than in normal term pigs, indicating a delayed development. The decrease in protein was not evenly distributed among the different organs. Muscle was more affected than the kidneys, which were more affected than the brain. Muscles of such small for gestational age pigs showed even less protein than muscles of fetuses with the same weight.

In analogy with the decreased liver protein synthesis due to lower quality and concentration of ribosomes in liver seen during postnatal protein undernutrition, the rate of incorporation of labelled thymidine into DNA/mg wet weight has been shown to be lower in intra-uterine growth-retarded rats (Roux, 1971a) produced through experimental uterine artery clamping (Wigglesworth, 1964). Incorporation was lower in liver, heart and lung, but not significantly lower in the cerebrum. The decline seems to be related to the age-dependent proportion of cells involved in the proliferation in each organ. In view of the differences seen in the proliferation phases of the different organs of different species these results arrived at through the study of experimental animals must be interpreted with great caution.

Prenatal metabolic adaptation

In hypertensive disorders during pregnancy associated with fetal growth retardation, the ratio between the cord plasma level and the mother's cubital vein plasma levels of essential amino acids is lower than under normal conditions (Lindblad, 1971). It has been suggested that the findings have some bearing on the growth retardation, being the consequence of a diminished supply of essential amino acids to the fetus. The metabolic situation of the small-for-dates newborn infant who has suffered from intra-uterine undernutrition might be more complex than that of mere substrate depletion, due to the unknown metabolic adaptation of the fetus to low nutrient supply.

There is a 'resistance to decline' of branched-chain amino acid levels in plasma during the immediate postnatal period of newborn growth-retarded infants of mothers with hypertension and of mothers from a very low socioeconomic group (Lindblad, 1971). A catabolism of labile protein cannot explain this finding, as the phenylalanine, tyrosine and urea concentrations of plasma were not increased during this period. The observation therefore suggests that there is, in these growth-retarded fetuses at birth, a decreased transport or utilisation of branched-chain amino acids. A temporary increase of branched-chain plasma amino acid concentrations is seen in starvation of adults (Adibi, 1968; Felig et al, 1969).

If there is in these newborn small-for-dates infants, a metabolic adaptation comparable to that of starvation (Lindblad, 1972), then the increased level of plasma alanine during the first hours of life (Lindblad, 1971) indicates an inhibited amino acid uptake or utilisation, rather than a decreased peripheral release of amino acids. As alanine is the main gluconeogenic precursor, the question arises if the small-for-dates baby with growth retardation before birth has an impaired gluconeogenic capacity. There are indications that newborn small-for-dates babies do not respond by enhanced hepatic glucose output upon intravenous or oral alanine feeding (Williams et al, 1975).

Normally, insulin levels are high in the fetus towards the end of gestation. Birth provokes a dramatic drop in the insulin : glucagon ratio in less than one hour (Girard et al, 1973). This may explain the normal rapid decrease of plasma amino acids seen immediately after birth in man (Lindblad, 1971). The early postnatal intensification of hepatic accumulation of amino acids, as described by Christensen and Clifford (1963), could also be explained by the perinatal decrease in the insulin : glucagon ratio.

Reisner et al (1973) have shown an unresponsiveness of blood glucose and plasma amino acids to glucagon in small-for-gestational-age newborn babies. This could explain the relative hyperalaninaemia seen immediately neonatally in small-for-gestational-age infants of mothers with pregnancy toxaemia and in newborn infants from a very low socioeconomic group (Lindblad, 1971). It remains to be seen if the mechanism behind the unresponsiveness of plasma amino acids to glucagon neonatally in the small-for-gestational-age newborn is due to low gluconeogenic enzyme system activity (alanine-2-oxoglutarate aminotransferase) during late fetal and early postnatal life, leading to the low plasma glucose levels indicated above and the, perhaps permanent, tendency to hypoglycaemia during postnatal life. If this is so, it would constitute an example of how the fetal environment could, through an extragenetic mechanism, permanently change the pattern of intermediate metabolism, or prove the existence of true 'metabolic imprinting' during early life.

SUMMARY

The teleological approach has lately led to some valuable hypotheses in the field of enzymatic development. New metabolic potentialities should 'make sense' (Greengard, 1971) in terms of the special physiological needs of the developing animal faced with an altered environment. The existence of an inhibitory embryonic environment should be considered. The deficiency of enzymatic activity in late fetal life could be a meaningful adaptation to intrauterine conditions, not an indication of biochemical immaturity. An example of this, described earlier in this chapter, could be the lack of cystathionase activity in human fetal liver (Gaull, 1973; Sturman and Gaull, 1974), or the low activity of ornithine aminotransferase and ornithine transcarbamylase as an adaptive inhibition that saves ornithine and arginine for protein synthesis during active growth (Räihä and Kekomäki, 1970).

The perinatal period of rapidly altering metabolism offers a useful model to test theories of metabolic control that may be fundamentally significant. At present, the dual control of hormones and starvation at birth is being given considerable attention. Does birth, through the relief of a repressive factor in the intra-uterine environment, trigger the enhanced activity of tryptophan oxygenase, tyrosine aminotransferase and argininosuccinate synthetase of newborn rats (Stawe, 1970)? Substrate evidently does not enhance activity until the enzyme protein appears. Adrenocortical hormones do not exhibit the same stimulating effects as seen in adult animals, while glucagon via liver cyclic AMP as a critical effector has a decisive influence on prenatal induction and regulation. It may be that some enzymes are induced by the birth process, while others are induced more directly by a 'clock control' (Greengard, 1971) and, after this, stimulated by hormonal effectors.

A substantial amount of experimental work has to be done to quantify the enzymatic activities in different organs as a function of age. It seems that enzymes are induced in 'clusters' (Greengard, 1971) as a spasmodic, stepwise process. This indicates that one stimulus may have several effects in many different metabolic pathways. Furthermore, little is known as to whether artificial enhancement of prenatal enzyme formation is still evident at birth and if hormones act in development at single, critical times effecting irreversible changes. These questions have to be answered before we can hope to produce precociously developed enzyme patterns for the therapy of perinatal disease and prematurity (Trolle, 1968; Greengard, 1971) like glucocorticoid treatment for the prevention of the respiratory distress syndrome of premature infants (Liggins and Howie, 1972). The great differences between enzymatic activity assays prenatally in vitro and in vivo stress the importance of in vivo experiments to establish firmer links between morphology, function and enzymatic activity. In view of the well established interspecies differences in enzymic differentiation (TAT—Sereni and Principi, 1965; Table 5.2; OKT—Kekomäki, Räihä and Bickel, 1969; cystathionase—Gaull et al, 1972; phenylalanine hydroxylase—Räihä, 1973), experimentation on human fetal tissues is necessary.

We must define normality before we can distinguish between delayed maturation and genetic anomalies. We would like to know if, analogous to early growth retardation, there are 'critical periods of development' when a fetal environmental factor may irrevocably change the biochemical development; gluconeogenesis from alanine has been dealt with here as a possible example of such a prenatal disadaptation.

True genetically determined errors of amino acid metabolism could, through nutritional mechanisms, cause the prenatal damage to the CNS which has been observed. There may be a genetic inability to supplement or 'justify' (Bessman, 1972) the amino acid environment of the brain. Deficiencies of the urea cycle could lead to arginine deficiency, and phenylketonuria to tyrosine deficiency in the growing brain. Could nonspecific mental retardation, especially in areas with widespread additional nutritional deficiency of the mothers, be explained by deficient synthesis of amino acids in heterozygous stages of genetic enzyme deficiencies?

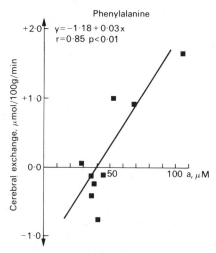

Figure 5.2. Cerebral exchange of phenylalanine (as measured by the difference between the arterial plasma level and the level of plasma collected simultaneously in the bulb of the internal jugular vein, multiplied by cerebral blood flow) in infants under general anaesthesia, and its correlation to the arterial plasma level. From Settergren, Lindblad and Persson (1976) with kind permission of the authors and the editor of *Acta Paediatrica Scandinavica*.

Statistical support for this hypothesis has been provided by Bessman (1972). What is the role of the amino acid synthesising systems in compensating for an abnormal maternal supply? Should arginine, tyrosine and perhaps cysteine (where all fetuses have low capacity for compensating deficiency) be supplemented to mothers in high-risk areas? A closely related problem which needs exploration in low socioeconomic groups is the relationship between intra-uterine infections, fetal nutrition and biochemical development.

The normal rates of fetal protein synthesis have to be established before we can provide indications for fetal and neonatal requirements (Lindblad, 1974). This is particularly urgent in view of the increasing practice of total intravenous feeding of newborn infants and premature babies, including the administration of amino acid solutions directly into the veins. This therapy in itself may provide an opportunity to correlate the knowledge of enzymatic immaturity derived from animal experiments with human conditions (Lindblad et al, 1976) (Figure 5.1). Even term infants may show disturbed plasma homeostasis of amino acids during total parenteral nutrition (Stegink and Baker, 1971; Das and Filler, 1973; Pildes et al, 1973). A phe/tyr ratio of 5:2 in plasma, instead of near unity as normal, has been reported to occur (Stegink and Baker, 1971). The metabolic immaturity of newborn infants, or the as yet largely unknown adaptation to an abnormal intra-uterine environment, may lead to increased arterial levels of several amino acids. This should be avoided, in view of the known effects on the CNS of amino acid imbalance during the perinatal period (Wong and Justice, 1972) and the fact that brain exchange is directly correlated with the arterial levels of amino acids in human infants (Settergren, Lindblad and Persson, 1976) (Figure 5.2). The brain uptake of amino acid in fetal sheep near term (2.02 ± 0.79 mg/100 g/min) is known to be correlated to the arterial level of the particular amino acid and not to the blood flow (Mann, 1970). In general, increases in blood levels cause a greater increase in immature brains (Lajtha and Piccoli, 1971). The safe administration of total parenteral nutrition to newborn immature babies requires further investigation of enzymatic maturity, with careful studies of amino acid tolerance at birth.

REFERENCES

Adamson, Y. R. & Bowden, D. H. (1975) Reaction of cultured adult and fetal lung to prednisolone and thyroxine. *Archives of Pathology*, **99**, 80–85.

Adibi, S. A. (1968) Influence of dietary deprivations on plasma concentration of free amino acids of man. *Journal of Applied Physiology*, **25**, 52–57.

Agrawal, H. C., Davis, J. M. & Hinwich, W. A. (1967) Postnatal changes in free amino acid pool of rabbit brain. *Brain Research*, **3**, 374–380.

Baintner, K. Jr (1973) Possible protein-absorptive ability in human fetuses. *Gastroenterology*, **65**, 695–696.

Barnabei, O. & Sereni, F. (1964) Cortisol induced increase of tyrosine-alpha-ketoglutarate transaminase in the isolated perfused rat liver and its relation to ribonucleic acid synthesis. *Biochimica et Biophysica Acta*, **91**, 239–247.

Bergstrand, C. G. & Czar, B. (1956) Demonstration of a new protein in serum from the human fetus. *Scandinavian Journal of Clinical and Laboratory Investigation*, **8**, 174.

Bessman, S. P. (1972) Genetic failure of fetal amino acid 'justification'. A common basis for many forms of metabolic, nutritional, and 'unspecific' mental retardation. *Journal of Pediatrics*, **81**, 834–842.

Bickel, H. & Souchon, F. (1955) Die Papierchromatographie in der Kinderheilkunde. *Archiv für Kinderheilkunde*, Supplement **31**, 1–151.

Cartwright, E. C., Connellan, J. M. & Dawks, D. M. (1973) Some properties of phenylalanine hydroxylase in human fetal liver. *Australian Journal of Experimental Biology and Medical Science*, **51**, 559–563.

Chapeville, F. & Fromageot, P. (1957) Formation de sulfite d'acide cystéique et de taurine à partir de sulfate par l'œuf embryonné. *Biochimica et Biophysica Acta*, **26**, 538–558.

Christensen, H. N. & Clifford, J. B. (1963) Early postnatal intensification of hepatic accumulation of amino acids. *Journal of Biological Chemistry*, **238**, 1743–1745.

Dancis, J. & Schafran, M. (1958) The origin of plasma proteins in the guinea pig fetus. *Journal of Clinical Investigation*, **37**, 1093–1099.

Dancis, J., Braverman, N. & Lind, J. (1957) Plasma protein synthesis in the human fetus and placenta. *Journal of Clinical Investigation*, **36**, 398–404.

Das, J. B. & Filler, R. M. (1973) Amino acid utilization during total parenteral nutrition in the surgical neonate. *Journal of Pediatric Surgery*, **8**, 793–799.

Dawkins, M. J. R. (1966) Biochemical aspects of developing function in newborn mammalian liver. *British Medical Bulletin*, **22**, 27–33.

Dickerson, J. W. T. & Widdowson, E. M. (1960) Clinical changes in skeletal muscle during development. *Biochemical Journal*, **74**, 247–257.

Doran, T. A., Benzie, R. J., Harkins, J. L., Owen, V. M. J., Porter, C. J., Thompson, D. W. & Liedgren, S. F. (1974) Amniotic fluid tests for fetal maturity. *American Journal of Obstetrics and Gynecology*, **119**, 829–837.

Edelman, C. M., Barnett, H. L. & Troupkan, V. (1960) Renal concentrating mechanism in newborn infants. *Journal of Clinical Investigation*, **39**, 1062.

Eiduson, S. (1971) Biogenic amines in the developing brain. *UCLA Forum in Medical Sciences*, **14**, 391–418.

Felig, P., Owen, O. E., Wahren, J. & Cahill, G. F. Jr (1969) Amino acid metabolism during prolonged starvation. *Journal of Clinical Investigation*, **48**, 584–594.

Fine, J. M., Imperato, C., Battistini, A. & Moretti, J. (1961) Immunological study of haptoglobins. Demonstration in cord blood of an incomplete form of haptoglobin. *Nouvelle Revue Francaise d'Hematologie*, **1**, 72–80.

Gan, J. C. & Jeffay, H. (1967) Origins and metabolism of the intracellular amino acid pools in rat liver and muscle. *Biochimica et Biophysica Acta*, **148**, 448–459.

Gaull, G. E. (1973) Sulphur amino acids, folate and DNA: metabolic inter-relationships during foetal development. In *Foetal and Neonatal Physiology* (Ed.) Comline, K. S., Cross, K. W., Dawes, G. S. & Nathanielsz, P. W. Cambridge: Cambridge University Press.

Gaull, G., Sturman, J. A. & Räihä, N. C. R. (1972) Development of mammalian sulfur metabolism: Absence of cystathionase in human fetal tissues. *Pediatric Research*, **6**, 538–547.

Gaull, G. E., von Berg, W., Räihä, N. C. R. & Sturman, J. A. (1973) Development of methyl-transferase activities of human fetal tissue. *Pediatric Research*, **7**, 527–533.

Gerbie, A. B., Melancon, S. B., Ryan, C. & Nadler, H. L. (1972) Cultivated epithelial-like cells and fibroblasts from amniotic fluid: their relationship to enzymatic and cytologic analysis. *American Journal of Obstetrics and Gynecology*, **114**, 314–320.

Girard, J. R., Cuendet, G. S., Marliss, E. B., Kervran, A., Rientort, M. & Assan, R. (1973) Fuels, hormones and liver metabolism at term and during the early postnatal period in the rat. *Journal of Clinical Investigation*, **52**, 3190–3200.

Gitlin, D. & Biasucci, A. (1969) Development of γG, γA, γM, β1C/β1A, C′1 esterase inhibitor, ceruloplasmin, transferrin, hemopexin, haptoglobin, fibrinogen, plasminogen, α_1-antitrypsin, orosomucoid, β-lipoprotein, α_2-macroglobulin, and prealbumin in the human conceptus. *American Journal of Clinical Investigation*, **48**, 1433–1446.

Gitlin, D., Perricelli, A. & Gitlin, G. M. (1972) Synthesis of α-foetoprotein by liver, yolk sac, and gastrointestinal tract of the human conceptus. *Cancer Research*, **32**, 979–982.

Gitlin, D., Kumate, J., Morales, C., Noriegan, L. & Arevalo, N. (1972) The turnover of amniotic fluid protein in the human conceptus. *American Journal of Obstetrics and Gynecology*, **113**, 632–645.

Gordon, H. H. & Marples, E. (1941) A defect in the metabolism of tyrosine and phenylalanine in premature infants. *Journal of Clinical Investigation*, **20**, 199–219.

Greengard, O. (1969) The hormonal regulation of enzymes in prenatal and postnatal rat liver. Effects of adenosyl-3′-5′-(cyclic)-monophosphate. *Biochemical Journal*, **115**, 19–25.

Greengard, O. (1971) The prematurely evoked synthesis of liver tryptophan oxygenase. *Proceedings of the National Academy of Sciences*, **68**, 1698–1701.

Greengard, O. & Dewey, H. K. (1967) Initiation by glucagon of the premature development of tyrosine aminotransferase, serine dehydratase and glucose-6-phosphatase in fetal liver. *Journal of Biological Chemistry*, **242**, 2986–2991.

Gresham, E. L., James, E. J., Raye, J. R., Battaglia, F. C., Makowski, E. L. & Meschia, G. (1972) Production and excretion of urea by the fetal lamb. *Pediatrics*, **50**, 372–379.

Henriksson, P., Hedner, U., Nilsson, I. M., Boehm, J., Robertson, B. & Lorand, L. (1974) Fibrin-stabilizing factor (Factor XIII) in the fetus and the newborn infant. *Pediatric Research*, **8**, 789–791.

Hirschfeld, J. & Lunell, N. O. (1962) Serum protein synthesis in foetus: haptoglobins and group specific components. *Nature*, **196**, 1220.

Jakubovic, A. (1971) Phenylalanine hydroxylating system in the human fetus at different developmental ages. *Biochimica et Biophysica Acta*, **237**, 469–475.

Johnson, T. C. (1968) Cell free protein synthesis by mouse brain during early development. *Journal of Neurochemistry*, **15**, 1189–1194.

Kaback, M. M., Leonard, C. O. & Parmley, T. H. (1971) Intrauterine diagnosis: comparative enzymology of cells cultivated from maternal skin, fetal skin, and amniotic fluid cells. *Pediatric Research*, **5**, 366–371.

Kapeller-Adler, R. & Hammad, W. A. (1972) A biochemical study on nucleic acids and protein synthesis in the human fetus and its correlation with relevant embryologic data. *Journal of Obstetrics and Gynaecology of the British Commonwealth*, **79**, 924–930.

Kaufman, S. (1971) The phenylalanine hydroxylating system from mammalian liver. *Advances in Enzymology and Related Subjects of Biochemistry*, **35**, 245–319.

Kekomäki, M. P., Räihä, N. C. R. & Bickel, H. (1969) Ornithine-ketoacid aminotransferase in human liver with reference to patients with hyperornithinemia and familial protein intolerance. *Clinica Chimica Acta*, **23**, 203–208.

Kekomäki, M., Seppälä, M. & Schwartz, A. L. (1971) Synthesis and release of plasma proteins by isolated perfused human fetal liver. *Pediatric Research*, **5**, 86.

Kekomäki, M., Seppälä, M., Elmholm, C., Schwartz, A. L. & Raivo, K. (1971) Perfusion of isolated human fetal liver: synthesis and release of α-fetoprotein and albumin. *International Journal of Cancer*, **8**, 150–258.

Koga, K. & Tamaoki, T. (1974) Developmental changes in the synthesis of α-fetoprotein and albumin in the mouse liver. Cell free synthesis by membrane-bound polyribosomes. *Biochemistry*, **13**, 3024–3028.

Koldovsky, O. (1970) Digestion and absorption during development In *Physiology of the Perinatal Period* (Ed.) Stawe, H. Vol. 1, pp. 379–415. New York: Appleton-Century-Crofts.

Koldovsky, O., Heringová, A., Jirsová, V., Kraml, J., Pelichová, H. & Uher, J. (1968) Development of enzymes and absorption processes in the small intestine of human fetus. In *Aspects of Prematurity and Dysmaturity* (Ed.) Jonxis, J. H. P., Visser, H. K. A. & Troelstra, J. A. Leiden: H. E. S. Stenfert Kroese N.V.

Koszalka, T. R., Jensh, R. & Brent, R. L. (1972) Creatinine metabolism in the developing rat fetus. *Comparative Biochemistry and Physiology, B: Comparative Biochemistry*, **41**, 217–229.

Krasilnikoff, P. A. (1967) The metabolism of albumin in normal and premature children. *Acta Paediatrica Scandinavica*, Supplement **177**, 33.

Kretchmer, N. & Greenberg, R. E. (1966) Some physiologic and biochemical determinants of development. *Advances in Paediatrics*, **14**, 201–251.

Kretchmer, N., Hurwitz, R. & Räihä, N. (1966) Some aspects of urea and pyrimidine metabolism during development. *Biology of the Neonate*, **9**, 187–196.

Kretchmer, N., Levine, S. Z., McNamara, H. & Barnett, H. L. (1956) Certain aspects of tyrosine metabolism in the young. I. The development of the tyrosine oxidizing system in human liver. *Journal of Clinical Investigation*, **35**, 236–244.

Lajtha, A. & Piccoli, F. (1971) Alterations related to the cerebral free amino acid pool during development. *UCLA Forum in Medical Sciences*, **14**, 419–446.

Larkin, L. H. & Stevens, A. R. (1972) Foetal and maternal RNA Labelled with ³H-cytidine. *Nature, New Biology*, **235**, 107–108.

Lev, R. & Orlie, D. (1972) Protein absorption by the intestine of the fetal rat in utero. *Science*, **177**, 552–523.

Levy, H. L., Shih, V. E., Madigan, P. M., Karolkewicz, V., Carr, J. R., Lum, A., Richards, A. A., Crawford, J. D. & MacCready, R. A. (1969) Hypermethioninemia with other hyperaminoacidemias; studies in infants on high protein diets. *American Journal of Diseases of Children*, **117**, 96–103.

Lichtenstein, A. (1931) Untersuchungen am Nabelschnurblut bei frühgeborenen und ausgetragenen Kindern mit besondere Berücksichtigung der Aminosäuren. *Zeitschrift für Kinderheilkunde*, **51**, 748–754.

Liggins, G. C. & Howie, R. N. (1972) A controlled trial of antepartum glucocorticoid treatment for prevention of the respiratory distress syndrome in premature infants. *Pediatrics*, **50**, 515–525.

Lind, T. (1971) Prenatal assessment of gestational age. In *Proceedings of the Second European Congress of Perinatal Medicine* (Ed.) Huntingford, P. J., Beard, R. W., Hytten, F. E. & Scopes, J. W. pp. 191–197. Basel: Karger.

Lindberg, T. (1966) Intestinal dipeptidases: characterization, development and distribution of intestinal dipeptidases of the human fetus. *Clinical Science*, **30**, 505–515.

Lindblad, B. S. (1971) The plasma aminogram in 'small for dates' newborn infants. In *Metabolic Processes in the Newborn Infant* (Ed.) Jonxis, J. H. P., Visser, H. K. A. & Troelstra, J. A. pp. 111–126. Leiden: H. E. Stenfert Kroese NV.

Lindblad, B. S. (1972) The short and light for dates newborn—an adaptation to prenatal protein–calorie undernutrition? *Pakistan Paediatric Journal*, **2**, 17–21.

Lindblad, B. S. (1974) Protein and amino acid metabolism and requirements in the neonatal period. *Acta Anaesthesiologica*, Supplement, **55**, 102–106.

Lindblad, B. S., Feychting, H., Persson, B. & Settergren, G. (1976) The blood levels of glucose, ketone bodies, lactate, pyruvate, free fatty acids, glycerol, triglycerides, amino acids and insulin during total parenteral nutrition of infants. Unpublished manuscript.

Lines, D. R. & Waisman, H. A. (1971) Placental transport of phenylalanine in the rat: maternal and fetal metabolism. *Proceedings of the Society for Experimental Biology and Medicine*, **136**, 790–793.

Machlin, L. J., Pearson, P. B. & Denton, C. A. (1955) The utilization of sulphate sulphur for the synthesis of taurine in the developing chick embryo. *Journal of Biological Chemistry*, **212**, 469–475.

Mann, L. I. (1970) Fetal brain metabolism and function. *Clinical Obstetrics and Gynecology*, **13**, 638–651.

Marks, N., Stern, F. & Lajtha, A. (1975) Changes in proteolytic enzymes and proteins during maturation of the brain. *Brain Research*, **86**, 307–322.

Mathews, J. & Partington, M. W. (1964) The plasma tyrosine levels of premature babies. *Archives of Disease in Childhood*, **39**, 371–378.

McCance, R. A. & Strangeways, W. M. B. (1954) Protein catabolism and oxygen consumption during starvation in infants, young adults and old men. *British Journal of Nutrition*, **8**, 21–32.

McLean, A., Marwick, M. J. & Clayton, B. E. (1973) Enzymes involved in phenylalanine metabolism in the human foetus and child. *Journal of Clinical Pathology*, **26**, 678–683.

Miller, S. A. (1969) Protein metabolism during growth and development. In *Mammalian Protein Metabolism* (Ed.) Munro, H. N. New York: Academic Press.

Monder, C. & Coufalic, A. (1975) Activities of tyrosine, alanine and aspartate aminotransferases of fetal rat liver in organ culture. *Enzyme*, **20**, 111–116.

Mori, M. & Iso, H. (1965) Study of protein biosynthesis in fetus and placenta II. Transfer of ^{35}S-methionine across the placenta and mechanism of protein biosynthesis in the fetus. *American Journal of Obstetrics and Gynecology*, **93**, 1172–1180.

Mukherjee, A. B., Hastings, C. & Cohen, M. M. (1973) Nucleic acid synthesis in various organs of developing human fetuses. *Pediatric Research*, **7**, 696–699.

Naeye, R. L., Blanc, W. & Paul, C. (1973) Effects of maternal nutrition on the human fetus. *Pediatrics*, **52**, 494–503.

Needham, J. (1931) *Chemical Embryology*. Cambridge: Cambridge University Press.

Nemeth, A. M. (1963) Biochemical events underlying the development and adaptive increase in tryptophan pyrrolase activity. In *Advances in Enzyme Regulation* (Ed.) Weber, G. Vol. I, pp. 57–60. New York: Pergamon Press.

Pascal, T. A., Gillam, B. M. & Gaull, G. E. (1972) Cystathionase: immunochemical evidence for absence from human fetal liver. *Pediatric Research*, **6**, 773–778.

Pildes, R. S., Ramamurthy, R. S., Cordero, G. V. & Wong, P. W. K. (1973) Intravenous supplementation of L-amino acids and dextrose in low-birth-weight infants. *Journal of Pediatrics*, **82**, 945–950.

Porter, P. N., Grishaver, M. S. & Jones, O. W. (1974) Characterization of human cystathionine β-synthase; evidence for the identity of human L-serine dehydratase and cystathionine β-synthase. *Biochimica et Biophysica Acta*, **364**, 128–139.

Potier de Courcy, G., Desmettre-Miguet, S., Macquart-Moulin, M. R. & Terroine, T. (1974) Enzymic changes of foetal and placental tissues of the rat in teratogenic riboflavin deficiency. *Journal of Embryology and Experimental Morphology*, **31**, 183–198.

Przyrenbel, H. & Bremer, H. J. (1972) Cystathionine in premature infants. *Clinica Chimica Acta*, **41**, 95–99.

Räihä, N. C. R. (1971) The development of some enzymes of amino acid metabolism in the human liver. In *Metabolic Processes in the Foetus and Newborn Infant* (Ed.) Jonxis, J. H. P., Visser, H. K. A. & Troelstra, H. E. pp. 26–34. Leiden: H. E. Stenfert Kroese N.V.

Räihä, N. C. R. (1973) Phenylalanine hydroxylase in human liver during development. *Pediatric Research*, **7**, 1–4.

Räihä, N. C. R. (1974) Biochemistry and nutrition of preterm infants. *Pediatrics*, **53**, 147–156.

Räihä, N. C. R. & Kekomäki, M. P. (1970) Factors involved in the development of ornithine-ketoacid aminotransferase activity in mammalian liver. In *Stoffwechsel des Neugeborenen* (Ed.) Jopping, G. & Wolf, H. Stuttgart: Hippokrates.

Räihä, N. C. R. & Kekomäki, M. (1975) Developmental aspects of amino acid metabolism in the human. In *Total Parenteral Nutrition; Premises and Promises* (Ed.) Ghadimi, H. pp. 199–211. New York: John Wiley.

Räihä, N. C. R. & Suihkonen, J. (1968) Development of urea-synthesizing enzymes in human liver. *Acta Paediatrica Scandinavica*, **57**, 121–124.

Räihä, N. C. R., Schwartz, A. L. & Lindroos, M. C. (1971) Induction of tyrosine-α-ketoglutarate transaminase in fetal rat and fetal human liver in organ culture. *Pediatric Research*, **5**, 70–76.

Reisner, S. H., Aranda, J. V., Colle, E., Papageorgiou, A., Schiff, D., Seriver, C. R. & Stern, L. (1973) The effect of intravenous glucagon on plasma amino acids in the newborn. *Pediatric Research*, **7**, 184–191.

Rose, W. C. & Wixom, R. L. (1955) The amino acid requirements of man. XII. The sparing effect of cystine on the methionine requirement. *Journal of Biological Chemistry*, **216**, 763–773.

Roux, J. M. (1971a) Decrease in the rate of the DNA synthesis in newborn rats with intrauterine growth retardation. *Biology of the Neonate*, **18**, 463–467.

Roux, J. M. (1971b) Nucleotide supply of the developing animal: role of the so called 'salvage pathway'. *Enzyme*, **15**, 361–377.

Rubino, A. (1975) Absorption of amino acids and peptides during development. In *Milk and Lactation. Modern Problems in Paediatrics* (Ed.) Kretchmer, N., Rossi, E. & Sereni, F. Basel: S. Karger.

Rutter, W. J. (1969) Independently regulated synthetic transitions in foetal tissues. In *Foetal Autonomy* (Ed.) Wolstenholme, G. E. W. & O'Connor, M. London: J. & A. Churchill.

Ryan, W. L. & Carver, M. J. (1966) Free amino acids of human foetal and adult liver. *Nature,* 212, 292–293.

Ryan, W. L. & Orr, W. (1966) Phenylalanine conversion to tyrosine by the human fetal liver. *Archives of Biochemistry and Biophysics,* 113, 684–685.

Schain, R. J., Carver, M. J., Copenhaver, J. H. & Underdahl, N. R. (1967) Protein metabolism in the developing brain: influence of birth and gestational age. *Science,* 156, 984–985.

Schimke, R. T. (1962) Adaptive characteristics of urea cycle enzymes in the rat. *Journal of Biological Chemistry,* 237, 459–468.

Schuit, K. E. & Dickie, M. W. (1973) Induction of enzyme activity during fetal development. The appearance of ornithine transcarbamylase activity in rat liver. *Biology of the Neonate,* 23, 171–179.

Sereni, F. & Luppis, B. (1968) Developmental changes in liver enzyme activities with special reference to the perinatal period of life. In *Aspects of Prematurity and Dysmaturity* (Ed.) Jonxis, J. H. P., Visser, H. K. A. & Troelstra, J. A. Leiden: H. E. Stenfert Kroese N.V.

Sereni, F. & Principi, N. (1965) The development of enzyme systems. *Pediatric Clinics of North America,* 12, 515–534.

Sereni, F. & Sereni, L. P. (1969) Spontaneous development of tyrosine aminotransferase in fetal liver cultures. *Advances in Enzyme Regulation,* 8, 253–267.

Sereni, F. & Sereni, L. P. (1971) Factors controlling biochemical development of foetal and newborn liver. In *Metabolic Processes in the Foetus and Newborn Infant* (Ed.) Jonxis, J. H. P., Visser, H. K. A. & Troelstra, J. A. pp. 40–50. Leiden: H. E. Stenfert Kroese N.V.

Sereni, F., Kenney, F. T. & Kretchmer, N. (1959) Factors influencing the development of tyrosine-β-ketoglutarate transaminase activity in rat liver. *Journal of Biological Chemistry,* 234, 609–612.

Settergren, G., Lindblad, B. S. & Persson, B. (1976) Cerebral blood flow and exchange of oxygen, glucose, ketone bodies, lactate, pyruvate and amino acids in infants. *Acta Paediatrica Scandinavica,* in press.

Simmons, M. A., Meschia, G., Makowski, E. L. & Battaglia, F. C. (1974) Fetal metabolic response to maternal starvation. *Pediatric Research,* 8, 830–836.

Singer, E. J., Hochstrasser, H. & Cerecedi, C. R. (1956) The tryptophan, leucine, and lysine content of the chick and mouse embryo during development. *Growth,* 20, 229–241.

Snyderman, S. E. (1970) Protein and amino acid metabolism. In *Physiology of the Perinatal Period* (Ed.) Stawe, H. Vol. I, pp. 441–456. New York: Appleton-Century-Crofts.

Snyderman, S. E., Boyer, A. & Holt, L. E. Jr (1959) The arginine requirement of the infant. *American Journal of Diseases of Children,* 97, 192–195.

Snyderman, S. E., Prose, P. H. & Holt, L. E. Jr (1959) Histidine, an essential amino acid for the infant. *American Journal of Diseases of Children,* 98, 459–460.

Southgate, D. A. T. (1971) The accumulation of amino acids in the products of conception of the rat and in the young animals after birth. *Biology of the Neonate,* 19, 272–292.

Stave, U. & Armstrong, M. D. (1973) Tissue free amino acid concentrations in perinatal rabbits. *Biology of the Neonate,* 22, 374–387.

Stawe, U. (1970) Enzyme development in the liver. In *Physiology of the Perinatal Period* (Ed.) Stawe, U. pp. 559–594. New York: Appleton-Century-Crofts.

Stegink, L. D. & Baker, G. L. (1971) Infusion of protein hydrolysates in the newborn infant: plasma amino acid concentrations. *Journal of Pediatrics,* 78, 595–602.

Stewart, R. J. C., Preece, R. F. & Sheppard, H. G. (1975) Twelve generations of marginal protein deficiency. *British Journal of Nutrition,* 33, 233–253.

Sturman, J. A. & Gaull, G. E. (1974) Polyamine biosynthesis in human fetal liver and brain. *Pediatric Research,* 8, 231–237.

Sturman, J. A. & Gaull, G. E. (1975) Taurine in the brain and liver of the developing human and monkey. *Journal of Neurochemistry,* in press.

Sugawa, T., Nakamura, K. & Ozaki, M. (1963) Studies on the amino acid and protein metabolism in fetal growth. III. Dynamics of free amino acids in the amniotic fluid and its nutritive role in the fetus. *Journal of the Japanese Obstetrical and Gynecological Society,* 10, 1–7.

Trolle, D. (1968) Phenobarbitone and neonatal icterus. *Lancet,* i, 251–252.

Unsworth, B. R. (1975) Rhodanese activity during the embryonic development of mouse liver and kidney. *Enzyme,* 20, 138–150.

Waisman, H. A. & Kerr, G. R. (1965) Amino acid and protein metabolism in the developing fetus and the newborn infant. *Pediatric Clinics of North America,* 12, 551–572.

Weber, R. (1965) *The Biochemistry of Animal Development,* Vol. I. *Descriptive Biochemistry of Animal Development.* New York: Academic Press.

Wicks, W. D. (1968) Induction of tyrosine α-ketoglutarate transaminase in fetal rat liver. *Journal of Biological Chemistry,* 243, 900–906.

Wicks, W. D. (1969) Induction of hepatic enzymes by adenosine 3′, 5′-monophosphate in organ culture. *Journal of Biological Chemistry*, **244**, 3941–3950.

Widdowson, E. M. (1964) Changes in the composition of the body at birth and their bearing on function and food requirements. In *The Adaptation of the Newborn Infant to Extra-uterine Life* (Ed.) Jonxis, H. J. P., Visser, H. K. A. & Troelstra, J. A. pp. 1–13. Leiden: H. E. Stenfert Kroese N.V.

Widdowson, E. M. (1971) Protein states of 'small for date' animals. In *Metabolic Processes in the Foetus and Newborn Infant* (Ed.) Jonxis, J. H. P., Visser, H. K. A. & Troelstra, J. A. pp. 165–174. Leiden: H. E. Stenfert Kroese N.V.

Widdowson, E. M. & Dickerson, J. W. T. (1960) The effect of growth and function on the chemical composition of soft tissues. *Biochemical Journal*, **77**, 30–43.

Wigglesworth, J. S. (1964) Experimental growth retardation in the foetal rat. *Journal of Pathology*, **88**, 1–13.

Williams, P. R., Fiser, R. J. Jr, Sperling, M. A. & Oh, W. (1975) Effects of oral alanine feeding on blood glucose, plasma glucagon and insulin concentrations in small-for-gestational-age infants. *New England Journal of Medicine*, **292**, 612–614.

Wilson, T. H. (1966) The development of vitamin B_{12} and amino acid absorption by the small intestine. *Biology of the Neonate*, **9**, 62–72.

Wong, P. W. K. & Justice, P. (1972) Effect of amino acid imbalance on polyribosome profiles and protein synthesis in fetal cerebral cortex. In *Advances in Experimental Medicine and Biology* (Ed.) Volk, B. W. & Aronson, S. M. pp. 163–174. New York: Plenum.

Zuckerman, H., Herschman, H. & Levine, L. (1970) Appearance of a brain specific antigen (S-100) during human fetal development. *Journal of Neurochemistry*, **17**, 247–251.

6

FETAL FAT METABOLISM

D. Hull

In lipid metabolism, as in many areas of biological enquiry, the fetus with its own complement of systems encapsulated within the mother poses a series of fascinating questions. Does the fetus receive or form its own lipids? Do maternal lipids pass unchanged through the membranes and cells of the placenta? Does placental metabolism influence the lipids available to the fetus? Do the factors which determine cellular uptake of lipids in the mother also determine lipid uptake by placental cells? In turn, does the fetus influence the rate of release of lipids by the placenta into its own circulation? What happens to the lipids in the fetal circulation? Can and does the fetus release lipids into its own blood stream? To these and many other key questions there are few answers.

Until recently the generally held view was that lipids do not cross the placenta in significant amounts and that the fetus synthesises its own. Evidence is accumulating that as a generalisation this is not true, although it may be a fair summary for some lipids under certain conditions.

After some introductory comments on lipids and adipose tissue, information will be discussed relating to:

1. Changes during pregnancy in maternal circulating lipids.
2. Entry of lipids into, and their metabolism by, the placenta.
3. Entry of lipids into the fetal circulation.
4. Uptake, utilisation and release of fatty acids by fetal tissue.

LIPIDS

Lipids are a heterogenous group of compounds with diverse biological roles which have in common a relative insolubility in water. This chapter is concerned primarily with those lipids which provide cellular energy and to a lesser extent with those involved in cellular structure.

Fatty acids are the lipid form metabolised by cells for energy. They are long single chains of carbon atoms of varying chain length and with a varying number of unsaturated bonds between the carbon atoms. At the end of the chain is a carboxyl group. The distribution of the various fatty acids in the free fatty acid compartment of one sample of blood from a woman

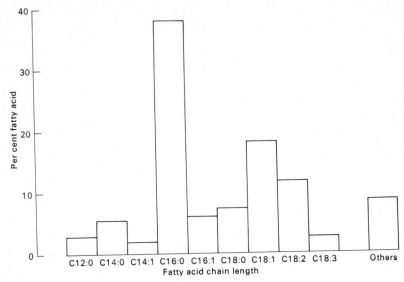

Figure 6.1. The distribution of fatty acids of different chain length with varying numbers of double bonds in the free fatty acid compartment of the plasma of a woman at term.

at term is shown in Figure 6.1. Palmitic acid (C16:0, i.e. 16 carbon atoms with no unsaturated bonds) is the commonest animal fatty acid. Indeed the majority of fatty acids have long chain lengths, with either none or only one unsaturated bond and they can be synthesised in the body from carbohydrate. The exceptions are the 'so-called' essential fatty acids—linoleic, linolenic and arachidonic acid. Since they contain more than one unsaturated bond they are often referred to as polyunsaturated fatty acids.

Excess nutrients, whether carbohydrates or fat, are stored by the body as triglyceride in adipose tissue stores. To form triglyceride, three molecules of fatty acid are esterified with one molecule of glycerol. Many of the structural lipids, the phospholipids and glycolipids, are

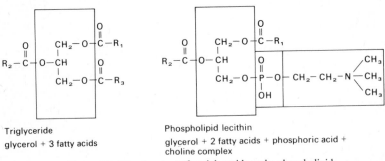

Figure 6.2. The structure of a triglyceride and a phospholipid.

also formed by esterification of glycerol, but in these lipids two fatty acid molecules are joined by a third complex molecule (Figure 6.2). These compounds linked with protein form cell membranes and the envelopes of subcellular structures.

Two important groups of compounds which are usually classed as lipids are steroids and prostaglandins. Both have major effects on body metabolism at very low concentrations, and they are of prime importance in reproductive biology. Their activities are discussed elsewhere (see Chapter 13).

ADIPOSE TISSUE

Adipose tissue is a highly specialised organ of energy storage and supply. It has the capacity to take up circulating plasma triglycerides, whether chylomicron from the bowel or endogenous triglycerides from the liver, and store them. It also converts glucose by lipogenesis to fatty acids. The release of fatty acids by adipose tissue is rapidly and delicately modulated by nervous and endocrine activity according to biological requirements in different physiological states. In the fetus this specialised organ does not develop until late gestation and many mammalian species do not lay down fat until after birth. The human fetus is unusual in that there is a large store of triglycerides in adipose tissue at birth, sufficient to maintain life for some weeks. Thus, the newborn human infant is not so dependent as other mammals on the early establishment of milk feeding.

Although the primary role of adipose tissue is the storage and supply of lipids, it has many secondary roles. Indeed, there may be many 'adipose tissues'. For example, the adipose tissue in the joint or sucking pad is a supporting or space-filling structure and may not release its stored lipid except in extremes of starvation, whereas adipose tissue in the abdominal cavity may be a depository of the lipid the body cannot hold within the actively functioning lipid storage and supply depots. The various distributions of adiposity in different clinical states (compare for example overeating obesity with Cushing's disease or the obesity of cretinism) also suggest that the adipose tissues do not respond in a uniform way. Of particular relevance to the newborn is brown adipose tissue, which has the specific capacity to produce heat to maintain thermal stability (Hull, 1974; Alexander, 1975). After birth the adipose tissue cells of the 'heat organ' appear to fill with fat and the tissue loses its capacity for thermogenesis.

FATTY ACIDS IN THE FETUS

The fetus needs fatty acids for structure, particularly for the rapidly growing brain; for storage, especially over the last third of gestation; and possibly for cellular energy. After birth the newborn infant readily metabolises fatty acids; indeed it must do so to survive. Not only do infants mobilise lipid energy reserves, they also, in milk, receive a mixed supply of nutrients with a high lipid content. The newborn appears to have little difficulty in metabolising fat; on the other hand, the capacity of the fetal tissues to oxidise lipids for cellular energy appears limited.

There are lipids in the fetal circulation, presumably travelling from one tissue to another. The question arises therefore whether the fetus controls its own energy supplies, and if so to what extent? What, for example, is the role of adipose tissue in the fetus? Is it the passive recipient of excess nutrients? Can the fetus be faced with excesses and, if so, under what circumstances? Under usual conditions one would not expect the fetus to be subject to intermittent nutrition or starvation, nor experience excitement, fear or cold or any of the other stimuli which activate the sympathetic nervous system and lead to lipolysis. Nevertheless, are there circumstances in which the fetus might mobilise its reserves?

Adipose tissue develops late in the phylogenetic as well as the ontogenetic scale, for it is found in birds and mammals, both free-roving higher animals. The lower animals store their triglyceride reserves in the liver. This suggests the possibility that in early fetal life the liver might act as a temporary lipid store. The placenta too could hold lipid temporarily to ensure that the fetal cells receive a regular supply of lipid.

LIPIDS IN THE MATERNAL CIRCULATION

To consider which lipids are available to the fetus, it is necessary to examine the lipid compartment in the maternal blood which bathes the placental cells. Lipids, being relatively insoluble in water, do not travel as such in the blood circulation; they are parcelled in a variety of ways with protein (Figure 6.3).

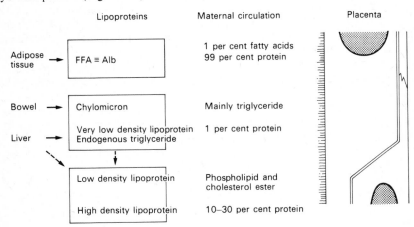

Figure 6.3. Components of lipoprotein in the maternal circulation.

Free fatty acids (FFA), which are carried in the blood bound to albumin, form less than one per cent of the lipid in circulation. Nevertheless, they are the vehicle by which fatty acids are transferred from adipose tissue to other cells. Their turnover is rapid with a half-life of about one minute. As a consequence, circulating concentrations rise and fall rapidly. For this reason single serum values are difficult to interpret. The rate of uptake by peripheral tissues appears to be related directly to perfusing concentrations. When fatty acids are available, glucose utilisation is suppressed. Circulating concentrations tend to indicate changes in lipolysis in adipose tissue.

In pregnancy lipid stores in maternal adipose tissue increase over the first two-thirds of gestation (Hytten and Leitch, 1971; Knopp, Wrath and Carroll, 1973). Towards the end of pregnancy lipolysis in adipose tissue increases and circulating FFA concentrations rise (for references see Robertson, Sprecher and Wilcox, 1968). Pain, fear, trauma, cold and anaesthesia all stimulate sympathetic nervous activity which in turn leads to rapid mobilisation of fatty acids, so it is not surprising to find raised levels during labour. Thus during labour or even during delivery by elective caesarean section the maternal side of the placenta contains blood rich in fatty acid.

Dietary fat travels from the bowel to the liver and peripheral tissues as chylomicron. The lipid is mainly triglyceride with small amounts of cholesterol and phospholipids. Chylomicrons are quickly cleared from the circulation by tissues requiring fat or by adipose tissue. Their uptake and clearance by peripheral tissues depend on the presence of a 'clearing factor', which is a lipoprotein lipase thought to be located in the lining of the peripheral tissue capillaries. The activity of this enzyme in different tissues varies with the biological stage. For example, it is more active in adipose tissue after a meal, in the mammary gland during lactation and in the muscle during exercise. The amount of chylomicron triglyceride in the circulation varies with the diet, and thus any changes in circulating concentrations which may occur during pregnancy will reflect principally changes in food intake.

However, even after a fast, triglyceride encapsulated in envelopes not unlike chylomicron but usually smaller, is found in the blood stream. This fraction is called very low density lipoprotein (VLDL) because of its behaviour on centrifugation, or pre-β-lipoprotein because of its characteristics on protein electrophoresis. This endogenous triglyceride is produced in the main by the liver, though small fractions may be produced by the bowel (Stout, 1973). Increased production follows high circulating FFA concentrations. Endogenous triglyceride is thought to be cleared by peripheral tissues in a similar manner to chylomicron. It is one channel by which lipid produced in the liver may be transferred to adipose tissue for storage.

In pregnancy the level of the fasting triglyceride increases towards term (Svanborg and Vikrot, 1965), but the cause of this increasing lipaemia has not been established. Studies on rats have shown that the rise is related to a fall in the activity of the adipose tissue clearing factor lipase. The activity in the diaphragm, heart and lungs is unchanged. The fall in fasting triglyceride levels after birth was associated with a rise in the clearing factor activity in the mammary gland (Robinson, 1967). The clearing factor activity in the circulation of women induced by heparin injection also decreases towards the end of pregnancy (Fabian et al, 1968). As pregnancy advances, there is increased production of lipolytic agents (e.g. human placental lactogen) and a rise in circulating FFA concentrations. Thus the increased flow of FFA into the liver could lead to an increase in the rate of endogenous triglyceride formation and, together with a fall in activity of tissue clearing factor lipase, explain the rise in fasting triglyceride concentrations in human pregnancy.

There have been a number of reports of women who develop high fasting triglyceride levels during pregnancy and have symptoms not unlike pancreatitis. The infants of these pregnancies have been reported to be normal, but there have been no reports of umbilical cord blood lipid concentrations in these cases. The one placenta studied showed numerous foam cells which were considered to be fat-filled macrophages lodged in the placenta on the maternal side (Nielsen, Jacobsen and Rolschau, 1973).

A larger and more constant serum lipoprotein compartment is formed by the fractions containing the majority of the circulating phospholipids, cholesterol and cholesterol ester. These are linked with apoprotein in various proportions and from their movement on ultracentrifugation may be divided into high density and low density lipoproteins (HDL and LDL). Their triglyceride content is around 10 per cent. The biological role of these fractions is uncertain. Their turnover time is much slower than that of either chylomicrons or FFA. There is some evidence to suggest that they are formed from chylomicron or endogenous triglyceride when the latter have transferred some of their triglyceride into peripheral tissues. The circulating concentrations of both fractions increase during human pregnancy (Knopp,

Wrath and Carrol, 1973), but not in all mammals: for example the cholesterol-containing compartments drop sharply to very low levels towards term in the rabbit. This occurs despite high cholesterol diets (Popjak, 1946; Zilzersmit, Hughes and Remington, 1972; Acebal et al. 1973). In monkeys, although concentrations of FFA and triglyceride may rise in the maternal blood towards term, other circulating lipid concentrations fall (Martin, Wolf and Meyer, 1971).

FATTY ACIDS AND THE PLACENTA

The fatty acid pools within placental cells might receive fatty acids from a number of directions (Figure 6.4).

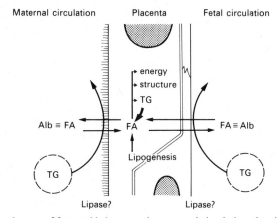

Figure 6.4. Possible exchanges of fatty acids between the maternal circulation, the placental cells and the fetal circulation. FA = fatty acids; TG = triglycerides.

1. They may be transferred from the mother's blood, either directly from the FFA fraction, or by breakdown of chylomicron or VLDL. Injection of labelled fatty acids into the maternal circulation of rats (Hummel et al, 1974), rabbits (Van Duyne, Havel and Felts, 1962; Elphick, Hudson and Hull, 1975), guinea-pigs (Hershfield and Nemeth, 1968; Kayden, Dancis and Money, 1969), sheep (Van Duyne et al, 1960) and monkeys (Portman, Behrman and Soltys, 1969) has demonstrated the rapid transfer of labelled fatty acids across the placenta and into the lipid fractions of the placental cells. Labelled chylomicron studies are more difficult to perform and interpret and the information to date relating to fatty acid uptake from chylomicron by the placenta is inconclusive (Hummel et al, 1974). If chylomicron and VLDL are to release fatty acid to placental cells, they must be broken down by a lipoprotein lipase. The enzyme has been shown to be present in homogenates of rat and human placental tissue (Mallov and Alousi, 1965). The placenta, however, faces two circulations and it has not yet been demonstrated whether it is on the maternal or fetal side or both.

2. The fatty acids may be formed by the placenta from glucose. Placental tissue of rat, rabbit and man has been shown to have the capacity to synthesise fatty acids. However, studies on human placentas in vitro from both early and late gestation have shown negligible levels of activity of acetyl-CoA-carboxylase, a key enzyme in fatty acid synthesis (Diamant

et al, 1975). The incorporation of labelled acetyl CoA into fatty acid was also limited. Both observations suggest that to have synthesis of fatty acid by the human placenta is unimportant, although the placental cells do appear to have the required enzyme systems (Sakvrai, Takagi and Hosoyan, 1969).

3. The placenta might maintain its own intracellular fatty acid pools from its own triglyceride store. Again, studies on placental cells in vitro have demonstrated that they do have a capacity to esterify fatty acids with glycerol to form triglyceride (Szabo, de Lellis and Grimaldi, 1973). This process is not suppressed by low glucose concentration or hypoxia. After injection of labelled palmitate into the doe or the fetal rabbit, label is found not only in the fatty acid fraction, but also in the structural fatty acids and the free triglyceride in the cells.

Histologists have reported lipid droplets in placental cells for many years; overfeeding with high cholesterol diet led to distension of the placenta with lipid. The triglyceride content of the human placenta is low, usually less than 0.5 g per cent wet weight (Younoszai and Haworth, 1969), whereas in rabbits and guinea-pigs it may be higher, between 2 and 10 g per cent wet weight. Both fetal rabbits and guinea-pigs also have high lipid contents in their livers and high circulating triglycerides towards the end of gestation. There are no reports of the factors influencing intracellular lipase activity in placental cells, and therefore whether and to what extent hydrolysis of triglyceride and release of fatty acids in the placenta are influenced by endocrine activity.

4. The placenta might receive fatty acid from the fetus. Human placental perfusion studies in vitro have demonstrated that the FFA perfusing the umbilical vessels enter and traverse the placenta (Szabo, Grimaldi and Jung, 1969; Dancis et al, 1973). Labelled palmitate injected into the fetus enters the placental lipid compartments as well as passing through to the maternal circulation. The present author knows of no study on whether or not circulating fetal triglyceride is a source of placental fatty acids.

In summary, evidence is accumulating that fatty acids may move easily in a variety of directions in the maternal–placental–fetal exchange. It might be expected that the net flow at any one time will depend amongst other things on previous supplies, on current concentrations in the maternal blood and on the rate of clearance by the fetus.

LIPIDS ENTERING THE UMBILICAL CIRCULATION

Fetal blood contains fatty acids, triglyceride, cholesterol and phospholipid, and as in adults, these are bound together into various lipoprotein fractions. The concentrations in general are lower in the fetus than in the mother, but not invariably so (for references see Robertson, Sprecher and Wilcox, 1968). This has led some investigators to conclude that lipids flow from mother to fetus down the gradient, whereas others, noting large maternal–fetal differences, concluded that the placenta was a barrier across which little or no transfer occurred. The general observation of average fetal concentrations lower than average maternal concentrations permits neither conclusion. On the other hand, a positive correlation between the maternal and the umbilical vein blood concentrations does demand some explanation. The simplest is that as the concentration in the maternal blood rises more enters the placenta, which in turn releases more into the fetal circulation. An alternative is that factors which stimulate a rise of a lipid fraction in the maternal blood have the same effect on the fetal systems. On current information it is difficult to visualise such a situation. A positive correlation has been demonstrated between maternal and fetal umbilical vein blood for FFA in rab-

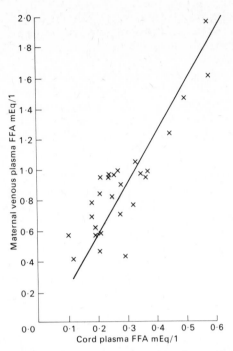

Figure 6.5. The relationship of blood plasma concentrations of free fatty acids in blood taken during elective caesarean section on women who had not gone into labour. y = 0.299, x + 0.03 (r = 0.79, n = 29, P < 0.001). From Elphick, Hull and Sanders (1976) with kind permission of the editor of *British Journal of Obstetrics and Gynaecology.*

bits (Elphick, Hudson and Hull, 1975), sheep (James, Meschia and Battaglia, 1971) and man (Whalley, Zuspan and Nelson, 1966; Sabata, Wolf and Lausmann, 1968; Elphick, Hull and Sanders, 1975).

Figure 6.5 illustrates information obtained at elective caesarean section (Elphick, Hull and Sanders, 1975). A positive correlation is present, but there is wide individual variation. This is perhaps not unexpected in the light of the rapid half-life of FFA in the maternal and fetal circulation, and the interposition of the placenta with its own metabolic demands between the two circulations. Also the uptake and rate of release in the two circulations are controlled individually and probably independently.

It might also be expected that the FFA concentration in umbilical blood leaving the placenta is related to the rate of uptake by the placenta of chylomicron and endogenous triglyceride from the maternal circulation. This is a difficult area of enquiry for circulating concentrations will not necessarily indicate rate of uptake. From limited data on women no correlation was found between maternal circulating triglyceride concentration and umbilical cord vein FFA concentrations.

In general, investigators have failed to find any significant correlation between maternal and fetal concentrations of VLDL, LDL and HDL (Bobok et al, 1974; Csako et al, 1974). Perhaps this too is not surprising and does not necessarily imply that the fetus does not receive cholesterol and phospholipids from the maternal blood stream. There is evidence that this does happen in animals from experiments using labelled substrates.

Some index of the rate of release of lipids *by the placenta* into the fetal circulation can be gained by measuring the difference between the concentration in the cord artery and vein. It does not necessarily follow from a positive venous–arterial difference that the fetus is receiving lipid from the mother. The lipid might be derived from the placenta or even the fetus itself. Thus the placenta could act on fetal circulating triglyceride and release free fatty acids. The existence of a positive correlation between maternal concentration and umbilical arteriovenous difference would be more suggestive that the lipid is derived directly from the mother.

Quantitative studies measuring both blood flow and umbilical arteriovenous differences in fetal sheep at mid-term showed that the net flow of FFA to the fetus was small (James, Meschia and Battaglia, 1971). Similarly quantitative studies of perfused placentas, although giving different values with different techniques, suggested that net flow to the fetus was well below fetal requirements (Dancis et al, 1973). On the other hand, arteriovenous differences

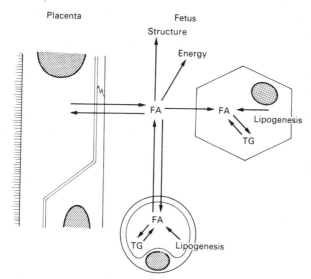

Figure 6.6. Possible exchanges of fatty acids between the placenta and the tissues of the fetus. FA = fatty acids; TG = triglycerides.

on cord blood taken after natural delivery or during elective caesarean section have consistently shown average values around +0.05 mEq/1, which with an assumed placental flow of 200 ml/kg fetal body weight indicates a net transfer of FFA to the fetus which would meet all its requirements of fatty acids for storage and structure (Sabata, Wolf and Lausmann, 1968; Persson and Tunnell, 1971; Elphick et al, 1975). However, in these enquiries little or no attention has been paid to the possible effect of fetal triglyceride concentrations on arteriovenous FFA differences. It must also be emphasised that the maternal FFA concentrations rise with excitement and pain, venepuncture, labour, anaesthesia and surgery, and thus arteriovenous differences in cord blood at birth may be very misleading.

It is important to digress for a moment to consider what factors might influence FFA release into the fetal circulation. The maternal system controls the rate of supply of fatty acids from adipose tissue into the blood stream according to maternal requirements. This is achieved by modulating the activity of the intracellular lipase in adipose tissue. Sympathetic nervous activity is the principal immediate mediator, but level of responsiveness may be influenced by various hormones including growth hormone, corticotrophin, glucagon and thyroxin. Insulin may also affect lipase activity, but it probably affects fatty acid release from adipose cells by other mechanisms as well (Hardman and Hull, 1972). The rate of FFA transfer across the placental membranes and cells may or may not be subject to similar controlling systems. Clearly the placenta will not be influenced directly by either the maternal or fetal sympathetic nervous system. Nor is there evidence to date that placental intracellular lipases are hormone-sensitive. Insulin, on the other hand, may influence transfer by acting more directly on the transport mechanisms. But if it does, it is important to determine whether it is fetal or maternal insulin which exerts the effect.

On average the umbilical arteriovenous difference of triglyceride obtained from cord blood at term after natural delivery has not differed significantly from zero. However, from the author's own experiences occasional pairs have given differences of such a magnitude that it is difficult to avoid the conclusion of Boyd and Wilson 40 years ago (Boyd and Wilson, 1935) that the placenta might take up or release triglyceride according to the prevailing conditions. It is an area requiring more careful and detailed investigations.

Again, measurement of arteriovenous differences of cholesterol have given different results. A recent study by Spellacy et al (1974) showed a consistent and impressive positive value suggesting that the placenta did supply cholesterol to the human fetus as has been demonstrated by other methods in animals. They also found a positive correlation between maternal vein and umbilical vein–artery blood cholesterol concentrations. This suggests a direct flow from mother to fetus; however, as noted previously, others did not find such a relationship. On the other hand, although the placenta contains the enzyme systems to convert acetate to cholesterol, studies in baboons in vivo (Khansi, Markatz and Solomon, 1972) and on perfused human placentas (Telegdy et al, 1970) indicated that the conversion rate was low. The placenta's high cholesterol content is presumably derived largely from the maternal blood stream. Just as the liver is a major site of cholesterol formation in the mother, it is probable that the liver is the important site of cholesterol formation in the fetus (Givner and Jaffe, 1971) and the cholesterol carried in the fetal blood stream to the cells of the body is of both maternal and fetal origin.

The placenta may well receive phospholipids like lecithin from the maternal circulation, but it can also form its own phospholipid (Karp, Sprecher and Robertson, 1973). In their studies on lipid release by the human placenta, Boyd and Wilson (1935) noted a significantly greater concentration of phospholipids, as well as cholesterol, in the umbilical cord vein than artery, but others have not confirmed this. In rabbits there is more convincing evidence that phospholipids formed in the placenta enter the fetal circulation (Bienzenski, Carrozza and Li, 1971).

LIPID PRODUCTION BY FETAL TISSUES AND RELEASE INTO THE FETAL CIRCULATION

Just as the placenta has the capacity to form fatty acid, phospholipid and cholesterol, so have a wide variety of fetal tissues, including the fetal liver, adipose tissue and brain (Yoshioka and Roux, 1972; Cook and Spence, 1974). Indeed it was the remarkable capacity of the fetal liver to form lipids from acetate and glucose that encouraged the suggestion that lipids do not cross the placenta to any degree. However, it is doubtful if the fetus any more than the mother can form the long-chain polyunsaturated fatty acids, the essential fatty acids. Just as the mother must receive these from the diet, so must the fetus receive them from the mother. Presumably they cross the placenta as such. There has been a considerable interest in the fetal concentrations of essential fatty acids. They have been found to form a higher fraction the total fatty acids in the fetus than they do in the mother, which led to the suggestion that they might be selectively transferred. Studies on isolated human placenta do not support selective transport of linoleic acid (Dancis et al, 1973), and infusion of labelled polyunsaturated fatty acids into guinea-pigs and rabbits does not suggest that they are handled differently from palmitate.

Feeding a diet high in polyunsaturated fatty acids had surprisingly little effect on the sheep fetal circulating fatty acid pattern (Scott, personal communication, 1974). On the other hand, the fatty acid profiles of rabbits, guinea-pigs and human fetuses did adjust to changes in a dietary intake by the mother (Sodërhjelm, 1953; Satomura and Sodërhjelm, 1962). Studies on second generation rats fed on diets with either high or low concentrations of essential fatty acids showed that the dietary content had little or no effect on the fatty acid composition of the brain phospholipids, but that the fatty acid patterns in the triglycerides of adipose tissue, liver and, presumably, blood reflected the fatty acid composition of the maternal diets (Alling et al, 1972). Whether the fetal circulating lipid fatty acid profile follows that of the fatty acid profile in the mother will depend on a wide variety of factors including nutrition, endocrine state and gestation. Dietary polyunsaturated fatty acids may prove to be a useful tool to explore further the time scale and rates of lipid exchanges between mother, placenta and fetus.

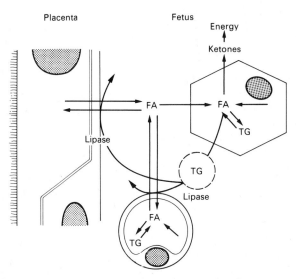

Figure 6.7. Diagrammatic illustration of some of the factors which might influence the circulating concentration of triglyceride in the fetus. FA = fatty acids; TG = triglycerides.

Fatty acids are readily produced by fetal liver, and adipose cells from glucose, acetate and pyruvate (Iliffe, Knight and Myant, 1973; Jones, 1973). In the liver the fatty acids might be utilised locally, or broken down to ketone bodies and released as such. Ketones have been shown to be a valuable source of cellular energy to many tissues and in particular to the developing brain (Dahlguist, Persson and Persson, 1972; Kraus, Schlenker and Schwedesky, 1974). However, studies on circulating ketones in late gestation in man have suggested that the majority in the fetal circulation are derived from the maternal circulation via the placenta, and the rate of ketone body production by fetal liver in vitro is not impressive (Lee and Fritz, 1971).

The liver might also discharge excess fatty acids as endogenous triglyceride. Fetal blood

does contain variable amounts of triglyceride, much of which is in the VLDL fraction. Oc
casionally plasma, which to the naked eye resembles milk, has been seen in fetal rabbit
Studies in guinea-pigs have demonstrated that the fetal liver is the source of this triglyceric
(Bohmer, Havel and Long, 1972). Various factors might lead to a raised triglyceride concen
tration in fetal blood, including maternal illness (hypertension and eclampsia) and feta
asphyxia (Tsang, Fallat and Glueck, 1974). In rabbits, fasting or cold exposure of the mothe
leads to a rise in the fetal triglyceride level. The simple explanation for these findings is tha
anything which causes a rise in fetal circulating FFA concentration leads to a secondary in
crease in triglyceride concentrations.

The factors influencing the production of endogenous triglyceride in the fetus compris
another area awaiting enquiry. But perhaps of more interest still is the fate of this lipid frac
tion. There are no reports on lipoprotein lipase activity in fetal tissues and it is not know
whether lipoprotein lipase activity varies with maternal conditions. Lipase activity has bee
reported in cord blood, so it must be present in some fetal tissues. The question arises as t
whether this triglyceride is taken up by adipose tissue and stored or taken up by the placent
and possibly discharged back into the mother. It is reasonable to wonder whether a hig
triglyceride concentration in the fetus influences the rate of FFA transfer across the placenta

The adipose tissue of the fetus not only makes fatty acids by lipogenesis from glucose,
can also clear fatty acids from the circulation. In fetal rabbits label is found in the triglycerid
fraction of adipose tissue extracts within five minutes of injection of labelled palmitate int
the fetal circulation. However, the possibility has not been excluded that the fatty acids wer
rapidly cleared by the liver, recirculated as triglyceride and then taken up by the adipocyte
Nevertheless, fetal adipose tissue in vitro readily incorporates labelled palmitate int
triglyceride.

Equally, fetal adipose tissue could also be the source of fetal circulating FFA. Studies o
fetal adipose tissue in vitro have demonstrated FFA release in the medium, the rate of whic
is greatly accelerated by the addition of noradrenalin which indicates the presence of an in
tracellular hormone-sensitive lipase (Elphick, Hudson and Hull, 1975).

Attempts to demonstrate lipolysis from fetal adipose tissue in vivo have been frustrated b
the complexity of the experimental models. FFAs with their rapid half life do not alway
show an increased concentration in the circulation following an infusion of noradrenaline c
adrenaline into fetal animals. However, the other product of lipolysis of triglyceride, glycero
is more stable, and a consistent rise in glycerol concentration has been observed after infu
sion of catecholamines into fetal sheep and rabbits (Dawkins, 1964; Comline and Silve
1972; Elphick et al, 1975).

There is also indirect evidence which suggests that fetal adipose tissue releases FFA. Fo
example, chronic hypoxia increased the rate of lipolysis in rabbit fetal brown adipose tissu
in vitro (Harding and Ralph, 1970). Asphyxia to the fetus causes a rise in both glycerol an
FFA concentrations suggesting that lipolysis is activated by increases in fetal sympatheti
activity or catecholamine concentrations. But it could equally be due to decreased utilisatio
or changes in placental transfer.

If labelled FFA is injected into the fetal rabbit, label appears in both the placental lipi
compartments and the maternal circulation within a matter of minutes. Although this onl
demonstrates exchange between mother and fetus, and not a net flow to the mother, it sti
points to the possibility that not only may fatty acids travel from mother to fetus, but unde
certain circumstances the reverse might occur. Concentrations of maternal FFA are not sub
ject to homeostatic control in the same way as circulating glucose; thus under normal con
ditions maternal FFA concentrations may fall to very low levels. It is reasonable to enquir
whether there is ever a net flow from fetus to mother. Examination of the relationshi
between maternal concentration and fetal umbilical and arteriovenous differences suggest

that this might occur at maternal concentrations of FFA below 0.3 mEq/l (Sabata, Wolf, and Lausman, 1968; Elphick et al, 1975).

UTILISATION OF FREE FATTY ACIDS BY THE FETUS

Fatty acids entering the fetal circulation, whether from placenta or fetal stores, have been demonstrated to enter the liver and adipose tissue and thus contribute to the triglyceride stores. Equally, these tissues may form fatty acids from glucose, amino acids and ketones. The fraction of the fatty acids in the triglyceride of the fetal stores which has been synthesised de novo may well depend on a variety of physiological conditions, e.g. maternal nutrition or duration of labour, and it may well vary during gestation. It may be that under usual circumstances in some species it is mainly formed from glucose, whereas in certain other conditions it may be largely derived from the mother. The widely held view that the human fetus forms most of its fatty acids from glucose under usual circumstances may or may not prove to be the case.

Fatty acids are readily taken up by the fetal tissues and incorporated into structural lipids. Fatty acid utilisation for energy is more difficult to study. Investigations on monkey fetal tissues in vitro suggest that their capacity to oxidise palmitate is fairly limited (Roux and Myers, 1974) and the activity of enzyme systems concerned with fatty acid oxidation is low in fetal tissues and rises rapidly after birth (Wolf et al, 1974). This contrasts with the activity of the enzymes concerned with synthesis of fatty acids, which have been shown to fall rapidly after birth in rabbits (Iliffe, Knight and Myant, 1973) and in man (Wolf et al, 1974).

CONCLUSION

This chapter is merely an introduction to a complex and fascinating aspect of fetal biology. Lipid metabolism in the placental–fetal unit is an area of growing interest. The clinical implications of these enquiries may be considerable. For example:

1. Any investigation into the effects of maternal malnutrition or faulty placental function requires that some consideration be given to their effects on lipid transfer across the placenta and the formation of lipids by placental and fetal tissues. Lipids are essential and major units of brain structure. One illustration is the finding that acute maternal starvation leads to a fatty liver in the fetus. This must not be interpreted as a pathological change in the liver cells (Edson, Hudson and Hull, 1975).

2. There has been an explosive interest in lipids in the amniotic fluid. They give some indication of the maturation of the fetal respiratory system. It would be of considerable value if more were known about the origins and the factors determining the rate of lipid production and release into amniotic fluid (Biezenski, 1973).

3. Maternal diabetes causes a disturbance in both lipid and glucose metabolism and both must be evaluated when different therapeutic approaches are assessed. It has been plausibly argued that the obesity in infants of diabetic mothers is due to excess transfer of fatty acids across the placenta (Szabo and Szabo, 1975).

4. The value of lipid analysis of cord blood to screen for inherited disorders of lipid

metabolism, which are far more common than phenylketonuria though not so responsive to dietary management, is being investigated in a number of centres, e.g. Kwiterovich (1974). Cord blood is easily obtained, but, for reasons given in this chapter, it may reflect maternal and placental as well as fetal metabolism (Tsang, Fallat and Glueck, 1974).

5. If the ultimate size of the adipose organ is determined by factors which influence its early growth and development, as many investigators have suggested, then far more must be known about triglyceride storage in the fetus if we are to influence its development in man.

In this chapter the results of recent investigations have generally been quoted. There are a number of excellent reviews available which also give references to earlier work; those by Robertson, Sprecher and Wilcox (1968), Harding and Ralph (1970), Myant (1970), Roux and Yoshioka (1970), Hahn (1972) and Wolf et al (1974) are of particular value.

REFERENCES

Acebal, C., Arche, R., Castro, J. & Municio, A. M. (1973) Effect of pregnancy and insulin administration on plasma lipid levels in the rabbit. *Steroid and Lipid Research*, **4**, 310–322.

Alexander, G. (1975) Body temperature control in mammalian young. *British Medical Bulletin*, **31**, 62–68.

Alling, C., Bruce, A., Karlsson, I., Sapia, O. & Svennerholm, L. (1972) Effect of maternal essential fatty acid supply on fatty acid composition of brain, liver, muscle and serum in 21-day-old rats. *Journal of Nutrition*, **102**, 773–782.

Biezenski, J. J. (1973) Origin of amniotic fluid lipids. 3. Fatty acids. *Proceedings of the Society for Experimental Biology and Medicine*, **142**, 1326–1328.

Biezenski, J. J., Carrozza, J. & Li, J. (1971) Role of placenta in fetal lipid metabolism. III. Formation of rabbit phospholipids. *Biochimica et Biophysica Acta*, **239**, 92.

Bobok, I., Casko, G., Csernyansky, H. & Ludmany, K. (1974) Lipids in maternal, cord and newborn blood serum. *Acta Paediatrica Academiae Scientiarum Hungaricae*, **15**, 95–100.

Bohmer, T., Havel, R. T. & Long, J. A. (1972) Physiological fatty liver and hyperlipemia in the fetal guinea pig: chemical and ultrastructural characterization. *Journal of Lipid Research*, **13**, 371–382.

Boyd, E. M. & Wilson, K. M. (1935) The exchange of lipids in the umbilical circulation at birth. *Journal of Clinical Investigation*, **14**, 7– 15.

Comline, R. S. & Silver, M. (1972) The composition of foetal and maternal blood during parturition in the ewe. *Journal of Physiology*, **222**, 233.

Cook, H. W. & Spence, W. M. (1974) Biosynthesis of fatty acids in vitro by homogenate of developing rat brain: desaturation and chain-elongation. *Biochimica et Biophysica Acta*, **369**, 129–141.

Csako, G., Csernyanszky, H., Bobok, I. & Ludmany, K. (1974) Lipoprotein fractions in maternal, cord and newborn serum. *Acta Paediatrica Academiae Scientiarum Hungaricae*, **15**, 101–108.

Dahlguist, G., Persson, U. & Persson, B. (1972) The activity of D-β-hydroxybutyrate dehydrogenase in fetal, infant and adult rat brain and the influence of starvation. *Biology of the Neonate*, **20**, 40.

Dancis, J., Jansen, V., Kayden, H. J., Schneider, H. & Levitz, M. (1973) Transfer across perfused human placenta. II. Free fatty acids. *Paediatric Research*, **7**, 192–197.

Dawkins, M. J. R. (1964) Changes in blood glucose and non-esterified fatty acids in the fetal and newborn man after injection of adrenaline. *Biology of the Neonate*, **7**, 160–166.

Diamant, Y. Z., Mayorek, N., Neuman, S. & Shafrir, E. (1975) Enzymes of glucose and fatty acid metabolism in early and term human placenta. *American Journal of Obstetrics and Gynecology*, **121**, 58–61.

Edson, J. L., Hudson, D. G. & Hull, D. (1975) Evidence for increased fatty acid transfer across the placenta during a maternal fast in rabbits. *Biology of the Neonate*, **27**, 50–55.

Elphick, M. C., Hudson, D. G. & Hull, D. (1975) Transfer of fatty acids across the rabbit placenta. *Journal of Physiology*, **252**, 29–42.

Elphick, M. C., Hull, D. & Sanders, R. R. (1976) Concentrations of free fatty acids in maternal and umbilical cord blood during elective Caesarean section. *British Journal of Obstetrics and Gynaecology*, in press.

Fabian, E., Stork, A., Kucerova, L. & Sponarova, I. (1968) Plasma levels of free fatty acids, lipoprotein lipase and fat heparin esterase in pregnancy. *American Journal of Obstetrics and Gynecology*, **100**, 904–907.

Givner, M. L. & Jaffe, R. B. (1971) Cholesterol biosynthesis in human fetal liver and adrenal. *Steroids*, **18**, 1–10.

ahn, P. (1972) Lipid metabolism and nutrition in the prenatal and postnatal period. *Current Concepts in Nutrition*, **1**, 99–124.

ardman, M. J. & Hull, D. (1972) Blood flow and fatty acid release by cervical adipose tissue of rabbits. *Journal of Physiology*, **235**, 1–8.

ershfield, M. S. & Nemeth, A. M. (1968) Placental transport of free palmitic and linoleic acids in the guinea pig. *Journal of Lipid Research*, **9**, 460–468.

ull, D. (1974) The function and development of adipose tissue. In *Scientific Foundations of Paediatrics* (Ed.) Davis, J. A. & Dobbing, J. Ch. 25. London: William Heinemann.

ummel, L., Schirrmeister, W., Zimmermann, T. & Wagner, H. (1974) Quantitative studies on the metabolism of placental triglycerides and phospholipids in the rat. *Acta Biologica et Medica Germanica*, **32**, 311–314.

ytten, F. E. & Leitch, I. (1971) *The Physiology of Human Pregnancy*, 2nd edition. Oxford, London, Edinburgh: Blackwell.

iffe, J., Knight, B. L. & Myant, N. B. (1973) Fatty acid synthesis in the brown fat and liver of foetal and newborn rabbits. *Biochemical Journal*, **134**, 341–343.

ames, E., Meschia, G. & Battaglia, E. C. (1971) A–V differences of free fatty acids and glycerol in the ovine umbilical circulation. *Proceedings of the Society for Experimental Biology and Medicine*, **138**, 823–826.

ones, C. T. (1973) The development of lipogenesis in the fetal guinea pig. In *Fetal and Neonatal Physiology. Proceedings of Sir Joseph Barcroft Centenary Symposium*, pp. 403–409. London: Cambridge University Press.

arp, W., Sprecher, H. & Robertson, A. (1973) Human placental phospholipid synthesis. *Biology of the Neonate*, **22**, 398–406.

ayden, H. J., Dancis, J. & Money, W. L. (1969) Transfer of lipids across the guinea pig placenta. *American Journal of Obstetrics and Gynecology*, **104**, 564–571.

hansi, F., Markatz, I. & Solomon, S. (1972) The conversion of acetate to cholesterol in the fetus of the baboon and the transfer of cholesterol from mother to fetus. *Endocrinology*, **91**, 6–12.

nopp, R. H., Wrath, M. R. & Carroll, C. J. (1973) Lipid metabolism in pregnancy. I. Changes in lipoprotein triglyceride and cholesterol in normal pregnancy and the effects of diabetes mellitus. *Journal of Reproductive Medicine*, **10**, 95–101.

raus, H., Schlenker, S. & Schwedesky, D. (1974) Developmental changes of cerebral ketone body utilization in human infants. *Hoppe-Seyler's Zeitschrift für Physiologische Chemie*, **355**, 164–170.

witerovich, P. O. (1974) Neonatal screening for hyperlipidaemia. *Pediatrics*, **53**, 455–458.

ee, P. K. & Fritz, I. B. (1971) Hepatic ketogenesis during develpment. *Canadian Journal of Biochemistry*, **49**, 599.

allov, S. & Alousi, A. A. (1965) Lipoprotein lipase activity of rat and human placenta. *Proceedings of the Society for Experimental Biology and Medicine*, **119**, 301–306.

artin, D. E., Wolf, R. C. & Meyer, R. K. (1971) Plasma lipid levels during pregnancy in the rhesus monkey, Macaca mulata 35957. *Proceedings of the Society for Experimental Biology and Medicine*, **138**, 638–641.

Myant, N. B. (1970) Lipid metabolism. In *Scientific Foundations of Obstetrics and Gynaecology* (Ed.) Philipp, E. E., Barnes, J. & Newton, M. London: William Heinemann.

ielson, F. H., Jacobsen, B. B. & Rolschau, J. (1973) Pregnancy complicated by extreme hyperlipaemia and foam-cell accumulation in placenta. *Acta Obstetrica et Gynecologia Scandinavica*, **52**, 83–89.

ersson, B. & Tunnell, R. (1971) Influence of environmental temperature and acidosis on lipid mobilization in the human infant during the first two hours after birth. *Acta Paediatrica Scandinavica*, **60**, 385–398.

opjak, G. (1946) Maternal and foetal tissue and plasma lipids in normal and cholesterol-fed rabbits. *Journal of Physiology*, **105**, 236–254.

ortman, O. W., Behrman, R. E. & Soltys, P. (1969) Transfer of free fatty acids across the primate placenta. *American Journal of Physiology*, **216**, 143–147.

obertson, A., Sprecher, H. & Wilcox, J. (1968) Free fatty acid patterns of human maternal plasma perfused placenta and umbilical cord plasma. *Nature*, **217**, 378–379.

obinson, D. S. (1967) The role of the clearing factor lipase in the removal of chylomicron triglycerides from the blood. In *Deuel Conference on Lipids on the Fate of Dietary Lipids*. p. 166.

oux, J. F. & Myers, R. E. (1974) In vitro metabolism of palmitic acid and glucose in the developing tissue of the rhesus monkey. *American Journal of Obstetrics and Gynecology*, **118**, 385–392.

oux, J. F. & Yoshioka, T. (1970) Lipid metabolism in the fetus during development. *Clinical Obstetrics and Gynaecology*, **13**, 595.

abata, V., Wolf, H. & Lausmann, S. (1968) The role of free fatty acids, glycerol, ketone bodies and glucose in the energy metabolism of the mother and fetus during delivery. *Biology of the Neonate*, **13**, 7.

akvrai, T., Takagi, H. & Hosoyan, N. (1969) Metabolic pathways of glucose in human placenta. Changes with gestation and with added 17-beta-estradiol. *American Journal of Obstetrics and Gynecology*, **105**, 1044–1054.

atomura, K. & Söderhjelm, L. (1962) Deposition of fatty acids in the newborn in relation to the diet of pregnant guinea pigs: a preliminary report. *Texas Reports in Biology and Medicine*, **20**, 671–679.

Söderhjelm, L. (1953) Fat absorption studies VI. The passage of polyunsaturated fatty acids though the placenta. *Acta Societatis Medicorum Upsaliensis,* **58,** 232–239.

Spellacy, W. N., Asbacher, L. V., Harris, G. K. & Buhi, W. C. (1974) Total cholesterol content in maternal and umbilical vessels in term pregnancies. *Obstetrics and Gynecology,* **44,** 661–665.

Stout, R. W. (1973) The physiology of triglyceride metabolism. *British Journal of Hospital Medicine,* **10,** 309–318.

Svanborg, A. & Vikrot, O. (1965) Plasma lipid fractions, including individual phospholipids at various stages of pregnancy. *Acta Medica Scandinavica,* **178,** 615.

Szabo, A. J. & Szabo, O. (1975) Placental free fatty acid transfer and fetal adipose tissue development: an explanation of fetal adiposity in infants of diabetic mothers. *Lancet,* **ii,** 498.

Szabo, A. J., de Lellis, R. & Grimaldi, R. D. (1973) Triglyceride synthesis by the human placenta. *American Journal of Obstetrics and Gynecology,* **115,** 257–262.

Szabo, A. J., Grimaldi, R. D. & Jung, W. F. (1969) Palmitate transport across perfused human placenta. *Metabolism,* **18,** 406–415.

Tsang, R. C., Fallat, R. W. & Glueck, C. J. (1974) Cholesterol at birth and age. *Pediatrics,* **53,** 458–471.

Telegdy, G., Weeks, J. W., Archer, D. F., Lerner, U., Wiqvistn, N. & Viczfalvsy, E. (1970) Acetate and cholesterol metabolism in the human foeto-placental unit at midgestation 1. 2. 3. *Acta Endocrinologica,* **63,** 91–133.

Van Duyne, C. M., Havel, R. J. & Felts, J. H. (1962) Placental transfer of palmitic acid-1-C^{14} in rabbits. *American Journal of Obstetrics and Gynecology,* **84,** 1069–1074.

Van Duyne, C. M., Parker, H. R., Havel, R. J. & Holm, L. W. (1960) Free fatty acid metabolism in fetal and newborn sheep. *American Journal of Physiology,* **199,** 987–990.

Whalley, W. H., Zuspan, F. P. & Nelson, G. H. (1966) Correlation between maternal and fetal plasma levels of glucose and free fatty acids. *American Journal of Obstetrics and Gynecology,* **94,** 419.

Wolf, H., Stave, U., Novak, M. & Monkus, E. F. (1974) Recent investigations on neonatal fat metabolism. *Journal of Perinatal Medicine,* **2,** 75–87.

Yoshioka, T. & Roux, J. F. (1972) In vitro metabolism of palmitic acid in human fetal tissue. *Paediatric Research,* **6,** 675–681.

Younoszai, M. K. & Haworth, J. C. (1969) Chemical composition of the placenta in normal, pre-term, term and intrauterine growth retarded infants. *American Journal of Obstetrics and Gynecology,* **103,** 262.

Zilzersmit, D. B., Hughes, L. B. & Remington, M. (1972) Hypolipidemic effect of pregnancy on the rabbit. *Journal of Lipid Research,* **13,** 750–755.

7

THE ENDOCRINE PANCREAS
OF THE PREGNANT MOTHER,
FETUS AND NEWBORN

F. A. Van Assche, J. J. Hoet and P. M. B. Jack

THE MATERNAL ENDOCRINE PANCREAS

Throughout pregnancy the mother must adapt to fulfil the metabolic requirements of the developing conceptus. The constant drain of nutrients across the placenta represents an ever-increasing challenge to maternal homeostatic mechanisms. However, during normal pregnancy, the maternal environment is kept relatively constant and the nutritional needs of the fetus are met without demanding any adaptation of the fetal secretory mechanisms prior to birth.

Ideally the major metabolic substrate of the growing fetus is glucose which is postulated to cross the placenta by facilitated diffusion (Howard and Krantz, 1967). Fetal blood glucose concentrations parallel those of the mother, whether the latter are basal levels or artificially elevated by a constant infusion or acute injection of glucose. A materno-fetal gradient is however maintained in normal pregnancies (Patterson, Philips and Wood, 1967; Raivo and Teramo, 1968; Schwartz, 1968; Adam et al, 1969; Obenshain et al, 1970). The developing fetus is therefore dependent on a well controlled maternal blood sugar level for a steady supply of glucose (de Gasparo and Hoet, 1971). Failure of the maternal control mechanisms may be hazardous to the unborn child as recent work in sheep has demonstrated that hyperglycaemia may be fatal to the slightly hypoxic fetus (Shelley, Bassett and Milner, 1975).

Carbohydrate metabolism is impaired to some extent in all women during pregnancy, probably due mainly to the increasing concentration of steroid and other hormones. Normally this is of little practical significance. However, in the established diabetic it is of considerable importance because of the adverse effects of abnormal glucose homeostasis on the fetal pancreas. There are many reports showing that glucose tolerance tested by either an intravenous or oral load is significantly impaired with advancing pregnancy (Burt, 1962; Picard et al, 1968; O'Sullivan et al, 1970; Campbell et al, 1971; Lind et al, 1973). From a teleological standpoint this finding is difficult to explain for there is no evidence to support the view that hyperglycaemia and marked variation in the maternal blood sugar is of any benefit to the fetus—in fact, all the evidence is to the contrary. Recently one group of women who had no features suggestive of a tendency to diabetes was studied by serial glucose determinations over a 24-hour period and a three-hour oral glucose tolerance test. These women were shown to have no significant alteration in the diurnal profiles of plasma glucose concentrations (Gillmer et al, 1975). The only indication of any glucose intolerance was a depression of preprandial and elevation of postprandial levels. From these results it can be concluded that the majority of women have a sufficient margin of glucose tolerance to maintain a stable blood sugar level throughout pregnancy. However, many women with normal blood sugar concentrations when non-pregnant develop a variable degree of intolerance that deteriorates with advancing pregnancy. The reasons for the development of this intolerance will be discussed below.

There is general agreement that the insulin released in response to a meal or a glucose challenge is greatly increased during pregnancy. This hypersecretion of insulin increases progressively from early to late pregnancy (Leake and Burt, 1962; Spellacy and Goetz, 1963; Bleicher, O'Sullivan and Freinkel, 1964; Spellacy, 1971). The significantly elevated insulin response in pregnant women during a glucose tolerance test is evident at 15 minutes, whereas the plasma glucose is only marginally higher at 30 minutes (Freinkel et al, 1974). This apparent insulin resistance in the peripheral tissues is probably a consequence of an alteration in the metabolism of free fatty acids (FFA). The usual fall in plasma FFA concentrations following glucose ingestion, observed in the non-pregnant state, is significantly less in late pregnancy. In addition there is a significant correlation between the insulinogenic response to glucose and the fasting FFA level (Freinkel et al, 1974). Short-lived increases in plasma triglycerides are the result of a glucose challenge in pregnancy. The rate of transport of triglycerides across the isolated human placenta is slow (Szabo, Grimaldi and Jung, 1969; Dancis et al, 1973) so this carbohydrate-induced triglyceridaemia could be a mechanism by which the mother excludes some glucose from the fetus during times of plenty. The retained glycerides could then be recalled as glycerol in times of fasting.

Changes in the second pancreatic hormone, glucagon, may also be altered as a result of pregnancy. Technical difficulties have however restricted studies on this hormone and data are sparse. Basal values of immunoreactive glucagon (IRG) following an overnight fast appeared unchanged when pregnant women were compared with nulliparous women of similar age group. On the other hand, the values of the pregnant group five to eight weeks postpartum were significantly lower than during pregnancy. The same women were presented with an oral glucose challenge between 30 and 40 weeks of gestation and again five to eight weeks postpartum (Freinkel et al, 1974). The characteristic decline in plasma glucagon concentration that coincides with the elevated plasma glucose level was significantly more pronounced during pregnancy than postpartum (Freinkel et al, 1974; Luyckx et al, 1975). This would appear to be another mechanism to 'facilitate anabolism' in the pregnant female. The enhanced inhibition of glucagon secretion would favour the insulin-induced retention and storage of dietary glucose (Freinkel et al, 1974).

The hyperinsulinism which is apparent in the pregnant human female is consistent with the heightened activity of the β-cell that has been observed in animal studies. In the rat, the endocrine pancreas of pregnancy shows significant hypertrophy of the islets of Langerhans. Both the total amount of endocrine tissue and the relative number of β-cells per islet are increased (Hellman, 1960; Van Assche, 1974). The higher insulin levels during pregnancy are related to the increased islet size and the increased number of β-cells (Saudek, Finkowski and Knopp, 1975). The absolute number of α-cells and argyrophilic cells per total pancreatic mass might also be increased since there is a three-fold increase in islet tissue. The argyrophilic cells are thought to represent somatostatin-secreting cells. Ultrastructural studies have demonstrated that the individual β-cells show morphological features of hyperactivity during pregnancy. Both the percentage of light β-granules and the volume of mitochondria are increased (Aerts and Van Assche, 1975).

The secretory capacity of the islets, assessed by in vitro studies, is enhanced as a result of pregnancy. Glucose, arginine and theophylline are effective stimulants of insulin secretion at lower concentrations during pregnancy than in the non-pregnant state. Glucagon and leucine are however ineffective in increasing the insulin released from the islets of pregnant rats (Green and Taylor, 1972). The failure of glucagon to stimulate insulin secretion could be because the adenyl-cyclase activity in the β-cell is already maximal and cannot be stimulated further (Malaisse, Malaisse-Lagae and Mayhew, 1967). The heightened sensitivity of the β-cell to glucose and an increased sensitivity of the membrane receptor for glucose may also be attributed to increased adenyl-cyclase activity (Matchinsky et al, 1971). Studies in the rat have revealed an increased glucose–insulin flux in the rat islet during pregnancy. This may be responsible for the facilitated inhibition of glucagon secretion and the low basal blood sugar levels that have been observed in human pregnancy (Saudek, Finkowski and Knopp, 1975).

Histological examination of the endocrine pancreas of the pregnant human at autopsy has produced similar results to those obtained in the pregnant rat. The pancreas from 17 pregnant women has been studied, 15 by Rosenlöcher (1932) and an additional two by Van Assche (unpublished observations, 1975). The increased islet size and number of β-cells observed would augment the total secretory capacity of the islets and be responsible for the hypersecretion of insulin observed during pregnancy.

Other hormones may be implicated in the changes of carbohydrate metabolism that are a consequence of pregnancy. The most obvious candidate is human placental lactogen (hPL) which is released in vast quantities from the placenta into the maternal circulation as pregnancy proceeds (Spellacy, 1969). hPL has similar metabolic actions to those reported for human growth hormone (hGH) and prolactin. All three hormones stimulate lipolysis and thus elevate plasma FFA concentrations. This lipolytic action could result in a resistance to the action of insulin in peripheral tissues and be indirectly responsible for the hyperinsulinism of pregnancy. However, studies on insulin-dependent diabetics during pregnancy have failed to demonstrate any correlation between the insulin requirement and the serum hPL concentrations (Spellacy and Cohn, 1973). These observations suggest that the metabolic changes of pregnancy cannot be attributed solely to hPL and the involvement of other factors must be considered. hGH is suppressed during pregnancy probably as a consequence of the hPL-induced elevation of FFA and can therefore be excluded from consideration. As previously stated, the inhibition of glucagon secretion by glucose is enhanced during pregnancy. Changes in this hormone cannot therefore account for the observed alterations in the peripheral actions of insulin. Although early studies reported greatly elevated levels of plasma glucocorticoids during pregnancy, subsequent studies have shown that this is due mainly to bound cortisol which is biologically inactive. Further investigations designed to measure the levels of free biologically active corticoids indicate a small but significant increase in their circulating levels (Doe et al, 1969). Even this modest rise in cortisol is likely to have metabolic consequences similar to those attributed to hPL above. There is evidence that steroids, such as oestrogens and progesterone, may cause an insulin resistance and, as a result, elevate both plasma glucose and insulin concentrations in the pregnant female (Kalkhoff et al, 1975). In addition, investigations on the metabolism of human placental tissue in vitro and in vivo have revealed an ability to remove insulin from the circulation and degrade it (Freinkel and Goodner, 1960). A continual breakdown of insulin such as this could cause the secretion of more insulin from the maternal pancreas to compensate. Such a mechanism might therefore account for an increased secretion of insulin but would not necessarily affect basal plasma glucose concentration. An alternative unproven explanation for the apparent insulin resistance of pregnancy may be that the insulin secreted is in some way itself less effective than in the non-pregnant state.

Pregnant women frequently fail to meet the increasing demand for insulin and gestational diabetes results. These subjects have lower insulin levels and elevated glucose levels (de Gasparo et al, 1969a; Hoet, 1969a; Gillmer et al, 1975). This inadequate insulin secretion may result from a failure of the islet tissue to hypertrophy and acquire the differential sensitivity associated with normal pregnancy. Such a failure has been shown to occur in the rat injected with the diabetogenic agent streptozotocin at the day of mating (Van Assche and Aerts, 1975). In pregnant women, whose insulin secretion fails to adapt and in which the insulin resistance is not met adequately, the resulting high maternal blood sugars and associated metabolic changes will prematurely challenge the secretory mechanisms of the fetal endocrine pancreas.

THE FETAL ENDOCRINE PANCREAS

Structural development

Various staining techniques have been used to differentiate between the β-cell and the other cells of the endocrine pancreas. The histological basis of these techniques is still obscure. The β-cell can be reliably identified but the other islet cells represent a heterogenous group whose components vary according to the staining method used. Classification of the cell types is clearer with the aid of electron micrographs (De Coninck et al, 1972). The insulin-secreting β-cells, the glucagon-secreting α-cells (the A_2 cells), the D cells (the A_1 cells), which have been reported to secrete both gastrin (Lomsky, Langr and Vortel, 1969) and somatostatin (Dubois et al, 1975), and a fourth cell type of unknown function can be identified.

Differentiated β-cells have been observed in the human fetus as early as 10 weeks of gestation and α-cells slightly earlier, from the ninth week (Like and Orci, 1972). Subsequent development of the fetal islets has been well documented by Robb (1961). The first stage (10 to 14 weeks) is characterised by small islets budding from the ducts. Some time between 10 and 16 weeks the endocrine tissue becomes independently vascularised and isolated from the ducts. From the 16th to the 20th week, bipolar islets develop with β and non-β-cells occupying opposite poles. Later in gestation the endocrine cells reorientate to form islets with the β-cells situated in the centre and the non-β-cells forming a 'mantle' round them. Some mature islets with β and non-β-cells intermingled are observed in late pregnancy.

Functional development

Insulin is present in the human fetal pancreas from eight to nine weeks of fetal life, indicating that synthesis and storage of the hormone begins at an early stage of intra-uterine life (Adam et al, 1969; Grillo and Shima, 1966). The pancreatic concentration increases in parallel with development. Fetuses of fairly well-controlled insulin-dependent diabetics have greater pancreatic insulin concentrations than control fetuses of comparable gestational age (Steinke and Driscoll, 1965; Rastogi, Letartre and Fraser, 1970). Insulin has been measured in fetal plasma from the 12th week of gestation (Adam et al, 1969; Obenshain et al, 1970). This insulin is entirely of fetal origin since it is generally agreed that the human placenta is either impermeable to insulin or that the amount transferred is physiologically insignificant (Adam et al, 1969).

The human placenta is also impermeable to glucagon (Adam et al, 1972; Johnston and Bloom, 1973). The concentration of pancreatic glucagon in the human fetus increases five-fold from the 10th to the 26th week of gestation and the hormone is present in fetal circulation from the eighth week (Assan and Boillot, 1973).

A different spectrum of stimuli is effective in raising fetal insulin secretion than in the newborn or adult. These differences have been the subject of investigations in utero and in vitro. Acute injections of glucose into fetuses at hysterotomy, between 16 and 20 weeks gestational age, were ineffective in elevating plasma insulin levels (Adam et al, 1969). However, the fetal hyperglycaemia caused by an infusion of glucose given to the mother over a two to four-hour period produced increases in fetal plasma insulin concentrations that were correlated with the fetal blood sugar but not with that of the mother (Obenshain et al, 1970). Later in pregnancy, before the onset of labour, the fetal insulin response to the maternal administration of glucose was individually variable with an occasional insulin peak at ten minutes (Oakley, Beard and Turner, 1972). The insulin secretory response appears to be determined by the duration rather than the degree of hyperglycaemia achieved. The conclusion can be drawn that the β-cell of the normal fetus born to a mother with normal glucose tolerance is capable of responding to a sustained glucose challenge with a sluggish and delayed rise in plasma insulin and that the response is greater at term than earlier in gestation.

Data obtainable in utero at hysterotomy have their limitations but studies on the premature newborn may give some insight into the functioning of the fetal islet. Grasso and his colleagues have made several studies on the insulin-secretory characteristics of the premature infant (Grasso et al, 1968, 1970, 1973, 1975; Reitano et al, 1971). These workers demonstrated that the ability to respond to an acute injection of glucose with a rise in insulin secretion could be induced by a non-stimulatory infusion of glucose over two hours. Infusions of arginine were also capable of inducing β-cell sensitivity to glucose. Insulin release was stimulated in the premature infant by either a mixture of essential amino acids or by arginine alone. The simultaneous infusion of glucose and arginine demonstrated that the two stimuli have a synergistic effect. A simultaneous infusion of glucose and a mixture of essential amino acids showed a similar synergism. An acute injection of glucagon caused a rapid rise in serum insulin concentration and the simultaneous infusion of independently non-stimulatory levels of theophylline and glucagon also caused a large progressive rise in insulin levels.

In a recent study, glucose tolerance and insulin secretion were compared in a group of very small preterm infants (26 to 33 weeks gestational age) and an older, larger group (34 to 40 weeks gestational age) during exchange transfusion (Cser and Milner, 1975). The insulin response to the glucose in the donor blood introduced via the umbilical artery was significant in the larger babies but insignificant in the premature infants although the rise in plasma glucose was similar in both groups. Following the transfusion there was a large increase in plasma insulin concentration in the older group and a smaller rise in the younger infants. However, in these very small infants the rate of glucose disappearance was greater. These data suggest that insulin does not directly affect the control of the normal plasma glucose concentrations in the normal healthy fetus until late gestation.

The premature infant does not respond to hyperglycaemia with a fall in glucagon levels (Massi-Benedetti et al, 1974). This is not attributable to incompetence of the secretory mechanisms which will respond to an infusion of arginine (Sperling et al, 1973).

In consideration of the controls of pancreatic hormone secretion, the functional activity of the fetal gastrointestinal tract should not be overlooked. By 14 weeks of gestation, taste buds are present in the human fetal tongue and swallowing of amniotic fluid has commenced (Davis and Potter, 1946; Bradley and Stern, 1967). The taste buds may convey information on the chemical composition of the amniotic fluid, such as the presence of glucose or amino acids, to the fetus resulting in the stimulation of hormonal factors (e.g. gastrointestinal glucagon) and the autonomic nervous system in the gut (Bradley and Mistretta, 1973). During the third trimester, the fetal lamb swallows between 250 to 500 ml of amniotic fluid per day. There is some evidence that swallowing is stimulated by an artificially elevated glucose concentration in the amniotic fluid (Bradley and Mistretta, 1973). In the fetal rat, acidification of the gastric juice increases from the 19th day of pregnancy, suggesting that the gastrointestinal tract is functionally competent in at least one aspect. The fetal stomach contains appreciable amounts of glucose that increase with gestational age. In the presence of a stable maternal blood glucose concentration the concentration of fetal plasma glucose, fetal plasma insulin and the percentage of β-cells in the fetal pancreas also increase from day 19 of gestation onwards. However, when the mother is starved in late pregnancy the fetal plasma glucose falls as does the glucose content of the amniotic fluid. The administration of glucose to the mother at 19.5 or 21.5 days increases the blood sugar and urine sugar of the fetus. This is accompanied by a rise in glucose concentration of the amniotic fluid and in the fetal stomach. Any increase in the absorption of glucose from the gastrointestinal tract as it becomes functionally competent or in the presence of an increased glucose load may stimulate gastrointestinal factors which may affect the fetal pancreas. The influence of gastrointestinal maturation on fetal pancreatic development, although at present speculative, merits further study. Studies during a single gastric administration of glucose in the fetal monkey in term pregnancy showed a moderate increase in plasma glucose while stomach emptying was verified and an insulin response failed to occur (Chez, Mintz and Hutchinson, 1973). The amount of glucose in the amniotic fluid and in the stomach might not be sufficient to stimulate the gastrointestinal tract at the different periods of pregnancy. However, more glucose could be absorbed normally through the gastrointestinal tract when it matures, as in the rat, or when it has a greater load than normal to cope with. Such an increased glucose absorption would induce an excessive percentage of β-cells and stimulate the insulin secretion. This would also explain the greater glycogen deposition in the rat liver at the end of pregnancy.

In vitro investigations using the techniques of organ culture and the incubation of fresh pieces of pancreas have shown that the basal release of insulin increases with advancing gestational age in the human fetus (Fujimoto and Williams, 1972; Ashworth, Leach and Milner, 1973). In agreement with the in vivo findings, glucose failed to stimulate insulin secretion in organ culture, in tissue culture or in incubated pieces of pancreas from fetuses between 12 and 16 weeks of gestation (Espinosa de los Monteros Mend, Driscoll and Steinke, 1970; Fujimoto and Williams, 1972; Milner, Ashworth and Barson, 1972; Leach, Ashworth and Milner, 1973). More recently it has been shown that human fetal islets grown in tissue culture were responsive to glucose if exposed to a high extracellular glucose concentration over the same period (Cser and Milner, 1976). This indication that the human fetal β-cell responds to chronic exposure to a high extracellular glucose concentration may have important consequences in the infant of the diabetic mother. Using fresh pieces of pancreas obtained from hysterotomy specimens the β-cell response to various stimuli has been investigated in fetuses ranging from 14 to 24 weeks of gestation and weighing between 50 and 625 g (Milner, Barson and Ashworth, 1971; Milner, Ashworth and Barson, 1972). Of the two amino acids studied, leucine was only effective as a stimulant of insulin release in fetuses weighing under 200 g, whereas arginine was stimulatory in larger fetuses. Particular attention was paid to stimuli that are thought to act by altering the intracellular concentration of cyclic AMP (cAMP). Theophylline, glucagon and dibutyryl cAMP were effective at all ages studied and in contrast to the mature pancreas did not require the presence of high extracellular glucose concentration. To exclude the possibility that the difference in the fetal pancreas was due to the breakdown of the large quantities of glycogen present in the fetal exocrine pancreas, theophylline was tested in the presence of mannoheptulose and 2-deoxyglucose. These inhibitors of glucose uptake and metabolism had no effect on the stimulation by theophylline, and also failed to depress basal release of insulin. The possibility that some other constituent of the incubation media, e.g. pyruvate, is stimulating insulin release from the fetal pancreas should be considered (Milner, Leach and Jack, 1975). Ionic stimuli of insulin secretion were effective at all ages.

In vivo and in vitro work indicates that glucose is not the most sensitive regulator of the basal pancreatic hormone secretion in the human fetus. Prior to the development of glucose sensitivity, amino acids may be one of the most important physiological controls of their secretion. In the normal, healthy fetus, basal glucose is disposed of in the absence of elevated plasma insulin levels or suppressed glucagon concentration. In pathological conditions however, involving prolonged hyperglycaemia, glucose sensitivity of the β-cell may be prematurely induced and glucose disposal rate will be enhanced (Mølsted-Pedersen and Jørgensen, 1972; Mølsted-Pedersen, 1974).

THE ENDOCRINE PANCREAS OF THE NEWBORN

Structural features

The normal neonatal endocrine pancreas is similar to that of the fetus in late pregnancy with predominantly 'mantle' islets (Robb, 1961; Van Assche, 1970). Mature islets are not common before the fourth year of life (Ferner and Stockenius, 1951). The islet volume is positively correlated with birthweight in normal infants and remains constant throughout the three months studied (Hultquist, 1971).

Functional features

At birth, the fetus must rapidly adapt from a relatively parasitic mode of life to an independent existence. Towards the end of gestation, preparations are made for this transition. There is a rapid accumulation of hepatic glycogen and an increase in the activity of the enzymes required for its mobilisation. Immediately after birth the neonate is normoglycaemic but the blood sugar level then falls as a consequence of the sudden severence of the maternal supply of glucose. Subsequently the blood glucose level rises, as glucose is provided by the fetal liver, and is maintained at a steady level (Cornblath and Reisner, 1965).

In the infant born to a mother with normal glucose tolerance the basal levels of insulin are low as compared to adult levels and do not increase when the fetal blood sugar is raised through glucose administration to the mother during parturition (Thomas, de Gasparo and Hoet, 1967). They are also comparatively stable over the first few days of extrauterine life (Joassin et al, 1967). In the immediate postnatal period the neonate is still relatively unresponsive to a glucose challenge. However after two hours of age the unfed newborn meets an intravenous glucose challenge with a biphasic insulin response (Isles, Dickson and Farquhar, 1968). The response to an oral glucose challenge is characterised by a gradual rise in plasma insulin concentration which remains elevated for a considerable time (Pildes et al, 1969). The prolonged elevation of insulin persists even after the blood glucose has declined. In contrast to the premature infant and the adult, the full-term infant two hours old has only a moderate insulin response to an arginine stimulus. The newborn infant therefore rapidly develops the ability to release insulin in response to a glucose stimulus.

Plasma glucagon levels are similar in maternal peripheral blood and the umbilical cord blood in normal term deliveries (Bloom and Johnston, 1972; Milner et al, 1973). At birth, there is no glucagon response to an elevated blood glucose. However, the glucagon secretory mechanisms are functional at birth as hypoxia can raise the plasma glucagon level (Johnston and Bloom, 1973). Glucose and insulin administered together are effective in lowering plasma glucagon levels (Luyckx et al, 1972). In the normal infant there is an increase in plasma glucagon two hours after birth (Bloom and Johnston, 1972). This rise may be related to splanchnic nerve stimulation, adrenal secretions or a change in gastrointestinal function.

THE INFANT OF THE DIABETIC MOTHER

Structural features

There is marked hyperplasia and hypertrophy of the pancreatic islets in infants born to mothers with reduced glucose tolerance (Cardell, 1953; Naeye, 1965; Van Assche, 1968; Van Assche, Gepts and de Gasparo, 1969; Van Assche and Gepts, 1971). These changes had been attributed to high maternal blood sugars and an increased glucose content of the amniotic fluid as early as 1920 before the hormonal significance of the islets was ascertained (Dubreuil and Anderodias, 1920). Similar histological features have been described in infants born to mothers whose diabetes only became overt in later life (Van Beeck, 1939; Woolf and Jackson, 1957).

The islets in the pancreas of the infant born to the diabetic mother are extremely vascular and numerous minute islets composed of only a few cells are observed (Van Assche, Gepts and de Gasparo, 1969; Hultquist, 1971). Growth of the islets may result from proliferation of islet cells, the continued production of endocrine cells from the exocrine matrix or a combination of both processes. It seems likely that the majority of the new endocrine cells are derived from the exocrine matrix, as little cell division is observed in the endocrine cell population (Wessels, 1964; Pictet and Rutter, 1972). Under conditions of islet hyperplasia in the pancreatic tissue of adult experimental animals, the peri-insular acinar cells show greater mitotic activity than those situated further from the islet or endocrine cells (Duff and Starr, 1944; Hughes, 1947; Hellerstrom et al, 1962; Hellman, Rothman and Hellerstrom, 1962; Kramer and Tan, 1968). The islet hypertrophy in the newborn of the diabetic woman is caused by an increase in the number of β-cells. In 30 per cent of cases, the pancreas of these infants showed infiltration of eosinophils in and around the islets. This infiltration was even found in the offspring of mothers that were not treated with insulin during pregnancy. These changes were positively correlated with the blood sugar level of the diabetic mother at delivery and are evident at the earliest age studied, 19 weeks of gestation (Cardell, 1953; Driscoll, Benirschke and Curtis, 1960; Van Assche, 1968; Van Assche, Gepts and de Gasparo, 1969; Van Assche et al, 1970; Van Assche and Gepts, 1971). Similar alterations in pancreatic histology have been observed in the offspring of rats with experimentally induced diabetes. In addition to an increased percentage of endocrine tissue, degranulation of the β-cells and a decrease in insulin content were found. The degree of degranulation and the reductions in insulin content were related to the severity of the experimental diabetes. In the fetal β-cell, glycogen deposits are present when the maternal blood sugar exceeds 300 mg/100 ml (Aerts and Van Assche, unpublished observations, 1975).

Hultquist (1971) has been able to demonstrate a correlation between the volume of the islets, the volume of the β-cells and the body weight of the newborn infant. The volume of islet tissue was also correlated with maternal glucose levels within six hours of delivery. Maternal and fetal blood glucose also appear to influence the size of the β-cell nucleus. These features were not related to birthweight in premature infants of less than 32 weeks gestational age. The association between maternal blood sugar, birthweight and the volume of islet tissue was less apparent when complications such as maternal ketonaemia or toxaemia were reported. This was also true when retinopathy was diagnosed (Hultquist, 1971). In the low birthweight infants born to mothers with vascular and renal complications, the total pancreatic mass was reduced due to a reduction in exocrine tissue, but a limited hypertrophy of the β-cells was still evident (d'Agostino and Bahn, 1963).

Functional features

Infants born to diabetic mothers may be either oversized, small-for-dates or have normal birthweight. The oversized infant will often be born to obese and hyperglycaemic mothers. Small-for-dates infants are often born to diabetic mothers with vascular complications where the placental blood supply is reduced and further constraints on fetal growth may be induced by maternal infections, or intra-uterine stress resulting from congenital malformation, intra-uterine infection or disease.

The concept that the prolonged exposure of the fetus of the diabetic pregnancy to hyperglycaemia stimulated the pancreas to produce excessive amounts of insulin was first proposed by Pedersen and his colleagues (1954). This hyperinsulinism must be secondary to the induction of glucose sensitivity in the fetal pancreas as a result of exposure to prolonged hyperglycaemic episodes. The insulin content of microdissected islets, in proportion to the number of β-cells, is increased in infants of diabetic mothers (de Gasparo et al, 1969b; Van Assche, Gepts and de Gasparo, 1969). This demonstrates that the intracellular stores of insulin are maintained by biosynthesis in the presence of a greatly increased hormone output. The increased insulin secretion results in lipogenesis, protein anabolism and an increase in cell number in many vital organs (Naeye, 1965). An insulin-induced increase in lipogenesis is, at least in part, responsible for the characteristic cherubic appearance of the overweight infant of the diabetic mother. In the high birthweight infant the insulin levels in cord blood are high and related to the excess weight (de Gasparo and Hoet, 1971) as is the percentage of islet tissue of the pancreas (Naeye, 1965). The administration of insulin to fetal rats and lambs in utero results in overweight newborn animals which resemble the overweight infant of the diabetic mother in the deposition of lipid and the retention of nitrogen (Picon, 1967; Liggins, 1974). The offspring of rats with mild experimental diabetes were also heavier than controls of comparable gestational age (Van Assche, unpublished observations, 1975).

Lipogenesis may also be enhanced by an increase in the placental transfer of FFA in the diabetic pregnancy (Szabo, 1975).

Human newborn infants with transient neonatal diabetes may represent the opposite case to the hyperinsulinism described above. There is evidence to suggest that many of these infants have delayed maturation of β-cell function (Ferguson and Milner, 1970; Pagliara, Karl and Kipnis, 1973). These infants are nearly always small-for-dates which may be due to the delay in the development of insulin secretion or a temporary resistance to the peripheral actions of insulin (Hill, 1974; Liggins, 1974).

Glucagon metabolism is also altered in the infant of the diabetic mother. The rise in plasma glucagon seen at two hours of age in the normal healthy infant does not occur in infants born to diabetic mothers. In contrast, small-for-dates babies have a significantly greater rise in plasma glucagon concentration (Johnston and Bloom, 1975). The elevated insulin levels present in the infant of the diabetic mother may be responsible for the suppression of glucagon secretion observed.

These observations suggest that insulin and glucagon are implicated in the regulation of fetal growth. Evidence for such a role has also been obtained at the cellular level. Experimental studies in the rat have shown that insulin stimulated the uptake of glucose, amino acid incorporation and the synthesis of protein by the fetal heart from day 16 of gestation onwards (Clark, 1971a, 1971b). The augmentation of growth of many tissues in vitro by insulin is well documented.

The determining factors in the adaptation of the fetal β-cell

The plasma levels of growth hormone are elevated in normal neonates but low in infants of diabetic mothers at birth. The data appear to indicate that the regulation of growth hormone secretion has been modified in infants of diabetic mothers (Westphal, 1967).

Studies on the endocrine pancreas of the anencephalic infant have demonstrated the importance of an intact hypothalamic–hypophyseal axis in the ability to respond to a premature glucose challenge. Two types of anencephalics can be recognised: those with a functional hypothalamic–hypophyseal connection and those without. The morphological and functional development of the endocrine pancreas is similar in anencephalic and normal infants if the mother has normal glucose tolerance. However, the hyperplasia and hypertrophy of the islets normally seen in the offspring of the diabetic mother are not present in the absence of an intact hypothalamic–hypophyseal axis (Van Assche, 1968; Van Assche, Gepts and de Gasparo, 1969; de Gasparo and Hoet, 1971).

These observations indicate that although the hypothalamus and pituitary are unnecessary for the normal development of the endocrine pancreas which has been confirmed in animal studies involving experimental decapitation (Van Assche, 1971; de Gasparo, Kolanowki and Hoet, 1974), they are essential for the increased multiplication of the fetal β-cell under the abnormal conditions imposed by a diabetic pregnancy. This effect may be directly under hypothalamic–hypophyseal control or mediated via the adrenal or thyroid glands. However, isolated adrenal insufficiency does not prevent β-cell hyperplasia (Hoet, Van Assche and Grasso, 1975). Growth hormone has been shown to sensitise the rat β-cell to secretagogues (Martin and Gagliardino, 1967) and the low growth hormone levels in the anencephalic infant (Grunt and Reynolds, 1970; Grumbach and Kaplan, 1973) may be important in this respect (Salazar et al, 1969; Van Assche, 1970, 1975; Hoet, Van Assche and Grasso, 1975). A cephalic influence on insulin output has been shown also to occur in the rabbit. Insulin output was however increased by decapitation and this increase was prevented by ACTH replacement (Jack and Milner, 1975).

Islets of Langerhans are also increased in size and number in the pancreas of erythroblastic infants and infants born with thalassaemia (Van Assche et al, 1970). Although the total amount of endocrine tissue, the insulin content of the pancreas and the insulin levels in the cord blood are all increased, there is no change in the proportion of β-cells per islet (Van Assche, 1970). Multiplication of the human fetal β-cell only occurs under conditions of glucose loading (Van Assche and Gepts, 1971). Increased mitotic activity has been observed in the fetal rat β-cell at the time of the normal rise in blood glucose concentrations from 30 to 80 mg/100 ml at 20 days gestational age. These changes coincided with an alteration in stomach pH from alkaline to acid, indicating an initiation of active transport mechanisms in the stomach mucosa. The adaptation of the insulin secretory mechanisms may possibly be related to the presence of glucose in the gastrointestinal tract (Hoet and Reusens, 1976).

The clinical consequences of abnormal pancreatic development

The fetus responds to a glucose challenge in utero by increasing the proportion of β-cells and as a result has an increased insulin secretory capacity and output. The adaptation to an abnormal intra-uterine environment with an increased insulin secretion will inhibit the maturation of pulmonary lecithin which is held responsible for the respiratory distress syndrome of these neonates (Smith et al, 1975). Further they have an increased risk of symptomatic hypoglycaemia after birth and are more prone to obesity and diabetes mellitus in later life (Farquhar, 1969; Shah and Farquhar, 1975). If the human β-cell is only capable of a finite number of cell divisions, as appears to be true in the rat (Logothetopoulos, 1972), an adverse intra-uterine environment resulting in β-cell hyperplasia could jeopardise the regenerative potential in later life. A reduced capacity for cell division in the β-cell population, in conjunction with normal β-cell development and function, may be one of the many factors determining the increased incidence of diabetes mellitus in individuals born to diabetic mothers. Unger and Orci (1975) have proposed that reduced β-cell secretory capacity in association with a persistent secretion of glucagon is responsible for the diabetic state.

Careful control of diabetic pregnancy is important not only for the infant but also for the future well-being of the mother. Infants born to diabetic mothers whose blood sugar levels have been carefully controlled with insulin throughout the pregnancy have less hyperplasia and hypertrophy of the pancreatic islets or none at all (Van Assche, 1970; Hultquist, 1971). Adequate maternal control also reduces clinical complications arising in the neonatal period (Persson, 1974, 1975). For the mother, pregnancy modifies maternal glucose homeostasis and failure to respond to the challenging needs of pregnancy with an increased number of β-cells and an enhanced insulin secretion may have serious consequences. Gestational diabetics not treated with insulin may show further deterioration of endocrine function, with associated vascular complications, years later, that the insulin-treated mother does not develop (O'Sullivan, Charles and Dandrow, 1971).

REFERENCES

Adam, P. A. J., King, K. C., Schwartz, R. & Teramo, K. (1972) Human placental barrier to I[125] glucagon early in gestation. *Journal of Clinical Endocrinology and Metabolism,* **34,** 772–782.
Adam, P. A. J., Teramo, K., Raiha, N., Gitlin, D. & Schwartz, R. (1969) Human foetal insulin metabolism early in gestation. Response to acute elevation of fetal blood glucose concentration and placental transfer of human insulin I[131]. *Diabetes,* **18,** 409–416.

Aerts, L. & Van Assche, F. (1975) Ultrastructural changes of the endocrine pancreas in pregnant rats. *Diabetologia*, 11, 285–289.

Ashworth, M. A., Leach, F. N. & Milner, R. D. G. (1973) Development of insulin secretion in the human foetus. *Archives of Disease in Childhood*, 48, 151–152.

Assan, R. & Boillot, J. (1973) Pancreatic glucagon and glucagon like material in tissues and plasma from human fetuses of 6–26 weeks old. *Pathologie et Biologie*, 21, 149–157.

Bleicher, S. J., O'Sullivan, J. B. & Freinkel, N. (1964) Carbohydrate metabolism in pregnancy. V. The interrelations of glucose, insulin and free fatty acids in late pregnancy and postpartum. *New England Journal of Medicine*, 271, 866–872.

Bloom, S. R. & Johnston, D. I. (1972) Failure of glucagon release in infants of diabetic mothers. *British Medical Journal*, iv, 453–454.

Bradley, R. M. & Mistretta, C. M. (1973) The sense of taste and swallowing activity in foetal sheep. In *Foetal and Neonatal Physiology, Proceedings of the Sir Joseph Barcroft Centenary Symposium*, pp. 77–81. Cambridge: Cambridge University Press.

Bradley, R. M. & Stern, I. B. (1967) The development of the human taste bud during the fetal period. *Journal of Anatomy*, 101, 743–752.

Burt, R. L. (1962) Glucose tolerance tests in pregnancy. *Diabetes*, 11, 277–228.

Campbell, N., Pyke, D. A. & Taylor, K. W. (1971) Oral glucose tolerance tests in pregnant women with potential diabetes, latent diabetes and glycosuria. *Journal of Obstetrics and Gynaecology of the British Commonwealth*, 78, 498–504.

Cardell, B. S. (1953) Hypertrophy and hyperplasia of the pancreatic islets in newborn infants. *Journal of Pathology and Bacteriology*, 66, 335.

Chez, R. A., Mintz, D. & Kutchinson, D. L. (1973) Carbohydrate metabolism in primate pregnancy. In *Proceedings of the 4th International Congress of Endocrinology, Washington D.C., June 1972*. Amsterdam: Excerpta Medica.

Clark, C. M. (1971a) Carbohydrate metabolism in the isolated fetal rat heart. *American Journal of Physiology*, 220, 583–588.

Clark, C. M. Jr (1971b) The stimulation by insulin of amino acid uptake and protein synthesis in the isolated fetal rat heart. *Biology of the Neonate*, 19, 379–388.

Cornblath, M. & Reisner, S. H. (1965) Blood glucose in the neonate and its clinical significance. *New England Journal of Medicine*, 273, 278–281.

Cser, A. & Milner, R. D. G. (1976) Glucose-stimulated insulin release from human foetal islets grown in tissue culture for 10 days. *Journal of Endocrinology*, 65, 57P.

Cser, A. & Milner, R. D. G. (1975) Glucose tolerance and insulin secretion in very small babies. *Acta Paediatrica Scandinavica*, 64, 457–463.

D'Agostino, A. N. & Bahn, R. C. (1963) A histopathologic study of the pancreas of infants of diabetic mothers. *Diabetes*, 12, 327–331.

Dancis, J., Jansen, V., Kayden, J., Schneider, H. & Levitz, M. (1973) Transfer across perfused human placenta. II. Free fatty acids. *Pediatric Research*, 7, 192–197.

Davis, M. E. & Potter, E. L. (1946) Intra uterine respiration of the human foetus. *Journal of the American Medical Association*, 131, 1194–1201.

De Coninck, J., Van Assche, F. A., Potvliege, P. R. & Gepts, W. (1972) The ultrastructure of the human islets. II. The islets of neonate. *Diabetologia*, 8, 326–333.

De Gasparo, M. & Hoet, J. J. (1971) Normal and abnormal foetal weight gain. In *Diabetes Mellitus. Proceedings of the Seventh Congress of the I.D.F.* (Ed.) Rodriguez, R. R. & Valance, J. pp. 667–676. Amsterdam: Excerpta Medica.

De Gasparo, M., Kolanowski, J. & Hoet, J. J. (1974) Insuline chez le foetus. *Biomedicine*, 21, 365–367.

De Gasparo, M., Malherbe, C., Gerard, C., de Hertogh, R., Thomas, K. & Hoet, J. J. (1969a) Insulin levels during pregnancy or obesity in normoglycemic women with a positive history of diabetes mellitus. *Hormone and Metabolic Research*, 1, 266–273.

De Gasparo, M., Van Assche, F. A., Gepts, W. & Hoet, J. J. (1969b) The histology of the endocrine pancreas and the insulin content in the microdissected islets of foetal pancreas. *Revue Française d'Etudes Cliniques et Biologiques*, 9, 904–906.

Doe, R. P., Dickinson, P., Zinneman, H. H. & Seal, U. S. (1969) Elevated non protein bound cortisol (NPC) in pregnancy or obesity in normoglycemic women with a positive history of diabetes mellitus. *Hormone and and Metabolism*, 29, 757–766.

Driscoll, S. G., Benirschke, K. & Curtis, G. W. (1960) Neonatal deaths among infants of diabetic mothers. *American Journal of Diseases of Children*, 100, 818–835.

Dubois, P. M., Paulin, C., Assan, R. & Dubois, M. P. (1975) Evidence for immunoreactive somatostatin in the endocrine cells of human foetal pancreas. *Nature*, 256, 731–732.

Dubreuil, G. & Anderodias, (1920) Ilots de Langerhans geants chez un nouveau-né issu de mère glycosurique. *Compte Rendu de la Société de Biologie*, 23, 1940–1941.

Duff, E. L. & Starr, H. (1944) Experimental alloxan diabetes in hooded rats. *Proceedings of the Society for Experimental Biology and Medicine*, **57**, 280–282.

Espinosa de los Monteros Mend, M. A., Driscoll, S. G. & Steinke, J. (1970) Insulin release from isolated human fetal pancreatic islets. *Science*, **168**, 1111–1112.

Farquhar, J. W. (1969) Prognosis for babies born to diabetic mothers in Edinburgh. *Archives of Disease in Childhood*, **44**, 36–40.

Ferguson, A. W. & Milner, R. D. G. (1970) Transient neonatal diabetes mellitus in sibs. *Archives of Disease in Childhood*, **45**, 80–83.

Ferner, H. & Stockenius, W. Jr (1951) Die cytogenese des Inselsystems beim Menschen. *Zeitschrift für Zellforschung*, **35**, 147.

Freinkel, N. & Goodner, C. J. (1960) Carbohydrate metabolism in pregnancy. 1. The metabolism of insulin by human placental tissue. *Journal of Clinical Investigation*, **39**, 116–131.

Freinkel, N., Metzger, B. E., Nitzan, M., Daniel, R., Surmaczynska, B. Z. & Nagel, T. (1974) Facilitated anabolism in late pregnancy. In *Diabetes Mellitus. Proceedings of the Eighth Congress of the I.D.F.* (Ed.) Malaisse, W. J., Pirart, J. & Vallance, J. pp. 478–488. Amsterdam: Excerpta Medica.

Fujimoto, W. Y. & Williams, R. H. (1972) Insulin from cultured human foetal pancreas. *Endocrinology*, **91**, 1133–1136.

Gillmer, M. D. G., Beard, R. W., Brooke, F. M. & Oakley, N. W. (1975) Carbohydrate metabolism in pregnancy. The diurnal plasma profile in normal and diabetic women. *British Medical Journal*, **iii**, 399–404.

Girard, J. R. & Marliss, E. B. (1974) Circulating fuels in late fetal and early neonatal life in the rat. In *Early Diabetes in Early Life* (Ed.) Camerini-Davalos, R. A. & Cole, H. S. p. 185. New York: Academic Press.

Grasso, S., Distefano, G., Messina, A., Vigo, R. & Reitano, G. (1975) Effect of glucose priming on insulin response in the premature infant. *Diabetes*, **24**, 291–294.

Grasso, S., Messina, A., Distefano, G., Vigo, R. & Reitano, G. (1973) Insulin secretion in the premature infant: response to glucose and amino-acids. *Diabetes*, **22**, 349–353.

Grasso, S., Messina, A., Saporito, N. & Reitano, G. (1970) Effect of theophylline, glucagon and theophylline plus glucagon in insulin secretions in the premature infant. *Diabetes*, **19**, 837–841.

Grasso, S., Saporito, N., Messina, A. & Reitano, G. (1968) Serum insulin levels in response to glucose and amino-acids in the premature infant. *Lancet*, **ii**, 755–756.

Green, I. C. & Taylor, K. W. (1972) Effects of pregnancy in the rat on the size and insulin secretory response of the islets of Langerhans. *Journal of Endocrinology*, **51**, 317–325.

Grillo, R. A. I. & Shima, K. (1966) Insulin content and enzyme histochemistry of the human foetal pancreatic islet. *Journal of Endocrinology*, **36**, 151–158.

Grumbach, M. N. & Kaplan, S. L. (1973) Ontogenesis of growth hormone, insulin, prolactin and gonadotrophin secretion in the human foetus. In *Foetal and Neonatal Physiology* (Ed.) Comline, K. S., Cross, K. W., Dawes, G. S. & Nathanielsz, P. W., pp. 462–487. Cambridge: Cambridge University Press.

Grunt, J. A. & Reynolds, D. W. (1970) Insulin, blood sugar and growth hormone levels in an anencephalic infant before and after intravenous administration of glucose. *Journal of Pediatrics*, **76**, 112–116.

Hellerstrom, C., Hellman, B., Brolin, S. & Larsson, S. (1962) In vitro incorporation of thymidine-H³ in the pancreas of normal and obese hyperglycemic mice. *Acta Pathologica et Microbiologica Scandinavia*, **54**, 1–7.

Hellman, B. (1960) The islets of Langerhans in the rat during pregnancy and lactation with special reference to the changes in the β and α cell ratio. *Acta Obstetrica et Gynecologica Scandinavica*, **39**, 331–342.

Hellman, B., Rothman, U. & Hellerstrom, C. (1962) Identification of a specific type of α-cell located in the central part of the pancreatic islets of the horse. *General and Comparative Endocrinology*, **2**, 558–564.

Hill, D. (1974) Citing Sherwood et al in discussion in *Size at Birth*. *Ciba Foundation Symposium 27* (Ed.) Elliott, K. & Knight, J., pp. 202–214. Amsterdam: Associated Scientific Publishers.

Hoet, J. J. (1969a) Nouvelles recherches sur le diabète de la gestation. *Mémoires de l'Académie Royale de Médecine de Belgique*, **8**, 121–186.

Hoet, J. J. (1969b) Normal and abnormal foetal weight gain. In *Foetal Autonomy. Ciba Foundation Symposium* (Ed.) Wohlstenholme, G. E. W. & O'Connor, M. pp. 186–213. London: Churchill.

Hoet, J. J. & Reusens, B. (1976) Étude de l'autonomie foetale et ses implications cliniques. *Bulletin de l'Académie Royale de Médecine de Belgique*, in press.

Hoet, J. J., Van Assche, F. A. & Grasso, S. (1975) Endocrine factors in islet maturation. In *Early Diabetes in Early Life* (Ed.) Camerini-Davalos, R. & Cole, H. S. p. 93. New York: Academic Press.

Howard, J. M. & Krantz, K. E. (1967) Transfer and use of glucose in the human placenta during in vitro perfusion and the associated effect of oxytocin and papaverine. *American Journal of Obstetrics and Gynecology*, **98**, 445–458.

Hughes, H. (1947) Cyclical changes in the islets of Langherans in the rat pancreas. *Journal of Anatomy*, **81**, 82–92.

Hultquist, G. T. (1971) Morphology of the endocrine organs in infants of diabetic mothers. In *Diabetes Mellitus* (Ed.) Rodriguez, R. R. & Valance, J. pp. 686–694. Amsterdam: Excerpta Medica.

Isles, T. E., Dickson, M. & Farquhar, J. W. (1968) Glucose tolerance and plasma insulin in new-born infants of normal diabetic mothers. *Pediatric Research,* **2,** 198–208.

Jack, P. M. B. & Milner, R. D. G. (1975) ACTH and the development of insulin secretion in the foetal rabbit. *Journal of Endocrinology,* **64,** 67–75.

Joassin, G., Parker, M. L., Pildes, R. S. & Cornblath, M. (1967) Infants of diabetic mothers. *Diabetes,* **16,** 306–311.

Johnston, D. I. & Bloom, S. R. (1973) Plasma glucagon levels in full term human infant and the effect of hypoxia. *Archives of Disease in Childhood,* **48,** 451–454.

Johnston, D. I. & Bloom, S. R. (1975) Neonatal glucagon response in infants of diabetic mothers. *Early Diabetes in Early Life* (Ed.) Camerini-Davalos, R. A. & Cole, H. S. p. 541. New York: Academic Press.

Kalkhoff, R. K., Costrini, N. V., Matute, M. L. & Kim, H. J. (1975) Metabolic modifications by the hormones of pregnancy. In *Early Diabetes in Early Life* (Ed.) Camerini-Davalos, R. A. & Cole, H. S. New York: Academic Press.

Kramer, M. F. & Tan, H. T. (1968) The peri-insular acini of the pancreas of the rat. *Zeitschrift für Zellforschung und Mikroskopische Anatomie,* **86,** 163–170.

Leach, F. N., Ashworth, M. A. & Milner, R. D. G. (1973) Insulin release from human foetal pancreas in tissue culture. *Journal of Endocrinology,* **59,** 65–79.

Leake, N. H. & Burt, R. L. (1962) Insulin-like activity in serum during pregnancy. *Diabetes,* **11,** 419–421.

Liggins, G. C. (1974) The influence of the fetal hypothalamus and growth. In *Size at Birth. Ciba Foundation Symposium 27* (Ed.) Elliott, K. & Knight, J. Amsterdam: Associated Scientific Publishers.

Like, A. A. & Orci, L. (1972) Embryogenesis of the human pancreatic islets. *Diabetes,* **21,** 511–534.

Lind, T., Billewicz, W. Z. & Brown, G. (1973) A serial study of changes occurring in the oral glucose tolerance test during pregnancy. *Journal of Obstetrics and Gynaecology of the British Commonwealth,* **80,** 1033–1039.

Logothetopoulos, J. (1972) Islet cell regeneration and neogenesis. In *Handbook of Physiology; Endocrinology; Endocrine Pancreas* (Ed.) Steiner, D. F. & Freinkel, N. pp. 67–76. Baltimore: Williams and Wilkins.

Lomsky, R., Langr, F. & Vortel, V. (1969) Immunohistochemical demonstration of gastrin in mammalian islets of Langerhans. *Nature,* **233,** 618–619.

Luyckx, A. S., Gerard, J., Gaspard, U. & Lefebvre, P. J. (1975) Plasma glucagon levels in normal women during pregnancy. *Diabetologia,* **11,** 549–554.

Luyckx, A. D., Massi-Benedetti, F., Falorni, A. & Lefebvre, P. (1972) Presence of pancreatic glucagon in the portal plasma of human neonates. *Diabetologia,* **8,** 296–300.

Malaisse, W. J., Malaisse-Lagae, F. & Mayhew, D. (1967) A possible role for the adenylcyclase system in insulin secretion. *Journal of Clinical Investigation,* **46,** 1724–1734.

Martin, J. & Gagliardino, J. J. (1967) Effect of growth hormone on the isolated pancreatic islets of rat in vitro. *Nature,* **213,** 630–631.

Massi-Benedetti, F., Caccomo, M. Z., Falorni, A. & Marini, A. (1974) Correlazioni endicrino-metaooliche nella matattia emolitica del neonata. *Proceedings of XVI Congresso Nazionale di Nipiologia, Riva del Garda, 1974.*

Matchinsky, F. M., Ellerman, J. E., Krzanowski, J., Kotler Brajtburg, J., Landgraf, R. & Fertel, R. (1971) The dual function of glucose in islets of Langerhans. *Journal of Biological Chemistry,* **246,** 1007–1011.

Milner, R. D. G., Ashworth, M. A. & Barson, A. J. (1972) Insulin release from human foetal pancreas in response to glucose, leucine and arginine. *Journal of Endocrinology,* **52,** 497–505.

Milner, R. D. G., Barson, A. J. & Ashworth, M. A. (1971) Human foetal pancreatic insulin secretion in response to ionic and other stimuli. *Journal of Endocrinology,* **51,** 323–332.

Milner, R. D. G., Leach, F. N. & Jack, P. M. B. (1975) Reactivity of the fetal islet. In *Carbohydrate Metabolism During Pregnancy and in the Newborn* (Ed.) Sutherland, H. & Stowers, J. Edinburgh: Churchill Livingstone.

Milner, R. D. G., Chouksey, S. K., Mickleson, K. N. P. & Assan, R. (1973) Plasma pancreatic glucagon and insulin:glucagon ratio at birth. *Archives of Disease in Childhood,* **48,** 241–242.

Mølsted-Pedersen, L. (1974) *Studies on Carbohydrate Metabolism in the Newborn Infants of Diabetic Mothers.* Thesis, Copenhagen.

Mølsted-Pedersen, L. & Jørgensen, K. R. (1972) Aspects of carbohydrate metabolism in newborn infants of diabetic mothers. *Acta Endocrinologica,* **71,** 115–125.

Naeye, R. L. (1965) Infants of diabetic mothers: quantitative morphologic study. *Paediatrics,* **35,** 980–989.

Oakley, N. W., Beard, R. W. & Turner, R. C. (1972) Effect of sustained maternal hyperglycaemia on the foetus in normal and diabetic pregnancies. *British Medical Journal,* **i,** 466–469.

Obenshain, S. S., Adam, P. A. J., King, K. C., Teramo, K., Raivio, K. O., Raiha, N. & Schwartz, R. (1970) Human fetal insulin response to sustained maternal hyperglycaemia. *New England Journal of Medicine,* **283,** 566–570.

O'Sullivan, J. B., Charles, D. & Dandrow, R. V. (1971) Treatment of verified prediabetics in pregnancy. *Journal of Reproductive Medicine,* **7,** 45–48.

O'Sullivan, J. B., Snyder, P. J., Sporer, A. C., Dandrow, R. V. & Charles, D. (1970) Intravenous glucose tolerance test and its modification by pregnancy. *Journal of Clinical Endocrinology and Metabolism*, **31**, 33–37.

Pagliara, A. S., Karl, I. E. & Kipnis, D. B. (1973) Transient neonatal diabetes: delayed maturation of the pancreatic beta-cell. *Journal of Paediatrics*, **82**, 97–101.

Patterson, P., Philips, L. & Wood, C. (1967) Relationship between maternal and fetal blood glucose during labor. *American Journal of Obstetrics and Gynaecology*, **98**, 938–945.

Pedersen, J., Bojsen-Moller, B. & Poulsen, H. (1954) Blood sugar in newborn infants of diabetic mothers. *Acta Endocrinologica*, **15**, 33–52.

Persson, B. (1974) Assessment of metabolic control in diabetic pregnancy. In *Size at Birth. Ciba Foundation Symposium 27* (Ed.) Elliott, K. & Knight, J. pp. 247–273. Amsterdam: Associated Scientific Publishers.

Persson, B. (1975) Glucose tolerance test in the newborn. *Carbohydrate Metabolism During Pregnancy and in the Newborn* (Ed.) Sutherland, H. & Stowers, J. p. 106. Edinburgh: Churchill Livingstone.

Picard, C., Ooms, H. A., Balsse, E. & Conrad, V. (1968) Effect of normal pregnancy on glucose assimilation, insulin and non-esterified fatty acid levels. *Diabetologia*, **4**, 16–19.

Picon, L. (1967) Effect of insulin on growth and biochemical composition of the rat fetus. *Endocrinology*, **81**, 1419–1421.

Pictet, R. & Rutter, W. J. (1972) Development of embryonic endocrine pancreas. In *Handbook of Physiology; Endocrinology; Endocrine Pancreas* (Ed.) Steiner, D. F. & Freinkel, N. pp. 25–66.

Pildes, R. S., Hart, R. J., Warner, R. & Cornblath, M. (1969) Plasma insulin responses during oral glucose tolerance test in newborn of normal and gestational diabetic mothers. *Paediatrics*, **44**, 76–83.

Raivo, K. O. & Teramo, K. (1968) Blood glucose of the human fetus prior to and during labour. *Acta Paediatrica Scandinavica*, **57**, 512–516.

Rastogi, G. K., Letartre, J. & Fraser, T. R. (1970) Immunoreactive insulin content of 203 pancreases from healthy mothers. *Diabetologia*, **6**, 445–446.

Reitano, G., Grasso, S., Distefano, G. & Messina, A. (1971) The serum insulin and growth hormone response to arginine and to arginine with glucose in the premature infant. *Journal of Clinical Endocrinology and Metabolism*, **33**, 924–928.

Robb, P. (1961) The development of the islets of Langerhans in the human foetus. *Quarterly Journal of Experimental Physiology*, **46**, 335–343.

Rosenlöcher, K. (1932) Die Veranderungen des Pankreas in der Schwangerschaft bei Mensch und Tier. *Archiv für Gynäkologie*, **151**, 567.

Salazar, H., McAulay, M. A., Charles, D. & Paido, M. (1969) The human hypophysis in anencephaly. 1. Ultrastructure of the pars distalis. *Archives of Pathology*, **87**, 201.

Saudek, C. D., Finkowski, M. & Knopp, R. H. (1975) Plasma glucagon and insulin in rat pregnancy. *Journal of Clinical Investigation*, **55**, 180–187.

Schwartz, R. (1968) Metabolic fuels in the foetus. *Proceedings of the Royal Society of Medicine*, **61**, 1231–1236.

Shah, M. P. K. & Farquhar, J. W. (1975) Children of diabetic mothers: subsequent weight. In *Early Diabetes in Early Life* (Ed.) Camerini-Davalos, & Cole, H. S. p. 587. New York: Academic Press.

Shelley, H. J., Bassett, J. M. & Milner, R. D. G. (1975) Control of carbohydrate metabolism in the fetus and the newborn. *British Medical Bulletin*, **31**, 37–43.

Smith, B. T., Giroud, C. P. J., Robert, M. & Avery, M. E. (1975) Insulin antagonism of cortisol action on lecithin synthesis by cultured fetal lung cells. *Journal of Pediatrics*, **87**, 953–955.

Spellacy, W. N. (1969) Human placental lactogen (HPL): The review of protein hormone important to obstetrics and gynaecology. *Southern Medical Journal*, **62**, 1054–1057.

Spellacy, W. N. (1971) Insulin and growth hormone measurements in normal and high risk pregnancies. In *Fetal Evaluation During Pregnancy and Labor* (Ed.) Crosignani, P. G. & Pardi, G. p. 110. New York: Academic Press.

Spellacy, W. N. & Cohn, J. E. (1973) Human placental lactogen levels and daily insulin requirements in patients with diabetes mellitus complicating pregnancy. *Obstetrics and Gynecology*, **42**, 330–333.

Spellacy, W. N. & Goetz, F. C. (1963) Plasma insulin in normal late pregnancy. *New England Journal of Medicine*, **268**, 988.

Sperling, M. A., Phelps, D., Delmater, D. V., Fisher, R. H. & Fisher, D. A. (1973) Islet cell function in the human newborn. *Pediatric Research*, **7**, 407.

Steinke, J. & Driscoll, G. G. (1965) The extractable insulin content of pancreas from fetuses and infants of diabetic and control mothers. *Diabetes*, **14**, 573–578.

Szabo, A. J. (1975) Fetal adipose tissue development: relationship to maternal free fatty acid levels. In *Early Diabetes in Early Life* (Ed.) Camerini-Davalos, R. & Cole, H. S. pp. 167–176. New York: Academic Press.

Szabo, A. J., Grimaldi, R. D. & Jung, W. F. (1969) Palmitate transport across perfused human placenta. *Metabolism*, **18**, 406–415.

Thomas, K., de Gasparo, M. & Hoet, J. J. (1967) Insulin levels in the umbilical vein and in the umbilical artery of newborns of normal and gestational diabetic mothers. *Diabetologia*, **3**, 299–304.

Unger, R. H. & Orci, L. (1975) The essential role of glucagon in the pathogenesis of diabetes mellitus. *Lancet*, **i**, 14–16.

Van Assche, F. A. (1968) A morphological study of the Langerhans islets of the fetal pancreas in late pregnancy. *Biologia Neonatorum*, **12**, 331–342.

Van Assche, F. A. (1970) *The Fetal Endocrine Pancreas. A Quantitative Morphologic Approach*. Thesis, Faculty of Medicine, Katholieke Universiteit Leuven.

Van Assche, F. A. (1971) Quantitative histology of the pancreas in decapitated and normal rat fetuses. *Hormone and Metabolic Research*, **3**, 285–286.

Van Assche, F. A. (1974) Quantitative morphologic and histoenzymatic study of the endocrine pancreas in non-pregnant and pregnant rats. *American Journal of Obstetrics and Gynecology*, **118**, 39–41.

Van Assche, F. A. (1975) The fetal endocrine pancreas. pp. 68–82, In *Carbohydrate Metabolism in Pregnancy and Newborn* (Ed.) Sutherland, H. & Stowers, J. pp. 68–82. Edinburgh: Churchill Livingstone.

Van Assche, F. A. & Aerts, L. (1975) Light and electron microscopic study of the endocrine pancreas of the rat during normal pregnancy and during diabetic pregnancy. *Diabetologia*, **11**, 381–289.

Van Assche, F. A. & Gepts, W. (1971) The cytological composition of the fetal endocrine pancreas. *Diabetologia*, **6**, 434–444.

Van Assche, F. A., Gepts, W. & de Gasparo, M. (1969) The endocrine pancreas in anencephalics. *Biologia Neonatorum*, **14**, 374–388.

Van Assche, F. A., Gepts, W., de Gasparo, M. & Renaer, M. (1970) The endocrine pancreas in erythroblastosis fetalis. *Biologia Neonatorum*, **15**, 176.

Van Beeck, C. (1939) Kan men aan een doodgeborene de diagnose diabetes mellitus der moeder stellen? *Nederlands Tijdschrift voor Geneeskunde*, **83**, 5973–5979.

Wessels, N. K. (1964) DNA synthesis, mitosis and differentiation in pancreatic acinar cells in vitro. *Journal of Cell Biology*, **20**, 415–433.

Westphal, O. A. (1967) Growth hormone levels in full-term normal infants, infants of diabetic mothers and in premature infants. *Acta Paediatrica Scandinavica*, Supplement **177**, 76–77.

Woolf, N. & Jackson, W. P. U. (1957) Maternal prediabetes and the foetal pancreas. *Journal of Pathology and Bacteriology*, **74**, 223–224.

8

THE FETUS OF THE DIABETIC

R. W. Beard and N. W. Oakley

Diabetes is a disease of particular interest as far as fetal development is concerned for it results in a naturally occurring disturbance of homeostasis that is variable but persistent throughout the whole of pregnancy. The exact cause of the fetal complications associated with the disease is not fully understood. Any disturbance of maternal metabolic homeostasis is liable to interfere with fetal development, which may well explain why untreated diabetes is associated in pregnancy with an increased incidence of abortion, fetal abnormality and perinatal mortality. Likewise, until shown otherwise, it is reasonable to assume that it is the disturbance of maternal carbohydrate metabolism that is most likely to be responsible for the tendency to fetal macrosomia, hypoglycaemia in the newborn and even some instances of fetal death in diabetic pregnancy.

In recent years there has been a dramatic improvement in the prognosis for the fetus and newborn of the diabetic mother. The reason for this improvement is not fully understood although it is probably due to improved medical management during pregnancy. In this chapter some aspects of what is known of normal and abnormal fetal metabolism and how the application of this knowledge can be applied to the care of the fetus of the diabetic will be discussed.

INCIDENCE OF DIABETES

In the community

In recent years attempts have been made throughout the world to determine the prevalence of diabetes. In the absence of any truly validated definition of diabetes, it can only be stated that prevalence rates vary widely between different racial and socioeconomic groups. If carbohydrate intolerance is defined as a two-hour oral glucose tolerance test (OGTT) value of more than 7.6 mmol/l (120 mg/100 ml) then the prevalence in Caucasian subjects in the USA and Britain may be as high as 15 per cent. This compares with a value of one to three per cent for individuals with definite diabetes (two-hour OGTT value greater than 11.1 mmol/l (200 mg/100 ml)).

Among pregnant women

Chemical (gestational) diabetes probably occurs in one to two per cent of pregnancies and overt diabetes in 0.1 to 0.2 per cent. The diabetogenic effect of pregnancy is thus more than counterbalanced by the youth of pregnant women, diabetes being largely a disease of the elderly. The appearance of carbohydrate intolerance for the first time in pregnancy is important for it may (1) persist after pregnancy, (2) reappear in a worse form in subsequent pregnancies, or (3) develop into clinical diabetes in later life. O'Sullivan et al (1966) reported that in a group of women studied for 15 years after pregnancy, 35 per cent of those in whom chemical diabetes was first detected in pregnancy subsequently developed clinical diabetes, as compared with two per cent in a control group.

FETAL COMPLICATIONS OF MATERNAL DIABETES

Perinatal mortality

Before the discovery of insulin, a viable pregnancy was unusual amongst young women who were fortunate enough to become pregnant. Relative infertility and abortion were common, while the perinatal mortality was high amongst women who reached the last three months of pregnancy. Joslin (1923) reported a fetal mortality of 44 per cent amongst a group of 108 personally supervised diabetics. The subsequent history of the disease has been fascinating

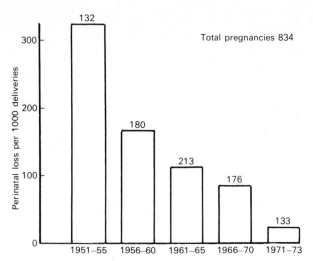

Figure 8.1. Distribution of perinatal mortality at King's College Hospital, London, 1951 to 1973. From Essex et al (1973) with kind permission of the authors and the editor of *British Medical Journal.*

because of the steady improvement in the prognosis for mother and fetus. This is well illustrated by the figures from King's College Hospital, London (Essex et al, 1973) shown in Figure 8.1.

Congenital abnormalities of the fetus

There is now little doubt from careful studies done in several centres (see Table 8.1) that there is a higher incidence of congenital abnormalities amongst infants of diabetic as compared with normal mothers. It can be seen that the overall incidence of abnormalities in both Copenhagen studies is three times that of a control group and slightly less than in the two British studies. The main source of the increase is amongst those infants with major defects. There is a striking similarity between the studies in the high incidence of major defects, many of which were fatal. The fact that these studies were done at a time when perinatal mortality was falling, the improvement being ascribed to better diabetic control in pregnancy, reveals that the problem of congenital abnormalities amongst diabetics is far from resolved.

There is considerable variation in the incidence of congenital abnormalities and one can only speculate on the possible causes for this. The actual care with which abnormalities are looked for plays an important part in the final reported incidence. It seems likely that in all the studies referred to, considerable care was taken to examine the infants at birth so that one must accept the difference in incidence as real. Yssing (1975) has recently reported that the incidence of abnormalities increases if the infants of diabetic mothers are followed up for several years after birth. If this is so, then the overall incidence of abnormalities associated with the disease is likely to be considerably higher than is currently recognised.

No specific defect is peculiar to diabetes, although Pedersen (1967) reported a higher incidence of congenital heart disease and severe skeletal deformity which Watson (1972) confirmed from data obtained at King's College Hospital. Both Yssing (1975) and Bibergeil (1975) have reported an increased incidence of neurological defect in the children of diabetic mothers. In the former series, neurological defects were found almost exclusively amongst growth-retarded babies born to mothers with a long history of diabetes. Bibergeil, on the

Table 8.1. *Summary of studies of congenital abnormalities occurring among the infants of diabetic mothers compared with a control group.*

| Study | Number | Malformations (per cent) | | |
		Major	Minor	Total
Pedersen, Tygstrup and Pedersen (1964)				
Diabetic	864	5.2 (2.1)	1.2	6.4
Normal	1212	1.2 (0.3)	0.9	2.1
Watson (1972)				
Diabetic	240			9.6
Normal	220			5.9
Pedersen (1975)				
Diabetic	1332	6.1 (2.4)	1.9	8.0
Normal	8789	1.6 (0.4)	1.2	2.8
Malins (1975)				
Diabetic	205	7.6 (4.4)	5.0	12.6
Normal	205	0 (0)	5.7	5.7

Figures in brackets refer to incidence of fetal malformations.

other hand, found evidence of intellectual impairment in schoolchildren that was not specifically related to the severity of the disease in the mother.

Little advance has been made in our understanding of how diabetes can give rise to developmental anomalies of the fetus since Pedersen reviewed the subject in 1967. The reason for this is undoubtedly on the one hand the laborious and time-consuming nature of epidemiological studies which must relate data collected in pregnancy to the behaviour of the offspring many years later, while on the other hand no suitable animal model is available which faithfully reproduces the metabolic disturbance that typifies diabetes in humans. A likely hypothesis is that the disturbance of metabolic homeostasis, which is the main feature of diabetes, results in an unfavourable environment for the developing embryo.

Fetal macrosomia and growth retardation

Many factors play a part in determining the size of a baby at birth (see Size at Birth, 1974) For this reason it is unwise to place too much emphasis on birthweight as an index of the effect of diabetes on the fetus.

Three types of fetal growth pattern are observed in diabetic pregnancy—excessive, normal and retarded. The overweight fetus (> 90th percentile) with a bloated appearance is so typical of diabetes that two babies of different diabetic mothers could be mistaken for identical twins. There has been much debate about the total body composition of these babies because of the clue such information could provide as to the cause of macrosomia. Pedersen in Copenhagen has been interested in this subject for many years and Table 8.2 is a summary of the findings of Osler (1965) working in his department. It can be seen that the mean weight of the babies of diabetic mothers, although the duration of pregnancy was only 37 weeks, was similar to the weight of the babies from non-diabetic mothers who were at term. The babies of the diabetics tended to be longer than the control babies, suggesting some skeletal overgrowth, but most noticeable is the excess of adipose tissue, muscle and bone thickness being unaffected. These data suggest that a growth-stimulating factor which specifically in-

Table 8.2. *Body composition of babies of diabetic mothers compared with control group of babies of non-diabetic mothers matched for gestation (group 1) and weight (group 2).*

	Infants of diabetic mothers	Infants of non-diabetic mothers Control 1	Control 2
Gestational age (days)	259	259	279
Birthweight (g)	3350	2700	3300
Length at birth (CR) (cm)	51.2	49.0	51.9
Subcutaneous fat thickness (mm)	11.2	7.5	8.1
Muscle thickness (mm)	16.1	16.0	17.7
Bone thickness (mm)	8.2	8.5	9.5

Adapted from Osler (1965) with kind permission of the author and the publisher (Amsterdam: Excerpta Medica).

creases fat deposits, such as insulin, could be responsible. In support of this view there is a considerable body of evidence (see Chapter 7) that the macrosomic fetus of the diabetic has hypertrophy of the pancreatic β-cells and hyperinsulinaemia, the significance of which will be discussed later in this chapter.

Fetal growth retardation is thought to be caused by diabetic angiopathy affecting the blood supply to the uterus, because it is seen most commonly amongst women with longstanding and complicated diabetes. This condition has not been investigated well enough to know whether these fetuses have hyperinsulinism. It is a question of some interest in view of the possible role of fetal insulin as a growth-promoting factor (Liggins, 1974).

Women with a mild form of diabetes or with well-controlled diabetes usually have babies whose weights fall within the normal weight for gestation range (10 to 90th percentile). The fact that treatment with insulin reduces the weight of babies has been confirmed in numerous studies both in severe (Pedersen, 1967; Oakley and Peel, 1968) and in very mild diabetes (O'Sullivan, Charles and Dandrow, 1971). The variability of treatment regimes between centres is such that it is not possible to generalise about the factors influencing the weight of the fetus of a diabetic mother. All that can be said is that with earlier diagnosis, the more liberal use of insulin for milder forms of the disease, and stricter control of the severe diabetic, the incidence of overweight babies has diminished. Persson (1974) notes that, in series published in 1953 by Lund and Weese and in 1970 by Morison, approximately one-third of the babies weighed more than 4000 g. In a more recent comparable series of 107 diabetic pregnancies published by Persson the incidence was only 19 per cent.

EFFECT OF DIABETES ON THE FETUS

The exact mechanism whereby growth of the fetus of the diabetic is affected is still a matter for speculation, but it seems likely that changes in the transplacental passage of substrates constitute the primary abnormality.

Carbohydrates (Figure 8.2)

Pedersen, Bojsen-Møller and Poulsen (1954) suggested that prolonged exposure of the fetus to hyperglycaemia (originating in the mother) triggers the normally quiescent fetal pancreatic β-cells into functional activity. This in turn leads to deposition of excessive amounts

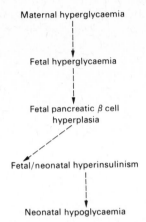

Maternal hyperglycaemia

Fetal hyperglycaemia

Fetal pancreatic β cell
hyperplasia

Fetal/neonatal hyperinsulinism

Neonatal hypoglycaemia

Figure 8.2. Maternal hyperglycaemia in fetal hyperinsulinism theory. Courtesy of Dr J. Pedersen.

of glycogen and conversion of glucose to triglycerides, thus increasing fetal adipose tissue. The evidence in favour of this theory is discussed in more detail in Chapter 7 and has also recently been reviewed by Pedersen (1975). The effect of diabetes on the pancreas is revealed histologically by β-cell hyperplasia, and biologically by the hyperinsulinaemia in umbilical cord and fetal scalp blood. The likely involvement of fetal insulin as the cause of excessive growth is suggested by the diminished growth of pancreatomised fetuses and of anencephalics with reduced pancreatic β-cell activity associated with an absent hypothalamic–pituitary system. This subject has been well reviewed by Adam (1971) and Milner, Leach and Jack (1975).

The weakness of the Pedersen theory lies in the fact that the weight of babies of diabetic mothers does not correlate well with estimations of mean maternal blood glucose during pregnancy (Karlsson and Kjellmer, 1972). In itself this evidence does not exclude the possibility that hyperinsulinism is the cause of fetal macrosomia as it is difficult to assess the mean glucose level to which any fetus is exposed during a particular pregnancy. Moreover, it may be that the surges of maternal blood glucose are more important than the mean concentration. Looked at in another way, if fetal insulin is an important cause of macrosomia, then it should have some relationship to fetal weight. Gillmer et al (1975a, 1975b) compared insulin concentration in the newborn two hours after birth with birthweight, but the correlation failed to reach a level of statistical significance possibly due to the small numbers of patients studied. Finally, before the Pedersen theory can be proven it is necessary to demonstrate that the fetus converts glucose to triglycerides, possibly as a means of disposing of excess glucose. Work in this area on animals may well not be applicable to man as important species differences in the conversion of glucose to free fatty acids (FFAs) by the liver and adipose tissue are known to exist. This is a subject that needs further investigation in the human fetus.

Lipids

In 1974 Szabo and Szabo suggested that the poor correlation between birthweight and the maternal glucose concentration in pregnancy could be explained by the transfer of excessive amounts of FFA from mother to fetus. This implies that fetal hyperinsulinaemia is not an essential prerequisite for the development of macrosomia of the fetus of the diabetic. The

Szabos' suggestion is attractive because FFAs can cross the placenta for use by the fetus as a source of energy. Moreover, plasma FFA levels are known to be increased in untreated diabetic pregnancy. The fact that insulin suppresses the lipogenic response of the diabetic mother, thus lowering the concentration of FFAs in the circulation, may be an explanation for the reduction in birthweight that follows the use of insulin in pregnancy. It is thus possible that both hyperlipidaemia and hyperglycaemia are contributory factors to the development of fetal macrosomia in diabetic pregnancy. However if, as the Szabos state, their theory provides an explanation for fetal macrosomia occurring in the absence of maternal hyperglycaemia, then it is necessary to demonstrate that hyperlipidaemia precedes the appearance of carbohydrate intolerance.

METABOLIC CONSIDERATIONS

Until recently much of the knowledge of fetal metabolism that was available was inferred from studies on immature fetuses delivered by hysterotomy, mature babies studied after the stress of delivery and on the newborn. Stress, either from the operative procedure or the change from the uterine to the external environment was a complication that made it impossible to be certain that the results were relevant to intra-uterine life. Equally, chronic catheter studies on animals such as the sheep and monkey, despite the advantage that the fetal environment is undisturbed, are of limited application to man because of species differences. In recent years the technique for collecting capillary blood from the scalp of the fetus has made possible the study of interrelationships between mother and fetus in their natural environment. By careful selection it is possible to study patients before the onset of labour, the only disturbance to the fetus being the rupture of the amniotic sac and the small incision into the skin of the fetal scalp.

An essential prerequisite for understanding the abnormal metabolic changes resulting from diabetes is a knowledge of the normal physiology. Equally it is impossible to interpret changes in the fetus without simultaneous study of the mother. Studies of this kind are still in their infancy because of the problems that are always encountered in human research, particularly when the fetus is involved. Thus it is important for the reader to recognise that while a number of questions have been answered, there are many posed by the data obtained that remain unanswered.

Placental transfer

The fetus is dependent on the mother for its nutrient supply and as a means of disposing of its waste products. Pregnancy leads to a preferential transfer of energy-yielding substrates from mother to fetus. Some of the more important pathways are shown in Figure 8.3. Associated with the drain of maternal energy products are hormonal changes which mobilise nutrients for the fetus at the expense of the mother, leading to what Freinkel (1965) has described as 'a state of accelerated starvation'. This is characterised by the metabolic changes associated with conversion from a glucose-utilising economy to one dependent on the catabolism of fat and protein. Triglycerides represent a particularly valuable form of stored energy to the mother as the placenta is impermeable to the large lipoprotein molecules. The triglyceride content of maternal lipoprotein increases during pregnancy, and fasting of the pregnant woman soon leads to ketonaemia as available glucose stores are exhausted and fat is

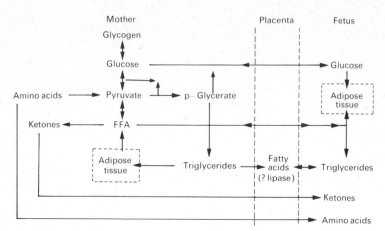

Figure 8.3. Diagram of placental transfer of energy-yielding substrates.

mobilised. Amino acids are also mobilised during pregnancy both for transfer to the fetus and as maternal glucose precursors.

If the fetus is to be preferentially supplied with nutrients by the mother it is vital that the placenta should be able to transfer energy-yielding substrates. It is evident from Figure 8.3 that glucose, amino acids, FFAs and ketones cross to the fetus. The transport of fats and amino acids is discussed in detail in Chapters 4, 5 and 6.

Glucose concentration in the normal (non-diabetic) pregnancy

In humans, unlike some animal species such as the sheep, the maternal–fetal (M–F) glucose relationship is normally close (Coltart et al, 1969), the M–F concentration difference under fasting conditions being only about 0.4 mmol/l (8 mg/100 ml of plasma). As the maternal hyperglycaemia increases, the fetal glucose concentration follows, remaining slightly below that of the mother, so that one may conclude that the fetal plasma glucose is dependent on the maternal concentration. As the latter rises the M–F difference remains small until a concentration of 10 to 12 mmol/l is reached, at which point the placental transport system is saturated and the fetal concentration will rise no further. The phenomenon, which is a characteristic of transport by facilitated diffusion, is not peculiar to man, having been observed in the guinea-pig by Krauer, Joyce and Young (1973). This finding is consistent with the observation that a change from poor to only fair control of diabetes is associated with little improvement in fetal loss, whereas the institution of very strict control has resulted in a perinatal mortality which is only slightly above that of the non-diabetic obstetric population.

Glucose concentration in the diabetic patient

The major difference between the normal and diabetic M–F glucose relationship is seen under fasting conditions (Figure 8.4). When the mother has diabetes the fasting fetal glucose values tend to be lower while the maternal values are higher than those found in normal pregnancy; the mean concentration difference among gestational diabetics being 1.5 mmol/l

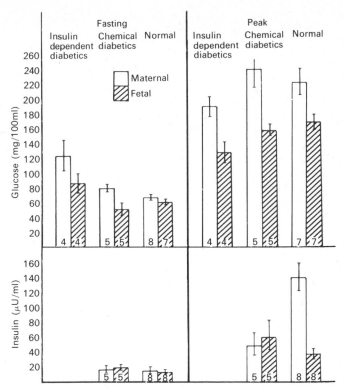

Figure 8.4. Histograms showing the relationship between the mean maternal and fetal concentrations of glucose in normal and diabetic patients (i) under fasting conditions and (ii) at peak levels of hyperglycaemia. Numbers at the bases of columns indicate size of study group. From Oakley, Beard and Turner (1972) with kind permission of the editor of *British Medical Journal*.

(27 mg/100 ml) as compared with 0.44 mmol/l (8 mg/100 ml) in normal pregnancies. Even under fasting conditions the fetus of the diabetic is relatively hyperinsulinaemic compared with the normal fetus, and it may well be that the increased metabolism and uptake of glucose consequent upon the fetal endogenous hyperinsulinism is sufficient to account for the greater M–F concentration difference in diabetic pregnancy. *This implies some ability on the part of the fetus to alter its own plasma glucose concentration in response to the prevailing glucose load, possibly by the secretion of insulin* (see also Chapter 9).

Placental transfer of other substances

Studies in man and numerous animal species have failed to demonstrate the transfer of insulin in either direction across the placenta (Adam, 1971). From a teleological point of view it would be surprising if insulin did cross the placenta, for glucose homeostasis by free equilibration with a large closely regulated maternal pool is a perfectly efficient method of maintaining a physiological fetal glucose level without participation of the fetal pancreas. Insulin can be regarded as a hormone evolved for maximum efficiency in a 'feast-and-fast' economy, quite unlike the situation of continuous substrate infusion that prevails in the fetus.

These comments also apply to other glucogenic hormones such as glucagon which does not cross from mother to fetus (Johnston et al, 1972). Human placental lactogen which is an insulin antagonist does not cross into the fetal circulation.

Fetal insulin response to glucose

Normal. Under fasting conditions Oakley, Beard and Turner (1972) found that the plasma immunoreactive insulin concentration of the fetus (12.7 µu/ml) is usually a little lower than that of the mother (15.1 µu/ml). The β-cells of the fetal pancreas contain insulin granules from as early as ten weeks gestation and the fact that insulin is present in the plasma at this stage of pregnancy is indicative of some secretory ability. It is not known whether the fetal pancreas ever becomes capable of responding to an acute glucose challenge such as occurs after a meal. Studies of the mature fetus of the non-diabetic mother suggest that it never develops an insulin response of such magnitude as the adult although the pattern of response, which may be biphasic or monophasic, is the same (Figure 8.5).

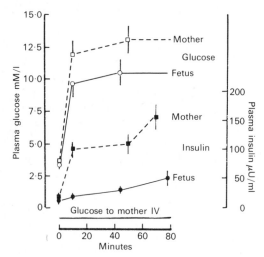

Figure 8.5. Effect of maternal glucose infusion on plasma glucose and insulin in seven normal pregnant women between 40 and 42 weeks gestation. From Oakley, Beard and Turner (1972) with kind permission of the editor of *British Medical Journal.*

Diabetic. Studies on the insulin response of the fetus of the diabetic have been limited to mild cases of diabetes not requiring insulin because of the interference with the measurement of insulin by antibodies which cross the placenta. Under fasting conditions the fetal concentration is variable and quite often the concentration is higher in the fetus than in the mother. Oakley, Beard and Turner (1972) reported mean values of 15.9 µu/ml in mothers with mild chemical diabetes and 19.2 µu/ml in their fetuses. Equally, the fetal insulin response to glucose loading is variable, the increase ranging from 20 to 900 per cent (Figure 8.6).

Although no close relationship between the M–F glucose differences and the concentration of insulin in fetal plasma has been found, the increased M–F gradient both under fasting conditions and during hyperglycaemia comparable to that produced in normal subjects may well be caused by endogenous hyperinsulinism. Glucose utilisation is dependent not only on the prevailing insulin concentration but also on such undetermined factors as the influence of insulin receptor sites.

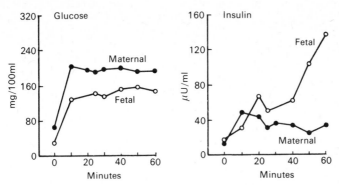

igure 8.6. Effect of maternal glucose infusion on plasma glucose and insulin in a woman with chemical diabetes ¹t 38 weeks gestation. From Oakley, Beard and Turner (1972) with kind permission of the editor of *British Medical Journal.*

ʾetal growth hormone

tudies on immature and mature fetuses (Turner, Schneelock and Paterson, 1971; Turner, ᴅakley and Beard, 1973) suggest that the response and regulation of growth hormone secre-ᵗion is similar to that of the adult. The mean growth hormone of the mature fetus of non-ᵈiabetic mothers was 32 ng/ml (range 11 to 59 ng/ml). The fetus of the diabetic mother ᵈiffered from the normal in having a significantly higher mean value of 47 ng/ml, and a ᵍreater depression of concentration when glucose was administered. It may be that growth ʰormone as an insulin antagonist plays some part in limiting the fetal hypoglycaemia ᵉsulting from endogenous hyperinsulinism and that fluctuating glucose levels in the fetus of a ᵈiabetic stimulate maturation of the normal pituitary response to hyperglycaemia earlier than ʰormal.

ᴹetabolic changes in the mother

ᵀhe importance of changes in concentrations of glucose, FFAs and amino acids in pregnant ᵂomen is that they may be regarded as specific adaptations by the mother to the needs of her ᵍrowing fetus. In response to profound changes in hormonal environment, levels of some ᵗubstrates such as FFAs alter, while others, such as glucose, remain remarkably constant. ᵀhis effect is well shown in Figure 8.7, which was obtained from studies done in early and ᵃgain in late pregnancy on normal women. It shows how remarkably stable the concentra-ᵗion of glucose remains over the 24-hour period, rarely exceeding 5.5 mmol/l (100 mg/100 ᵐl) both in early and late pregnancy. In order to maintain this constancy of glucose in late ᵖregnancy, it is apparent that the pregnant woman has to secrete nearly twice as much in-ˢulin as she did in early pregnancy. A similar response can be seen following the 50 g OGTT. These findings demonstrate the additional demands that are made by pregnancy on the ᵐaternal pancreas, and it is not difficult to appreciate how any inherent tendency to ᵈiminished islet cell function will be unmasked by pregnancy, leading to a variable degree of ᶜhemical diabetes.

Chemical diabetes may develop in pregnancy as a result of inadequate insulin secretion, as ˢhown in Figure 8.8, or an increase in insulin resistance. It results not only in a higher ᵃbsolute mean diurnal glucose concentration but also greater fluctuation, particularly during ᵗhe day. Insulin-dependent diabetics rely on administered insulin to maintain euglycaemia,

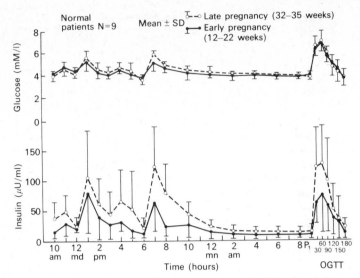

Figure 8.7. Plasma glucose and insulin concentrations during diurnal profile and oral glucose tolerance tests in nine normal (non-diabetic) women studied in early and late pregnancy. From Gillmer et al (1975a, b) with kind permission of the editor of *British Medical Journal*.

and Figure 8.9 reveals how a group of 13 pregnant diabetics, who are well controlled by modern standards, have marked fluctuations in plasma glucose during the day with a tendency to hypoglycaemia at night. Hypoglycaemia is most marked at 04.00 hours and hyperglycaemia at 10.00 hours, after breakfast. The daytime findings are virtually identical with those of Persson and Lunell (1975) who studied normal and diabetic women over an eight-hour period (08.00 to 16.00 hours) in the last three months of pregnancy.

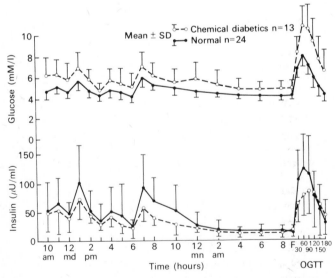

Figure 8.8. Plasma glucose and insulin concentrations during diurnal profile and oral glucose tolerance tests in 24 normal and 13 chemical diabetic women studied during the last trimester of pregnancy. From Gillmer et al (1975a, b) with kind permission of the editor of *British Medical Journal*.

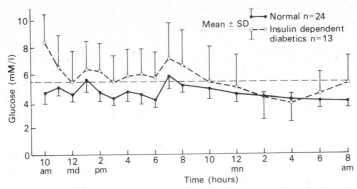

Figure 8.9. Diurnal glucose concentrations in 13 insulin-dependent diabetics and 24 women with normal glucose tolerance studied between 32 and 35 weeks of pregnancy. From Gillmer et al (1975a, b) with kind permission of the editor of *British Medical Journal*.

Persson and Lunell (1975) studied FFAs (Figure 8.10), glycerol and beta-hydroxybutyrate in the same way. They found that the concentrations of these substances are interdependent, the absolute concentration being increased amongst the diabetics. In non-diabetics the post-breakfast fall in lipid concentration was greater than in diabetics; insulin-dependent diabetics showed evidence of suppressed lipid mobilisation in the afternoon, reflecting the expected effects of administered depot insulin.

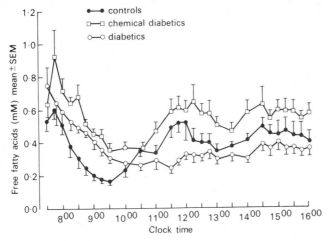

Figure 8.10. Mean free fatty acid concentration ($\pm$ s.e.m.) in healthy control, chemical diabetic and insulin dependent diabetic mothers studied over eight hours in the last three months of pregnancy. From Persson and Lunell (1975) with kind permission of the authors and the editor of *American Journal of Obstetrics and Gynecology*.

PROGNOSTIC VALUE OF GLUCOSE TOLERANCE TESTS

The diagnosis of diabetes and assessment of the severity of the disease is based on certain arbitrary limits of the glucose tolerance test, notably those of the British Diabetic Association, of Fajans and Conn (1965) in non-pregnant subjects and those of O'Sullivan and

Mahan (1964) for pregnant women. These have been well discussed by Hadden (1975
These limits have been determined in the usual manner by obtaining values from a large por
ulation and using an upper limit to distinguish between the normal and diabetic groups. Th
limitation of this approach is that it does not take into account the possibility that mino
degrees of intolerance, that would not be considered abnormal in non-pregnant subjects
may in pregnancy adversely affect the fetus. Molsted-Pedersen (1972) found that fetal weigh
showed a close positive correlation with disappearance rate of glucose not only in babies o
diabetic mothers but also in those whose mothers had, by definition, normal carbohydrat
tolerance. If pancreatic β-cell function of the baby at birth is determined solely by the car
bohydrate tolerance of the mother, then clearly we will have to look more closely at mino
deviations from normal tolerance. What is required is a test for use in pregnancy that gives th
clinician some idea of the effect the maternal diabetes is having on the fetus; but before this ca
be achieved a suitable fetal end-point is required in order to assess the significance of any suc
test.

If the Pedersen hyperglycaemia/hyperinsulinaemia theory is correct, then it would seen
reasonable to use the glucose and insulin concentration of the newborn shortly after birth a
an end-point against which to compare various indices of maternal carbohydrate tolerance
Table 8.3 summarises the results of such a comparison in which 10 chemical diabetic and 2

Table 8.3. *Correlation between maternal and newborn carbohydrate tolerance indices.*

	Neonatal incremental K	Neonatal plasma glucose at 2 hours
Oral glucose tolerance test		
total area	0.678[a]	−0.690[a]
2-hour glucose	0.593[a]	−0.620[a]
incremental index	0.571[a]	−0.591[a]
Diurnal plasma glucose		
mean 24-hour	0.456[b]	−0.409[c]
mean daytime	0.473[b]	−0.451[b]
peak values	0.502[b]	−0.513[b]
range over 24 hours	0.444[c]	−0.471[b]

From Gillmer et al (1975a, b) with kind permission of the editor of *British Medical Journal.*

[a] $p < 0.001$.
[b] $p < 0.005$.
[c] $p < 0.05$.

normal women were studied. The neonatal incremental K value (McCann et al, 1966) is a
measure of glucose assimilation by the newborn in the first two hours after birth. The maternal index that best identified babies with a two-hour plasma glucose of < 1.78 mmol/l (30
mg/100 ml), all of whom had elevated plasma insulin levels, was the total area of a three-hour
OGTT of more than 45 area units using mmol/l of glucose (800 using mg/100 ml). Although
correlation of the two-hour OGTT value was nearly as good, the scatter of individual values
was much greater, making it definitely inferior as a predictive indicator of the effect of
diabetes on the baby. These results lend support to the hyperglycaemia/hyperinsulinaemia
theory, but it is still not possible to say what function of glucose metabolism triggers the fetal
pancreas into premature activity. Grasso (1973) has shown that the pancreas of premature

newborn babies can be sensitised by exposure to a glucose infusion with a concentration as low as 6.1 mmol/1 (110 mg/100 ml) for up to two hours. A comparison of diurnal plasma glucose results with the metabolic performances of the newborn of both normal and mildly diabetic women suggests that the peak glucose values in the 24-hour period correlate best with the subsequent disposal of glucose by the newborn—the higher the peak in the mother the more rapid the fall of glucose in the newborn immediately after birth (Gillmer et al, 1975a, 1975b). When this finding is viewed in conjunction with the fact that an artificial challenge like the glucose tolerance test also correlates well with the metabolic performance of the fetus, it may well be that the 'variability' of maternal glucose rather than the basal concentration of glucose is the critical factor in determining whether fetal hyperinsulinism develops or not. Thus, intermittent surges of hyperglycaemia in diabetic mothers after meals or consequent upon poor diabetic control may be a more important determinant of whether fetal hyperinsulinism develops or not than the mean concentration of glucose to which the fetus is exposed.

The limitation of this whole approach is that the ability to predict whether a fetus will develop endogenous hyperinsulinism does not necessarily mean that all the other fetal and neonatal complications can be equally well predicted pari passu. An alternative approach to the use of the total area of a glucose tolerance test as a predictive indicator is the insulin response to a glucose load. Recently Edstrom and Thalme (1975) have reported that infants of mothers with a normal glucose tolerance test but a low insulin response ('low insulin responders') are liable to develop chemical diabetes at a later stage of pregnancy and also to have large babies. This is an important observation for it may provide the clue that will enable clinicians to detect 'prediabetes'.

CAUSES OF PERINATAL DEATH

It has been said that fetal and neonatal deaths in diabetic pregnancy cannot be ascribed to any single cause. However, certain types of death are peculiar to diabetes and if they are to be prevented it is important to describe the particular clinical features of these deaths.

The pattern of perinatal death is illustrated in a study by Evans et al (1972) in Melbourne who reported on a series of 93 pregnant diabetics, most of whom were insulin-requiring. There were 12 perinatal deaths (perinatal mortality 130 per thousand deliveries) of whom four were fetal and eight neonatal. Two of the fetuses which died had evidence of placental insufficiency for some time before death, and two died unexpectedly in the manner classically associated with diabetes. All eight babies who died after birth, of whom six were premature, developed fetal respiratory distress.

Placental insufficiency

Placental insufficiency occurs most commonly in women with severe diabetes of long standing, often with evidence of vascular complications. The management of these patients is the same as for any case of fetal growth retardation, that is, by serial biparietal cephalometry and oestriol measurements followed by premature delivery if there is evidence of serious deterioration of the condition of the fetus. The determination of pulmonary function of the baby by estimating the lecithin : sphingomyelin ratio in the amniotic fluid is a valuable adjunct to management if delivery is considered before term.

Unexpected fetal death

Unexpected fetal death occurs most commonly in the poorly controlled diabetic. It is often associated with hydramnios and/or a fetus that feels large for the duration of pregnancy. The death is not typically asphyxial in origin. Not only are the baby and placenta large but the accepted tests of fetal and placental function indicate continuing growth of both the fetus and placenta (Gillmer and Beard, 1975). Two theories have been put forward to explain the deaths of these babies:

Fetal hyperglycaemia. Studies in the sheep (Shelley, Bassett and Milner, 1975) have shown that a doubling of the normal glucose concentration results in a small but definite increase in the plasma lactate of the fetus. With increasing hyperglycaemia the lactate accumulates because of the low capacity for oxidative metabolism of certain fetal tissues such as the brain and liver. Shelley has suggested that lactacidaemia is of little consequence to the well oxygenated healthy fetus but may lead to fetal death when it occurs in association with hypoxia. In man, the condition of the fetus is known to deteriorate if the fetus is exposed to prolonged or excessive hyperglycaemia (Anderson, Cordero and Hon, 1970). It may be that the fetus of the diabetic is at risk from this condition, although fetal hypoxia is no more common in diabetic than normal pregnancies.

Fetal hypoglycaemia. Hypoglycaemia is only of consequence to the newborn if it is profound and prolonged, when it may lead to death from brain damage. The fetus is normally plentifully supplied with glucose by the mother, so that hypoglycaemia at first sight appears as an unlikely cause of death. However, recent evidence, already referred to, does suggest that under certain conditions the fetus may be subjected to severe hypoglycaemia. Diurnal studies on pregnant diabetic mothers have shown that on occasions, particularly in the early hours of the morning, blood glucose may fall as low as 2 mmol/l (36 mg/100 ml). In view of this and also the observation that when the mother is fasting the fetus of the diabetic may become hypoglycaemic, it may be that occasionally the combination of maternal hypoglycaemia and fetal hyperinsulinism leads to profound fetal hypoglycaemia resulting in intra-uterine death. Unfortunately there are no histological studies available on the brain of macrosomic stillbirths of diabetic mothers to test this hypothesis. However, there is sufficient evidence from studies of pregnant diabetics to show that nocturnal hypoglycaemia is common and should be avoided if possible.

Respiratory distress of the newborn

It is generally thought that the newborn of the diabetic tends to be more deficient in pulmonary surfactant than the normal baby. Gluck and Kulovich (1973) found that lecithin appeared earlier than normal in the amniotic fluid of severe diabetics. Usher, Allen and McLean (1971) have questioned this concept by ascribing the high incidence of respiratory distress amongst infants of diabetics to the tendency of obstetricians to deliver diabetics prematurely by caesarean section. Tchobroutsky (personal communication, 1975) has demonstrated that lecithin appears in the amniotic fluid of treated diabetics at the same time and in the same quantities as in normals.

Hypoglycaemia, hypocalcaemia and hyperbilirubinaemia

These are occasional causes of neonatal death which can be avoided if the paediatrician is aware that they are complications of diabetic pregnancy.

Congenital abnormalities

Congenital abnormalities are significant and persistent causes of intra-uterine or neonatal death.

PROBLEMS OF MANAGEMENT OF THE PREGNANT DIABETIC

Management is a subject that has been dealt with exhaustively in obstetric textbooks and which has been summarised by Brudenell (1975). However, because of the paucity of information about the fetus of the diabetic, a relatively empirical approach has been adopted towards certain aspects of obstetric and diabetic management which will be reviewed in the light of recent work, some of which has been described in this chapter.

Reducing the incidence of congenital defects

Although the cause of congenital defects associated with diabetes is not known with certainty, it seems likely that the abnormal metabolic environment of the embryo at the time of implantation and in the first three months of pregnancy is an important factor. If this is so, then clearly it is important that the diabetic state is well controlled at the time of conception. To achieve this it is necessary for young women who are diabetic to be educated about the importance of planning their pregnancies. They should consult their physicians as soon as they stop contraception so that a treatment regime can be planned to ensure that the diabetes is well under control both at the time of conception and during the early weeks of pregnancy.

Early detection of diabetes in pregnancy

Screening for diabetes should become one of the routine procedures at the antenatal booking visit. Unfortunately the detection of glycosuria or the selection of potential diabetics cannot be relied upon to detect all cases of mild chemical diabetes. O'Sullivan (1975) has described a simple screening system whereby plasma glucose is estimated on a sample of blood collected one hour after 50 g oral glucose load, which does not require any preparation such as an overnight fast. A value of approximately 7.8 mmol/l (140 mg/100 ml) or more indicates the need for a full OGTT.

Regulation of diabetes

There is now a considerable body of evidence suggesting that insulin therapy, even in mild cases of chemical diabetes, reduces the incidence of fetal macrosomia. There is also direct evidence that insulin may be responsible for a reduction in perinatal mortality. Clearly it would be impracticable to advocate the use of insulin for every case of mild carbohydrate intolerance, but on the available evidence it is reasonable to propose that if it proves difficult to maintain the diurnal plasma glucose below 5.5 mmol/l (100 mg/100 ml) by diet then insulin therapy should be started. Oral hypoglycaemics have considerable advantages over insulin, but their use is not favoured in pregnancy because they cross the placenta with the likelihood of inducing fetal hyperinsulinism.

The place of the diurnal profile described by Gillmer et al (1975a, 1975b) has as yet not been established, but it seems likely that it will provide a useful yardstick to determine the effectiveness of therapy. Obviously it would be impractical to perform diurnal profiles at frequent intervals, but the occasional test would provide a useful check on the degree of control achieved over 24 hours. It should be used after regulation of the plasma glucose has been established in the usual manner by adjusting insulin dosage on the basis of four preprandial blood samples. When optimal control is attempted particular attention should be paid to (1) avoiding the post-breakfast peak by giving sufficient soluble insulin in the morning dose and (2) ensuring that nocturnal hypoglycaemia does not occur by limiting the amount of long-acting insulin given in the evening and also by providing sufficient calories overnight. Although hospitalisation in the last trimester is expensive and interferes with home life, there is no doubt that it enables the best possible degree of diabetic control to be achieved. However, such good results have been achieved by outpatient care of pregnant diabetics (Wright, Dixon and Joplin, 1968) that it should be possible to adopt a flexible policy. A sensible patient with a normal pregnancy who is well controlled may be treated as an outpatient, being seen at weekly intervals after 28 weeks from the first day of the last menstrual period. The patient whose diabetes is difficult to control or who has any abnormality of pregnancy such as fetal growth retardation, hydramnios or pre-eclamptic toxaemia should be admitted until delivery.

Delivery

It has been the practice in many centres to advocate caesarean section for all but those with the mildest form of diabetes, despite the fact that Spellacy (1972) demonstrated that perinatal mortality was the same regardless of whether the baby was delivered vaginally or by caesarean section. Nevertheless, fetal distress occurs more commonly amongst diabetics and if vaginal delivery is to be undertaken fetal monitoring must be used. A recent report (Beard and Brudenell, 1975) showed that, between 1971 and 1973, despite the fact that the majority of diabetic patients were delivered vaginally using the protocol shown in Table 8.4, there

Table 8.4. *Outline of regime for vaginal delivery of insulin-dependent diabetics following induction of labour.*

Day of Delivery	07.00	Estimate plasma glucose.
	08.00	i.v. 8 per cent glucose infusion + $\frac{1}{5}$N saline at 300 ml/hour. i.v. 25 g glucose given stat. Half usual morning dose of insulin.
	08.30	Estimate plasma glucose.
	09.00	Rupture membranes. Apply electrode to fetal scalp. Obtain fetal blood sample for pH measurement. Insert epidural catheter. Start continuous FHR monitoring. Start i.v. oxytocin (2mu/min) by infusion pump.
	11.30	Estimate plasma glucose. Determine regime for 4-hourly soluble insulin and i.v. glucose regime, and then start regime.
	18.00	If good labour progresses and diabetes well controlled, allow labour to continue. If not, then consider delivery by caesarean section.

were no intrapartum losses. It is tempting to ascribe the improved perinatal mortality shown for these years in Figure 8.1 to vaginal delivery, but similar results have been obtained in centres with considerable experience of diabetic pregnancy, such as that of Persson in Stockholm, where caesarean section is the routine method of delivery for all but mild cases of diabetes. What the King's College Hospital results do show is that vaginal delivery can be made as safe for the diabetic as the non-diabetic.

The timing of delivery is probably of more critical importance than the route of delivery. In most centres the major perinatal problems arise in the neonatal rather than the intra-uterine period. Thus prematurity should be avoided at all costs, and every attempt should be made to wait until the lecithin content of amniotic fluid is within the limits of normal pulmonary function for the newborn. Dexamethasone may be used to improve fetal pulmonary maturation, but it should be realised that high doses of steroids increase insulin resistance leading to loss of diabetic control. It should only be administered under strict control, preferably with insulin given by continuous intravenous infusion, the dosage being adjusted according to the results of frequent glucose estimations.

REFERENCES

Adam, P. A. J. (1971) Control of glucose metabolism in the human fetus and newborn infant. In *Advances in Metabolic Disorders* (Ed.) Levine, R. & Luft, F. pp. 184–278. New York, London: Academic Press.

Anderson, G. G., Cordero, L. & Hon, E. H. (1970) Hypertonic glucose infusion during labour. *Obstetrics and Gynecology*, **36**, 405–414.

Beard, R. W. & Brudenell, J. M. (1975) Fetal monitoring in diabetic pregnancy. In *Early Diabetes in Early Life. Proceedings of the 3rd International Symposium on Early Diabetes, Madeira, 1974* (Ed.) Camarini-Davalos, R. A. In press.

Bibergeil, H. (1975) Complications arising from diabetes in human pregnancy. In *Early Diabetes in Early Life. Proceedings of the 3rd International Symposium on Early Diabetes, Madeira, 1974* (Ed.) Camarini-Davalos, R. A. In Press.

Brudenell, J. M. (1975) Care of the clinical diabetic woman in pregnancy and labour. In *Carbohydrate Metabolism in Pregnancy and the Newborn* (Ed.) Sutherland, H. W. & Stowers, J. M. pp. 221–229. London: Churchill-Livingstone.

Brudenell, J. M. & Beard, R. W. (1972) Diabetes in pregnancy. In *Clinics in Endocrinology and Metabolism*, Vol. 1, No. 3 (Ed.) Pyke, D. pp. 673–695. London: W. B. Saunders.

Coltart, T. M., Beard, R. W., Turner, R. C. & Oakley, N. W. (1969) Blood glucose and insulin relationships in the human mother and fetus before onset of labour. *British Medical Journal*, **iv**, 17–19.

Edstrom, K. & Thalme, B. (1975) Infants of mothers with a high and of mothers with a low insulin response to glucose infusion. Glucose tolerance and insulin response and clinical appearance during early neonatal period. *Journal of Perinatal Medicine*, **3**, 21–33.

Essex, N. L., Pyke, D. A., Watkins, P. J., Brudenell, J. M. & Gamsu, H. R. (1973) Diabetic pregnancy. *British Medical Journal*, **iv**, 89–93.

Evans, J. H., Taft, H. P., Rome, R. M. & Brown, J. B. (1972) Oestriol excretion in the pregnancy complicated by diabetes mellitus. *Australian and New Zealand Journal of Obstetrics and Gynaecology*, **12**, 95–101.

Fajans, S. S. & Conn, J. S. (1965) Prediabetes, subclinical diabetes and latent clinical diabetes. Interpretation, diagnosis and treatment. In *On the Nature and Treatment of Diabetes* (Ed.) Leibel, B. S. & Wrenshall, G. A. International Congress Series, **84**, 641–656. New York: Excerpta Medica Foundation.

Freinkel, N. (1965) Effects of the conceptus on maternal metabolism during pregnancy. In *On the Nature and Treatment of Diabetes* (Ed.) Leibel, B. S. & Wrenshall, G. A. International Congress Series, **84**, 679–691. New York: Excerpta Medica Foundation.

Gillmer, M. D. G. & Beard, R. W. (1975) Fetal and placental function in diabetic pregnancy. In *Carbohydrate Metabolism in Pregnancy and the Newborn* (Ed.) Sutherland, H. W. & Stowers, J. M. pp. 168–194. London: Churchill-Livingstone.

Gillmer, M. D. G., Beard, R. W., Brooke, F. M. & Oakley, N. W. (1975a) Carbohydrate metabolism in pregnancy. Part I. Diurnal plasma glucose profile in normal and diabetic women. *British Medical Journal*, **iii**, 399–402.

Gillmer, M. D. G., Beard, R. W., Brooke, F. M. & Oakley (1975b) Carbohydrate metabolism in pregnancy. Part II. Relationship between maternal glucose tolerance and glucose metabolism in the newborn. *British Medical Journal*, **iii**, 402–404.

Gluck, L. & Kulovich, M. V. (1973) Lecithin/sphingomyelin ratios in normal and abnormal pregnancy. *American Journal of Obstetrics and Gynecology*, **115**, 539–544.

Grasso, S. (1973) *Presentation to Diabetic Pregnancy Study Group, Bruges, 1973.*

Hadden, D. R. (1975) Glucose tolerance tests in pregnancy. In *Carbohydrate Metabolism in Pregnancy and the Newborn* (Ed.) Sutherland, H. W. & Stowers, J. M. pp. 19–41. London: Churchill-Livingstone.

Johnston, D. I., Bloom, S. R., Green, K. R. & Beard, R. W. (1972) Failure of the placenta to transfer pancreatic glucagon. *Biologia Neonatorum*, **21**, 375–380.

Joslin, E. P. (1923) *The Treatment of Diabetes Mellitus*, 3rd edition. Philadelphia: Lea and Febiger.

Karlsson, K. & Kjellmer, I. (1972) The outcome of diabetic pregnancies in relation to the mother's blood sugar level. *American Journal of Obstetrics and Gynecology*, **112**, 213–220.

Krauer, F., Joyce, J. & Young, M. (1973) The influence of high maternal plasma glucose levels and maternal blood flow on the placental transfer of glucose in the guinea pig. *Diabetologia*, **9**, 453–456.

Liggins, G. C. (1974) The influence of the fetal hypothalamus and pituitary on growth. In *Size at Birth. Ciba Foundation Symposium 27* (Ed.) Elliot, K. & Knight, J. pp. 165–183. London: Ciba Foundation.

Lund, C. J. & Weese, W. H. (1953) Glucose tolerance and excessively large babies in non-diabetic mothers. *American Journal of Obstetrics and Gynecology*, **65**, 815–832.

McCann, M. L., Chan, C. H., Katigbak, E. B., Kotchen, J. M., Lekly, B. F. & Schwartz, R. (1966) Effects of fructose on hypoglucosemia in infants of diabetic mothers. *New England Journal of Medicine*, **275**, 1–7.

Milner, R. D. G., Leach, F. N. & Jack, P. M. B. (1975) Reactivity of the fetal islet. In *Carbohydrate Metabolism in Pregnancy and the Newborn* (Ed.) Sutherland, H. W. & Stowers, J. M. pp. 83–104. London: Churchill-Livingstone.

Molsted-Pedersen, L. (1972) Aspects of carbohydrate metabolism in newborn infants of diabetic mothers I. *Acta Endocrinologica*, **69**, 174–188.

Morison, J. E. (1970) *Fetal and Neonatal Pathology*, 3rd edition, pp. 153–157. London: Butterworth.

Oakley, N. W., Beard, R. W. & Turner, R. C. (1972) Effect of sustained maternal hyperglycaemia on the fetus in normal and diabetic pregnancies. *British Medical Journal*, **i**, 466–469.

Oakley, W. G. & Peel, J. H. (1968) Pregnancy. In *Clinical Diabetes and its Clinical Basis* (Ed.) Oakley, W. G., Pyke, D. A. & Taylor, K. W. pp. 624–662. Oxford: Blackwell.

Osler, M. (1965) Structural and chemical changes in infants of diabetic and prediabetic mothers. In *On the Nature and Treatment of Diabetes Mellitus* (Ed.) Leibel, B. S. & Wrenshall, G. A. International Congress Series, **84**, 692–699. Amsterdam: Excerpta Medica.

O'Sullivan, J. B. (1975) Prospective study of gestational diabetes and its treatment. In *Carbohydrate Metabolism in Pregnancy and the Newborn* (Ed.) Sutherland, H. W. & Stowers, J. M. pp. 195–204. London: Churchill-Livingstone.

O'Sullivan, J. B. & Mahan, C. M. (1964) Criteria for the oral GTT in pregnancy. *Diabetes*, **13**, 278–285.

O'Sullivan, J. B., Charles, D. & Dandrow, R. V. (1971) Treatment of verified prediabetics in pregnancy. *Journal of Reproductive Medicine*, **7**, 21–24.

O'Sullivan, J. B., Gellis, S. S., Dandrow, R. V. & Tenney, B. D. (1966) The potential diabetic and her treatment in pregnancy. *Obstetrics and Gynaecology*, **27**, 683–689.

Pedersen, J. (1952) Course of diabetes during pregnancy. *Acta Endocrinologica*, **9**, 34–364.

Pedersen, J. (1967) *The Pregnant Diabetic and her Newborn*. Copenhagen: Munksgard.

Pedersen, J. (1975) Fetal macrosomia. In *Carbohydrate Metabolism in Pregnancy and the Newborn* (Ed.) Sutherland, H. W. & Stowers, J. M. pp. 247–273. London: Churchill-Livingstone.

Pedersen, J., Bojsen-Møller, B. & Poulsen, H. (1954) Blood sugar in newborn infants of diabetic mothers. *Acta Endocrinologica (Copenhagen)*, **15**, 33–52.

Pedersen, M., Tygstrup, I. & Pedersen, J. (1964) Congenital malformations in newborn infants of diabetic women. *Lancet*, **ii**, 1124–1126.

Persson, B. (1974) Assessment of metabolic control in diabetic pregnancy. In *Size at Birth. Ciba Foundation Symposium 27* (Ed.) Elliot, K. & Knight, J. pp. 247–273. London: Ciba Foundation.

Persson, B. & Lunell, N. O. (1975) Metabolic control in diabetic pregnancy. Variations in plasma concentrations of glucose, free fatty acids, glycerol, ketone bodies, insulin and human chorionic somatomammotropin during the last trimester. *American Journal of Obstetrics and Gynecology*, **122**, 737–745.

Shelley, H. J., Bassett, J. M. & Milner, R. D. G. (1975) Control of carbohydrate metabolism in the fetus and newborn. In *Perinatal Research* (Ed.) Nathanielsz, P. W. *British Medical Bulletin*, **31**, 37–43.

Size at Birth (1974) *Ciba Foundation Symposium 27* (Ed.) Elliot, K. & Knight, J. London: Ciba Foundation.

Soler, N. & Malins, J. (1976) Diabetes and pregnancy—congenital malformations. In *Proceedings of the Fifth European Congress of Perinatal Medicine, Uppsala, 1976*. In press.

Spellacy, W. N. (1972) Diabetes mellitus complicating pregnancy. In *Davis Gynaecology and Obstetrics*. pp. 1–14. Maryland: Harper and Row.

Szabo, A. J. & Szabo, O. (1974) Placental free fatty acid transfer and fetal adipose tissue development. An explanation of fetal adiposity in infants of diabetic mothers. *Lancet*, **iii**, 498–499.

Turner, R. C., Oakley, N. W. & Beard, R. W. (1973) Human fetal plasma growth hormone prior to the onset of labour. *Biologia Neonatorum*, **22**, 169–176.

Turner, R. C., Schneelock, B. & Paterson, P. (1971) Changes in plasma growth hormone of the human fetus following hysterotomy. *Acta Endocrinologica*, **66**, 577–586.

Usher, R. H., Allen, A. C. & McLean, F. H. (1971) Risk of respiratory distress syndrome related to gestational age, route of delivery and maternal diabetes. *American Journal of Obstetrics and Gynecology*, **111**, 826–832.

Watson, C. (1972) *Late Prognosis of Children born to Diabetic Mothers*. MD thesis, London.

Wright, A. D., Dixon, H. G. & Joplin, G. F. (1968) Diabetes and latent diabetes in pregnancy (Ed.) Clayton, S. G. *British Medical Bulletin*, **24**, 25–31.

Yssing, M. (1975) Long term prognosis of children of mothers diabetic when pregnant. In *Early Diabetes in Early Life. Proceedings of the 3rd International Symposium on Early Diabetes, Madeira, 1974* (Ed.) Camarini-Davalos, R. A. & Cole, H. S. pp. 575–593. New York: Academic Press.

9

FETAL GLUCOSE METABOLISM

John M. Bassett and Colin T. Jones

Early investigations on the respiratory quotient (RQ) during pregnancy (Bohr, 1931) suggested a fetal value of one. This was taken to imply that carbohydrate is almost the sole metabolic fuel for fetal metabolism. Similar conclusions were drawn from studies on exteriorised fetal sheep (Alexander, Britton and Nixon, 1966). The RQ is a very indirect estimate of metabolism and at best can give only a broad indication of a range of compounds that may be metabolised. Recently direct measurement of umbilical arteriovenous differences of glucose and oxygen have suggested that tissue respiration in fetal sheep involves a substantial component from compounds other than glucose (Battaglia and Meschia, 1973). Thus, while glucose may be very important for the maintenance of brain and heart function, the oxidation of compounds such as amino acids may be of equal importance in the other tissues.

It is likely that the mechanisms controlling the maintenance and utilisation of fetal blood glucose are qualitatively similar to those of the adult, although the supply of glucose across the placenta, the low rate of glucose production by fetal liver and kidney and the high rate of fetal growth imply major quantitative differences between the fetus and adult. These may vary substantially from species to species. In the rat fetus for example the development of glucose homeostasis probably takes place at birth, while in more mature fetuses, such as sheep or guinea-pigs, it may occur during the latter stages of gestation.

Information on the regulating mechanisms of glucose homeostasis in the fetus falls into three categories:

1. Studies of the enzyme pathways involved in glucose utilisation and production.
2. The in vitro measurement of glucose metabolism and its regulation by fetal tissues.
3. The factors regulating blood glucose concentration in the intact fetus.

The rat has been used extensively as a model for fetal development and detailed information in all three areas is limited for other species. However, the rat may not be typical for species with longer gestation, such as man. The development in recent years of chronic cannulation methods giving prolonged access to the fetal circulation has made possible the study of glucose homeostasis of long gestational fetuses in normal 'resting' in utero conditions (see Chapter 10).

The object of this chapter is to discuss briefly such information in an attempt to define factors in the regulation of fetal glucose metabolism and to highlight areas for further investigation. The development of glycogen stores in fetal tissues has been reviewed extensively by Dawes and Shelley (1968) and will not be discussed in detail.

CELLULAR METABOLIC PATHWAYS

Pathways of glucose production

In adult life the plasma glucose concentration is maintained through dietary intake or de novo glucose production by the liver and kidney (Krebs, 1964). The balance between glucose consumption by muscle and brain or glucose production by liver and kidney is largely controlled by insulin and glucagon (Hales, 1967), glucose consumption being stimulated during feeding with a diet high in carbohydrates and gluconeogenesis being stimulated between feeds. Under normal conditions in fetal life, a maintained supply of glucose is received across the placenta from the maternal circulation. Thus the need to produce glucose via gluconeogenesis for the maintenance of the blood glucose concentration is not so important in fetal as in adult life (Ballard, 1971). This probably explains why in short-gestation species such as rat and rabbit the gluconeogenic enzymes are absent from, or present in low activity in, the fetal liver (Greengard, 1970, 1971; Usatenko, 1970) and glucose synthesis is not detected at significant rates until after birth (Ballard and Oliver, 1963, 1965; Yeung and Oliver, 1967; Vernon, Eaton and Walker, 1968). In addition, the aminotransferases responsible for the initial metabolism of amino acids for gluconeogenesis are also present in low activity in the fetal rat liver. In contrast, gluconeogenesis has been detected in the fetal rat kidney (Zorzoli, Turkenkopf and Mueller, 1969). Substantial activity of the gluconeogenic enzymes has been detected in the liver of the sheep, pig, guinea-pig, monkey and human fetus (Aurricchio and Rigollo, 1960; Ballard and Oliver, 1965; Dawkins, 1966; Raiha and Lindros, 1969; Mersmann, 1971; Jones and Ashton, 1972, 1976; Kirby and Hahn, 1973). Gluconeogenesis at significant rates has been demonstrated in vitro in the human, guinea-pig and sheep fetal liver (Villee, 1954; Ballard and Oliver, 1965; Jones and Ashton, 1976). The changes in in vitro gluconeogenesis from lactate by slices of the fetal guinea-pig liver are shown in Figure 9.1a. Thus in species with a long gestation that have been investigated, a pathway for de novo glucose synthesis is present in the fetal liver, although its functional significance remains to be established. If significant rates of glucose synthesis do occur in these species in vivo, then it may reflect an inability of the maternal circulation to maintain an adequate supply of glucose. The fetal demands on maternal glucose supply may be very large; in the pregnant sheep it has been suggested that the pregnant uterus represents 70 per cent of the glucose metabolism of the ewe (Setchell et al, 1972). Thus with a large fetal:maternal weight ratio late in gestation the fetus may be required to produce some of its own glucose. It has been suggested from rat studies that the 'reduced state' of the fetal liver associated with the low fetal arterial Po_2 is partly responsible for the low fetal liver gluconeogenesis (Ballard and Philippidis, 1971). This

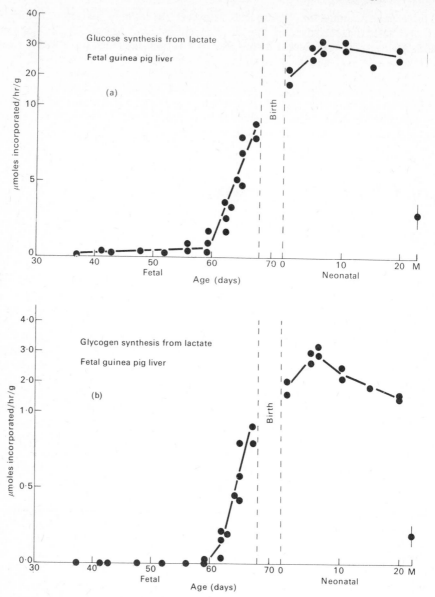

Figure 9.1. The synthesis of glucose and glycogen by liver slices of the fetal and neonatal guinea-pig. The incorporation of ^{14}C lactate (5 mmol/l) into (a) glucose and (b) glycogen was measured.

is not universally true since the liver of the fetal guinea-pig is not in a reduced state compared with that of the adult (Faulkner and Jones, 1976a). In conclusion, studies are required on the intact fetus of several species to establish the possible contribution of fetal gluconeogenesis to glucose supply.

Pathways of glucose utilisation

Glucose consumption in adult tissues is controlled largely by tissue permeability (Randle et al, 1964), glucose phosphorylation (Ballard, 1965; Scrutton and Utter, 1968), availability of alternative substrates (Randle, 1964) and the distribution of the cardiac output. In some adult tissues, particularly muscle, permeability to glucose is controlled by insulin (Hales, 1967). In the fetus there is evidence that the glucose permeability barrier is not fully developed (Guidotti and Foa, 1961; Clark, 1971), although insulin still exerts a large effect on glucose utilisation (page 164). In the adult non-ruminant liver glucose is phosphorylated by glucokinase, an enzyme that increases its phosphorylation rate with physiological increases in blood glucose, and hexokinase, an enzyme that works at maximum rate at physiological glucose concentrations (Walker, 1966). Thus the rate of glucose uptake by the adult liver can be modified by alterations in blood glucose. In the fetus glucokinase has not been detected in any tissues studied (Walker, 1963; Ballard and Oliver, 1964; Walker and Holland, 1965), and glucose phosphorylation is likely to limit uptake and glycolysis (Hommes, 1971), except possibly in those tissues such as muscle with a glucose permeability barrier. Thus fetal liver is unlikely to respond to changes in blood glucose except through alterations in the hepatic circulation. If guinea-pig fetal liver is completely perfused in vitro, it may represent as much as 10 per cent of the fetal glucose consumption (Jones and Faulkner, unpublished observations).

The provision of alternative substrates such as fatty acids normally reduces glucose utilisation in adult tissues such as cardiac muscle (Randle, 1964). The poor ability of such fetal tissues to oxidise metabolites like fatty acids suggests that the control of glucose metabolism by alternative substrates is quantitatively less significant in the fetus (Wittels and Bressler, 1965; Warshaw, 1972). In the adult, peripheral vasoconstriction or vasodilation could have major effects on glucose utilisation. While such vascular responses occur in the fetus to preserve glucose supply to the brain (Dawes, 1968; Rudolph and Heymann, 1974), about 50 per cent of the fetal cardiac output goes to the placenta, so their effects on glucose turnover in the fetus are likely to be less pronounced. In summary, the differing tissue permeability to glucose, the nature of glucose phosphorylation, the oxidation of alternative substrates and the circulation in the fetus indicate that the factors influencing fetal glucose turnover are likely to be substantially different from those in the adult. Some quantitative information is available on glucose turnover in fetal sheep (Setchell et al, 1972), but more detailed information is required on glucose consumption and production under a range of conditions.

The tissue control of the pathways of glucose utilisation changes substantially during development. While glucose is a major substrate for fetal respiration, its function in providing precursors for the synthesis of lipids, protein and nucleic acids for rapid growth is probably of equal importance. Glycolysis controls this precursor supply and in fetal tissues activities of the glycolytic enzymes used for the maintenance of high rates of glucose utilisation are normally relatively high (Burch et al, 1963; Walker, 1963; Hommes and Wilmink, 1968; Sydow, 1969; Hommes, 1971; Faulkner and Jones, 1975a, b, c, 1976b). This is associated with high activity of the pentose phosphate pathway and high rates of lactate and fatty acid production. Such metabolic patterns are characteristic of rapidly growing tissues. Towards term a fall in fatty acid synthesis and pentose phosphate pathway activity usually occurs in the fetal liver coincident with increases in tissue glycogen (Dawes and Shelley, 1968). It seems unlikely that such alterations in the pathways of glucose utilisation are alone responsible for the changes in glycogen deposition. Other changes such as an increase in the activity of I-glycogen synthetase (Schwartz and Rall, 1973) and an increase in pituitary and adrenal activity (Jost, 1966; Monder and Coufalik, 1972) are involved. During the period of glycogen deposition some of the glycogen may originate not from plasma glucose but from gluconeogenic precursors such as lactate (Figure 9.1b). Late in gestation glycogen can be an important source of glucose in response to short-term demands such as hypoxia (Shelley, 1973).

Endocrine control mechanisms

The endocrine factors controlling fetal carbohydrate metabolism are poorly understood. Primarily two types of approach to their study have been made. Attempts to determine the hormones responsible for the appearance of key enzymes or metabolic pathways have been directed either to the effects of large quantities of the hormone administered directly to the fetus (Greengard, 1970, 1971) or to the removal of endocrine glands (Jost, 1966). While a range of hormones induces the premature appearance of several enzymes, including those involved in gluconeogenesis, such experiments are of limited value until similar hormonal changes can be demonstrated to occur normally in utero. They have been useful in demonstrating the appearance of liver hormone-sensitive adenylcyclase. The effects of endocrine gland removal on glycogen deposition (Jost, 1966) are of more physiological interest, but more than one hormone is removed by such procedures. Some naturally occurring changes, such as the increase in fetal plasma corticosteroids close to term, occur at a time when tissue glycogen concentrations and the activity of gluconeogenic enzymes are increasing. Detailed information on whole organ hormone sensitivity is required, although

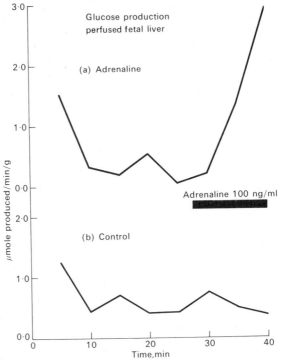

Figure 9.2. The effect of adrenaline on glucose production by the fetal guinea-pig liver. The liver of an (a) 63-day fetus and (b) 61-day fetus was perfused (11 to 12 ml/min) for 30 min with Krebs bicarbonate buffer (2 mmol/l glucose) then for a further 15 min with buffer alone (b) or buffer containing adrenaline (100 ng/ml). Courtesy of Drs Jones and Faulkner.

there is evidence that carbohydrate production or consumption by the fetal muscle (Britton and Blade, 1970; Bocek, Young and Beatty, 1973; Clark, Beatty and Allen, 1973) or liver (Eisen, Goldfine and Glinsmann, 1973; Figure 9.2) are influenced by adrenaline or insulin. In addition, hormone binding sites have been detected in the fetal liver plasma membranes of a number of species (Kelly et al, 1974). Information is required on the quantitative nature of the metabolic responses of individual fetal organs to a variety of changes in endocrine state.

In summary, fetal carbohydrate metabolism is probably dominated by the need for rapid growth and its control is rapidly changing as the tissue pathways undergo large changes and alterations in sensitivity to circulating hormones. The extent to which the fetus is able to switch its metabolism away from glucose utilisation at times when glucose is in short supply remains to be established. Indirect measurements (Battaglia and Meschia, 1973) suggest that this ability is well developed in the mature fetal sheep.

REGULATION OF THE FETAL BLOOD GLUCOSE CONCENTRATION

Placental supply of glucose

Glucose in the fetus is obtained principally by placental transfer from the mother. This occurs rapidly by a stereospecific facilitated diffusion process (Widdas, 1961) and it is evident that the rate at which glucose is obtained by the fetus depends greatly on the maternal concentration and the gradient across the placenta. In all species examined glucose concentrations of undisturbed fetuses in good condition are far lower (half to one-third) than those of the mother (Dawes and Shelley, 1968; Shelley, 1973). Furthermore, there is compelling evidence from studies on chronically cannulated lambs (James et al, 1972; Shelley, 1973; Bassett and Madill, 1974a) confirming the existence of a close relationship between maternal and fetal plasma glucose concentrations (Dawes and Shelley, 1968).

Conclusive evidence on the quantitative aspects of glucose transfer from mother to fetus and on the utilisation of glucose in the various compartments of the conceptus is still lacking. However, studies of umbilical arteriovenous glucose concentration differences, maternal arterial glucose concentrations and measurements of umbilical blood flow using antipyrine (James et al, 1972) provide evidence that glucose uptake by the fetal lamb in utero is positively related to the maternal arterial glucose concentration and to the maternal–fetal arterial glucose concentration difference. More recent studies have shown that maternal starvation rapidly reduces the maternal arterial glucose concentration and the maternal–fetal concentration difference (Bassett and Madill, 1974a; Simmons et al, 1974), so reducing fetal glucose uptake (Boyd et al, 1973). In addition, measurements of the glucose:oxygen quotient suggest that the maximum possible contribution to fetal respiration of glucose from the placenta is around 50 per cent and that this decreases to less than 20 per cent on starvation (Tsoulos et al, 1971; Boyd et al, 1973), thus implying that decreases in fetal plasma glucose concentration in maternal fasting involve not only a reduction in glucose uptake by the fetus but also the use of alternative substrates in fetal respiration. In these circumstances some glucose may be derived from gluconeogenesis in the fetal liver and kidney.

It is apparent that the maternal plasma glucose concentration and the maternal–fetal glucose gradient play a major role in determining the supply of glucose to the fetus. However, many questions remain. In particular, it is desirable to know how generally applicable the sheep results may be to other species. It is also of importance to know whether, as was formerly thought, fetal glucose uptake is a passive reflection of the maternal glucose concentration or whether the gradient can be actively regulated by fetal homeostatic mechanisms controlling the fetal blood glucose concentration and the tissue utilisation of glucose.

Fetal blood glucose homeostasis

Blood glucose homeostasis in postnatal life is largely achieved by endocrine and neuroendocrine regulatory mechanisms. It is therefore pertinent to consider whether similar mechanisms are involved during fetal life. To examine such regulatory mechanisms it is important to carry out observations on undisturbed intact fetuses. The fetal sheep with chronically implanted vascular catheters is currently the only satisfactory model in which these conditions have been attained. The use of these preparations has led to increasing evidence that the fetal endocrine system regulates glucose metabolism.

Glucose utilisation—the role of insulin

Insulin is the most important hormone regulating glucose utilisation in the adult; it is now evident that it is also of major importance during fetal life. The insulin-secreting β-cells of the islets of Langerhans develop relatively early in gestation (Clark and Rutter, 1972) (see Chapter 7 for fuller discussion of pancreatic development). Further, there is little doubt that insulin is present in plasma and that active insulin secretion occurs during fetal life in species of short (Milner, 1969; Cohen and Turner, 1972; Girard, 1974) and long gestation (Mintz, Chez and Horger, 1969; Bassett and Thorburn, 1971; Kaplan, Grumbach and Shepard, 1972). Insulin at physiological concentrations increases fetal glucose utilisation in several species and thereby lowers blood glucose (Picon and Moutané, 1968; Chez et al, 1970; Colwill et al, 1970; Shelley, 1973). This is particularly well illustrated by the studies of Shelley (1973) on fetal lambs, where insulin infusion at rates up to 2.5 mg/min progressively reduced the fetal plasma glucose concentration (Figure 9.3). The continued and, in this situation, possibly increased influx of glucose across the placenta must minimise the observed fall in blood glucose produced by the insulin infusion. Despite this, the clearcut effects of insulin indicate that insulin increases glucose utilisation by the fetus and possibly placenta. This and the close interrelation between fetal blood insulin and glucose levels (see below) indicates that insulin plays an important role in regulating fetal glucose utilisation and blood concentration. Interference with insulin action by administration of anti-insulin serum did not significantly alter blood glucose in fetal lambs during acute studies (Alexander et al, 1970), but destruction of fetal lamb pancreatic β-cells with streptozotocin at 119 days evidently does lead to increased plasma glucose concentration (Shelley, 1975).

In postnatal life glucose is the major regulator of insulin release. However, much in vivo and in vitro evidence points to immaturity of mechanisms regulating glucose stimulation of insulin release from fetal pancreas (Asplund, Westman and Hellerstrom, 1969; Mintz, Chez and Horger, 1969; Milner, Ashworth and Barson, 1972; Bassett et al, 1973; Milner et al, 1975). Consequently it has been questionable whether the fetal plasma glucose concentration could be a regulator of insulin release in utero. Indeed if the blood glucose lowering effect of insulin in the fetus is an important means of maintaining the maternal fetal glucose gradient and fetal glucose uptake, it might be advantageous if glucose were not the major regulator of insulin release. Amino acids may stimulate insulin release from the fetal pancreas more readily than glucose (Milner, Ashworth and Barson, 1972; Milner et al, 1975), but other studies suggest that fetal insulin secretion does not respond readily to amino acid

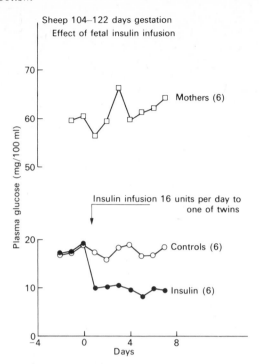

Sheep 104–122 days gestation
Effect of fetal insulin infusion

Mothers (6)

Insulin infusion 16 units per day to one of twins

Controls (6)

Insulin (6)

Plasma glucose (mg/100 ml)

Days

Figure 9.3. Mean arterial plasma glucose concentrations in six pairs of chronically catheterised twin lambs and their mothers 104 to 122 days gestation (□). One twin of each pair (●) was given a continuous slow infusion of insulin. The control twin (O) received saline. Modified from Shelley (1973).

stimulation (Mintz, Chez and Horger, 1969; Lernmark and Wenngren, 1972; Chez et al, 1974; Fiser et al, 1974). However, there is now substantial evidence that glucose can regulate insulin release during fetal life, despite the mass of in vitro evidence against this from a variety of species. This has been most clearly demonstrated in fetal sheep. Like early in vivo studies on sheep (Willes, Manns and Boda, 1969), in vitro studies failed to demonstrate consistently stimulation of insulin release by glucose, unless caffeine was also present (Bassett et al, 1973). However, more recent in vivo studies on the effects of continuous glucose infusions into chronically cannulated lambs in utero have shown that glucose can stimulate insulin release (Bassett and Thorburn, 1971; Shelley, 1973; Bassett and Madill, 1974b; Fiser et al, 1974), so that during prolonged infusions to the fetus, plasma insulin and glucose concentrations are closely correlated (Bassett and Madill, 1974b), even though the acute insulin secretory response to change in glucose concentration, so characteristic of the postnatal response, is absent. Perhaps the most striking finding of these studies has been that glucose can regulate insulin release in the fetal lamb over the physiological concentration range, concentrations which would be regarded as non-stimulatory in postnatal life (Bassett et al, 1973; Shelley, 1973). Confirmation that these findings are physiologically important has come from the observation by Shelley (1973) and Bassett and Madill (1974) that fetal lamb plasma glucose and insulin concentrations are strongly correlated when the only factor influencing maternal and fetal plasma glucose levels was variable nutrition (Figure 9.4).

It now seems clearly established, therefore, in sheep that the circulating glucose and insulin levels of the fetus are closely interrelated. There can be little doubt about the fetal origin of this interrelation, since insulin does not cross the placenta in this species (Alexander et al,

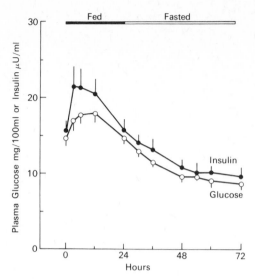

Figure 9.4. The effect of maternal food intake on fetal plasma glucose (◯) and fetal plasma insulin (●) in 11 chronically catheterised fetal lambs 104 to 130 days gestation. (◯) arithmetic mean concentration, (●) geometric mean concentration. Vertical bars present ± s.e.m. From Bassett and Madill (1974a) with kind permission of the editor of *Journal of Endocrinology*.

1972). In vitro studies (Bassett, unpublished observations, 1975) suggest that glucose could regulate insulin release in this species during most of the last two-thirds of gestation. There is now also evidence for glucose regulation of insulin release in utero in the fetuses of short gestation species such as the rat (Girard, 1974). The observations on sheep (Bassett et al, 1973) suggest that the absence of acute insulin secretory responses to large increases in blood glucose concentration is no criterion by which to judge the overall interrelation of glucose and insulin concentrations in the fetus in utero. The absence of plasma insulin responses to high rates of glucose infusion into monkey and human infants at term (Mintz, Chez and Horger, 1969; Oakley, Beard and Turner, 1972) cannot be regarded as conclusive evidence that glucose does not regulate insulin release in utero. Whether or not insulin secretion from the fetal pancreas is capable of responding to changes in glucose concentration, chronic elevation of the fetal glucose concentration as in uncontrolled diabetes, either naturally occurring as in women (Oakley, Beard and Turner, 1972) or streptozotocin-induced as in monkeys (Mintz, Chez and Hutchinson, 1972), can lead to adaptive increases in the fetal insulin secretory response to administered glucose. So clearly some interrelation exists in these species. While many of the observations discussed require confirmation, there can be little doubt that insulin–glucose interrelations play a very important part in determining the fetal blood glucose concentration and utilisation rate. Much more information about the control of insulin release by metabolites other than glucose and about insulin-sensitive pathways of glucose metabolism in fetal tissues is required before the full significance of the insulin–glucose relation can be fully assessed.

Glucose production—glucagon and catecholamines

The role of hormone mechanisms promoting glucose influx and restricting glucose efflux from the blood during fetal life is far less certain. With transplacental transfer of glucose as he source of this metabolite for the fetus, the maternal glucose concentration and possibly he fetal insulin level may be the major regulators of glucose influx. Fetal mobilisation of its glycogen stores, particularly near term, is one alternative way in which the fetus could augment its glucose supply when placental transfer is inadequate. However, as mentioned previously, the extent to which fetal glycogenolysis or gluconeogenesis can contribute to maintenance of the fetal plasma glucose concentration is unknown. Blood glucose could also be increased through a reduction in plasma insulin levels and thereby in glucose utilisation by insulin-sensitive tissues.

In postnatal life glucagon and the catecholamines adrenaline and noradrenaline are the hormones most concerned in the regulation of glycogenolysis and gluconeogenesis. Glucagon is present during fetal life and has been shown to be capable of increasing the fetal glucose concentration close to term in rats (Hunter, 1969) and during the last third of gestation in monkeys (Mintz, Chez and Horger, 1969) and sheep (Bassett and Thorburn, 1971).

High concentrations of glucagon are present in the fetal pancreas almost from the beginning of pancreatic organogenesis (Pictet and Rutter, 1972) and this hormone is present in plasma for much of gestation in man (Assan and Boillot, 1971) and sheep (Alexander et al, 1971; Fiser et al, 1974). Girard (1974) reported high glucagon concentrations in rat plasma, but the insulin–glucagon ratio was also high and, in consequence, fetal metabolism may be dominated by insulin rather than glucagon. Maternal undernutrition decreased fetal insulin and increased glucagon concentration in rats. However, experiments with monkeys (Chez et al, 1974) and sheep (Fiser et al, 1974) have indicated that fetal glucagon is unresponsive to

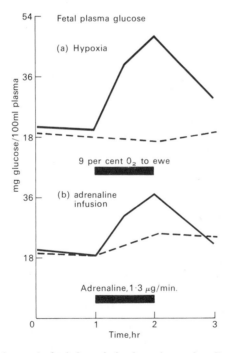

Figure 9.5. Plasma glucose changes in fetal sheep during hypoxia or adrenaline infusion. A fetal sheep (127 days) was (a) made hypoxic by administration of 9 per cent O_2 + 3 per cent CO_2 in N_2 to the pregnant ewe or (b) given a direct infusion of adrenaline (1.3 mg per min) via the jugular vein. The data are plotted as the blood glucose changes observed without (——) or with (– – –) an infusion of phentolamine (100 mg per min) into the fetal jugular vein. Courtesy of Drs Jones and Ritchie.

stimulation by amino acids or by hypoglycaemia. In contrast, the in vitro perfused fetal sheep pancreas will release glucagon in response to amino acid stimulation (Bassett, unpublished observations, 1975. The effects of cholinergic and adrenergic stimulation on glucagon secretion in the fetus have received little study, although these are important regulators of glucagon release in the immediate postnatal period (Bloom, Edwards and Vaughan, 1974) and in adult life (Woods and Porte, 1974). However, Girard (1974) has recently shown that adrenergic and cholinergic agents stimulate glucagon release in the fetal rat. Despite this, the contribution of glucagon to fetal blood glucose regulation remains uncertain, and additional information on the role of glucagon in the fetus is urgently required.

Changes in circulating catecholamine levels or in direct sympathetic stimulation of the liver may also be important components in the mechanisms controlling fetal blood glucose. In the fetal sheep both hypoxia and adrenaline infused at rates giving blood concentrations similar to those observed in hypoxia (Jones and Robinson, 1975) produce a rise in plasma glucose which can be blocked by phentolamine (Figure 9.5). Inhibition of insulin secretion occurs in both these situations and can be overcome by phentolamine (Woods and Porte, 1974). This suggests that inhibition of insulin release during fetal hypoxia may be largely responsible for the changes in blood glucose seen in this situation. However, the catecholamines may also stimulate glucagon release (Shelley, Bassett and Milner, 1975) as they do in the fetal rat (Girard, 1974), but the role of glucagon in mediating the changes in glucose during hypoxia has not been elucidated.

Other hormones

Other hormones such as glucocorticoids and growth hormone play a role in blood glucose regulation after birth through their anti-insulin actions and stimulation of glucose production. Fetal plasma contains very high concentrations of growth hormone throughout much of gestation in sheep (Bassett, Thorburn and Wallace, 1970), monkey (Mintz, Chez and Horger, 1969) and human (Kaplan, Grumbach and Shephard, 1972). Cortisol or corticosterone concentrations in fetal plasma may also rise to high levels in several species just before term (Challis and Thorburn, 1975). Surprisingly, there is no unequivocal evidence for any hyperglycaemic or anti-insulin action of either in the fetus, though it does appear that the glucocorticoids may be involved in bringing about the changes in hepatic enzymes before birth.

It is evident that blood glucose regulation during fetal life, or at least the latter part of it, involves functional endocrine regulatory mechanisms just as postnatal regulation does. Additional measurements of blood metabolite and hormone concentrations should clarify the present uncertainty.

DISCUSSION

The contribution of glucose to fetal metabolism as a whole or in individual tissues still cannot be defined precisely. Clearly it is substantially influenced by alterations in maternal nutrition, e.g. a fall is associated with maternal starvation. Nutritional factors producing such changes are likely to be numerous, although alterations in blood glucose could be responsible for modification in the rates of fetal glucose metabolism. Evidence from uptake and hormone studies shows that, at least in species with a longer gestation, glucose utilisation by the fetus is dependent both on the size of the maternal–fetal gradient across the placenta and also on the fetal insulin secretory responses to changes in glucose delivery to the fetal compartment. Alterations in the supply of glucose across the placenta are amplified by the associated changes in fetal insulin levels. This suggests that insulin plays a major role in determining fetal growth and may explain both the increased fetal growth seen in maternal diabetes and the growth retardation seen in fetal hypoinsulinism (Liggins, 1974). The stimulatory effects of insulin on amino acid utilisation give further support to this view.

Identification of which individual tissues are responsible for the responses to insulin awaits further information on their hormonal sensitivity. The importance of other hormones in fetal glucose homeostasis remains to be established, although the high insulin: glucagon ratio (Girard, 1974) further supports the dominant role of insulin in fetal glucose homeostasis. However, control of fetal glucose utilisation by insulin may be overriden in some circumstances. Short periods of hypoxia, for instance, suppress insulin secretion and glycogen mobilisation occurs. Together these changes produce a rise in fetal blood glucose concentration and are partly responsible for a diversion of glucose away from the insulin-sensitive tissues. It is possible that similar alterations in glucose metabolism produced by changes such as prolonged fetal hypoxia may produce reductions in fetal growth (Alexander, 1964). In conclusion, it is evident that the coarse control of fetal glucose utilisation and fetal growth is probably exerted by the input of glucose across the placenta. The fine control of the pathways of fetal glucose utilisation and fetal growth, however, are probably largely determined by the actions of fetal insulin and its interaction with other hormones. To understand fully the regulation of fetal growth, it will be essential to elucidate the fetal glucose homeostatic mechanisms in man and in experimental animals.

REFERENCES

Alexander, D. P., Britton, H. G. & Nixon, D. A. (1966) Observations on the isolated foetal sheep with particular reference to the metabolism of glucose and fructose. *Journal of Physiology*, **185**, 382–399.

Alexander, D. P., Assan, R., Britton, H. G. & Nixon, D. A. (1971) Glucagon in the foetal sheep. *Journal of Endocrinology*, **51**, 597–598.

Alexander, D. P., Britton, H. G., Cohen, N. M. & Nixon, D. A. (1970) The response of the sheep foetus and the young lamb to anti-insulin serum. *Biology of the Neonate*, **15**, 142–155.

Alexander, D. P., Britton, H. G., Cohen, N. M. & Nixon, D. A. (1972) The permeability of the sheep placenta to insulin. Studies with the perfused placental preparation. *Biology of the Neonate*, **21**, 361–368.

Alexander, G. (1964) Studies on the placenta of the sheep (Ovis aries L.); effect of surgical reduction in the number of caruncles. *Journal of Reproduction and Fertility*, **7**, 307–322.

Asplund, K., Westman, S. & Hellerstrom, C. (1969) Glucose stimulation of insulin secretion from the isolated pancreas of foetal and newborn rats. *Diabetologia*, **5**, 260–262.

Assan, R. & Boillot, J. (1971) Pancreatic glucagon and glucagon-like material in tissues and plasma from human foetuses 6–26 weeks old. In *Metabolic Process in the Fetus and Newborn Infant* (Ed.) Jonxix, J. H. P., Visser, H. K. A. & Troekstra, J. J. A. pp. 210–219. Leiden: H. E. Stenfert Kroese.

Aurricchio, S. & Rigillo, N. (1960) Glucose 6-phosphatase activity of the human foetal liver. *Biology of the Neonate*, **2**, 146–151.

Ballard, F. J. (1965) Glucose utilisation in mammalian liver. *Comparative Biochemistry and Physiology*, **14**, 437–443.

Ballard, F. J. (1971) Carbohydrates. In *Physiology of the Perinatal Period* (Ed.) Stave, U. Vol. 1, pp. 417–440. New York: Appleton–Century Croft, Meredith Corporation.

Ballard, F. J. & Oliver, I. T. (1963) Glycogen metabolism in embryonic chick and neonatal rat liver. *Biochimica et Biophysica Acta*, **71**, 578–588.

Ballard, F. J. & Oliver, I. T. (1964) Ketohexokinase, isoenzymes of glucokinase and glycogen synthesis from hexoses in neonatal rat liver. *Biochemical Journal*, **90**, 261–268.

Ballard, F. J. & Oliver, I. T. (1965) Carbohydrate metabolism in liver from fetal and neonatal sheep. *Biochemical Journal*, **95**, 191–200.

Ballard, F. J. & Philippidis, H. (1971) The development of gluconeogenic functions in the rat liver. In *Regulation of Gluconeogenesis* (Ed.) Soling, H. D. & Willms, B. pp. 66–81. Stuttgart: Georg Thieme Verlag.

Bassett, J. M. & Madill, D. (1974a) The influence of maternal nutrition on plasma hormone and metabolite concentrations of foetal lambs. *Journal of Endocrinology*, **61**, 465–477.

Bassett, J. M. & Madill, D. (1974b) Influence of prolonged glucose infusion on plasma insulin and growth hormone concentrations of foetal lambs. *Journal of Endocrinology*, **62**, 299–309.

Bassett, J. M. & Thorburn, G. D. (1971) The regulation of insulin secretion by the ovine foetus *in utero*. *Journal of Endocrinology*, **50**, 59–74.

Bassett, J. M., Thornburn, G. D. & Wallace, A. L. C. (1970) The plasma growth hormone concentration of the foetal lamb. *Journal of Endocrinology*, **48**, 251–263.

Bassett, J. M., Madill, D., Nichol, D. H. & Thorburn, G. D. (1973) Further studies on the regulation of insulin release in foetal and post-natal lambs. The role of glucose as a physiological regulator of insulin release *in utero*. In *Foetal and Neonatal Physiology, Barcroft Centenary Symposium* (Ed.) Comline, R. S., Cross, K. W., Dawes, G. S. & Nathanielsz, P. W. pp. 351–359. London: Cambridge University Press.

Battaglia, F. C. & Meschia, G. (1973) Foetal metabolism and substrate utilisation. In *Foetal and Neonatal Physiology, Barcroft Centenary Symposium* (Ed.) Comline, R. S., Cross, K. W., Dawes, G. S. & Nathanielsz, P. W. pp. 382–397. London: Cambridge University Press.

Bloom, S. R., Edwards, A. V. & Vaughan, N. J. A. (1974) The role of the autonomic innervation in the control of glucagon release during hypoglycaemia in the calf. *Journal of Physiology*, **236**, 611–623.

Bocek, R. M., Young, M. K. & Beatty, C. H. (1973) Effect of insulin and epinephrine on the carbohydrate metabolism and adenylate cyclase activity of rhesus fetal muscle. *Pediatric Research*, **7**, 787–793.

Bohr, C. (1931) The respiration and heat production of the embryo. In *Chemical Embryology* (Ed.) Needham, J., Vol. II, pp. 728–729. London: MacMillan.

Boyd, R. D. H., Morris, F. H., Meschia, G., Makowski, E. L. & Battaglia, F. C. (1973) Growth of glucose and oxygen uptakes by fetuses of fed and starved ewes. *American Journal of Physiology*, **225**, 897–902.

Britton, H. G. & Blade, M. (1970) The incorporation of radioglucose into glycogen in foetal and neonatal rat diaphragm *in vitro*: the effect of insulin. *Biology of the Neonate*, **16**, 370–375.

Burch, H. B., Lowry, O. H., Kuhlman, A. M., Skerjance, J., Diamont, E. J., Lowry, S. R. & Von Dippe, P. (1963) Changes in patterns of enzymes of carbohydrate metabolism in developing rat liver. *Journal of Biological Chemistry*, **238**, 2267–2273.

Challis, J. R. G. & Thorburn, G. D. (1975) Prenatal endocrine function and the initiation of parturition. *British Medical Bulletin*, **31**, 57–62.

Chez, R. A., Mintz, D. H., Horger, E. O. & Hutchinson, D. L. (1970) Factors affecting the response to insulin in the normal subhuman pregnant primate. *Journal of Clinical Investigation*, **49**, 1517–1527.

Chez, R. A., Mintz, D. H., Epstein, M. F., Fleischman, A. R., Oakes, G. K. & Hutchinson, D. L. (1974) Glucagon metabolism in non-human primate pregnancy. *American Journal of Obstetrics and Gynecology*, **120**, 690–694.

Clark, C. M. (1971) Carbohydrate metabolism in the isolated fetal rat heart. *American Journal of Physiology*, **220**, 583–588.

Clark, C. M., Beatty, B. & Allen, D. O. (1973) Evidence for delayed development of the glucagon receptor of adenylate cyclase in the fetal and neonatal rat heart. *Journal of Clinical Investigation*, **52**, 1018–1025.

Clark, W. R. & Rutter, W. J. (1972) Synthesis and accumulation of insulin in the fetal rat pancreas. *Developmental Biology*, **29**, 468–481.

Cohen, N. M. & Turner, R. C. (1972) Plasma insulin in the fetal rat. *Biology of the Neonate*, **21**, 67–111.

Colwill, J. R., Davis, J. R., Meschia, G., Makowski, E. L., Beck, P. & Battaglia, F. C. (1970) Insulin-induced hypoglycemia in the ovine fetus *in utero*. *Endocrinology*, **87**, 710–715.

Dawes, G. S. (1968) *Foetal and Neonatal Physiology*. Chicago: Yearbook Medical Publishers.

Dawes, G. S. & Shelley, H. J. (1968) Physiological aspects of carbohydrate metabolism in the fetus and newborn. In *Carbohydrate Metabolism and its Disorders* (Ed.) Dickens, W. F., Randle, P. J. & Whelan, W. J. Vol. II, pp. 87–121. London, New York: Academic Press.

Dawkins, M. J. R. (1966) Biochemical aspects of developing functions in newborn mammalian liver. *British Medical Bulletin*, **22**, 27–33.

Eisen, H. J., Goldfine, I. D. & Glinsman, W. H. (1973) Regulation of hepatic glycogen synthesis during fetal development: roles of hydrocortisone, insulin and insulin receptors. *Proceedings of the National Academy of Sciences*, **70**, 3454–3457.

Faulkner, A. & Jones, C. T. (1975a) Pyruvate kinase isoenzymes in tissues of the developing guinea pig. *Archives of Biochemistry and Biophysics*, **170**, 228–241.

Faulkner, A. & Jones, C. T. (1975b) Pyruvate kinase isoenzymes in tissues of the human fetus. *Federation of European Biochemical Societies Letters*, **53**, 167–169.

Faulkner, A. & Jones, C. T. (1975c) Changes in the activity of some glycolytic enzymes during the development of the guinea pig. *International Journal of Biochemistry*, **6**, 789–792.

Faulkner, A. & Jones, C. T. (1976a) Metabolite concentrations in the liver of the adult and developing guinea pig and the control of glycolysis in vivo. *Archives of Biochemistry and Biophysics*, in press.

Faulkner, A. & Jones, C. T. (1976b) Hexokinase isoenzymes in tissue of the adult and developing guinea pig. *Archives of Biochemistry and Biophysics*, **175,** in press.

Fiser, R. H., Erenberg, A., Sperling, M. A., Oh, W. & Fisher, D. A. (1974) Insulin–glucagon substrate interrelations in the fetal sheep. *Pediatric Research*, **8,** 951–955.

Girard, J. R. (1974) Factors affecting the secretion of insulin and glucagon by the rat fetus. *Diabetes*, **23,** 310–317.

Greengard, O. (1970) *Biochemical Action of Hormones* (Ed.) Litwack, G. pp. 53–87. New York, London: Academic Press.

Greengard, O. (1971) Enzymic differentiation in mammalian tissues. *Essays in Biochemistry*, **7,** 159–205.

Guidotti, G. G. & Foa, P. P. (1961) Development of an insulin-sensitive glucose transport system in chick embryo hearts. *American Journal of Physiology*, **201,** 869–872.

Hales, C. N. (1967) Some actions of hormones in the regulation of glucose metabolism. *Essays in Biochemistry*, **3,** 73–104.

Hommes, F. A. (1971) Development of enzyme systems in glycolysis. In *Metabolic Processes in the Foetus and Newborn Infants* (Ed.) Jonxis, J. H. P., Visser, H. K. A. & Troekstra, J. A. pp. 3–10. Leiden: Kroese, N. V.

Hommes, F. A. & Wilmink, C. W. (1968) Developmental changes of glycolytic enzymes in rat brain, liver and skeletal muscle. *Biology of the Neonate*, **9,** 183–193.

Hunter, D. J. S. (1969) Changes in blood glucose and liver carbohydrate after intrauterine injection of glucagon into foetal rats. *Journal of Endocrinology*, **45,** 367–374.

James, E. J., Raye, J. R., Gresham, E. L., Makowski, E. L., Meschia, G. & Battaglia, F. C. (1972) Fetal oxygen consumption, carbon dioxide production and glucose uptake in a chronic sheep preparation. *Pediatrics*, **50,** 361–371.

Jones, C. T. & Ashton, I. K. (1972) The development of some enzymes of gluconeogenesis in the liver and kidney of the fetal guinea pig. *Biochemical Journal*, **130,** 23–24.

Jones, C. T. & Ashton, I. K. (1976) The appearance, properties, and functions of gluconeogenic enzymes in the liver and kidney of the guinea pig during fetal and early neonatal development. *Archives of Biochemistry and Biophysics*, **174,** 506–524.

Jones, C. T. & Robinson, R. O. (1975) Plasma catecholamines in foetal and adult sheep. *Journal of Physiology*, **248,** 15–33.

Jost, A. (1966) Problems of fetal endocrinology: the adrenal glands. *Recent Progress in Hormone Research*, **22,** 541–569.

Kaplan, S. L., Grumbach, M. M. & Shephard, T. H. (1972) The ontogenesis of human fetal hormones. l. Growth hormone and insulin. *Journal of Clinical Investigation*, **51,** 3080–3093.

Kelly, P. A., Posner, B. I., Toshio, T. & Friesen, H. G. (1974) Studies of insulin, growth hormone and prolactin binding: ontogenesis, effects of sex and pregnancy. *Endocrinology*, **95,** 532–539.

Kirby, L. & Hahn, P. (1973) Enzyme induction in human fetal liver. *Pediatric Research*, **7,** 75–81.

Krebs, H. A. (1964) Gluconeogenesis. *Proceedings of the Royal Society*, **159B,** 545–564.

Lernmark, A. & Wenngren, B. I. (1972) Insulin and glucagon release from the isolated pancreas of foetal and newborn mice. *Journal of Embryology and Experimental Morphology*, **28,** 607–614.

Liggins, G. C. (1974) The influence of the fetal hypothalamus and pituitary on growth. In *Size at Birth*, CIBA Foundation Symposium 27, pp. 165–183. Amsterdam: Associated Scientific Publishers.

Mersmann, H. J. (1971) Glycolytic and gluconeogenic enzyme levels in pre- and postnatal pigs. *American Journal of Physiology*, **220,** 1297–1302.

Milner, R. D. G. (1969) Plasma and tissue insulin concentrations in foetal and post-natal rabbits. *Journal of Endocrinology*, **43,** 119–124.

Milner, R. D. G., Ashworth, M. A. & Barson, A. J. (1972) Insulin release from human foetal pancreas in response to glucose, leucine and arginine. *Journal of Endocrinology*, **52,** 497–505.

Milner, R. D. G., Leach, F. N., Ashworth, M. A., Cser, A. & Jack, P. M. B. (1975) Development of pathways of insulin secretion in the rabbit. *Journal of Endocrinology*, **64,** 349–361.

Mintz, D. H., Chez, R. A. & Horger, E. O. (1969) Fetal insulin and growth hormone metabolism in the subhuman primate. *Journal of Clinical Investigation*, **48,** 176–186.

Mintz, D. H., Chez, R. A. & Hutchinson, D. L. (1972) Subhuman primate pregnancy complicated by streptozotocin induced diabetes mellitus. *Journal of Clinical Investigation*, **51,** 837–847.

Monder, C. & Coufalik, A. (1972) Influence of cortisol on glycogen synthesis and gluconeogenesis in fetal rat liver in organ culture. *Journal of Biological Chemistry*, **247,** 3608–3617.

Oakley, N. W., Beard, R. W. & Turner, R. C. (1972) Effect of sustained hyperglycaemia on the fetus in normal and diabetic pregnancies. *British Medical Journal*, i, 466–469.

Picon, L. & Moutane, M. (1968) Glycémies foetale et maternelle chez la ratte à divers stade de la gestation. Action de l'insuline injectée au foetus sur la glycémie. *Comptes Rendus d'Academie des Sciences*, **267,** 860–863.

Pictet, R. & Rutter, W. J. (1972) Development of the embryonic endocrine pancreas. In *Handbook of Physiology; Section 7, Endocrinology*; Vol. 1., *Endocrine Pancreas* (Ed.) Steiner, D. F. & Freinkel, N. Ch. 2, pp. 25–66. Washington D.C.: American Physiological Society.

Raiha, N. C. R. & Lindros, K. O. (1969) Development of some enzymes involved in gluconeogenesis in human liver. *Annales Medicinae Experimentalis et Biologiae Fenniae*, **47**, 146–148.

Randle, P. J. (1964) Fuel and power in the control of carbohydrate metabolism in mammalian muscle. *Symposium of the Society for Experimental Biology*, **18**, 129–155.

Randle, P. J., Garland, P. B., Hales, C. N., Newsholme, E. A., Denton, R. M. & Pogson, C. I. (1964) Interaction of metabolism and the physiological role of insulin. *Recent Progress in Hormone Research*, **22**, 1–44.

Rudolph, A. M. & Heymann, M. A. (1974) Foetal and neonatal circulation and respiration. *Annual Review of Physiology*, **36**, 185–207.

Schaub, J., Gutmann, I. & Lipport, H. (1972) Developmental changes of glycolytic and gluconeogenic enzymes in fetal and neonatal rat liver. *Hormone and Metabolic Research*, **4**, 110–115.

Schwartz, A. L. & Rall, T. W. (1973) Hormonal regulation of glycogen metabolism in neonatal rat liver. *Biochemical Journal*, **134**, 985–993.

Scrutton, M. C. & Utter, M. F. (1968) The regulation of glycolysis and gluconeogenesis in animal tissues. *Annual Review of Biochemistry*, **37**, 249–302.

Setchell, B. P., Bassett, J. M., Hinks, N. T. & Graham, N. McC. (1972) The importance of glucose in the oxidative metabolism of the pregnant uterus and its contents in conscious sheep with some preliminary observations on the oxidation of fructose and glucose by fetal sheep. *Quarterly Journal of Experimental Physiology*, **57**, 257–266.

Shelley, H. J. (1973) The use of chronically catheterized foetal lambs for the study of foetal metabolism. In *Foetal and Neonatal Physiology, Barcroft Centenary Symposium* (Ed.) Comline, R. S., Cross, K. W., Dawes, G. S. & Nathanielsz, P. W. pp. 360–381. London: Cambridge University Press.

Shelley, H. J. (1975) Insulin and the control of plasma glucose in chronically catheterised foetal lambs. *Journal of Physiology*, **252**, 66–67P.

Shelley, H. J. Bassett, J. M. & Milner, R. D. G. (1975) Control of carbohydrate metabolism in the foetus and newborn. *British Medical Bulletin*, **31**, 37–43.

Simmons, M. A., Meschia, G., Makowski, E. L. & Battaglia, F. C. (1974) Fetal metabolic response to maternal starvation. *Pediatric Research*, **8**, 830–836.

Sydow, V. G. (1969) Hexokinase- und Phosphofructokinase Activät in Geweben der Ratte während der prä- und postnatalen Entwicklung. *Hoppe-Seyler's Zeitschrift für Physiologische Chemie*, **350**, 263–268.

Tsoulos, N. G., Colwill, J. R., Battaglia, F. C., Makowski, E. L. & Meschia, G. (1971) Comparison of glucose, fructose and O_2 uptakes by fetuses of fed and starved ewes. *American Journal of Physiology*, **221**, 234–237.

Usatenko, M. S. (1970) Hormonal regulation of phosphoenol pyruvate carboxykinase activity in liver and kidney of adult animals and formation of this enzyme in developing rabbit liver. *Biochemical Medicine*, **3**, 298–310.

Vernon, R. G., Eaton, S. W. & Walker, D. G. (1968) Carbohydrate formation from various precursors in neonatal rat liver. *Biochemical Journal*, **110**, 725–731.

Villee, C. A. (1954) The intermediary metabolism of human fetal tissues. In *Cold Spring Harbour Symposium on Quantitative Biology*, **14**, 186–199.

Walker, D. G. (1963) On the presence of two soluble glucose-phosphorylating enzymes in adult liver and the development of one of these after birth. *Biochimica et Biophysica Acta*, **77**, 209–226.

Walker, D. G. (1966) The nature and function of hexokinases in animal tissues. *Essays in Biochemistry*, **2**, 33–67.

Walker, D. G. & Holland, G. (1965) The development of hepatic glucokinase in the neonatal rat. *Biochemical Journal*, **97**, 845–854.

Warshaw, J. B. (1972) Cellular energy metabolism during fetal development. IV. Fatty acid activation, acetyl transfer and fatty acid oxidation during development of the chick and rat. *Developmental Biology*, **28**, 537–544.

Widdas, W. F. (1961) Transport mechanisms in the fetus. *British Medical Bulletin*, **17**, 107–111.

Willes, R. F., Manns, J. G. & Boda, J. M. (1969) Insulin secretion by the ovine fetus *in utero*. *Endocrinology*, **84**, 520–527.

Wittels, B. & Bressler, R. (1965) Lipid metabolism in the newborn heart. *Journal of Clinical Investigation*, **44**, 1639–1646.

Woods, S. C. & Porte, D. (1974) Neural control of the endocrine pancreas. *Physiological Reviews*, **54**, 596–619.

Yeung, D. & Oliver, I. T. (1967) Development of gluconeogenesis in neonatal rat liver: effect of premature delivery. *Biochemical Journal*, **105**, 1229–1233.

Zorzoli, A., Turkenkopf, J. J. & Mueller, V. L. (1969) Gluconeogenesis in developing rat kidney cortex. *Biochemical Journal*, **111**, 181–185.

10

FETAL ENERGY METABOLISM

Marian Silver

FETAL ENERGY REQUIREMENTS

The fetus, unlike the neonate or adult, requires little or no energy for movement, digestion, or temperature regulation. Its metabolism must, however, provide for continued growth and development, and allow reserves of glycogen and fat to be accumulated. Periodic fetal activity, such as breathing, swallowing, etc., probably accounts for relatively little energy expenditure compared with the requirements of those organs and tissues which are metabolically active throughout fetal life.

Efficient placental exchange mechanisms are of course essential for the provision of adequate supplies of oxygen and nutrients to the fetus and for the elimination of waste materials like carbon dioxide and urea. These transfer processes in turn depend upon the maintenance of the blood supply on either side of the placenta throughout gestation, particularly during the period of rapid fetal growth that occurs in many species in the last few weeks before birth.

The whole subject of placental exchange, particularly with respect to blood gases, has been extensively examined in recent years, and a number of reviews covering both experimental and theoretical aspects are available (Meschia, Battaglia and Bruns, 1967; Metcalfe, Bartels and Moll, 1967; Dawes, 1968; Longo, Hill and Power, 1972; Silver, Steven and Comline, 1973; Comline and Silver, 1974a, 1975). A detailed analysis of the factors affecting uterine and umbilical blood flow distribution and regulation is also beyond the scope of this chapter. However, some of the problems associated with the measurement of uterine and umbilical blood flows will be considered, since an accurate assessment of these is fundamental to any study involving quantitative observations on rates of uptake and utilisation by the fetus and by the utero-placental tissue.

EXPERIMENTAL TECHNIQUES

In order to estimate the metabolism and substrate utilisation of the fetus in any given species, it is necessary to determine its rate of oxygen consumption and its uptake of different metabolic fuels. This immediately imposes technical limitations on the use of small laboratory animals, since it is virtually impossible to obtain simultaneous samples of umbilical arterial and venous blood without serious impairment of flow. Furthermore, since anaesthesia and surgery may affect both umbilical and uterine blood flows and metabolism the use of acute experiments for the evaluation of energy balance in the fetus in any species is not very satisfactory.

Studies on conscious animals with indwelling catheters have so far been confined to the larger domestic animals, notably sheep. In ruminants and the horse it is possible to insert catheters into the umbilical vein and artery of the fetus and into the main uterine vein and a convenient artery of the mother, and to maintain such preparations for several weeks (Meschia et al, 1965; Comline and Silver, 1970; Silver, Steven and Comline, 1973). The difficulties and limitations of the chronically catheterised fetus and mother are considered in Chapter 12.

In such experimental preparations the sampling of arterial and venous blood from uterine and umbilical circulations is not difficult, but, since blood flow rates are very high, the actual arteriovenous (A–V) differences to be measured are inevitably small and may even be beyond the limits of the methods available. Battaglia and Meschia (1973) have drawn attention to these difficulties. Some of the ways in which they have been overcome will be considered later.

The measurement of uterine and umbilical blood flow in the conscious animal is not easy. Flow meters can be used only on uterine vessels, and although they are ideal for demonstrating rapid changes, measurements from one or even both middle uterine arteries probably underestimate total flow. All other methods of measurement are indirect, based on various modifications of the Fick principle. They have the disadvantage that steady-state conditions are required for measurement, that an incorrectly placed catheter can lead to erroneous results, and that a number of corrections and assumptions must be made in such determinations. Probably the most reliable of these methods is the steady state diffusion method of Meschia et al (1967b), whereby the fetus is constantly infused with an inert freely diffusible material (antipyrine). Once equilibrium conditions are obtained (40 min to one hour) any number of flow measurements may be made by measuring the umbilical and uterine A–V difference in antipyrine. Since the rate of infusion (Rf) into the fetus is approximately equal to the rate of loss into the uterine circulation, blood flow = Rf/(A–V).

A number of corrections to the numerator in the equation allows a more accurate assessment of flow but does not normally reduce the value by more than five per cent. Absolute flows are obtained with the method and can only be converted to flow/kg by weighing the fetus and uterus. Thus flow related to tissue weight can only be estimated in a chronic preparation.

A second widely used method is the diffusion equilibrium method of Huckabee et al

1972), which enables single estimations of uterine and/or umbilical flow to be made. The measurement takes about 20 min to make but neither the *amount* of test material delivered to the organ nor its weight need be determined. This is achieved by estimating the tissue water concentration (which is equal to blood water concentration) at the end of the period over which flow is being measured. An A–V difference is created by infusing antipyrine for a short (five to seven-min) period; by the end of the 20-min test period the A–V difference has disappeared and the blood and tissue concentrations [C] are sufficiently close to substitute blood concentration as the numerator in the Fick equation, so that flow can be expressed in ml/kg tissue perfused/min. The blood flow is calculated from the expression:

$$\frac{|C|}{\int([A] - [V])dt}$$

where $\int([A] - [V])$ is the integrated A − V difference and t is the time for equilibrium to be established. Obviously the smaller the total A–V difference the greater the blood flow.

Another problem exists in the uterine circulation, since blood flow is distributed to endometrium, myometrium and placenta, and it is only the blood flow in the latter which is relevant to the transfer of gases and nutrients to the fetus. However, measurements of relative flows to these areas may be made by determining the distribution of radioactively labelled microspheres (Makowski et al, 1968a). A relatively small number of spheres 15 to 25 μm in diameter are injected into the left ventricle or upper aorta and these become completely trapped in the capillary beds throughout the body. Since there is no recirculation of the spheres, the amount of radioactivity present in any organ or tissue will be proportional to its blood flow. If the total radioactivity in the arterial blood during injection of the microspheres is also measured, then the blood flow rate to the tissue can be determined. Such studies in sheep have shown that 85 per cent or more of the total uterine blood flow goes to the placenta in late gestation (Makowski et al, 1968a).

It may be argued that in the chronic preparation the presence of the catheters within the umbilical and uterine vessels will seriously impede the local circulation and cause some general decrease in flow. This seems less likely to occur in the larger animals, particularly when cord vessels are catheterised directly as in the horse (Comline et al, 1975) or approached from a primary cotyledon with its vessels converging on the cord, as in the cow (Comline et al, 1974). In view of these flow problems it is essential that the chronically catheterised fetus be monitored carefully; this not only applies to its oxygenation and acid–base balance but also to the plasma concentration of various key metabolites, e.g. glucose, lactate, urea, etc., which should be related to levels in the maternal circulation. Furthermore, the general well-being and nutritional state of the mother must obviously be within normal limits for the species.

No truly comparable studies on the primate fetus have been made. In monkeys and baboons either acute experiments or semichronic preparations (with the mother sedated) have been used (Table 10.1), while in humans it is only possible to obtain umbilical cord blood samples during caesarean section or at the end of labour—these can scarcely be considered representative of the human fetus in utero.

UMBILICAL AND UTERINE BLOOD FLOW

In the sheep, uterine and umbilical blood flows keep pace with the growth of the uterus and fetus throughout the latter half of gestation, i.e. the rates of flow when expressed per unit

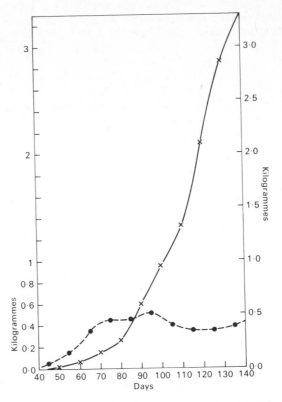

Figure 10.1. Average growth–weight curve for sheep fetuses x-x-x, and for placental cotyledons ········· From Barcroft (1946) by kind permission of the publishers (Oxford: Blackwell).

weight of tissue remain unchanged (within rather wide limits) during this period (for references see Comline and Silver, 1974a). These findings are particularly remarkable when it is remembered that in this species there is no enlargement of the placenta after 60 to 70 days gestation (Figure 10.1), so that the actual rate of blood flow through both fetal and maternal placental tissue must increase enormously during the second half of pregnancy. By contrast, the placenta in many other species, including man, continues to enlarge slightly as term approaches and hence blood flow rate through the placental vasculature may not increase so dramatically as in the ruminants. Nevertheless, values for *total* uterine and umbilical blood flow increase substantially in all species examined, although the precise mechanisms by which these changes are brought about are still a matter for speculation. Clearly, the overall increase in umbilical blood flow with age is related to the gradual rise in arterial blood pressure and cardiac output of the fetus as it increases in size (Dawes, 1968). Maternal cardiac output also rises during pregnancy, while uterine vascular resistance becomes very low and it is possible that these changes are brought about by alterations in the hormonal climate of the animal. Whether the gradual rise in fetal and maternal placental blood flow is also under endocrine control, perhaps via local hormonal changes within the placenta (Barron, 1970), has yet to be shown experimentally, although indirect evidence along these lines is convincing (Meschia, 1974).

Since absolute values for uterine and umbilical blood flow increase during gestation, total blood flows through these two circulations are normally related to the weight of the uteru

Table 10.1. *Summary of uterine and umbilical blood flow data.*

Uterine blood flow (ml/kg/min)

Species	Flow	Preparation[a]	Method[b]	Reference
Sheep	248	CC	DE	Huckabee et al, 1972
	282	A	SSD	Meschia et al, 1967b
Goat	354	CC	DE	Cotter, Blechner and Prystowsky, 1969
	277	A	DE	Huckabee et al, 1961
Cow	315	CC	DE	Silver and
	295	A	SSD	Comline, 1975a
Mare	312	CC	DE	
	290	A	DE/SSD	
Rhesus monkey	100	sedated	SSD	Parer et al, 1968
	114	sedated	SSD	Meschia et al, 1967a
	210	CC	SSD	
	140	semi-sedated	SSD	Cotter and Little, 1970
Human	110	A (caesarean)	DE	Blechner, Stenger and Prystowsky, 1974

Umbilical blood flow (ml/kg/min)

Species	Flow	Preparation[a]	Method[b]	Reference
Sheep	170	A	EM flow meter	Dawes and Mott, 1964
	176	A	M	Makowski et al, 1968b
	199	CC	M	Faber and Green, 1972
	221	A	SSD	Rudolph and Heymann, 1970
	175	CC	SSD	James et al, 1972
Cow	232	CC	DE	Silver and
	184	A	SSD	Comline, 1975a
Mare	171	CC	DE	
	113	A	SSD/DE/M	
Rhesus monkey	208	A	SSD	Behrman et al, 1970
Baboon	104	A	SSD	Fisher et al, 1972

[a] CC = chronically catheterised; A = anaesthetised.
[b] DE = diffusion equilibrium; SSD = steady state diffusion; M = labelled microspheres; EM = electromagnetic.

and its tissue contents or to the fetus respectively. A summary of recent data for ruminants horse and primate is given in Table 10.1, and the methods of measurement and the type o preparation used are also indicated. It will be seen that values for uterine blood flow in th various domestic animals are of the same order, whereas those for primates are lower. Apar from the obvious disadvantages of using sedated animals, the variable venous drainage of th primate uterus may give misleading results (Battaglia, Makowski and Meschia, 1970).

Umbilical blood flows are lower than uterine flows whether expressed in absolute terms c per unit weight. In the sheep no consistent differences have been found between the value observed in conscious animals and those from acute anaesthetised preparations in which th fetus has been kept under good conditions in utero (Table 10.1). On the other hand exteriorisation of the fetus can result in a drastic fall in umbilical flow (Heymann an Rudolph, 1967). A number of different methods have been used to measure umbilical flow i the sheep, but it seems unlikely that the wide range of values obtained is due solely t differences in technique, since large variations may be observed in the same animal, wherea two different methods tested simultaneously on the same animal can give identical result (Rudolph and Heymann, 1967). In the larger animals anaesthesia and surgery appeared t have a somewhat deleterious effect on umbilical blood flow (Table 10.1), since the value obtained in acute experiments were consistently lower than those from chronicall catheterised cows and mares. It is unfortunate that the umbilical flows reported for primate were in acute anaesthetised preparations; data obtained at birth in the human are als variable (75 to 140 ml/kg/min), as might be expected (see Stembera, Hodr and Janda, 1965 It is thus virtually impossible to gauge the normal range of umbilical blood flow rates i primates during late gestation.

OXYGEN UPTAKE OF THE FETUS AND UTERO-PLACENTAL TISSUE

Exchange mechanisms

The problems associated with the transfer of oxygen from mother to fetus have probabl received more attention than any other aspect of fetal physiology (for references see Comlin and Silver, 1975). In addition to the mechanisms which affect the passage of any freel diffusible molecule across the placental barrier, e.g. rates of supply and removal (blood flow) vascular architecture, placental usage, there are some special features which help to ensur that an adequate supply of oxygen reaches the fetus under both normal and abnormal con ditions. These include (1) an oxygen affinity which is generally higher than that of the mother (2) a capacity to increase the oxygen carrying power of the blood and (3) the ability to effect redistribution of the circulation so that blood flow to essential areas (brain, heart, placenta) i maintained or increased at the expense of flow to other areas.

The presence of a high blood oxygen affinity in the fetus deserves some explanation, par ticularly since the difference between maternal and fetal P_{50} may be only 1 to 2 mm Hg (i horse) or 10 to 25 mm Hg (in sheep, cow, pig, human). ($P_{50} = O_2$ tension at which blood is 5(per cent saturated, at pH 7.4.) In the latter species there is a large transplacental Po_2 gradien and all the evidence suggests that gas exchange is not very efficient (perhaps because of th vascular arrangement and flow patterns found in these types of placenta). By contrast, in th horse the exchange areas have a unique type of microcirculation (Silver, Steven an

Comline, 1973) and transplacental Po_2 gradients are extremely small. Thus, in the fetal foal, little increase in blood oxygen saturation would be achieved by a leftward shift of its oxyhaemoglobin equilibrium curve, since the umbilical venous blood is already about 80 per cent saturated at an oxygen affinity close to that of the mother. On the other hand, in those species in which umbilical venous Po_2 rarely rises above 35 to 40 mm Hg (e.g. ruminants, pigs), it is essential that the oxygen affinity is high so that blood returning to the fetus is at least 70 to 80 per cent saturated (Comline and Silver, 1974b).

The Po_2 of fetal *arterial* blood is generally maintained just above the normal P_{50} for the species. This ensures that maximum unloading of oxygen at the tissues will occur with minimum changes in tension. Under stable resting conditions in utero there is no reason to suppose that the oxygen supply to the fetus is inadequate, or that the tension at which it is carried is too low. There is in fact little evidence to suggest that any great changes in umbilical venous Po_2 can be effected by the fetus, although it has some capacity to increase the *amount* of oxygen transferred. Thus, during fetal hypoxaemia, whether acute or chronic, the fetal oxygen-carrying capacity of the blood rises and cardiovascular regulation ensures that the blood flow to non-essential areas is decreased, while placental flow is maintained (for references see Dawes, 1968; Comline and Silver, 1974a). However, it is probable that neither of these mechanisms is particularly active during a normal, non-eventful pregnancy. Meschia et al (1965) showed that the oxygen capacity in chronically catheterised sheep and goat fetuses remained stable as term approached, although the values were raised on the day after operation. It seems, therefore, that only under conditions in which fetal oxygen supply may be in jeopardy, is the oxygen-carrying power of its blood increased, as for example during anaesthesia or surgery, during acute hypoxia or after exposure to high altitude, or during the terminal stages of parturition (Comline and Silver, 1974a).

Similarly, the reflex cardiovascular readjustments which may occur in the fetus in response to hypoxaemia would also appear to be short-term defence mechanisms. The whole basis of the redistribution of the fetal circulation under these conditions was elegantly shown by Dawes and his colleagues in acute experiments on the fetal lamb (Dawes et al, 1969). That such changes in organ blood flow also occur in the non-anaesthetised fetus in response to maternal hypoxia has now been demonstrated by Cohn et al (1974) using labelled microspheres to show changes in fetal blood flow distribution.

Fetal and placental oxygen consumption

Provided that measurements of the A–V differences in oxygen across the umbilical and uterine circulations are made at the same time as estimations of blood flow rate, then the actual amount of oxygen used by the uterus as a whole and that taken up by the fetus may be compared.

In a number of species, an inverse relationship between the A–V difference in oxygen and the blood flow rate has been observed both in the uterine and umbilical circulations (Crenshow et al, 1968; Parer et al, 1968; Silver and Comline, 1976), so that the actual oxygen consumption remains within a relatively narrow range despite wide fluctuations in blood flow. Table 10.2 summarises the data available for oxygen consumption of the whole uterus and for the fetus alone in the various species under consideration.

Uterine uptake is generally higher than that of the fetus, and if the relative weights of the fetus and utero-placental mass are known, it is possible to calculate the oxygen consumption of the latter (Table 10.2). As might be expected utero-placental uptake, whether measured directly (Meschia et al, 1967b) or calculated (Comline and Silver, 1975) is high compared with that of the fetus. If the distribution of blood flow to the placental and non-placental tissues is determined using the labelled microsphere technique (Makowski et al, 1968a), then estimates of the oxygen uptake of these tissues can be made. This information is as yet only available for the sheep, and here it appears that placental oxygen consumption may be as high as 30 to 35 ml/kg/min, while the remaining uterine oxygen uptake is only one-tenth of this (Comline and Silver, 1974a).

The values for fetal oxygen consumption in the different species are surprisingly uniform (Table 10.2). However, variations may occur within a species even under stable chronic conditions. Battaglia and Meschia (1973) have shown that in twin pregnancies the fetal oxygen

Table 10.2. *Mean values for oxygen consumption of the fetus and of the uterus and contents during late gestation in different species.*

Species	Mean O_2 consumption (ml/kg/min)			Reference
	Uterus, fetus and placenta	Fetus	Utero-placental mass	
Sheep[b]	10.4			Huckabee et al, 1972
Sheep and goat [a]	9.9	7.1	14.1	Meschia et al, 1976b
Sheep and goat [b]		8.5		Crenshaw et al, 1968
Sheep [b]		6.0		James et al, 1972
Cow [b]	8.0	6.8	11.0[c]	Comline and
Mare [b]	8.5	7.5	10.0[c]	Silver, 1975.
Monkey [b]	6.10			Cotter and Little, 1970
Monkey [a]		7.0		Behrman et al, 1970

[a] Acute experiments.
[b] Chronic experiments with implanted catheters.
[c] Calculated from weight data giving a fetal to uterine weight ratio of 6:4.

uptake appears to be lower (6.53 ± 0.27 ml/kg/min) than that of singleton fetuses under identical conditions (7.85 ± 0.26 ml/kg/min). It seems probable that a lower oxygen consumption may be characteristic of fetuses with some degree of growth retardation—whether this is due to placental insufficiency or other causes.

During acute oxygen deprivation of the fetus, its oxygen utilisation may be markedly reduced. Some years ago Dawes and colleagues showed that maternal hypoxaemia led to a decrease in fetal oxygen consumption in the exteriorised, anaesthetised fetus (see Dawes 1968). Since we now know that reflex cardiovascular readjustments can result in very restricted peripheral blood flows (to limbs, lungs, etc.) in the chronically catheterised fetus (Cohn et al, 1974), it is more than likely that during any conditions resulting in inadequate placental exchange, total fetal oxygen uptake will be decreased. Inevitably, in those tissues to which blood flow is drastically reduced, some anaerobic respiration will occur. Eventually the fetus will become acidotic due to excess lactate production in these tissues and, unless placental exchange is greatly improved, deterioration of the fetus will result, since lactic acid is probably metabolised only under conditions of good oxygenation and little appears to be transferred directly across the placenta into the maternal circulation (see Shelley, 1973; Silver, Steven and Comline, 1973; Burd et al, 1975).

Fetal tissue oxygen uptake

As yet there have been few studies on the oxygen uptake of different organs and tissues even in the normal, well oxygenated fetus, although differential blood flow measurements (Cohn e al, 1974) have indicated that a very wide range may be found, from 270 ml/100 g/min in the adrenal to 60 ml/100 g/min in lung. Recent investigations by Makowski et al (1972) on fetal cerebral blood flow and oxygen uptake in the lamb, have shown that the oxygen consumption of this tissue (4.0 ml/100 g/min) is of the same order as that found in adult human brain (3.5 ml/100 g/min). This high rate of metabolism is maintained by a high cerebral blood flow of 100 to 120 ml/100 g/min, i.e. twice that of the adult. Clearly, fetal cerebral oxygenation is dependent on adequate control of the blood supply to this area, for even a slight reduction in flow at the low arterial oxygen concentration normally found in the fetus may jeopardise cerebral metabolism. In this context it is particularly interesting that Cohn et al (1974) have shown that during fetal hypoxaemia cerebral blood flow almost doubles and myocardial flow increases still more, although total cardiac output remains unchanged under these conditions. Whether these changes in flow are sufficient to maintain cerebral oxygen consumption at the normal rate during hypoxaemia has yet to be demonstrated in the conscious animal.

FETAL AND UTERO-PLACENTAL SUBSTRATE UTILISATION

Glucose has always been assumed to be the major or even the only metabolic fuel of the fetus, but the evidence for this view is very indirect and recent work on the conscious sheep and its fetus suggests that other substrates must be examined carefully for their importance in fetal metabolism before its energy balance can be computed (Battaglia and Meschia, 1973). These authors looked particularly at the evidence for fetal uptake and utilisation of glucose and other sugars, ketoacids, free fatty acids (FFA) and glycerol; they also investigated the energy available from amino acid catabolism. These studies, together with relevant data from other species, including the evidence for acetate and lactate utilisation and any information on utero-placental uptakes, will be briefly reviewed before assessing the contribution made by each to the overall metabolism of the fetus.

Glucose

The importance of an adequate supply of glucose to the pregnant animal has long been recognised. In ruminants particularly, the uterus may well utilise most of the available glucose, so that poor nutrition can easily retard fetal growth and result in ketosis and pregnancy toxaemia (Kronfeld, 1958; Reid, 1968). The high rate of glucose uptake by the pregnant uterus was emphasised by the experiments of Setchell et al (1972) who showed that at least 70 per cent of the total glucose metabolism of the pregnant ewe could be accounted for by uterine uptake.

Early experiments on the exteriorised fetus showed that it could utilise large amounts of glucose but the conditions in these preparations varied and maternal concentrations were rarely measured (see Crenshaw, 1970). It was not until the advent of the chronically catheterised fetus that the relationship between maternal and fetal glucose concentrations was examined in detail in the sheep (Comline and Silver, 1970; Battaglia and Meschia, 1973; Shelley, 1973; Silver, Steven and Comline, 1973). It was shown that fetal plasma concentrations were dependent upon the maternal levels (Figure 10.2), although fetal values were generally only about one-third or one-quarter of those in the mother.

It is perhaps unfortunate that so much attention should have been focused on the sheep. In this species maternal plasma glucose concentrations may fall to 30 to 40 mg/100 ml without

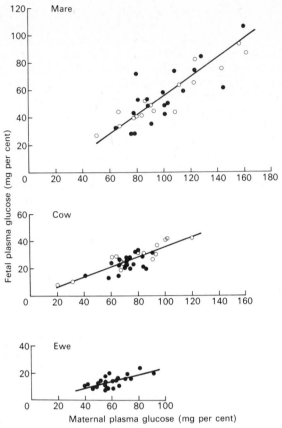

Figure 10.2. The relation between maternal and fetal plasma glucose levels in mare, cow and sheep. ●, values from conscious animals; o, values from anaesthetised preparations. Two to three values are given for each experiment. From Silver et al (1973) with kind permission of the publishers (Cambridge: Cambridge University Press).

obvious detriment to either mother or fetus, but under these circumstances fetal plasma glucose levels become extremely low. In view of the high utero-placental uptake, it is possible that this takes precedence over the fetus, so that during periods when maternal glucose falls the fetal uptake is diminished and the fetus becomes relatively hypoglycaemic (see page 188). On the other hand, when maternal concentrations are artificially raised by infusion, fetal values plateau at concentrations between 40 and 60 mg/100 ml suggesting that some limit to fetal uptake may have been reached (Shelley, 1973; Silver, Steven and Comline, 1973).

The relationship between fetal and maternal glucose concentrations in the sheep may be compared with that found in the cow and horse (Figure 10.2). Although the cow is another species of ruminant, its plasma glucose concentrations appear to be maintained at much higher levels (60 to 85 mg/100 ml) and fetal concentrations are likewise higher than those in lambs. The horse, like the pig and primate, has a high basal plasma glucose concentration in the adult, and fetal plasma glucose is normally about 60 to 70 per cent of the maternal value in all these species. Whether the passage of glucose across the placental barrier takes place by facilitated diffusion, as suggested by Widdas (1961), would seem to require more direct experimental evidence. Recent experiments on the transfer of different sugars across the sheep placenta (Boyd et al, 1976) have suggested that some form of facilitated ansfer exists. On the other hand, in those species with a high maternal plasma glucose, acental transfer seems to occur more readily, or at any rate the high maternal concen-ations apparently ensure an adequate supply for both utero-placental and fetal uptake. In uman and monkey, fetal plasma glucose may rise extremely high during maternal yperglycaemia, but it is not yet clear whether a limit to diffusion from mother to fetus may e reached (see Oakley, Beard and Turner, 1972; Chez et al, 1975).

In Table 10.3 mean uterine and fetal glucose uptakes in sheep, cow and horse may be com-ared. In all these species the fetal uptake of glucose is much lower than that of the uterus as a hole. Utero-placental usage was estimated in the same way as its oxygen consumption (see able 10.2) using a weight ratio of utero-placental mass: fetus of 4:6 (obtained from acute xperiments). Obviously much of the high utero-placental uptake must be due to placental tilisation, for the placenta is not just an organ for exchange but contains endocrine tissue hich is likely to have a high rate of metabolism. The evidence of Setchell et al (1972) iggests that a considerable proportion of the glucose removed by the uterus is not oxidised nd may well be used for glycogen storage or other synthetic processes.

Table 10.3. *Mean values ($\pm$ s.e.m.) for glucose uptake of the uterus, fetus and the utero-placental mass during late gestation in different species (conscious animals).*

pecies	Mean glucose consumption (mg/kg/min)			Reference
	Uterus and tissue contents	Fetus	Utero-placental mass	
heep	11.1 (4)	—	—	Setchell et al, 1972
		3.1 ± 0.3 (22)	—	James et al, 1972
		4.6	—	Crenshaw, 1970
ow	9.0 ± 0.8 (6)	5.2 ± 0.3 (6)	15^a	Silver and
lare	10.9 ± 1.1 (4)	6.8 ± 0.6 (4)	17^a	Comline, 1975a

Estimated using the weight ratio of 6:4 for fetus: utero-placental mass.
Number of observations given in parenthesis.

In the sheep the uptake of glucose by the chronically catheterised fetus is generally lower han the values of 5 to 10 mg/kg/min reported for acute anaesthetised preparations (see Crenshaw, 1970). It is probable that raised ACTH, corticosteroid and catecholamine levels a both ewe and fetus might, in part, account for a high fetal glucose uptake in acute xperiments. Nevertheless, it is difficult to understand why fetal glucose uptake in the sheep nder normal resting conditions in utero should be quite so low. Battaglia and Meschia 1973) found a range of fetal uptake between 1 and 6 mg/kg/min, which appeared to be elated to the maternal arterial glucose concentration. Over the maternal blood concentra-on range of 20 to 55 mg/100 ml (ca 35 to 70 mg/100 ml plasma) there was no indication nat a maximum fetal uptake had been reached. In general, the values for twins were lower han for singleton lambs at the same maternal concentration. These studies are at variance /ith the findings of Crenshaw (1970), who used similar chronic preparations and could find o relationship between fetal glucose uptake and maternal concentrations; both seemed in-ependently variable.

In both cows and horses values for fetal uptake lay within a relatively narrow range (Table 0.3) and there was no evidence for any dependence of fetal uptake upon maternal arterial oncentrations; this is shown for the cow in Figure 10.4. Further experiments under con-itions of maternal hypoglycaemia are clearly required, but the available evidence suggests hat in the cow an uptake of about 5.0 mg/kg/min is maximal for this species (Comline and ilver, 1976).

No comparable investigations have been made in the subhuman primate and only limite data from cord samples taken during labour or caesarean section are available for th human. Here, like the results from acutely anaesthetised lamb preparations, the A–V glucos differences are in general fairly high (Sabata, Wolf and Lausmann, 1968); if a low umbilic blood flow rate of 80 to 100 ml/kg/min is assumed (see Stembera, Hodr and Janda, 1965 the uptake of glucose by the human fetus during labour may be in the region of 7 to 1 mg/kg/min. This high uptake may well be related to the maternal hyperglycaemia which ca occur during labour. In addition, plasma cortisol and catecholamines in the fetus may t elevated at birth; inevitably such observations made during parturition tell us little about th normal metabolism of glucose by the human fetus in utero.

Fructose

In the fructogenic species (ruminant, horse, pig) there is always a high concentration of fruc tose in the fetal plasma. This sugar is produced in the placenta and its concentration is depen dent on the plasma glucose concentration in both the mother and fetus (Comline and Silve 1970). It is virtually confined to the fetus and its fluids, with no transfer back into the mate nal circulation, but there is little or no evidence for its utilisation in any of the species studie Very small amounts of fructose appeared to be metabolised in acute, anaesthetise preparations (Alexander et al, 1969) and similar conclusions were reached by Setchell et a (1972) using chronically catheterised fetuses. They looked at the fate of ^{14}C from labelle fructose and glucose injected into the fetus, and found some incorporation of both sugar into glycogen and CO_2 but neither sugar could account for more than a fraction of the CC production. These experiments are open to a number of criticisms (Shelley, 1973), and it possible that the low rate of fetal glucose utilisation observed by these authors was partly du to inadequate uptake. In a different type of investigation, A–V differences in both fructos and glucose were examined in chronically catheterised sheep fetuses (Tsoulos et al, 1971 These authors could find no evidence for any detectable umbilical A–V difference in fructos whether the ewes were fed or starved, whereas fetal A–V glucose differences were diminishe by about 60 per cent during starvation.

In both cows and horses no consistent umbilical A–V differences in fructose have bee observed (Silver and Comline, 1975b). It would seem therefore that this sugar, which is pre sent in such high concentrations in the fetal plasma and the amniotic and allantoic fluids, ha a very low turnover and a very limited metabolism in the fetus.

Amino acids

The uptake of amino acids and the very specialised mechanisms involved in their transfe from mother to fetus are discussed in detail in Chapter 4. Amino acids are not only require for the formation of new protein but they may also be deaminated and subsequentl metabolised or incorporated into glycogen or fat. There is at present no information on th relative importance of these pathways in the fetus, but measurements of the production an placental transfer of urea allow some estimation of the extent of amino acid catabolism in th fetus. In all animals examined fetal plasma urea concentrations are higher than those of th mother (Battaglia and Meschia, 1973). The feto-maternal urea concentration gradient in th sheep appears to be constant over a wide range of maternal concentrations and implies steady diffusion of urea from the fetal to maternal circulation (Figure 10.3). In order to es timate the actual amount of urea transferred, the conventional Fick methods cannot b

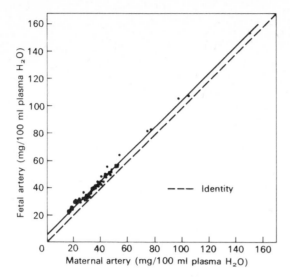

re 10.3. Relationship of fetal arterial urea concentration to the concentration of urea in maternal blood.
rvations made on sheep, four or more days after surgery. From Battaglia and Meschia (1973) with kind permission of the authors and the publisher (Cambridge: Cambridge University Press).

lied since the A–V urea difference across the umbilical circulation is below the limits of
surement. This difficulty has been overcome by measuring the transplacental clearance
rea (Gresham et al, 1972). Since urea clearance (Cu) is defined as follows:

$$Cu = \frac{\text{urea excretion rate}}{(Ua) - (Ma)}$$

measurement of Cu and the urea concentrations in the umbilical artery (Ua) and the
ernal artery (Ma) allows the urea excretion rate to be calculated. In the sheep under quiet
ing conditions, mean values for urea clearance (19.0 and 20.5 ml/kg/min) obtained by
independent methods agreed within five per cent of each other and since the artery-to-
ry urea concentration difference was 3.6 mg/100 ml, the mean excretion rate of urea was
4 ± 0.3 mg/kg/min (or 0.36 g urea N_2/kg/day). This value is four times that found in the
nal adult sheep. Gresham et al (1972) estimated that in the sheep about 40 per cent of the
l nitrogen which crosses the placenta from mother to fetus is returned to the mother as
a. Since the amount of oxygen required for deamination can be calculated from indirect
orimetry, the contribution made by amino acid breakdown to fetal metabolism can be
essed.
imilar information is not yet available for the other domestic animals or for the human,
ough urea clearance in subhuman primates (Battaglia et al, 1968) does not appear to be
different (15 ml/kg/min) from that in the sheep. However, the (Ua) − (Ma) urea concen-
ion difference in the human fetus at term is lower (2.5 mg/100 ml) than in sheep so that
excretion rate may be estimated at 0.38 mg/kg/min (Battaglia and Meschia, 1973). In
horse and cow the artery-to-artery urea concentration differences between fetus and
her are also low (1 to 2 mg/100 ml), so that even if a clearance value as high as 20
kg/min is assumed for these species, the urea excretion rate is likely to be only 0.2 to 0.4
kg/min, i.e. a lower rate of fetal amino acid catabolism than has been found in the sheep.

Free fatty acids and glycerol

Comparatively little is known about the mechanisms which affect the transfer of FFA and glycerol across the placenta (Hull, 1975). The relationship between fetal and maternal FFA concentrations and the possible uptake of these substrates by the fetus have, however, been examined in a few species. In ruminants FFA concentrations in the fetus are invariably low and do not appear to be related to maternal levels (Silver, Steven and Comline, 1973). Attempts to raise FFA concentrations in fetal ruminants have largely failed. For example, injections of catecholamines into the fetus resulted in very small increases in fetal plasma FFA (Comline and Silver, 1972), whilst elevation of maternal values by starvation led to very slight increases in the fetal plasma concentrations of both FFA and glycerol (see Battaglia and Meschia, 1973). The latter authors could find no detectable umbilical A–V differences in FFA and only very small differences in glycerol in their sheep. They concluded that neither FFA nor glycerol could contribute significantly to the metabolism of the fetal sheep; the same would appear to be true for the fetal calf (Comline and Silver, 1976).

   In the horse, primate, rat and rabbit, fetal plasma FFA concentrations are much higher and are more closely related to values in the maternal circulation (see Chapter 6). Detectable umbilical A–V differences have been reported for the rabbit (Hull, 1975) and for the human during labour where high maternal FFA concentrations are found (Sheath et al, 1972). However, measurements during delivery have doubtful relevance to conditions in the undisturbed fetus in utero. In any event Sabata, Wolf and Lausmann (1968) and Sheath et al (1972) conclude that FFA and glycerol uptake by the fetus contributes little towards its metabolic needs compared with glucose utilisation.

   In the mare maternal plasma FFA concentrations are extremely labile but no consistent differences in FFA across the umbilical circulation in chronically catheterised fetuses could be found (Silver and Comline, 1975a). It would seem, therefore, that although the passage of some FFA from mother to fetus occurs during gestation and can be demonstrated using labelled materials (see Hull, 1975) the magnitude of this transfer is small, so that fetal utilisation is comparatively unimportant in terms of energy production.

Other possible substrates for fetal utilisation

Since glucose uptake by the fetus is much diminished during starvation in the ewe (Tsoulos et al, 1971), these authors sought other possible substrates which might have some importance in supplying energy to the fetus. Morriss et al (1974) investigated the umbilical uptake of acetoacetate and β-OH butyrate, since these metabolites are known to increase in the maternal blood during starvation. Small but significant umbilical A–V differences in both substances could be detected, but it was found that the actual amounts removed by the fetus, whether under normal or starvation conditions, could contribute little to its oxidative metabolism.

   The possibility that volatile fatty acids might be used by the fetus has been re-examined in the ruminant (Comline and Silver, 1976). Acetate in particular plays an important part in the metabolism of the adult ruminant and some years ago Pugh and Scarisbrick (1955) showed, in acute experiments on sheep, that very small umbilical A–V differences in acetate were present at artificially elevated maternal levels. In a different type of experiment Alexander, Britton and Nixon (1967) reported that the isolated perfused sheep fetus removed 2 to 5 mg acetate/kg/min from the perfusate; glucose uptakes in comparable preparations were 3 to 8 mg/kg/min.

   Since no information was available for chronically catheterised animals, the relationship tween fetal and maternal acetate concentrations and the uptakes, if any, by the fetus and erus were investigated in the conscious cow in late gestation (Comline and Silver, 1976). was found that acetate concentrations in the fetal blood were related to maternal levels in a anner similar to that described for glucose in the ruminant (Figure 10.2); fetal values were nerally one-third to one-quarter those of the mother over a maternal range of 2 to 10 g/100 ml blood. Measurable A–V differences in acetate across both uterine and umbilical rculation were found. The mean value for uterine uptake in six cows was 5.0 ± 0.6 g/kg/min while the corresponding figure for the fetus was 1.7 ± 0.6 mg/kg/min; utero- acental uptake (by calculation) was 10 mg/kg/min. It was noticed that, unlike fetal glucose otake in the cow, acetate utilisation by the fetus appeared to be related to the maternal terial concentration (Figure 10.4); thus in some animals fetal uptake was below 1 g/kg/min; in another with a maternal arterial concentration of 9 mg/100 ml, fetal uptake as 3.5 mg/kg/min. These findings indicate that the fetal uptake of acetate may make a small ut significant contribution to its energy balance, but further studies on both sheep and cows, nd on non-ruminant species, are required before the role of acetate in fetal metabolism can be ut on a definite quantitative basis.

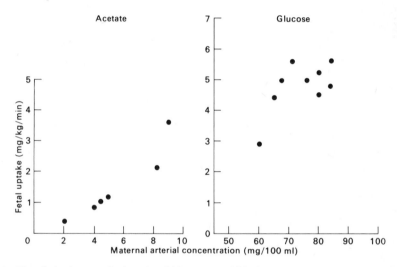

igure 10.4. The relation between fetal uptake of (a) acetate and (b) glucose and the concentrations of these sub- rates in the maternal arterial blood in the cow (chronic preparations) during late gestation. From Comline and Silver (1976) by kind permission of the editor of *Journal of Physiology*.

Recently Burd et al (1975) have provided evidence that lactate may be a possible substrate or oxidation in the fetal lamb. They found small but highly significant A–V differences in ctate concentration across both umbilical and uterine circulations. Since the highest lactate alues were found in the *venous* blood from these two circulations, a placental release of lac- te, with a significant uptake by the fetus, was strongly implicated. This finding is difficult to econcile with the apparent inability of the fetus to metabolise large amounts of endogenous- produced lactate. It is well known that once fetal plasma lactate concentrations rise, as for xample during a short hypoxic episode, the original concentrations are not restored for any hours (Shelley, 1973). Further observations on both ruminants and other species are learly required, and it would also be of considerable interest to know whether lactate utilisa- on by the fetus is increased during maternal starvation, since fetal glucose uptake under ese circumstances is reduced (Tsoulos et al, 1971).

ENERGY BALANCE IN THE FETUS

If the amount of oxygen consumed by the fetus is compared with the amount of substrate utilised, the contribution made by each substrate to the total energy balance of the fetus may be assessed. In fact, if measurements of the A–V difference in oxygen and substrate are measured in identical samples on a molar basis the energy quotient can be determined without the necessity for blood flow measurement (Tsoulos et al, 1971). Thus the contribution to total oxygen consumption made by aerobic glucose metabolism in the sheep fetus is calculated by the following equation:

$$\text{Glucose}:O_2 \text{ quotient} = \frac{6 \times \Delta \text{ glucose}}{\Delta O_2}$$

where Δglucose and ΔO_2 are the umbilical A–V differences measured simultaneously.

The value for this quotient in normal fed sheep is 0.4 to 0.5 (Tsoulos et al, 1971; Battaglia and Meschia, 1973), which means that glucose metabolism in the sheep fetus can account for only 40 to 50 per cent of its total oxygen consumption. This finding dispels the widely held view that glucose is virtually the sole source of energy in the fetus. In their search for other possible metabolic fuels, Battaglia and Meschia showed that amino acid catabolism could account for a further 25 per cent of the oxygen usage by the sheep fetus but that other substrates examined made relatively insignificant contributions to the energy balance in this species. However, their recent observations on lactate uptake suggest that the remaining 25 per cent of the fetal oxygen consumption can be accounted for by the utilisation of this substrate.

These findings for the sheep may be compared with data calculated in a similar manner for the fetal calf and foal. In the calf the mean value for the glucose oxygen quotient was found to be 0.57 (Comline and Silver, 1976), indicating that glucose utilisation in this species is somewhat higher than in the sheep, perhaps because maternal plasma glucose concentrations were uniformly high in this series of animals. In addition, the acetate:oxygen quotient in the fetal calf, though variable (0.16 ± 0.06, n = 7) could well account for at least 10 to 20 per cent of its oxygen consumption. If we assume that amino acid catabolism is less than that found in the fetal lamb (on the basis of the lower feto-maternal urea differences), it will perhaps account for 10 per cent of the oxygen uptake. The remaining 10 to 30 per cent oxygen may well be used in the metabolism of lactate since, like the sheep, there is a small but significant V–A difference in lactate across the umbilical circulation of the calf (Comline and Silver, 1976).

In the horse, glucose plays a much more important role in fetal metabolism (Silver and Comline, 1975a), since the glucose:oxygen quotient is much higher in this species (0.7). The evidence for acetate and lactate utilisation in the fetal foal is still somewhat equivocal, but it is possible that the combined metabolism of all the other known substrates could explain the remaining 30 per cent of the oxygen uptake of the equine fetus. In the human, metabolism is also primarily based on glucose and fetal uptake of this substrate is probably high. Sabata, Wolf and Lausmann (1968) have reviewed possible energy sources in the human fetus and conclude that glucose must be the main metabolic fuel, but the data available are extremely sparse and only relate to conditions during labour.

Although the oxygen consumption of the normal fetal lamb in utero would appear to be approximately balanced by its uptake of different substrates, a reduction in food intake by the ewe results in a drastic fall in fetal glucose uptake, despite the fact that oxygen consumption remains unchanged (Tsoulos et al, 1971). Under these circumstances, what metabolic fuels are available to the fetus? At present it is only possible to speculate that increased amino acid catabolism, lactate usage or endogenous glycogen breakdown from fetal liver and muscle stores may occur together with a limited uptake of ketoacids, glycerol and even fructose.

It is perhaps legitimate at this point to raise the question of whether conditions in the chronically catheterised fetus of an apparently well-fed animal are always optimal, particularly in a twin pregnancy, and to what extent such a fetus may use its previously established reserves during the period of catheterisation. If for any reason the nutrient supplies to the fetus are limited (perhaps due to inadequate maternal intake or placental impairment), it is difficult to see how normal fetal growth and metabolism can continue to be maintained and how reserves can be built up. As a result the lamb at birth may be smaller and perhaps weaker than normal; this is not an entirely infrequent occurrence in catheterised animals.

Carbon and nitrogen balance in the fetus

In the sheep fetus, carcass analyses at different stages of gestation have enabled the amounts of carbon and nitrogen accumulated in the fetus per day to be estimated (Battaglia and Meschia, 1973). Since the amounts passed back into the maternal circulation can be measured, the total carbon or nitrogen crossing the placenta from mother to fetus can be assessed. Gresham et al (1972) showed that 0.6 g N/kg was accumulated in the fetus each day, while 0.36 g/kg was eliminated back to the mother as urea; thus the total amount of nitrogen transferred across the placenta to the fetus was 0.96 g N/kg/day.

The carbon balance was calculated in a similar manner. James et al (1972) showed that 3.15 g C/kg/day was accumulated and 4.64 g/kg/day was excreted, either as carbon dioxide or as urea; i.e. in the lamb during late gestation as much as 7.7 g C/kg enters the fetus daily. However, according to their figures for glucose uptake in this species, glucose will supply on average 1.76 g C/kg/day; the remaining 77 per cent must, therefore, come from other sources. Battaglia and Meschia (1973) rejected the assumption that all of this carbon could be supplied in the form of amino acids since the resultant C:N ratio of 6.1 would be much higher than that for an average protein (3.3).

If, however, we assume that both acetate and lactate are utilised by the sheep fetus, this could explain much of the apparent carbon deficit. For example, a fetal uptake of 1 to 3 mg acetate/kg/min would amount to 0.58 to 1.7 g C/kg/day, while an uptake of lactate of 2.8 mg/kg/min would supply 1.6 g C/day; this brings the known carbon uptake to between 4 and 5 g/day. The remainder might well be transferred as amino acids, for the C:N ratio under these circumstances would be between 3 and 4.

The accumulation of carbon in the fetus during growth means that assessment of its energy balance by means of RQ measurement is not really possible. James et al (1972) calculated that the mean RQ of their lamb fetuses near term was 0.94 ± 0.01. At first sight this might seem indicative of a predominantly carbohydrate metabolism, but they point out that since nearly half the total carbon entering the fetus is retained, RQ values per se can give virtually no information about the type of fuel used by the fetus. There is thus no short-cut method for the assessment of fetal metabolism.

Special tissue requirements

There is little or no information about the metabolism of individual fetal tissues and their specific substrate requirements, if any. In the adult there are certain tissues, notably brain, which normally utilise only glucose.

Recent studies on the relative rates of uptake of glucose and oxygen by the fetal brain have shown that glucose uptake is sufficient to supply all the metabolic needs of the fetal brain; the mean glucose/oxygen quotient for this tissue was 1.1 (Makowski et al, 1972). These experiments suggest that the metabolism of the fetal brain does not differ significantly from that of adult human brain. However, the sheep fetus must supply both oxygen and glucose to this tissue at far lower concentrations than are found in man, and during hypoxia or maternal starvation the margin of safety must decrease to limits which are almost incompatible with its continued aerobic glucose metabolism.

These findings on the metabolic requirements of the fetal brain prompted an investigation into the substrate utilisation of a different type of tissue. Morris et al (1973) examined the glucose and oxygen uptake of the hind limbs in fetal lambs and found that the glucose:oxygen quotient increased with the availability of substrate, i.e. at relatively high fetal arterial glucose concentrations (15 to 20 mg/100 ml) the glucose:oxygen was always greater than 1; the range of values found was 0.2 to 1.7. Thus in well-fed ewes, the fetal limb glucose uptake always exceeded the oxidative metabolism in the tissue. These results do not, however, exclude the possibility that other substrates may be used by the limb, nor that some of the glucose removed may be used anaerobically or for glycogen synthesis or growth.

CONCLUSIONS

The foregoing account of fetal energy metabolism and substrate utilisation illustrates both the usefulness and limitations of animal experiments when applied to problems of human fetal physiology. Thus, despite some anomalies we now have a reasonable picture of the major sources of energy available to the ruminant fetus and some information along these lines for the fetal foal. Nevertheless, to extrapolate from these two groups to the human or to other mammals is scarcely justifiable, for although any fetus may be supplied with glucose, amino acids, FFA, acetate, ketoacids, lactate and other metabolites, the actual amount of each nutrient which may be used for metabolism and growth probably varies widely in different species.

It is unfortunate that in the human, virtually all the available information is confined to the observations made during the terminal stages of labour (Stembera, Hodr and Janda, 1965; Sabata, Wolf and Lausmann, 1968; Sheath et al, 1972). This is a period when the hormonal climate of both mother and fetus is very different from that found during the latter part of gestation. These endocrine changes together with the increased activity of the sympathetic and central nervous systems which may occur during parturition are scarcely consistent with normal basal metabolism in either mother or fetus.

Experiments on substrate utilisation do not appear to have been carried out on subhuman primates, although there is little doubt that monkeys and baboons are more suitable models for comparison with man than the ruminant or horse. Unfortunately, the technical difficulties associated with the insertion and maintenance of umbilical vascular catheters in these species are immense. Furthermore, their agility and ingenuity make sedation almost obligatory, but its effect on fetal and maternal metabolism is not known. There is obviously a great need for an experimental preparation which is hormonally and metabolically similar to the human, with a fetus and a placenta comparable with that found in primates, so that data more applicable to man can be obtained under normal resting conditions in utero.

REFERENCES

Alexander, D. P., Britton, H. G. & Nixon, D. A. (1967) Acetate metabolism in the isolated sheep foetus. *Journal of Physiology,* **190,** 295–308.

Alexander, D. P., Britton, H. G., Cohen, N. M. & Nixon, D. A. (1969) Foetal metabolism. In *Foetal Autonomy, Ciba Foundation Symposium,* pp. 95–113. London: J. & A. Churchill.

Barcroft, J. (1946). *Researches on Prenatal Life.* Oxford: Blackwell.

Barron, D. H. (1970). In *Prenatal Life: Biological and Clinical Perspectives* (Ed.) Mack, H. C. pp. 109–127. Detroit, Michigan: Wayne State University Press.

Battaglia, F. C. & Meschia, G. (1973) Foetal metabolism and substrate utilization. In *Foetal and Neonatal Physiology, Barcroft Centenary Symposium* (Ed.) Comline, R. S., Cross, K. W., Dawes, G. S. & Nathanielsz, P. W. pp. 382–397. London: Cambridge University Press.

Battaglia, F. C., Makowski, E. L. & Meschia, G. (1970) Physiologic study of the uterine venous drainage of the pregnant rhesus monkey. *Yale Journal of Biology and Medicine,* **42,** 218–228.

Battaglia, F. C., Behrman, R. E., Meschia, G., Seeds, A. E. & Bruns, P. D. (1968) Clearance of inert molecules, Na and Cl ions across the primate placenta. *American Journal of Obstetrics and Gynecology,* **102,** 1135–1143.

Behrman, R. E., Lees, M. H., Peterson, E. N., de Lannoy, C. W. & Seeds, A. E. (1970) Distribution of the circulation in the normal and asphyxiated fetal primate. *American Journal of Obstetrics and Gynecology,* **108,** 956–969.

Blechner, J. N., Stenger, V. G. & Prystowsky, H. (1974) Uterine blood flow in women at term. *American Journal of Obstetrics and Gynecology,* **120,** 633–640.

Boyd, R. D. H., Haworth, C., Stacey, T. E. & Ward, R. H. T. (1976) Permeability of the sheep placenta to unmetabolized polar non-electrolytes. *Journal of Physiology,* **256,** 617–634.

Burd, L. I., Jones, Douglas M. Jr, Simmons, M. A., Makowski, E. L., Meschia, G. & Battaglia, F. C. (1975) Placental production and foetal utilisation of lactate and pyruvate. *Nature,* **254,** 710–711.

Chez, R. A., Mintz, D. H., Reynolds, W. A. & Hutchinson, D. L. (1975) Maternal–fetal plasma glucose relationships in late monkey pregnancy. *American Journal of Obstetrics and Gynecology,* **121,** 938–940.

Cohn, H. E., Sachs, E. J., Heymann, M. A. & Rudolph, A. M. (1974). Cardiovascular responses to hypoxemia and acidemia in fetal lambs. *American Journal of Obstetrics and Gynecology,* **120,** 817–824.

Comline, R. S. & Silver, M. (1970) Daily changes in foetal and maternal blood of conscious pregnant ewes, with catheters in umbilical and uterine vessels. *Journal of Physiology,* **209,** 567–586.

Comline, R. S. & Silver, M. (1972) The composition of foetal and maternal blood during parturition in the ewe. *Journal of Physiology,* **222,** 233–256.

Comline, R. S. & Silver, M. (1974a) Recent observations on the undisturbed foetus in utero and its delivery. In *Recent Advances in Physiology* (Ed.) Linden, R. J. pp. 406–454. London: J. & A. Churchill.

Comline, R. S. & Silver, M. (1974b) A comparative study of blood gas tensions, oxygen affinity and red cell 2,3-DPG concentrations in foetal and maternal blood in the mare, cow and sow. *Journal of Physiology,* **242,** 805–826.

Comline, R. S. & Silver, M. (1975) Placental transfer of blood gases. *British Medical Bulletin,* **31,** 25–31.

Comline, R. S. & Silver, M. (1976) Some aspects of foetal and utero-placental metabolism in cows with indwelling umbilical and uterine vascular catheters. *Journal of Physiology,* in press.

Comline, R. S., Hall, L. W., Lavelle, R. B., Nathanielsz, P. W. & Silver, M. (1974) Parturition in the cow: endocrine changes in animals with chronically implanted catheters in the foetal and maternal circulations. *Journal of Endocrinology,* **63,** 451–472.

Comline, R. S., Hall, L. W., Lavelle, R. B. & Silver, M. (1975) The use of intra-vascular catheters for long term studies on the mare and fetus. *Journal of Reproduction and Fertility,* Supplement 23, 583–588.

Cotter, J. R. & Little, W. A. (1970) Uterine blood flow and oxygen consumption of the pregnant uterus of *Macaca mulatta. American Journal of Obstetrics and Gynecology,* **106,** 1191–1195.

Cotter, J. R., Blechner, J. N. & Prystowsky, H. (1969) Blood flow and oxygen consumption of pregnant goats. *American Journal of Obstetrics and Gynecology,* **103,** 1098–1101.

Crenshaw, C. (1970) Fetal glucose metabolism. *Clinical Obstetrics and Gynecology,* **13,** 579–585.

Crenshaw, C., Huckabee, W. E., Curet, L. B., Mann, L. & Barron, D. H. (1968) A method for the estimation of the umbilical blood flow in unstressed sheep and goats with some results of its applications. *Quarterly Journal of Experimental Physiology,* **53,** 65–75.

Dawes, G. S. (1968) *Foetal and Neonatal Physiology.* Chicago, Illinois: Year Book Medical Publishers.

Dawes, G. S. & Mott, J. C. (1964) Changes in O_2 distribution and consumption in foetal lambs with variations in umbilical blood flow. *Journal of Physiology,* **170,** 524–540.

Dawes, G. S., Duncan, S. L. B., Lewis, B. V., Merlet, C. L., Owen-Thomas, J. B. & Reeves, J. T. (1969) Hypoxaemia and aortic chemoreceptor function in foetal lambs. *Journal of Physiology*, **201**, 105–116.

Faber, J. J. & Green, T. J. (1972) Foetal placental blood flow in the lamb. *Journal of Physiology*, **223**, 375–394.

Fisher, D. E., Paton, J. B., Peterson, E. N., De Lannoy, C. W. & Behrman, R. E. (1972) Umbilical blood flow, fetal oxygen consumption and placental diffusion clearance of antipyrine in the baboon. *Respiration Physiology*, **15**, 141–150.

Gresham, E. L., James, E. J., Raye, J. R., Battaglia, F. C., Makowski, E. L. & Meschia, G. (1972) Production and excretion of urea by the fetal lamb. *Pediatrics*, **50**, 372–379.

Heymann, M. A. & Rudolph, A. M. (1967) Effect of exteriorisation of the sheep fetus on its cardiovascular function. *Circulation Research*, **21**, 741–745.

Huckabee, W. E., Crenshaw, C., Curet, L. B. & Barron, D. H. (1972) Uterine blood flow and oxygen consumption in the unrestrained pregnant ewe. *Quarterly Journal of Experimental Physiology*, **57**, 12–23.

Huckabee, W. E., Metcalfe, J., Prystowsky, H. & Barron, D. H. (1961) Blood flow and oxygen consumption of the pregnant uterus. *American Journal of Physiology*, **200**, 274–278.

Hull, D. (1975) Storage and supply of fatty acids before and after birth. *British Medical Bulletin*, **31**, 32–36.

James, E. J., Raye, J. R., Gresham, E. L., Makowski, E. L., Meschia, G. & Battaglia, F. C. (1972) Fetal O_2 consumption, CO_2 production, and glucose uptake in a chronic sheep preparation. *Pediatrics*, **50**, 361–371.

Kronfeld, D. S. (1958) The fetal drain of hexose in ovine pregnancy toxemia. *Cornell Veterinarian*, **48**, 394–404.

Longo, L. D., Hill, E. P. & Power, G. G. (1972) Theoretical analysis of factors affecting placental O_2 transfer. *American Journal of Physiology*, **222**, 730–739.

Makowski, E. L., Meschia, G., Droegemueller, W. & Battaglia, F. C. (1968a) Distribution of uterine blood flow in the pregnant sheep. *American Journal of Obstetrics and Gynecology*, **101**, 409–412.

Makowski, E. L., Meschia, G., Droegemueller, W. & Battaglia, F. C. (1968b) Measurement of umbilical arterial blood flow to the sheep placenta and fetus in utero. *Circulation Research*, **23**, 623–631.

Makowski, E. L., Schneider, J. M., Tsoulos, N. G., Colwill, J. R., Battaglia, F. C. & Meschia, G. (1972) Cerebral blood flow, oxygen consumption, and glucose utilization of fetal lambs in utero. *American Journal of Obstetrics and Gynecology*, **114**, 292–301.

Meschia, G. (1974) Effect of estrogens on uterine blood flow. In *Perinantal Pharmacology: Problems and Priorities*, pp. 109–112. New York: Raven Press.

Meschia, G., Battaglia, F. C. & Bruns, P. D. (1967) Theoretical and experimental study of transplacental diffusion. *Journal of Applied Physiology*, **22**, 1171–1178.

Meschia, G., Behrman, R. E., Hellegers, A. E., Schruefer, J. J., Battaglia, F. C. & Barron, D. H. (1967a) Uterine blood flow in the pregnant rhesus monkey. *American Journal of Obstetrics and Gynecology*, **97**, 1–7.

Meschia, G., Cotter, J. R., Breathnach, C. S. & Barron, D. H. (1965) The hemoglobin, oxygen, carbon dioxide and hydrogen ion concentrations in the umbilical bloods of sheep and goats as sampled via indwelling plastic catheters. *Quarterly Journal of Experimental Physiology*, **50**, 185–195.

Meschia, G., Cotter, J. R., Makowski, E. L. & Barron, D. H. (1967b) Simultaneous measurement of uterine and umbilical blood flows and oxygen uptakes. *Quarterly Journal of Experimental Physiology*, **52**, 1–12.

Metcalfe, J., Bartels, H. & Moll, W. (1967) Gas exchange in the pregnant uterus. *Physiological Reviews*, **47**, 782–838.

Morriss, F. H. Jr, Boyd, R. D. H., Makowski, E. L., Meschia, G. & Battaglia, F. C. (1973) Glucose/oxygen quotients across the hindlimb of fetal lambs. *Pediatric Research*, **7**, 794–797.

Morriss, F. H., Boyd, R. D. H., Makowski, E. L., Meschia, G. & Battaglia, F. C. (1974) Umbilical V–A differences of acetoacetate and β-hydroxybutyrate in fed and starved ewes. *Proceedings of the Society for Experimental Biology and Medicine*, **145**, 879–883.

Oakley, N. W., Beard, R. W. & Turner, R. C. (1972) Effect of sustained maternal hyperglycaemia on the fetus in normal and diabetic pregnancies. *British Medical Journal*, i, 466–469.

Parer, J. T., de Lannoy, C. W., Hoversland, A. S. & Metcalfe, J. (1968) Effect of decreased uterine blood flow on uterine oxygen consumption in pregnant macaques. *American Journal of Physiology*, **100**, 813–820.

Pugh, P. D. S. & Scarisbrick, R. (1955) Acetate uptake by the foetal sheep. *Journal of Physiology*, **129**, 67P.

Reid, R. L. (1968) The physiopathology of under-nourishment in pregnant sheep with particular reference to pregnancy toxemia. *Advances in Veterinary Science*, **12**, 163–238.

Rudolph, A. M. & Heymann, M. A. (1967) Validation of the antipyrine method for measuring fetal umbilical blood flow. *Circulation Research*, **21**, 185–190.

Rudolph, A. M. & Heymann, M. A. (1970) Circulatory changes during growth in the fetal lamb. *Circulation Research*, **26**, 289–299.

Sabata, V., Wolf, H. & Lausmann, S. (1968) The role of free fatty acids, glycerol, ketone bodies and glucose in the energy metabolism of the mother and fetus during delivery. *Biology of the Neonate*, **13**, 7–17.

Setchell, B. P., Bassett, J. M., Hinks, N. T. & Graham, N. M. (1972) The importance of glucose in the oxidative metabolism of the pregnant uterus and its contents in conscious sheep with some preliminary observations on the oxidation of fructose and glucose by the fetal sheep. *Quarterly Journal of Experimental Physiology*, **57**, 257–266.

Sheath, J., Grimwade, J., Waldron, K., Bickley, M., Taft, P. & Wood, C. (1972) Arteriovenous non-esterified fatty acids and glycerol differences in the umbilical cord at term and their relationship to fetal metabolism. *American Journal of Obstetrics and Gynecology,* **113,** 358–362.

Shelley, H. J. (1973) The use of chronically catheterized foetal lambs for the study of foetal metabolism. In *Foetal and Neonatal Physiology, Barcroft Centenary Symposium* (Ed.) Comline, R. S., Cross, K. W., Dawes, G. S. & Nathanielsz, P. W. pp. 360–381. London: Cambridge University Press.

Silver, M. & Comline, R. S. (1975a) Transfer of gases and metabolites in the equine placenta: a comparison with other species. *Journal of Reproduction and Fertility,* Supplement 23, 589–594.

Silver, M. & Comline, R. S. (1975b) Fetal and placental O_2 consumption and the uptake of different metabolites in the ruminant and horse during late gestation. In *Third Oxygen Transport to Tissue Symposium* (Ed.) Reneau, D. D. & Grote, J. New York: Plenum Press. In press.

Silver, M., Steven, D. H. & Comline, R. S. (1973) Placental exchange and morphology in ruminants and mare. In *Foetal and Neonatal Physiology, Barcroft Centenary Symposium* (Ed.) Comline, R. S., Cross, K. W., Dawes, G. S. & Nathanielsz, P. W. pp. 245–271. London: Cambridge University Press.

Stembera, Z. K., Hodr, J. & Janda, J. (1965) Umbilical blood flow in healthy newborn infants during the first minutes after birth. *American Journal of Obstetrics and Gynecology,* **91,** 568–574.

Tsoulos, N. G., Colwill, J. R., Battaglia, F. C., Makowski, E. L. & Meschia, G. (1971) Comparison of glucose, fructose and O_2 uptakes by fetuses of fed and starved ewes. *American Journal of Physiology,* **221,** 234–237.

Widdas, W. F. (1961) Transport mechanisms in the foetus. *British Medical Bulletin,* **17,** 107–111.

11

WATER AND MINERAL EXCHANGE BETWEEN MATERNAL AND FETAL FLUIDS

R. J. Barnes

Previous reviews of fetal water and electrolyte exchange have been concerned mainly with the results of experiments using anaesthetised preparations. There is no doubt that such acute experiments provide much valuable information, but the disturbance of the maternal diet and fluid intake prior to surgery and the disturbance of maternal hormone balance, notably antidiuretic hormone (ADH) and corticosteroid release, in response to surgical stress may distort the equilibrium between maternal and fetal fluid compartments.

The aim of this chapter is to present the existing information about fetal fluid and electrolyte balance, placing particular emphasis on information obtained using chronically catheterised ewes and their fetuses, but it must be clearly noted that extrapolation from information obtained using a species with a syndesmochorial placenta to the primate with a haemochorial placenta may not be justifiable. Where possible comparable information about the human fetus will be presented and where particularly useful experiments have been performed with other species these will also be discussed.

THE MAGNITUDE OF THE FETAL ACCUMULATION OF WATER AND CERTAIN MINERALS

At term the human fetus weighs approximately 3.5 kg and the sheep fetus weighs a similar amount (perhaps 3.2 kg in the Welsh mountain sheep). Table 11.1 shows the mineral composition of the human fetus at term (McCance and Widdowson, 1951), and the similar compositions of fetal sheep tissues (see Barcroft, 1946) suggest that the accumulation of minerals by the sheep fetus is of the same order of magnitude. These values are very important because they define the limits of the disequilibria between the maternal and fetal plasma over the total period of intra-uterine growth.

Table 11.1. *Composition of the fetus at term.*

Substance	Human	Sheep
Water	2550 g	2400 g
Sodium	243 mEq/l	220 mEq/l
Chloride	160 mEq/l	144 mEq/l
Potassium	150 mEq/l	135 mEq/l
Calcium	28.2 g	25.4 g
Phosphorus	16.2 g	14.6 g
Magnesium	0.76 g	0.68 g
Iron	260 mg	234 mg
Zinc	52 mg	47 mg
Copper	10.7 mg	9.6 mg

These figures are taken from McCance and Widdowson (1951) for the human and the figures for the sheep fetus are calculated on the assumption of a similar composition of the lean body mass of the fetus. Analysis of individual tissues (see Barcroft, 1946, for references) supports this assumption. A direct weight for weight proportionality cannot be assumed as the human fetus contains a higher percentage of fat (16 per cent at term) than the sheep fetus (less than 8 per cent by difference using the figures given by Barcroft).

The maximum rate of growth of the sheep fetus is about 80 g/day at 115 days of gestation. This represents a daily transplacental net flux of 60 g water towards the fetus. Measurements of uterine blood flow at this gestational age suggest a total uterine flow of at least 700 ml/min, so that the calculated mean arteriovenous difference for water across the uterine circulation is only 0.06 μl/ml. This difference is undetectable by conventional methods of analysis and yet water is the substance which crosses the placenta in greatest amount. Similar calculations made for other substances such as sodium or calcium show that conventional methods of chemical analysis are unlikely to be of use in the estimation of transplacental fluxes of these electrolytes. Mellor (1970), Mellor and Slater (1971, 1972) and Barnes, Comline and Silver (unpublished observations, 1975) could find no significant or consistent differences between the electrolyte concentrations in maternal peripheral plasma and uterine vein plasma in the sheep. It is possible that umbilical arteriovenous concentration differences for electrolytes might exist if significant electrolyte exchange between the fetal and maternal fluids occurs at sites other than the placental exchange area. There is no detectable arteriovenous difference in osmolality across the sheep umbilical circulation (Meschia, Battaglia and Barron, 1957), but few other studies report electrolyte concentrations measured simultaneously across the umbilical circulation. The available evidence suggests that the major part of the exchange of water and electrolytes between mother and fetus takes place across the placenta in both human and sheep, but the possibility of alternative routes for exchange must still be kept in mind. A small unidirectional movement of ions by, for example, the fetal membranes could significantly affect the overall balance where net fluxes are so small. The chorio-allantoic membrane of the pig fetus is capable of transporting sodium out of the allantois into the maternal extracellular fluid (Crawford and McCance, 1960) and this could occur in other species. The complexity of the structure of the human amnion (see Bourne, 1970) suggests an active but as yet undefined role for this membrane.

PLACENTAL PERMEABILITY

A knowledge of the permeability of the placenta to water and solutes is essential to the understanding of overall fetal mineral balance. The use of radioactively labelled ions has facilitated the study of this aspect of placental function. Meschia, Battaglia and Bruns (1967) used a modification of the diffusion equilibrium technique to study transplacental diffusion of water, sodium, chloride, urea and antipyrine. Infusion of a test substance into the fetus leads eventually to an equilibrium condition in which the transplacental diffusion of that substance is equal to the rate of infusion. Meschia, Battaglia and Bruns (1967) showed that the transplacental movement of tritiated water under these conditions was limited by the rates of fetal placental blood flow. The same was true for antipyrine to which the placenta presented no significant barrier. Urea movement across the placenta was partly limited by placental permeability, while sodium and chloride diffusion was greatly limited by a low placental permeability. Even in the presence of very large fetal to maternal gradients for radioactive sodium or chloride, there was no detectable difference between the levels of radioactivity in the umbilical artery and vein. After two hours of infusion of these substances, there was no detectable rise in the radioactivity in the uterine venous blood. Thus, in the sheep, the placenta is relatively permeable to water and relatively impermeable to ions. The available results in humans (Vosburgh et al, 1948) are comparable with those in sheep, but ion diffusion is not quite as severely limited.

Longo, Hill and Power (1972) have analysed theoretical aspects of respiratory metabolite exchange across the placenta. It is clear that the observed equilibrium for placental diffusion of even highly diffusible substances is the result of the interaction of an extremely complex set of variables. The problems arising from intraplacental shunting of blood away from exchange areas, from the difficulties of estimation of the true concentration gradients at the capillary beds and from the unequal feto-maternal perfusion ratios which may occur in different parts of the placenta are discussed. It would appear that the experimental assessment of transplacental diffusion is required for each species in which the investigation of feto-maternal fluid exchange is contemplated, as no universally acceptable model has yet been constructed.

While it is clear that water is freely diffusible across all the types of placenta so far examined and that proteins do not cross the placental barrier by diffusion in any species, the influence of molecular size and ionic charge upon placental permeability to other substances has not been examined in detail. That there are major differences in placental permeability to such substances is shown by the observation that mannitol does not cross the sheep placenta in significant amounts but it does cross the rabbit placenta in amounts sufficient to raise the osmolality of the fetal fluids (vide infra, Faber, 1972).

TRANSPLACENTAL CONCENTRATION DIFFERENCES FOR WATER AND SOME MINERALS AND THE MOVEMENT OF THESE SUBSTANCES ACROSS THE PLACENTA

Mean maternal and fetal plasma concentrations of different electrolytes in late gestation in sheep, and where available in humans, are presented in Table 11.2. There is some argument about whether there are consistent feto-maternal concentration differences for sodium in the sheep, but the figures presented here support the concept that fetal and maternal ions are not freely exchangeable. If the observation of a transplacental potential difference, whereby the fetus is 50 mV negative to the mother, is taken into account then the observed transplacental differences represent a far from equilibrium condition (Table 11.2). The relative impermeability of the placental barrier to ions and smaller molecular weight substances is thus emphasised. This relative impermeability has certain implications for the movement of water across the placenta. The high permeability of the placental barrier to water has already been discussed. The extent to which the dissolved solutes contribute osmotic forces which might be involved in water movements across the placenta will depend upon the permeability of the placenta to these substances. The simplest concept of transplacental movement of water would be that water flows across the placenta partly under the influence of hydrostatic and partly under the influence of osmotic forces. If the placenta were totally impermeable to solutes then the osmotic forces acting could be computed by measurement of the vapour pressures of the maternal and fetal blood samples at 37°C. If the placenta were freely permeable to all small molecules below the molecular weight of, for example, 50 000, then the colloid osmotic pressures would be the effective osmotic forces acting across the placenta. It is also clear that the exact contribution of each solute will depend upon the characteristics of the placenta under investigation. The overall balance can only be determined experimentally.

In the sheep the total osmotic pressure difference measured across the placenta by freezing point determination in fetal and maternal bloods is perhaps 3 mosmol/kg water, which represents a pressure of 57 mm Hg at 37°C. The colloid osmotic pressure difference between the two bloods is only 4 mm Hg, so that non-colloids are contributing an appreciable amount of the difference. Faber and Green (1972) infused hypertonic solutions of sodium chloride and mannitol into the maternal circulation of chronically catheterised ewes in which the fetus had also been catheterised. The changes in haematocrit, sodium concentration, potassium concentration and total osmolality were followed in both maternal and fetal circulations. The initial adjustment of osmotic balance across the sheep placenta was due entirely to the movement of water. Similar experiments in rabbits showed that in this species also the initial restoration of equilibrium was due to water movement, although subsequently there was some movement of mannitol into the fetus from the maternal circulation. From these experiments it can be concluded that water does indeed move across the placenta under the influence of osmotic forces and that crystalloids may contribute to these forces.

It has also been shown (Faber, 1972) that hydrostatic forces act to transfer water between maternal and fetal fluid compartments in the sheep. The human placenta is probably more like the rabbit placenta in its response to osmotic change, since it is relatively more permeable to small molecular weight substances and ions (vide infra).

The transplacental redistribution of water in response to hydrostatic and osmotic forces has been established and it is clear, from other studies, that transplacental fluxes of water are far in excess of the net flux estimated from fetal growth measurements. The use of heavy water for the study of transplacental water flux (see, for example, Flexner and Gellhorn, 1942) showed that water flux from mother to fetus is up to 500 times in excess of that

Table 11.2. *The composition of fetal and maternal plasmas at term in the sheep and the human together with some of the expected fetal concentrations if the two plasmas were in electrochemical equilibrium.*

Substance	Human			Sheep		
	Maternal	Fetal		Maternal	Fetal	
		Found	Calculated		Found	Calculated
Sodium	138 mEq/l	139 mEq/l	138 mEq/l	145 mEq/l	139 mEq/l	327 mEq/l
Potassium	4.6 mEq/l	6.4 mEq/l	4.6 mEq/l	5.5 mEq/l	5.7 mEq/l	12.8 mEq/l
Chloride	107 mEq/l	108 mEq/l	107 mEq/l	106 mEq/l	105 mEq/l	46.3 mEq/l
Bicarbonate				26.5 mM/l	25.2 mM/l	
Phosphate	3.8 mg per cent	14.9 mg per cent		7.8 mg per cent	7.4 mg per cent	
Calcium	10.2 mg per cent	11.9 mg per cent		9.2 mg per cent	12.1 mg per cent	
Iron	60–80 µg per cent	160 µg per cent				
Total osmolality	299.7 mosmol				297 mosmol	
Colloid osmotic pressure	29 mm Hg	25 mm Hg		20.5 mm Hg	17.5 mm Hg	

These figures are derived from sources mentioned in the text.

required for growth. It is highly probable that an analogous situation to that which occurs in tissue capillary beds occurs at the placenta. Fluid may be expected to enter the exchange capillaries at the venous end and to leave at the arterial end under the influence of the hydrostatic and osmotic forces. Large total fluxes would then occur with only a small net flux of water towards the fetus, caused by the accumulation in the fetus of small amounts of osmotically active substances such as sodium, i.e. expanding the intracellular fluid volume. The observation by Faber, Hart and Poutala (1968) that the vascular endothelium makes little contribution to the resistance to diffusion of water, chloride, urea and sodium across the rabbit placenta suggests that the main barrier to diffusion lies elsewhere. The exact position of this placental diffusion barrier is unknown.

The movement of ions across the placenta is less clearly documented than the movement of water. One problem is that, in contrast to the position across the cell membrane or even across the kidney tubule, there is no one ion which is distributed according to electrochemical equilibrium. In the human the observed potential difference at term (Mellor et al, 1969; Mann, personal communication, 1967) is very small, perhaps 2 mV, fetus positive. It is possible that the observed potential difference depends upon the interaction of too many factors for simple analysis. The only reported attempt to alter the potential difference across the placenta by the manipulation of transplacental concentration differences is that of Stulc et al (1972) in guinea-pigs. A rise in maternal potassium concentration lowered the transplacental potential difference and a rise in fetal potassium raised the potential difference, but the behaviour of the potential was not explicable in terms of the Nernst equation. In general the origin of transplacental potential differences is known in only two species. In the pig it may be due to active transport of sodium out of the fetus across the chorio-allantoic membrane and in the rabbit it is almost certainly due to the reabsorption of sodium from the allantoic fluid by the fetal stomach (Wright, 1962). In the rabbit there is no true transplacental potential difference (between maternal and fetal extracellular fluids) but only a potential difference between the maternal or fetal extracellular fluid and the amniotic cavity.

TRANSPLACENTAL MOVEMENT OF INDIVIDUAL ION SPECIES

Sodium

Evidence presented already suggests that the sheep placenta is relatively impermeable to sodium. That sodium is not distributed according to its electrochemical gradient strengthens this belief (Table 11.2). The majority of workers consider that fetal sheep plasma has a lower sodium concentration than maternal plasma and this, together with the observation that the fetal plasma is electrically negative with respect to the maternal, has led to the suggestion that sodium is actively pumped out of the fetus into the maternal extracellular fluid. This hypothesis has not been properly tested in sheep, but elegant in vitro studies in the pig have shown that the chorio-allantoic membrane of the pig fetus is capable of transporting sodium before 65 days of gestation (Crawford and McCance, 1960). A potential difference was generated across the membrane in vitro with the fetal side electrically negative. Short-circuit current measured across the membrane was equal to that predicted from measured net sodium flux. The rate of pumping of the sodium depended upon the concentration of potassium on the maternal side and upon the P_{CO_2} of the bathing fluid. An unknown inhibitor in allantoic fluid was also demonstrated. Unfortunately radioactive isotopes were not available to these workers, so that the information they obtained was not as complete as would otherwise have been possible. Further work on this tissue may reveal information, not only about the unidirectional ion fluxes, but also about the possible involvement of the sodium pump in the transport of other substances across the chorio-allantoic membrane. The value of a mechanism which pumps sodium out of the fetus is not clear; whether it generates a potential gradient down which other ions can move passively, is involved in the transport of other substances across the placenta, or is involved in the maintenance of fetal vascular volume and osmotic equilibrium are purely matters for speculation.

In the sheep the potential difference across the placenta appears to be generated in the cotyledons (Mellor, 1970). There is no detectable electrical activity across the fetal membranes in vitro. In the monkey (Friedman et al, 1959) most of the water exchange between amniotic fluid and the mother takes place through the fetal circulation, while at least some of the sodium exchange between the two is probably explicable in terms of an alternative route of transfer. According to Hutchinson et al (1959), at least some of the water exchange in the human between the mother and the amniotic cavity takes place directly without the water passing through the fetal compartment but it is not known whether the same is true of amniotic fluid sodium.

The net flux of sodium into the fetus each day is only a few milliequivalents. This could be accounted for by transplacental diffusion, even with the limitation of permeability which occurs across the sheep placenta. The possibility that other routes of sodium transfer between mother and fetus may be important should still be entertained.

Chloride

Very little is known about the accumulation of chloride in the fetus. The argument that little net transplacental flux is necessary for fetal growth still applies, but there is no way in which simple diffusion could account for the movement from mother to fetus. The fetal plasma chloride concentration is slightly less than maternal (see Table 11.2), but at equilibrium the expected value of chloride in fetal plasma would be about 46 mEq/l, because of the 51 mV potential difference across the placenta. It is highly likely that chloride is actively transported into the fetus, but whether this is a placental mechanism or occurs at some other site is not clear.

Potassium

The potassium gradient across the placenta shows that potassium also is not in equilibrium between the fetal and maternal compartments. The studies of Faber and Green (1972) showed that the placenta is not highly permeable to potassium in the sheep, since osmotic adjustment did not involve transplacental movement of potassium. Here, while the concentration difference across the placenta is in favour of the movement of potassium ions out of the fetus, the electrochemical equilibrium is in favour of the movement of potassium ions into the fetus (at equilibrium a fetal plasma potassium concentration of about 13 mEq/l would be expected). The assumption may be made that slow diffusion of potassium across the placental barrier may be sufficient to account for the fetal accumulation. It is interesting to note that the transport of sodium across the pig chorio-allantoic membrane is dependent upon the presence of potassium ions on the maternal side (Crawford and McCance, 1960). If this is also true of the mechanism responsible for generating the electrical potential across the sheep placenta then the movement of potassium into the fetus may be partly due to active transport in exchange for sodium.

Calcium

The magnitude of the ionised calcium gradient across the placenta is difficult to determine. Although it is clear, in most species, that the total calcium in fetal plasma is at a higher concentration than in maternal plasma, the transplacental difference in ionised and diffusible un-ionised calcium is more difficult to assess. Delivoria-Papodopoulos et al (1967) examined total, protein-bound and ultrafilterable calcium in both sheep and human plasma, and their data are presented in Table 11.3. From this information it would seem that the feto-maternal

Table 11.3. *The calcium content of fetal and maternal plasmas in sheep and human.*

	Human (at term)	Sheep (at term)
Total calcium	F 5.96 ± 0.45 mEq/l M 5.11 ± 0.68 mEq/l	F 6.78 ± 0.64 mEq/l M 4.23 ± 0.37 mEq/l
Bound calcium	F 2.13 ± 0.33 mEq/l M 2.20 ± 0.36 mEq/l	F 1.89 ± 0.29 mEq/l M 1.42 ± 0.08 mEq/l
Ultrafilterable calcium	F 3.83 ± 0.40 mEq/l M 2.91 ± 0.46 mEq/l	F 4.89 ± 0.41 mEq/l M 2.81 ± 0.23 mEq/l

F = fetal; M = maternal.

These data are derived from the work of Delivoria–Papodopoulos et al (1967), who quote the results in mEq/kg plasma water. To convert to mg per cent the figures are multiplied by 2. For explanation of table see text.

concentration difference in total calcium is almost entirely accounted for by ultrafilterable calcium in man, while both protein-bound and ultrafilterable calcium contribute to the feto-maternal concentration difference in the sheep. There is no significant difference between the calcium binding per gram of protein in the fetal or maternal plasma of the human, but in the sheep the fetal plasma proteins have a much higher binding capacity earlier in pregnancy which declines towards adult levels as the fetus matures.

Iron

The higher fetal plasma iron concentrations in late gestation in man and sheep could come either from the active uptake of iron across the placenta from maternal plasma iron stores or from the phagocytosis of red cells by the placenta, with degradation of the maternal haem and release of the contained iron into the fetal circulation. Nylander (1953) summarised evidence that the source of fetal iron in the rat is entirely from transferrin and more recent work has confirmed this in the rat, rabbit, guinea-pig and human. There is significant storage of iron as ferritin in the rat placenta and it is believed that ferritin formation is involved in the active transplacental movement of iron in this species. Recently it has been shown that there is maturation of a system for binding iron in the cell membranes of rat placental cells at the same time as the maximum rates of iron transfer are occurring in vivo (Mansour, Schulert and Glasser, 1972). In cats at least some of the transplacental iron transfer is of iron derived from maternal haem (Baker and Morgan, 1973).

In summary, apart from free permeability to water, in sheep and to some degree in all species the placental barrier acts as a somewhat leaky protection to the fetal plasma against changes in the maternal plasma electrolyte environment. It allows the relatively small net fluxes required for fetal growth, yet provides the possibility of relative fetal autonomy in regulation of its own mineral environment.

THE COMPOSITION AND FORMATION OF FETAL FLUIDS

The volumes of fetal fluids measured either acutely (sheep) or by dilution techniques (human) are presented in Table 11.4. In both these species there is an increase in the amount of amniotic fluid during late gestation to a plateau at about 100 to 115 days in the sheep and about

Table 11.4(a). *The volume of the fetal fluids at different gestational ages in the sheep.*

Fluid	Gestational age and weight			
	60 days 100 g	85 days 350 g	115 days 1400 g	145 days 3500 g
Amniotic	170 ml	550 ml	620 ml	360 ml
Allantoic	170 ml	180 ml	440 ml	750 ml
Blood		60 ml	260 ml	710 ml

Table 11.4(b). *The volume of the amniotic fluid at different gestational ages in the human.*

Fluid	Gestational age and weight			
	15 weeks	30 weeks 1600 g	37 weeks 3000 g	40 weeks 3550 g
Amniotic	200 ml	850 ml	800 ml	400 ml

Data from Barcroft (1946), Malan, Malan and Curson (1937) and Gadd (1970).

30 to 37 weeks in the human. Thereafter the volume of amniotic fluid declines in both species, somewhat more rapidly in the human than in the sheep. The allantoic fluid volume in the sheep rises towards term; there is no comparable fluid compartment in the human fetus.

Using chronically catheterised fetuses Mellor and co-workers have studied gestation trends in fetal fluid composition (Mellor, 1970; Mellor and Slater, 1971). Amniotic fluid composition in the sheep showed progressive changes between about 70 days and term. Following recovery from surgery the total osmolality declined from about 295 mosmol/kg to about 270 mosmol/kg at term. Sodium fell from 135 mEq/l to 95 mEq/l, while potassium rose slowly from 5 mEq/l at 70 days to 10 mEq/l at about 139 days and then more rapidly to 15 to 20 mEq/l during the last seven days of gestation. Chloride concentrations remained fairly steady at about 110 mEq/l until about 130 days of gestation, then fell to about 8. mEq/l over the next 14 days. Urea concentrations rose progressively from 4 mmol l to 1. mmol/l over the time course of the experiment.

Allantoic fluid composition showed more dramatic changes over the last part of gestation. Between 85 days and term the osmolality rose from 270 mosmol/kg to 295 mosmol/kg while at the same time the sodium concentration *fell* from 85 to 20 mEq/l. An equally dramatic *rise* in allantoic fluid potassium occurred from about 20 mEq/l at 85 days to about 85 mEq/l at term. Chloride showed a slight rise from 12 to 20 mEq/l at this time, while urea remained fairly steady at 5 to 10 mmol/l. The amino acid concentration of the allantoic fluid, much higher than that of the amniotic fluid (40 mmol/l compared with 2 mmol/l), fell from 85 days (55 mmol/l) to 115 days (35 mmol/l) and then remained fairly steady apart from a slight rise in the last week of gestation. Other osmotically active components were not estimated. These results on chronically catheterised sheep differ markedly from observations on acutely operated sheep. The fetal fluids are much less hypotonic (Alexander et al, 1958a), but the main gestational trends do correspond. Mellor and Slater (1973) have suggested that the withholding of food from animals may influence allantoic fluid composition, while surgical stress may be important in the production of low osmotic pressures in the fluids at operation. They have discussed the changes in ionic composition of the fetal fluids following recovery from surgery, the major changes being a rise in allantoic fluid sodium concentration and a fall in amniotic potassium concentration in the postoperative period (the latter change being much more marked in younger fetuses). Mellor and Slater (1973) have pointed out that they did not observe low sodium concentrations in allantoic fluid in a series of experiments on anaesthetised sheep (Mellor, 1970), and attribute this to the lack of starvation of these animals before surgery. However, it must also be noted that the animals from the chronically operated series were given 60 to 75 mg progesterone intramuscularly before surgery (24 hours) and the possibility that this might influence fetal fluid composition must be kept in mind (see Alexander and Williams, 1968).

The observation of a transplacental potential difference between mother and fetus was first made by Barron and co-workers who observed a fetal electronegativity in acute experiments after 60 days of gestation in the goat (Meschia, Wolkoff and Barron, 1958), and also in sheep, (Barron et al, unpublished data, 1975). The potential difference increased until about 110 days of gestation and then declined towards term with an abrupt fall to zero shortly before parturition. These workers could find no potential difference between the fetal fluid sacs and the fetal plasma and they attributed the potential difference entirely to the activity of the placental layers. Two more recent studies in acute preparations (Widdas, 1961; Mellor, 1970) have found that there is a transplacental potential difference in goats and sheep which does not vary with gestational age between 60 days and term. Mellor also demonstrated a potential difference between the fetal extracellular fluid and the amniotic and allantoic fluid sacs in acutely anaesthetised sheep. There was a progressive decline in the potential difference between the fetus and the amniotic fluid during later gestation and a similar decline in the potential difference between the maternal extracellular fluid and the amniotic sac also occurred (Table 11.5). The allantoic fluid potentials did not vary with gestational age. There

Table 11.5. *The potential difference across the placenta between the maternal and fetal extracellular fluids (ECF) and between the fetal ECF and the fetal fluid sacs in the sheep at different gestational ages.*

Gestational age	Potential difference between maternal and fetal ECF	Potential difference between the fetal ECF and amnion	Potential difference between the fetal ECF and allantois
76 days	−45 mV	−26 mV	−33 mV
95 days	−60 mV	−41 mV	−47 mV
109 days	−47 mV	−12 mV	−40 mV
124 days	−49 mV	−4 mV	−48 mV
136 days	−47 mV	−8 mV	−27 mV
140 days	−47 mV	−1 mV	−32 mV

hese data are derived from Mellor (1970). Some of the figures given are averages of the range which Mellor ound in individual experiments, but the main trends which he observed are shown here. Principally there is a ecline with gestational age of the fetal ECF to amniotic fluid potential difference, while there are no clear estational trends in the other potential differences. This is in contrast to the observation of Meschia, Wolkoff and arron (1958) in goats, where they could detect no potential difference between the fetal ECF and amniotic or llantoic fluid. Meschia, Wolkoff and Barron also noted a decline in the transplacental potential difference during estation. This divergence in results remains unexplained.

is no obvious relationship between any of these potential differences and ionic distribution. Mellor and Slater (1971) suggested that these results implied equilibrium between the amniotic fluid and both maternal and fetal plasmas, while the allantoic fluid was in equilibrium with fetal plasma only. It should be remembered that the *proof* of equilibrium depends upon demonstration of alterations in the potential difference following alterations in ionic distribution between the two compartments in accordance with the predictions of the Nernst equation. It should also be borne in mind that the impermeability of the fetal membranes to ions, as already discussed, and the constant addition of fluids to and removal of fluids from the fetal sacs by mechanical flow could significantly contribute to the observed disequilibria of these substances. The sources of the amniotic and allantoic potentials between fetus and fluid sacs must remain as yet unresolved. It is conceivable that the fetal urinary tract could be responsible for the production of the potential difference between the fetal extracellular fluid and fluid sacs. In some species, e.g. rabbit, the potential difference between mother and amnion is dependent upon the potential difference across the fetal stomach wall, but this does not appear to be true for the sheep (for reference see Mellor, 1970).

In the human, amniotic fluid is slightly hypotonic to fetal and maternal plasmas. There is a slight decline in sodium (140 to 104 mEq/l) and osmolality (268 to 252 mosmol/kg water) over the period from 24 to 40 weeks. There is no gestational trend in potassium concentration (4.2 to 6.6 mEq/l) (Cassady and Barnett, 1968). It is interesting that Mellor et al (1969) could find no transplacental potential difference in the term infant and only a very small (2 mV amnion positive) potential difference between the maternal extracellular fluid and the amnion. However, the potential differences at earlier gestational ages in the human have not been measured.

THE SOURCES OF FETAL FLUIDS IN LATER GESTATION

The changes in volume and composition of the fetal fluids throughout gestation are the result of a number of processes which add fluid to the sacs and remove fluid from them. Much of the evidence presented so far suggests that the fetal fluid balance is relatively autonomous and that the major determinants of both volume and composition of fluids must be looked for in the fetus itself. There are four obvious sites at which secretion and absorption of fetal fluid might occur, the respiratory system, the urinary system, the alimentary system and in addition there could be some exchange between the amniotic fluid and fetal blood through the fetal skin. Each of these will be considered in turn.

Fetal skin

In mature fetuses of both sheep and humans the integument is well developed. In the sheep fetus, hair is found in increasing amounts from about the 100th day. It is unlikely that this mature epithelium will be involved in significant exchange of electrolyte across its full thickness. However, in the earlier fetus, France (1974) has shown that the fetal sheep skin is capable of transporting sodium from amnion to fetal side. This property is present until after 90 days, but later gestational ages have not been examined. It is possible that this ability of the younger fetus represents a totipotency of function which disappears as the epithelium becomes more specialised. How far this ability modifies the composition of the amniotic fluid in vivo is difficult to assess, but the flux ratio for sodium in these fetuses was 1.256 in favour of sodium uptake from the amniotic fluid; at this time the amniotic fluid volume would have been about 500 ml. Whether this represents a significant factor in the equilibrium of the fetus with its amniotic fluid can only be decided by further quantitative estimation of the ionic fluxes.

Respiratory system

Communication between the amniotic fluid and the tracheobronchial tree has been well documented. The constant production of lung liquid in the fetus has been shown both in pathological specimens and in the normal sheep fetus. The human and the sheep fetus make respiratory movements, in utero, leading usually to small fluid movements between amnion and lung but sometimes to gushes of up to 40 ml of fluid from the lung (Dawes, 1973). Reynolds (1953) has shown that the fetal buccal cavity secretions can amount to 15 ml/hour, while Dawes (1973) suggests that net outward movement of fluid from the trachea can amount to 100 ml/kg fetus/day near term. The mechanisms of lung liquid formation and absorption have been investigated by Strang and colleagues (for references see Egan, Olver and Strang, 1975).

The alimentary canal

The demonstration that the fetal human in utero swallows amniotic fluid was made many years ago by radiographic methods and has since been confirmed by inulin tracer studies (see Jeffcoate and Scott, 1959). It has been estimated that the human fetus can swallow up to 500 ml of fluid each day.

In the sheep fetus there is ample evidence of swallowing in utero. Using chronically implanted electromagnetic flow meters Bradley and Mistretta (1973) have shown that the fetal sheep may swallow up to 500 ml fluid per day. The fetal stomach is capable of absorbing sodium against a concentration gradient making it highly likely that this is an important route of fetal fluid reabsorption (Wright, 1974). There is no evidence that the fetal gut acts as a source of supply of fluids or electrolytes to the amniotic cavity.

The fetal urinary tract

The observation that the fetus produces a hypotonic urine together with the observation that the fetal fluids are hypotonic led to the suggestion (Jacqué, 1903) that fetal urine might contribute to the formation of fetal fluids in older fetuses. Earlier studies of fetal renal function were of acutely anaesthetised and catheterised fetuses delivered into warm saline baths (Alexander et al, 1958b) or catheterised in utero but maintained under anaesthesia (Smith et al, 1966). More recently chronically catheterised fetuses have been used (Gresham et al, 1972).

There are four possible sites of catheterisation for chronic studies of fetal urine production: the pelvis or ureter, the bladder, the urethra or the urachus. Each presents certain problems. Chronic catheterisation of the ureter inevitably leads to hyponephrosis of the kidney on that side (Barnes, Comline and Silver, unpublished data, 1975) possibly because of interference with the pressure characteristics of the ureteric flow. In utero, ureteric peristalsis expels the preformed urine from the renal pelvis. Blockage of the ureteric catheter results in hypertrophy of the ureter. Catheterisation of the bladder enables the sampling of urine daily from the fetus, but does not allow the estimation of the volume of urine production unless the urachus and urethra are tied off to prevent leakage. It has the added disadvantage that the bladder mucosa is easily damaged and a fetal laparotomy is required for catheter insertion. This technique has been very successfully used by Mellor and Slater (1973). Urethral catheterisation has been used successfully by Buddingh et al (1971) and urachal catheterisation by Gresham et al (1972), but in the former case the entry of urine into the amnion is impaired, while in the latter case the entry into the allantois is cut off.

The author's experience and that of Buddingh et al (1971) is that continuous drainage of fetal urine leads to fetal death, or premature delivery, in about nine days. In only two of 20 sheep did urine drainage continue to normal full term, and it is possible that in both these animals the urine had not been completely drained. The return of urine to the amniotic cavity led to fetal survival to term in 18 of 20 fetuses (Buddingh et al, 1971).

Essentially the results from all types of chronic study are similar. The fetus produces a hypotonic urine. 500 ml of urine may be produced in 24 hours. The main osmotic constituents are fructose and sodium. Glucose is almost completely reabsorbed even in the younger fetuses and the urine is protein-free.

Complete drainage of urine from the fetus for up to 18 days (Gresham et al, 1972; Barnes et al, unpublished observations, 1975) leads to an almost total lack of fetal fluids at subsequent caesarian section. It is clear that the fetal urine makes a very significant contribution to the volume of both fetal fluid sacs in the sheep and in view of the oligohydramnios associated with renal agenesis this is probably also true in the human. The fetal kidney could provide a way for the fetus to regulate the volume of its fetal fluids, in association with the recirculation of fluid and electrolytes produced by fetal swallowing. The rates of fetal urine production (200 to 500 ml/day) are of the same order of magnitude as the rates of fetal swallowing.

In both the fetal lamb and the human the process of nephrogenesis is almost complete at birth and in man it is usually complete by the 36th week of gestation (Macdonald and Emery, 1959). In the sheep fetus histological studies have suggested that the metanephric kidney may have started to function by the 40th day of gestation, so that after about 55 days, when the mesonephros has degenerated, the urine obtained from sheep fetuses is almost certainly completely metanephric in origin (Davies, 1950; Davies and Davies, 1950). It seems probable that most of the differences between adult and fetal kidney in later gestation in both sheep and human will be due to functional rather than anatomical causes.

Blood supply to the fetal kidney

The normal functioning of the adult kidney depends upon the stabilisation of renal blood flow and glomerular filtration within the range of normal arterial pressure—the phenomenon of autoregulation. It also depends upon the distribution of the blood supply between the medulla and cortex such that the countercurrent multiplication system of the loop of Henle is not short-circuited by excessive medullary blood flow. In the fetus the arterial blood pressure is about 40 to 50 mm Hg, well below the adult autoregulatory range, and it would not be surprising if autoregulation were absent.

The measurement of fetal renal blood flow is difficult; it cannot be assumed that para-aminohippurate (PAH) clearance will reflect effective renal plasma flow and the use of flow meters on the renal artery cannot be considered to provide representative values for the normal fetus. Probably the most useful technique will be that of microsphere injection and indeed this has been used with some success. It has the added advantage that it will enable the investigator to assess regional blood flows as well as total renal blood flow (a discussion of the use of microspheres is given in Chapter 10). No complete study of renal blood flow has been conducted. The information which is available suggests that there is a relatively high resistance to flow in the fetal lamb kidney (Vaughan et al, 1968) and that resting renal blood flows are of the order of 160 ml/min/100 g tissue (Rudolph and Heymann, 1967; Beguin, Dunnihoo and Quilligan, 1974). The fetal kidney receives only two per cent of the cardiac output compared with the normal 25 per cent in the adult. This is probably due to the demands of the umbilical circulation. Until the relative proportions in which the blood flows through the medulla and cortex are known the assessment of tubular maturity, and especially of the functioning of the ascending limb of the loop of Henle, cannot be complete.

PAH clearance studies for the estimation of renal blood flow have been used in both acute and chronic preparations. In the acutely anaesthetised preparation, Alexander and Nixon (1961) found that the clearance of PAH varied from 1.2 to 1.5 times that of inulin compared to 6.4 in the adult. They pointed out that this could reflect either an immaturity of the secretory function or a deficiency of blood flow around the secretory elements. In chronically catheterised sheep fetuses Gresham et al (1972) found creatinine clearance ratios of the same order as those found for PAH in the acute preparation, but Buddingh et al (1971) observed inulin: PAH clearance ratios of 1:1, suggesting that the urinary PAH might be entirely derived from filtration. Estimation of glomerular filtration in the newborn puppy using ^{14}C-inulin (Kleinman and Lubbe, 1972) suggested that autoregulation did not occur. One further point which may have some bearing on these investigations is that if, as seems likely, the fetal secretory mechanisms are immature, then the greatest care must be exercised in the use of such substances as PAH, because saturation of the tubular capacity to handle these substances will result in a correlation between inulin clearance and clearance of these substances and will not indicate the true mechanism of their excretion by the kidney.

In summary, it can be said that renal blood flows are low in the fetus compared with the adult and represent a smaller percentage of the cardiac output.

Glomerular filtration

Little is known about the pressure relationships involved in glomerular filtration in the fetus, but the pressure relationships must be very different from those of the adult. In the adult glomerular filtration depends upon an imbalance between the hydrostatic pressures across the glomerular membrane and the osmotic forces of the non-filtered colloids. In the fetus the maximum available hydrostatic pressure is perhaps 40 to 50 mm Hg and, if colloids are excluded from the ultrafiltrate, this is opposed by an oncotic pressure of perhaps 15 mm Hg. It is likely that the much lower values of glomerular filtration in the fetus partly result from this much lower filtration pressure.

The classical method of inulin clearance has been used by several groups of workers to investigate glomerular filtration in sheep fetuses. The most consistent finding has been that the mature fetus has a lower filtration rate than the newborn lamb or the adult. Values of about 1 ml/kg were obtained in chronic preparations by Gresham et al (1972) and values of 1 to 4 ml/min for total glomerular filtration rate (GFR) have been found by Buddingh et al (1971), which are comparable with Gresham et al (1972) on a weight basis. In acute preparations Alexander et al (1961) report a decline in clearance from 2.4 ml/kg/min at 61 days gestation to 0.4 ml/kg/min at 142 days, compared with 2 ml/kg/min in adult sheep. Buddingh et al (1971) report that inulin clearance rises significantly in the last 15 days of gestation, which agrees with the acute experiments of Smith et al (1966). Alterations in blood flow following exteriorisation of the fetus by Alexander et al (1958a) may partly explain the discrepancies.

The absence of autoregulation in the newborn puppy has already been mentioned, and it is likely that autoregulation does not occur in the fetus.

Secretory and absorptive functions

The production of hypotonic urine by the sheep fetus can only be the result of selectively greater reabsorption of solutes than of water by the kidney. In the adult the only region of the kidney in which hypotonic tubular fluid is produced is the ascending limb of the loop of Henle and the early distal tubule. Very little is known about the function of the different regions of the renal tubule in the fetus, but it is possible that the final dilution of the fetal urine depends upon active processes in the loop of Henle and impermeability to water of the distal convoluted tubule and collecting duct. The possible role of antidiuretic hormone (ADH) in this mechanism will be discussed, but the low resting concentrations of ADH reported in the chronically catheterised fetus (Alexander et al, 1974) would be compatible with this hypothesis.

Dye secretion studies on pieces of nephron in vitro suggest that certain proximal tubular secretory functions are present as early as 14 weeks in the human fetus and until the discrepancies between the results of PAH studies are resolved it is reasonable to assume some secretory function of the proximal tubule for this substance also.

The majority of investigators have examined total renal function using inulin clearance as an index of glomerular filtration of electrolytes and small solutes and estimating the fractional reabsorption of the filtered substances. In chronically catheterised fetuses the sodium reabsorption was between 96.5 and 99.5 per cent of the filtered load (Gresham et al, 1972). Glucose is rarely found in the fetal urine and the reabsorptive mechanism for this substance must be present. Fructose, on the other hand, contributes significantly to the osmolality of the fetal urine; it may reach concentrations as high as 1000 mg/100 ml compared with 60 mg/100 ml in fetal lamb plasma.

Gestational trends in urine composition

The studies of Buddingh et al (1971), Gresham et al (1972), Mellor and Slater (1973), and the author's own observations show that there are no major trends in urine composition, apart from those immediately after surgery, until very late in gestation in the fetal lamb. Mellor and Slater (1973) report a slight fall in total osmolality, sodium, chloride and fructose concentrations from 70 days to about 135 days of gestation. Throughout gestation the fetus produces a hypotonic urine with sodium as the major osmotic component and fructose (in the sheep) as the next most important osmotic constituent. It is not until the last week or so of gestation that major changes in osmolality and composition occur. Urine flow rates in the chronically catheterised fetus are higher than in the acute experiments, but there is no systematic study which might indicate a gestational trend. There are quite large differences between animals in flow rates and moderately large differences even in the same individual. One study (Buddingh et al, 1971) suggests a circadian rhythm in urine flow and free water clearance.

During the last seven days before parturition there is a rise in the osmolality and in the concentrations of fructose and electrolytes in the urine (Figure 11.1). Perhaps the most striking change is in the sodium: potassium ratio, the rise in potassium being proportionally greater than that of sodium. In Mellor and Slater's study this rise in potassium begins gradually about 14 days before term and becomes more pronounced in the last seven days. The alteration in urine composition is not accompanied by major changes in the electrolyte composition of fetal plasma. It does not occur in chronically hypophysectomised fetuses at similar gestational ages (Barnes et al, unpublished data, 1975) suggesting an association between these urine changes and the onset of parturition. The most likely explanation is that the urine

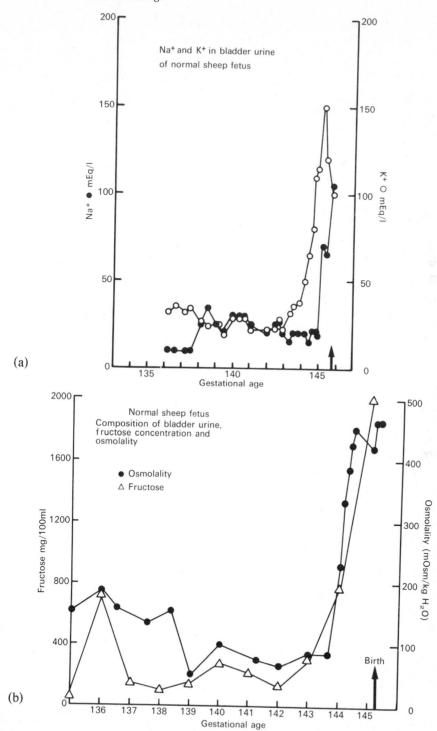

Figure 11.1. The composition of fetal urine collected continuously through a urachal catheter in a normal sheep fetus from 135 days to term. (a) Potassium○and sodium●concentrations, and (b) fructose concentration▲and osmolality●are illustrated.

changes reflect the alterations in the endocrine secretions of the fetus which occur at about this time. In particular, alterations in the levels of ADH may be expected to influence the osmolality and it is of interest that the maximum osmolality achieved towards term (perhaps 450 mosmol/kg H_2O) is not increased by the injection of ADH. Alexander et al (1974) have recently shown that there is a rise in fetal ADH from very low levels (less than 3.5 μu/ml) to very high levels (up to 40 μu/ml) at parturition in the sheep. A similar high level of ADH in cord blood has been reported in the human (Chard et al, 1971). The alteration in the sodium:potassium ratio of the urine might be expected to result from the rising levels of cortisol reported preceding parturition, but the role of aldosterone in induction of these changes requires investigation.

The lack of an obvious gestational trend in urine composition and flow before the last few days of gestation contrasts quite markedly with the observations in acute preparations, but changes seen at surgery for chronic implantation of catheters may help to explain the differences. In all studies there is a rise in osmolality between the onset of surgery and the end of operation. This rise is not related to gestational age after 120 days and is very much greater in normal fetuses than in hypophysectomised ones (Figure 11.2). Unfortunately simultaneous measurements of urine osmolality and ADH levels have not been made in the chronic preparation, but it is a reasonable working hypothesis that the rise in fetal urine osmolality depends upon alterations in fetal ADH secretion in response to the stress of anaesthesia and surgery. This mechanism could be responsible for the gestational trends reported over a wider age range by Alexander and Nixon (1961).

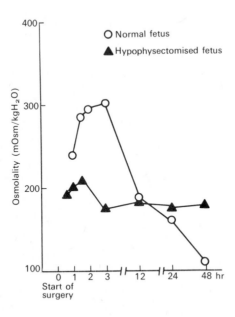

Figure 11.2. The rise in osmolality of fetal urine in a normal fetus following surgery contrasted with that of a hypophysectomised fetus following surgery.

THE RENIN–ANGIOTENSIN SYSTEM

The renin–angiotensin system in the fetus has been excellently reviewed by Mott (1975). That the system is functional in the fetus has been shown by Mott and co-workers (see Mott, 1975, for references). The responsiveness of the system to changes in vascular volume of as little as three per cent suggests that the renin–angiotensin system may be ideally suited to help maintain vascular volume and blood pressure in the fetus. The removal of both kidneys leads to a fall in blood pressure in both newborn lambs and rabbits, and it is possible that the role of the renin–angiotensin system in the fetus and newborn is closely concerned with the maintenance of blood pressure within stable limits. In the adult renin release can be provoked by many stimuli and the relative importance of these different stimuli in the control of renin release by the fetal kidney remains to be determined.

The renin–angiotensin system in the fetus may also regulate aldosterone secretion by the adrenal cortex. This warrants further investigation since both renin and aldosterone levels are elevated in cord blood of the human and sheep at birth. Whether the rise in renin (and angiotensin) precedes the rise in aldosterone or whether both are the result of some other process occurring during parturition remains to be determined.

THE INTRAFETAL CIRCULATION OF FLUID

The relationship of the fetus to its fluid sacs is illustrated diagrammatically for the sheep (Figure 11.3a) and the human fetus (Figure 11.3b). The fetus exists in dynamic equilibrium with its fluids. From about 80 days of gestation the flow of urine into the amniotic sac probably increases, while the flow of urine into the allantoic sac of the sheep decreases but does not cease altogether. This observation is based upon a comparison of gestational trends in amniotic and allantoic fluid composition with the composition of simultaneously formed urine (Mellor and Slater, 1971, 1972). Parallel changes in allantoic fluid and urine sodium and potassium concentrations suggest that other influences on allantoic fluid composition either act in parallel with the influences on urine composition or are relatively unimportant. The less clear correlation between urine and amniotic fluid compositions suggests that other independent influences on amniotic fluid composition are relatively important (e.g., tracheal fluid formation).

The measurement of the bulk flows into and out of the fetal fluid sacs is essential before a proper analysis of the relationships between the different fluid compartments of the fetus can be made. Until this information is available the role of the fetal membranes will remain confused. The supply of fluid to and removal of fluid from the amniotic cavity are both clearly documented, but what happens to fluid entering the allantoic sac in the sheep is still unknown.

CONCLUSIONS

The limitation of free movement of ions by the placental barrier allows the fetus to exist in a very different mineral environment from that of the maternal tissues, while at the same time

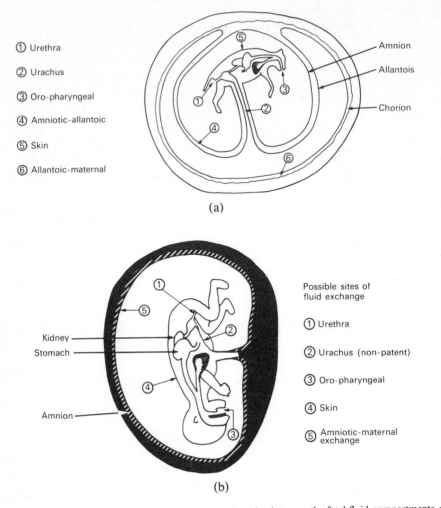

Figure 11.3. A diagrammatic representation of the relationships between the fetal fluid compartments of the sheep fetus (3a) and the human fetus (3b) with an indication for each of the possible sites at which fluid exchange between their respective fluid compartments might occur.

allowing the relatively small net fluxes of ions which are required for the process of fetal growth. Except in a few specific cases, it is not yet known which ions are treated actively and which passively by the placenta, nor is it known how the active processes are regulated. It is tempting to speculate that the control of the fetal fluid compartments is achieved through the fetus's own endocrine system and that this endocrine system also influences the movement of ions and water across the placenta. The fetal kidney plays a central role in the regulation of the fetal fluid volumes and compositions. The application of more sophisticated surgical and analytical techniques to the chronically catheterised preparation may help to explain some of the difficulties which are still apparent about the relationships between the fetal fluid compartments and the membranes which surround them.

REFERENCES

Alexander, D. P. & Nixon, D. A. (1961) The foetal kidney. *British Medical Bulletin,* **17,** 112–117.

Alexander, D. P., Bashore, R. A., Britton, H. G. & Forsling, M. L. (1974) Maternal and foetal arginine vasopressin in the chronically catheterised sheep. *Biologia Neonatorum,* **25,** 242–248.

Alexander, D. P., Nixon, D. A., Widdas, W. F. & Wohlzogen, F. X. (1958a) Gestational variations in the composition of the foetal fluids and foetal urine in the sheep. *Journal of Physiology,* **140,** 1–13.

Alexander, D. P., Nixon, D. A., Widdas, W. F. & Wohlzogen, F. X. (1958b) Renal function in the sheep foetus. *Journal of Physiology,* **140,** 14–22.

Alexander, G. & Williams, D. (1968) Hormonal control of amniotic and allantoic fluid volume in ovariectomised sheep. *Journal of Endocrinology,* **41,** 477–485.

Baker, E. & Morgan, E. H. (1973) Placental iron transfer in the cat. *Journal of Physiology,* **232,** 485–501.

Barcroft, J. B. (1946) *Researches on Pre-natal Life.* Oxford: Blackwell.

Beguin, F., Dunnihoo, D. R. & Quilligan, E. J. (1974) Effect of carbon dioxide elevation on renal blood flow in the fetal lamb in utero. *American Journal of Obstetrics and Gynecology,* **119,** 630–637.

Bernstine, R. L. (1970) A chronic renal model for the fetus. *Laboratory Animal Care,* **20,** 949–956.

Bourne, G. (1970) The membranes. In *Scientific Foundations of Obstetrics and Gynaecology* (Ed.) Philipp, E. E., Barnes, J. & Newton, M. pp. 181–185. London: William Heinemann.

Bradley, R. M. & Mistretta, C. M. (1973) The sense of taste and swallowing activity in foetal sheep. In *The Sir Joseph Barcroft Centenary Symposium* (Ed.) Comline, R. S., Cross, K. W., Dawes, G. S. & Nathanielsz, P. W. pp. 77–81. Cambridge: Cambridge University Press.

Buddingh, F., Parker, H. R., Ishizaki, G. & Tyler, W. S. (1971) Long term studies of the functional development of the fetal kidney in sheep. *American Journal of Veterinary Research,* **32,** 1993–1998.

Cassady, G. & Barnett, R. (1968) Amniotic fluid electrolytes and perinatal outcome. *Biologia Neonatorum,* **13,** 155–174.

Chard, T., Hudson, C. N., Edwards, C. R. W. & Boyd, N. R. H. (1971) The release of oxytocin and vasopressin by the human foetus during labour. *Nature,* **234,** 352–354.

Cloete, J. H. L. (1939) Prenatal growth in the merino sheep. *Onderstepoort Journal of Veterinary Science,* **13,** 417–558.

Crawford, J. D. & McCance, R. A. (1960) Sodium transport by the chorioallantoic membrane of the pig. *Journal of Physiology,* **151,** 458–471.

Davies, J. (1950) The blood supply of the mesonephros of the sheep. *Proceedings of the Zoological Society of London,* **120,** 95–112.

Davies, J. & Davies, D. V. (1950) The development of the mesonephros of the sheep. *Proceedings of the Zoological Society of London,* **120,** 73–93.

Dawes, G. S. (1973) Breathing and rapid eye movement sleep before birth. In *The Sir Joseph Barcroft Centenary Symposium* (Ed.) Comline, R. S., Cross, K. W., Dawes, G. S. & Nathanielsz, P. W. pp. 49–62. Cambridge: Cambridge University Press.

Delivoria-Papodopoulos, M., Battaglia, F. C., Bruns, P. D. & Meschia, G. (1967) Total, protein bound and ultrafilterable calcium in maternal and fetal plasmas. *American Journal of Physiology,* **213,** 363–366.

Egan, E. A., Olver, R. E. & Strang, L. B. (1975) Changes in non-electrolyte permeability of alveoli and the absorption of lung liquid at the start of breathing in the lamb. *Journal of Physiology,* **244,** 161–180.

Faber, J. J. (1972) Regulation of fetal placental blood flow. In *Respiratory Gas Exchange and Blood Flow in the Placenta. A Symposium* (Ed.) Longo, L. D. & Bartels, H. DHEW No. (NIH) pp. 73–361. Bethesda, Maryland: NIH.

Faber, J. J. & Green, T. J. (1972) Foetal placental blood flow in the lamb. *Journal of Physiology,* **223,** 375–393.

Faber, J. J., Hart, F. M. & Poutala, A. C. (1968) Diffusional resistance of the innermost layer of the placental barrier of the rabbit. *Journal of Physiology,* **197,** 381–393.

Flexner, L. B. & Gellhorn, A. (1942) Comparative physiology of placental transfer. *American Journal of Obstetrics and Gynecology,* **43,** 965–974.

France, V. M. (1974) Sodium uptake by the skin of the foetal sheep. *Journal of Physiology,* **240,** 27P.

Friedman, E. A., Gray, M. J., Hutchinson, D. L. & Plentl, A. A. (1959) The role of the monkey foetus in the exchange of the water and sodium of the allantoic fluid. *Journal of Clinical Investigation,* **38,** 961–970.

Gadd, R. L. (1970) The liquor amnii. In *Scientific Foundations of Obstetrics and Gynaecology* (Ed.) Phillip, E. E., Barnes, J. & Newton, M. pp. 254–259. London: William Heinemann.

Gresham, E. L., Rankin, J. H. G. , Makowski, E. L., Meshia, G. & Battaglia, F. C. (1972) An evaluation of fetal renal function in a chronic sheep preparation. *Journal of Clinical Investigation,* **51,** 149–156.

Hutchinson, D. L., Gray, M. J., Plental, A. A., Alvarez, H., Caldeyro-Barcia, R., Kaplan, B. & Lind, J. (1959) The role of the foetus in the water exchange of amniotic fluid of normal and hydramniotic patients. *Journal of Clinical Investigation,* **38,** 971–980.

Jacqué, L. (1903) De la genère des liquides amniotique et alantoidien; cryoscopie et analyses chimiques. *Mémoire. Courantes de l'Academie Royale Belgique*, **63**, 3–117.

Jeffcoate, T. N. A. & Scott, J. S. (1959) Polyhydramnios and oligohydramnios. *Canadian Medical Association Journal*, **80**, 77–86.

Kleinman, L. I. & Lubbe, R. J. (1972) Factors affecting the maturation of glomerular filtration rate and renal plasma flow in the new born dog. *Journal of Physiology*, **223**, 395–409.

Longo, L. D., Hill, E. P. & Power, G. G. (1972) Theoretical aspects of analysis of factors affecting placental oxygen transfer. *American Journal of Physiology*, **222**, 730–739.

Macdonald, M. S. & Emery, J. L. (1959) The late intrauterine and postnatal development of human glomeruli. *Journal of Anatomy*, **93**, 331–340.

Malan, A. I., Malan, A. P. & Curson, H. H. (1937) The influence of age on (a) amount and (b) nature and composition of the allantoic and amniotic fluids of the merino ewe. *Onderstepoort Journal of Veterinary Science*, **9**, 205–221.

Mansour, M. M., Schulert, A. R. & Glasser, S. R. (1972) Mechanism of placental iron transfer in the rat. *American Journal of Physiology*, **222**, 1628–1633.

McCance, R. A. & Widdowson, E. M. (1951) Composition of the body. *British Medical Bulletin*, **7**, 297–306.

Mellor, D. J. (1970) Distribution of ions and electrical potential differences between mother and foetus at different gestational ages in goats and sheep. *Journal of Physiology*, **207**, 133–150.

Mellor, D. J. & Slater, J. S. (1971) Daily changes in amniotic and allantoic fluid during the last three months of pregnancy in conscious, unstressed ewes with catheters in their foetal fluid sacs. *Journal of Physiology*, **217**, 573–604.

Mellor, D. J. & Slater, J. S. (1972) Daily changes in foetal urine and relationships with amniotic and allantoic fluid and maternal plasma during the last two months of pregnancy in conscious, unstressed ewes with chronically implanted catheters. *Journal of Physiology*, **227**, 503–525.

Mellor, D. J. & Slater, J. S. (1973) The composition of maternal plasma and foetal urine after feeding and drinking in chronically catheterised ewes during the last two months of pregnancy. *Journal of Physiology*, **234**, 519–532.

Mellor, D. J., Cockburn, F., Lees, M. M. & Blagden, A. (1969) Distribution of ions and electrical potential differences between mother and foetus in the human at term. *Journal of Obstetrics and Gynaecology of the British Commonwealth*, **76**, 993–998.

Meschia, G. (1955) Colloidal osmotic pressure of fetal and maternal plasmas of sheep and goats. *American Journal of Physiology*, **181**, 1–8.

Meschia, G., Battaglia, F. C. & Barron, D. H. (1957) A comparison of the freezing points of fetal and maternal plasmas of sheep and goats. *Quarterly Journal of Experimental Physiology*, **42**, 163–170.

Meschia, G., Battaglia, F. C. & Bruns, P. D. (1967) Theoretical and experimental study of transplacental diffusion. *Journal of Applied Physiology*, **22**, 1171–1178.

Meschia, G., Wolkoff, A. S. & Barron, D. H. (1958) Difference in electrical potential across the placenta of goats. *Proceedings of the National Academy of Sciences*, **44**, 483–485.

Mott, J. C. (1975) Place of the renin–angiotensin system before and after birth. *British Medical Bulletin*, **31**, 44–50.

Nylander, G. (1953) On the placental transfer of iron. An experimental study in the rat. *Acta Physiologica Scandinavica*, **29**, Supplement 107.

Reynolds, S. R. M. (1953) A source of amniotic fluid in the lamb: the naso-pharyngeal and buccal cavities. *Nature*, **172**, 307–308.

Rudolph, A. M. & Heymann, M. A. (1967) The circulation of the fetus in utero. Methods for studying the distribution of blood flow, cardiac output and organ blood flow. *Circulation Research*, **21**, 163–184.

Smith, F. G. Jr, Adams, F. H., Borden, M. & Hilburn, J. (1966) Studies of renal function in the intact fetal lamb. *American Journal of Obstetrics and Gynecology*, **96**, 240–246.

Stulc, J. J., Rietveld, W. J., Soeteman, D. W. & Verspille, A. (1972) The transplacental potential difference in guinea pigs. *Biologia Neonatorum*, **21**, 130–147.

Vaughan, D., Kirschbaum, T. H., Bersentes, T., Dilts, P. V. Jr & Assali, N. S. (1968) Fetal and neonatal response to acid loading in the sheep. *Journal of Applied Physiology*, **24**, 135–141.

Vosburgh, G. J., Flexner, L. B., Cowie, D. B., Hellman, L. M., Proctor, N. K. & Wilde, W. S. (1948) The rate of renewal in woman of the water and sodium of the amniotic fluid as determined by tracer techniques. *American Journal of Obstetrics and Gynecology*, **56**, 1156–1159.

Widdas, W. F. (1961) Transport mechanisms in the foetus. *British Medical Bulletin*, **17**, 107–111.

Wright, G. H. (1962) Net transfers of water, sodium, chloride and hydrogen ions across the gastric mucosa of the rabbit foetus. *Journal of Physiology*, **163**, 281–293.

Wright, G. H. (1974) Electrical impedance, ultrastructure, and ion transport in foetal gastric mucosa. *Journal of Physiology*, **242**, 661–672.

12

THE FETAL THYROID

Peter W. Nathanielsz

The purpose of this chapter is to review the role of the thyroid gland in fetal development. Absence of the thyroid gland at birth, or hypofunction of the fetal thyroid, have long been known to impair fetal development. The extent of this impairment, the nature of the tissue and organ systems involved and the reversibility of the lesions caused by the deficiency are areas of considerable dispute. Difficulties in locating the consequences of thyroid deficiency precisely are the direct result of the complex role that the thyroid hormones play in conjunction with other important growth-promoting and developmental factors, both nervous and endocrine. Human fetal endocrine function will never be capable of investigation in the same manner as in experimental animals. We therefore have to consider how the various data available from controlled animal experiments correlate with the information obtained in the human. Human material is invariably obtained from abortion, premature delivery or postnatal cord blood from term deliveries. As such it is not necessarily representative of the undisturbed physiological state in utero. This somewhat obvious observation must be stated in view of the number of publications which refer to neonatal cord blood concentrations as *fetal* values. The most common experimental models are the rat, and the chronically catheterised fetal sheep preparation with indwelling vascular catheters, which is ideally suited to investigation of fetal endocrine mechanisms (see page 221).

THE IMPORTANCE OF THE FETAL THYROID IN DEVELOPMENT

For convenience we may consider the role of the thyroid hormones (TH)* as being to exert control on (a) fetal growth and (b) tissue differentiation. Growth may be defined as any permanent increase in size resulting from an increase either in mean cell size or in the number of cells as a result of mitosis. Differentiation, in contrast, is the development of the specific characteristics of different tissues from initial cell lines, all of which have the same genetic material.

Fetal growth

The clearest demonstration that fetal thyroid hormones play a role in development comes from observations in experimental species in which the fetus can be thyroidectomised in utero. Objections exist to experimental preparations in which propylthiouracil (PTU) has been administered to the pregnant animal in order to decrease both maternal and fetal thyroid function. Although PTU does cross the placenta and interferes with TH production in the fetal thyroid, PTU also has actions on peripheral tissues (Escobar and Escobar, 1961) and inevitably maternal thyroid function will also be impaired. Fetal decapitation or hypophysectomy will affect the circulating concentrations of several growth-promoting hormones. For this reason consideration will only be given to studies of surgical removal of the fetal thyroid. As well as experiments with fetal sheep, data obtained using the newborn rat as an experimental model will be included. Not only is this a simple, cheap and ubiquitous laboratory animal, but it is now clear that certain developmental phases which occur in utero in the human and sheep are similar to those taking place in the first two to three weeks of extra-uterine life in the rat. This difference in timing of critical developmental phases is true for many systems, particularly those concerned with maturation of brain–endocrine relationships (Brown-Grant, 1973). It is thus important at the outset to note that both the nature of the developing systems which require TH and the critical periods over which TH have an important role to play in development may vary in different species.

   Overall body size is considered to be little affected by gross fetal TH deficiency in utero in several species (Jost, 1959; Hamburgh, Lynn and Weiss, 1964). However, the physiological significance of these observations must be assessed carefully. Firstly, as we shall see, effects do manifest themselves in specific organ systems and it is therefore important to look at more precise and discriminating features than overall growth. Secondly, the clinical literature is inevitably anecdotal, uncontrolled (in respect of paired data from as near equivalent subjects lacking only the TH deficiencies) and often deficient in actual measurement of relevant hormone values. Thus in one paper often quoted to show that normal fetal growth occurs in the

---

* Throughout this chapter the abbreviation TH will be used for thyroid hormones whenever it is only intended to refer to the endocrine function of the thyroid hormones without differentiating specifically between thyroxine and triiodothyronine. When it is intended to refer specifically to thyroxine, the abbreviation T4 will be used. Triiodothyronine will be referred to as T3.

absence of fetal TH, body proportions within the normal range are described for an infant born with holoacephalus (Pennel and Kukral, 1946). Although no trace of a head was found, it is impossible to state that the growth of this particular individual had not been at least marginally impaired, there being no individual control. Similarly, there may have been some TH available (even if only of maternal origin) at early, critical phases of growth. We shall return to these problems when considering differentiation. Although in such cases there are usually no macroscopically visible thyroid remnants, it is very necessary to make hormone measurements. In the past this has not been done. It is also uncertain whether normal growth can occur in the presence of lower fetal plasma TH concentrations than those required for normal tissue differentiation and maturation.

It is almost impossible to produce an experimental preparation in which both maternal and fetal compartments are free of TH at an early stage of pregnancy. Such an animal would in any case be very unphysiological. The experimental investigation of the role of TH in growth and differentiation has therefore necessarily been confined to the later phases of pregnancy and the early neonatal phase in the rat. More information related to a possible role of maternal TH is required.

In the studies on polytocous species such as the rat and rabbit, born at a relatively immature stage of development, decapitation in utero does not impair fetal growth. It must, however, be remembered that in these species the plasma half-life of TH is of the order of 12 to 24 hours and the half-life of TH already bound to tissues is certainly longer. In addition, when it is considered that the circulating plasma of most animals contains a reservoir of protein-bound TH equal to several days of thyroid secretion, it is difficult to interpret the effects of removal of the thyroid gland alone unless an adequate time interval has elapsed for clearance of the TH pool. This is obviously impossible in animals with short gestation periods. Similar considerations apply to experiments involving removal of the pituitary for whose hormonal secretions the above points also pertain. In all approaches to these problems it is therefore necessary to attempt to quantitate the degree of thyroid deficiency at the tissue level. It is becoming increasingly clear that considerations involving tissue responsiveness and the development of hormone receptors are likely to affect the level of activity of hormones in the fetus.

The best study of the effect of TH on growth is that in the thyroidectomised fetal lamb (Hopkins and Thorburn, 1972). Thyroidectomy at 0.55 of term resulted in body weight of 33 per cent of normal at delivery. The major effects observed were shortening of the limbs. In conjunction with the caveats expressed above regarding other experimental data, this work allows us to conclude that complete fetal thyroid deficiency, with no other primary endocrine defects, for an adequate period of time in the latter part of pregnancy, results in marked impairment of growth in the sheep. It is probable that TH play a similar role in the human. Many of the developmental stages which occur in utero in the human and sheep are postnatal in the rat, a species in which postnatal hypothyroidism produced by administration of PTU to the pups from the day of birth causes impairment of growth after 15 days (Nicholson and Altman, 1972).

Differentiation

Bone and integument

Observations on thyroidectomised fetal sheep (Hopkins and Thorburn, 1972) show clearly that prolonged fetal hypothyroidism produces abnormal development of bone and the integument. The retardation of ossification and the lamellation of the bone shaft were more marked when fetal thyroidectomy was performed at 0.55 of term than 0.63. In the neonatal rat, thyroidectomy at birth results in delay of appearance of ossification centres and a decrease in their size. In other studies in the rat, neonatal hypothyroidism has been shown to affect longitudinal bone growth and to slow development of the bones of the skull. These deficiencies can be reversed by the administration of TH (Becks et al, 1950).

Nervous system

Thyroid deficiency in the adult results in impairment of brain function and eventually in histologically demonstrable lesions. These manifestations are fully reversible. In the human neonate the age of onset of hypothyroidism is a feature of cardinal importance. The hypothyroid human baby requires immediate treatment and responds well to TH administration at birth. It is generally considered that early treatment prevents the appearance of permanent damage. The initial requirement for TH is approximately thyroxine 15 μg/kg body weight daily. Treatment should be monitored by measurement of the plasma hormone concentrations produced at different dose levels. It is preferable if plasma T3 and T4 concentrations are followed at different dose levels. If hypothyroidism only occurs after the age of two years, the necessity for immediate treatment to avoid long-term damage is less acute (Smith, Blizzard and Wilkins, 1957).

The existence of a critical phase of influence of TH on neural development has been well monitored in the rat (Eayrs, 1961). The degree of cerebral impairment produced by thyroidectomy of the newborn rat decreased with increasing age at thyroidectomy. When thyroidectomy was delayed until day 25, there was no detectable effect on performance. If replacement therapy was delayed until after day 24 it was not possible to reverse the impairment of nervous function. An adequate understanding of the cellular basis of these manifestations of TH deficiency is not yet possible (see next section). Neonatal hypothyroidism results in a decreased intensity of cerebral vascular connections in the rat (Eayrs, 1954). These changes may be the primary defect or alternatively they may reflect a decreased invasion of nervous tissue by blood vessels as a result of depression of brain development.

One example of a critical period of brain development is the demonstration by Best, Duncan and Best (1969) that excess administration of TH to the newborn rat in the first two weeks of life results in permanent impairment of growth and a resetting of the level of activity of the thyroid axis (see page 227). The high levels of TH result in permanent reduction of pituitary and plasma thyrotropin (TSH) concentrations (Bakke and Lawrence, 1966; Azizi et al, 1974). Similarly, a short period of hypothyroidism in the neonatal period can also result in irreversible alteration of the feedback system (Bakke, Gellert and Lawrence, 1970).

Surfactant

Lambs thyroidectomised in utero at about 0.55 of term die within hours of birth (Hopkins and Thorburn, 1972). This observation is in keeping with the demonstration that T4 injections into fetal rabbits accelerate the appearance of pulmonary surfactant (Wu et al, 1973). In the sheep, the critical period for the development of pulmonary surfactant is 120 to 130 days. It is clear that glucocorticoids play an important role in this process (Avery, 1975). Three fetal lambs thyroidectomised at 130 days gestation did not demonstrate respiratory distress at birth and survived for at least 10 days without TH replacement (Nathanielsz and Thomas, unpublished observations, 1975). It is therefore possible that TH are necessary for the initial differentiation of the systems responsible for initiation of surfactant production but not maintenance of synthesis thereafter. Alternatively when thyroidectomy was performed at 130 days gestation, even though plasma TH concentrations were below the limits of detection, tissue activity may have persisted for the period of observation, a further 30 days.

IN VITRO STUDIES AND EFFECTS ON SUBCELLULAR SYSTEMS

A recent review of the action of TH at the cellular level commences with the honest statement that "After nearly 30 years of intensive research we do not yet know how to explain the physiological actions of thyroid hormones in terms of molecular mechanisms" (Tata, 1974). One of the major problems is to define the actions of TH which are of a catabolic nature in contrast to those which are anabolic. This is of importance both in cases of natural pathology and in those experiments in which the pharmacology of TH has been investigated by the use of massive unphysiological doses of TH administered to experimental animals. Thyrotoxicosis, a pathological experiment of nature, leads to marked catabolism which does not initially appear to have much relation to our present consideration of the effects of TH on growth.

One basic difference between the effects of anabolic and catabolic doses of T3 has been demonstrated by Tata (1964). Although both effects result in increased basal metabolic rate (BMR) and oxygen utilisation, the anabolic doses produce their effects with a much longer latency. This observation may be of considerable importance in the intact animal, in which TH will have to act in the presence of other synergistic and antagonistic hormones. Anabolic and catabolic doses of TH produce different effects on phosphorylation ratios in liver cells of thyroidectomised rats, but, as with the previously mentioned effects, the latency with anabolic effects is much longer.

TH cause an increase in messenger RNA synthesis and an even greater increase in ribosomal RNA synthesis in liver. The number of ribosomes is increased. In liver cells, the effects of growth hormone, TH and testosterone are additive (Widnell and Tata, 1966). These functional changes may be related to the observations of reorganisation of ribosomal distribution within the cell which occurs after TH-induced metamorphosis in the tadpole. T3-induced metamorphosis converts the cell appearance from one in which the hepatic ribosomes exist in small groups around simple vesicular membranes into a more complex organised pattern with aggregates of ribosomes attached to a clearly differentiated double lamellar reticulum (Tata, 1967a, b). These are the types of cellular changes which would be expected to occur in connection with increased protein synthesis. Other less striking though potentially significant biochemical changes can be induced by TH, such as stimulation of phospholipid for membrane synthesis (Kaiser and Bygrave, 1969).

Using different methods of investigation—predominantly radioactive tracers—it has been demonstrated that the steroid hormones localise initially within the cell nucleus and produce similar stimulation of synthesis of important cellular proteins. The specificity whereby cells distinguish different hormonal instructions to their activity depends upon the hormone–receptor complex. TH binding occurs to most cellular fractions; no specific binding protein has yet been isolated.

MORPHOLOGICAL MATURATION OF THE THYROID AXIS

Many excellent reviews are available which describe the evolution of the endocrine thyroid from a pharyngeal diverticulum which releases its secretion into the gastrointestinal tract (Fisher and Dussault, 1974). The embryological differentiation of the gland in the mammal follows a similar series of steps in all mammalian species studied to date.

Initially the thyroglossal duct grows caudally from its site of origin at the junction of the anterior two-thirds and posterior third of the tongue. This duct gives rise to the primitive thyroid which is composed of solid cords of cells. Colloid droplets appear at the apices of the cells. Subsequently colloid is extruded between the cells to produce the typical follicular appearance. These features of embryology explain several minor pathological aberrations such as the localisation of thyroid cell rests along the track taken by the thyroid in its descent into the neck. Similarly they throw light on the relationship of the thyroid gland cells which produce TH to both the parathyroid cells, which develop from the dorsal wings of the third and fourth pharyngeal pouches and give rise to the parathyroid glands which produce the hypercalcaemic factor, parathormone. Cells derived from the last pharyngeal pouch (the ultimobranchial body) produce a plasma calcium lowering hormone, calcitonin. In many species these cells come to lie within the substance of the thyroid, the parafollicular (C) cells. In this case the hormone produced is more correctly called thyrocalcitonin. In the human, thyroglobulin production begins at about six weeks gestational age, colloid formation at eight weeks, and iodothyronines appear at 12 weeks. In the sheep these landmarks are reached at approximately 50, 52 and 70 days.

THE THYROID AXIS IN THE ADULT MAMMAL

The major links, neural and endocrine, in the thyroid axis of the adult mammal are shown in Figure 12.1. It is important to discuss the system at four levels of activity: the target tissues of

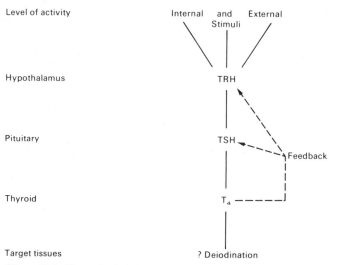

Figure 12.1. The major links in the hypothalamic–pituitary–thyroid axis.

TH; the function of the thyroid gland itself; the pituitary; and finally the hypothalamus. There are probably two sites of feedback of TH: at the hypothalamic and at the pituitary level. The effects of TH on their target tissues during fetal development have been discussed above. It is now necessary to consider the dynamic and quantitative aspects of the hypothalamic–hypophyseal–thyroid–target tissue axis (HHTT axis) in development.

THE CHRONICALLY CATHETERISED FETAL SHEEP MODEL

Following the introduction by Meschia et al (1965) of surgical methods for the implantation and long-term maintenance of patency of indwelling vascular catheters in the umbilical vessels of fetal sheep, the endocrinology of the fetus has been one of the features of fetal physiology extensively investigated by several groups of workers. The use of various surgical procedures on the fetus, such as thyroidectomy, hypophysectomy, adrenalectomy and nephrectomy, together with catheterisation of fetal and maternal vessels, has permitted the sequential study of a single fetus in which controlled endocrine modifications have been introduced. The use of labelled tracer hormones or hormone precursors together with sensitive radioimmunoassay techniques has enabled the accumulation of much quantitative data regarding the function of the HHTT axis. These techniques enable the experimenter to avoid many of the criticisms mentioned in the chapter opening.

Data referred to here produced by the author and his colleagues have been obtained from samples taken from catheters advanced into the fetal aorta and inferior vena cava after insertion via tarsal vessels. All preparations were in dated, single-mated pregnancies and 48 hours were allowed to elapse after surgery before any experiment was commenced. This is almost certainly the minimum period which should be allowed for several reasons. First, anaesthesia increases the permeability of the placenta to steroid hormones (Nathanielsz et al, 1972). Many investigators have demonstrated that various physiological parameters are changed in the days immediately post-surgery. Forty-eight hours post-surgery the frequency of fetal breathing movements has returned to within the normal range, although it is probably five days before complete normality is restored (Dawes, 1973). Fetal antidiuretic hormone concentrations are elevated after surgery (Alexander et al, 1974). Maternal and fetal plasma electrolyte concentrations require about three days to stabilise postoperatively (Mellor and Slater, 1971). The recovery period from fetal catheterisation is also accompanied by changes in fetal metabolism and similar examples could be quoted for features of carbohydrate and urea metabolism (Shelley, 1973).

There are, therefore, many problems in the interpretation of data from preparations that have been recently exposed to surgery. It is also important to state the eventual outcome of the preparation from which the data were obtained. Whilst the stability of different preparations will remain a matter for discussion, the best indications of fetal well-being available at the present time are normal blood values for fetal oxygen and carbon dioxide tension and pH. Other variables such as fetal plasma glucose concentration are also useful in assessing fetal condition. The aim for suitable preparations for a sequential study should be the birth of a healthy live lamb near the expected date, preceded by a rise in fetal plasma cortisol concentration of the normal extent and time course after a period of stable fetal plasma cortisol of a week or more. Even when all these various details are observed there are other important constraints upon fetal investigations. For example, it has been demonstrated that repeated fetal blood sampling can affect the fetal renin–angiotensin system before changes in fetal haematocrit occur (Mott, 1975). Introduction of catheters into blood vessels may alter local vascular reactivity, change peripheral resistance characteristics within the whole circulation or simply occlude a segment of the circulation by virtue of the size of the catheters. A more detailed consideration of problems associated with the use of the fetal sheep preparation to investigate fetal endocrinology is given elsewhere (Nathanielsz, 1976).

EXPERIMENTAL OBSERVATIONS

Plasma thyroxine and TSH concentrations

Observations in experimental animals

Fetal lamb plasma cortisol concentrations rise in the last few days of intra-uterine life (Basset and Thorburn, 1969; Comline et al, 1970). A similar, though less pronounced, increase has been demonstrated in the fetal calf (Comline et al, 1974). The significance of these fetal endocrine changes in the processes of parturition is discussed in Chapter 13. Figure 12.2 contains a summary of the data obtained for various important thyroid hormones. In both the lamb and calf this period can be divided arbitrarily into four stages. A steady state of fetal plasma cortisol, T4, T3 and TSH exists more than seven or eight days before birth (Stage I).

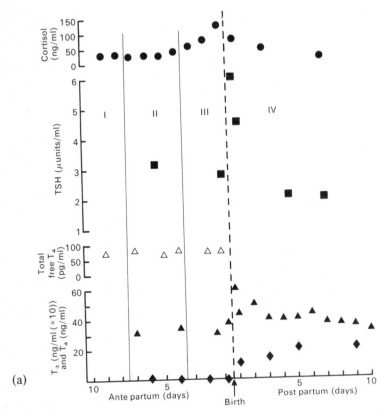

There is then a short transition stage (II) before the cortisol rise, during which the various fetal and maternal endocrine changes discussed in Chapter 13 are occurring (Stage III). The final stage is the postdelivery stage (Stage IV) with which we are not concerned here. It is probable that when more information is available Stage III and Stage IV will require further subdivision.

During Stage I, observations are available from three different centres which show that

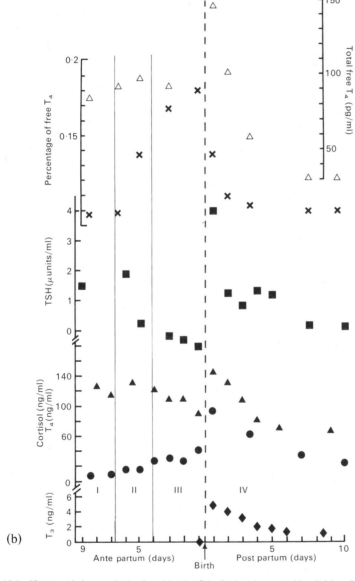

Figure 12.2. Hormonal changes in the thyroid axis of the fetal and neonatal lamb (a) and calf (b). Stages I, II, III and IV as described in text. X = percentage of free thyroxine (T4); Δ = total free T4; ■ = thyroid-stimulating hormone (TSH); ▲ = T4; ● = cortisol; ◆ = tri-iodothyronine (T3). Modified from Nathanielsz (1975) and reproduced with kind permission of the editor of *British Medical Bulletin*.

fetal plasma T4 concentrations vary between 45 and 100 ng/ml (Hopkins and Thorburn, 1972; Erenberg and Fisher, 1973; Nathanielsz, Silver and Comline, 1973). This variation in values is demonstrated in all reports to date and probably represents individual animal variation, since during this period (between 110 and 114 days of gestation) published results showing data from individual fetuses sampled sequentially show remarkably steady values. In individual animals the concentration of dialysable T4 is also steady at 30 to 100 pg/ml (Nathanielsz, Silver and Comline, 1973).

Before considering the changes during Stages II and III, it is useful to relate Stage I to values found in the immediate postnatal period (Stage IV). The increased neonatal T4 concentrations may be caused by the stress effect of labour itself. In the light of these observations great care must be taken in the interpretation of cord blood values from the human and experimental animal. Very exact timing is necessary and, in any event, newborn values must not be taken as a direct indication of fetal concentrations.

In the bovine, fetal plasma T4 concentrations decrease during Stage III, after the increase in fetal plasma cortisol (Figure 12.2b). During this phase the percentage of circulating fetal T4 that is dialysable increases from approximately 0.1 to 0.2 per cent. Total plasma T4 falls proportionately, with the result that total free T4, the physiologically important moiety of circulating T4, remains constant. Fetal plasma TSH drops to undetectable levels over the last three days of intra-uterine life. This decrease in TSH results in a fall in total plasma T4 concentration that has a half-life of about five to six days. The half-life of T4 in the newborn calf is two days, and it is therefore probable that fetal T4 secretion is not completely turned off in the last days of gestation. Premature induction of delivery by the administration of either ACTH or cortisol to the bovine fetus produces a similar fall in plasma TSH and T4 concentrations (Nathanielsz et al, 1974). Plasma T3 does not rise before delivery in either normal or induced delivery. However, samples were not taken in the last few hours (see sheep data below).

In thyroidectomised calves, 17 to 22 days old, Thomas, Abel and Nathanielsz (1974) demonstrated that simultaneous infusion of cortisol and T4 has a greater inhibitory effect on plasma TSH concentrations than infusion of the same dose of T4 alone. This effect comes on within four hours and is not accompanied by a significant increase in circulating plasma T3 concentrations. This observation enables us to put forward an explanation of the changes seen in the fetal calf. It would appear that increased fetal cortisol secretion in some way potentiates the inhibitory effect of circulating T4 on TSH. The HHTT axis then functions at lower T4 concentrations. This resetting has not been completed before the stress of delivery overcomes the inhibition of TSH secretion to cause the rise in Stage IV.

In the fetal sheep, Thorburn et al (1972) propose that the fall they demonstrate in fetal plasma T4 precedes the increase in fetal plasma cortisol and they put forward the interesting suggestion that these thyroid changes reflect a maturational change of the hypothalamus which plays an important role in the processes leading to delivery in this species. Their observations that fetal plasma TSH did not fall in this period of falling fetal T4 concentration suggest that the thyroid is changing its sensitivity to TSH (Thorburn and Hopkins, 1973; Hopkins, Wallace and Thorburn, 1975).

Thomas et al (unpublished observations, 1975) have shown that the induction of premature delivery in the fetal lamb, by infusing cortisol at 130 days gestation for four days to produce an increase in fetal plasma cortisol which mimics the normal rise at delivery, causes a fall in fetal plasma T4 concentrations and an increase in fetal plasma T3. These results are similar to those described above when parturition is induced in the fetal calf.

The author would bring together these considerations of the interrelationship of the fetal thyroid and adrenocortical axes in the following fashion. The prime event is the increase in fetal plasma cortisol concentrations. Under certain conditions, the increased cortisol activity either enhances the inhibitory feedback of T4 or alternatively acts directly on the fetal thyroid and there follows a fall in fetal plasma TSH and T4 concentrations. These events occur during spontaneous delivery of calves born a little prematurely (261 to 283 days) or in cortisol induction of delivery in the bovine at 270 days gestation or in the lamb at 130 days. Mature fetal lambs may possibly demonstrate this fall only in the presence of iodine deficiency. Alternatively, there may be breed differences. In any event, from experimentally induced delivery the thyroid changes appear to be secondary to the cortisol changes. The possible role of T3 in these situations is discussed in the section on plasma triiodothyronine concentrations.

Observations in the human

Placental permeability to T4 and T3 is probably low in the human, as it is in the sheep (Fisher, Lehmann and Lackey, 1964; Dussault et al, 1969). As mentioned earlier, hormonal concentrations in cord blood of fetuses removed by hysterotomy must be interpreted with care; they do not necessarily reflect the values in the undisturbed human fetus. Fisher et al (1970) have demonstrated that total fetal plasma T4 rises steadily through gestation and this rise is at least in part due to high circulating plasma thyroxine binding globulin (TBG) concentrations. Fetal TBG concentrations in the human rise during pregnancy because oestrogen concentrations are high; this is not so in the sheep. The phase of neonatal thyroid hyperactivity in the human (Fisher et al, 1969) is very similar to Stage IV (Figure 12.2a) in the sheep, suggesting that the sheep is a good experimental model for studying the activity of the thyroid gland in the perinatal period. Neonatal thyroid hyperactivity is only partially caused by stimulation of the newborn by exposure to cold. Warming infants in the first few hours of life does not significantly reduce the postnatal plasma TSH rise (Fisher and Odell, 1969).

Kinetic data

Isotopically labelled T4 and T3 have been used for the investigation of fetal distribution volumes and turnover rates for T4 and T3 in the sheep (Fisher et al, 1973; Nathanielsz et al, 1974) and the monkey (Koch et al, 1966). Whereas the data obtained from T4 studies are probably valid, great care must be exercised in interpreting results from single injection experiments with T3. As discussed, circulating plasma T3 reflects both thyroidal T3 secretion and generation within the tissues. Therefore, calculation of kinetic data as a result of the exogenous administration of a single injection of T3 may be of little physiological significance. Distribution volumes in kinetic studies are calculated from the extrapolation of plasma concentrations of the tracer achieved. After single injections of T3, distribution volumes in the ewe considerably exceed 1 l/kg and in the fetus approach 8 l/kg. Therefore, exogenously administered T3 must be concentrated in some tissues of the body. Since fetal plasma T3 concentrations are generally below the limits of assay sensitivity, it is only possible to express total daily turnover of the fetal T3 *blood pool* in terms of maximum amounts. Values obtained are therefore stated as 'less than'. Fetal T4 turnover is much more rapid than in the ewe (by a factor of 8), whereas absolute fetal T4 only a little over double that in the mother. Placental transport of T4 in both directions is also minimal (Koch et al, 1966; Erenberg and Fisher, 1973; Nathanielsz et al, 1974).

Plasma triiodothyronine in the fetus

Observations in experimental animals

It is now clear that an overall view of thyroid function in certain clinical states requires information on the circulating concentration of T3 (Bellabarba, Benard and Langlois, 1972). From the outset it is important to note that T3 in the plasma is derived from two sources. The thyroid gland secretes both T4 and T3 directly into the blood. T3 is also produced in the peripheral tissues by the monodeiodination of T4. T3 appears in the plasma of thyroidectomised adult animals injected with T4; there are however many difficulties in assessing the proportion of T3 produced in the tissues which eventually finds its way back into the blood.

The observation that circulating plasma T3 concentration is very low in the chronically maintained sheep fetus (Erenberg and Fisher, 1973; Nathanielsz, Silver and Comline, 1973) and the calf fetus (Nathanielsz et al, 1974) in the presence of high rates of T4 production demonstrates that the thyroid axis in these species is functioning in a different fashion in the fetus and the adult. However, it is not yet possible even in the adult to quantify the proportion of circulating plasma T3 that is of thyroid origin and the proportion that is produced by deiodination in the tissues. It is therefore difficult to interpret the low circulating plasma T3 concentrations in the fetus. Several possible explanations may be put forward.

1. Thyroidal T3 secretion is less in the fetus than the newborn, which demonstrates a massive rise of T3 in the first few hours of life (Figure 12.2). Fisher et al (1973) demonstrated that thyroid gland homogenates from human fetuses have the same T4:T3 ratio as adults. Massive stimulation of the thyroid with TSH will increase the plasma T3:T4 ratio in the adult animal. When fetal and five-day-old lamb plasma TSH concentrations are elevated by the administration of TRH (thyrotrophin releasing hormone), the increase in plasma T4 concentrations is similar, but the rise in T3 in the fetus is much less than that in the five-day-old lamb (Nathanielsz et al, unpublished observations, 1975). This evidence suggests that there may be deficiency in the secretion of T3 by the fetal thyroid. It is interesting to speculate whether the rise in fetal cortisol increases the ability to secrete T3 in response to TSH, since the TSH rise at birth is accompanied by a rapid increase in T3. It is important to obtain more data on the effects of acute and long-term fetal administration of TSH on the fetal thyroid both in vivo and in vitro.

2. Peripheral conversion of T4 to T3 may be deficient in the fetus. If this is so, then the fetus demonstrates a qualitatively different mechanism of action of T4. T3 replacement will prevent hypothyroidism in the thyroidectomised adult animal. The effect of T3 replacement should be studied in the thyroidectomised fetus. Since fetal plasma TSH concentrations increase after thyroidectomy (Thorburn and Hopkins, 1973), a simple system would be to test the negative feedback effect of T3 in the fetus as a method of assessing T3's action on at least one fetal target tissue.

3. The ability of T3 generated in the peripheral tissues of the fetus to leak back into the blood may be less than in the adult.

4. The fetus may have pathways for further rapid degradation of T3.

Any of the last three mechanisms would explain the observation that after the injection of radioactively labelled T4 into the sheep fetus, the rate of appearance of labelled T3 in the fetal plasma is much slower than in the adult (Fisher and Dussault, 1974). This aspect of fetal thyroid function is a fascinating area requiring further research. Certainly the massive rise in neonatal T3 concentrations must be of thyroid origin, since it is too rapid to be the result of peripheral deiodination of T4 secreted at delivery.

Chopra, Sack and Fisher (1976a) have suggested that the fetus may deiodinate T4 at the 5 position initially, thereby producing 3′, 5′,3-triiodothyronine (reverse T3, rT3) rather than as n the adult where monodeiodination generally occurs at the 5′ position in the outer ring to ield 3,5,3′ -triiodothyronine (T3). These authors have demonstrated high rT3 plasma concentrations in the fetal sheep and in newborn human cord blood (Chopra, Sack and Fisher, 976b). Such a qualitative difference in peripheral deiodination might account for several of he differences between fetal and adult thyroid function. Further work is necessary to show hat rT3 does have an endocrine function in the sheep and human fetus related to T3 and T4. or a more detailed discussion of the possible significance of rT3 in the fetus see Nathanielsz 1976).

Observations in the human

Human plasma T3 concentrations are low in cord blood (500 pg/ml) (Hüfner et al, 1973). To late no values are available for the human fetus and, although samples comparable to those n the chronically catheterised lamb or calf cannot be obtained, it would be of interest to obain data from human scalp blood samples in utero and at caesarian section, if possible comaring them with simultaneous cord blood concentrations.

Possibility of placental transport of triiodothyronine from mother to fetus

Much of the literature relating to placental permeability to T3 in both the human and in experimental animals reports experiments performed before assay methodology for T3 had peen placed on a secure basis (Raiti et al, 1967). Fisher et al (1972) using kinetic studies in the pregnant sheep calculated that very limited materno-fetal transfer of T3 did occur but that it contributed less than one per cent of the total production of thyronine (i.e. T4 + T3) within he fetal compartment. Data obtained from human neonatal cord blood must be interpreted with caution, since changes in placental permeability may occur with placental separation and the physiological and endocrine mechanism in the newborn human infant are not the same as would exist in the steady state in the human fetus in utero. Dussault et al (1969) attempted to study this problem by repeated administration of large doses of T3 to pregnant women for up to three weeks before delivery with subsequent measurements of cord blood T3 concentrations. Not only were the doses of T3 pharmacological but the same author reports later on 'the contribution of methodological artifacts to the measurement of T3 concentration in serum' as they were at that time (Fisher and Dussault, 1971). It is the opinion of the author of this chapter that there is no sound evidence to believe that the human fetus is not, like the sheep, autonomous in all aspects of thyroid physiology, including T3 during the later stage of gestation.

Hypothalamic control of TSH secretion by the fetus

Thorburn and Hopkins (1973) have compared the effect of fetal hypophysectomy or pituitary stalk section on fetal plasma TSH concentrations in the sheep. After stalk section TSH is depressed to about half the concentration observed in control animals, thereby suggesting that in the normal sheep fetus, adenohypophyseal TSH secretion is the result of both a degree of autonomous activity and some hypothalamic drive. Fetal sheep plasma TSH concentrations are higher than the maternal concentrations (Thorburn and Hopkins,

1973; Thomas et al, 1975). Nevertheless, administration of TRH provokes a three-fold increase in plasma TSH of fetuses of only 132 days gestation (Thomas et al, 1975). It is quite clear that there is a considerable degree of reserve capacity of TSH secretion in the fetus and this is consistent with the observation of Thorburn and Hopkins (1973) that fetal thyroidectomy results in a four to five-fold increase in TSH in 10 days.

Possible roles of the placenta

The placenta is a source of various glycoprotein and other protein hormones at different periods of gestation. A placental TSH has been described and characterised in the human (Hennen, Pierce and Freychet, 1969). Other workers have been unable to demonstrate a placental TSH (Odell, Wilber and Utiger, 1967). In view of the low level of thyroid activity reported by Thorburn and Hopkins (1973) in the hypophysectomised fetus, it is unlikely that a placental TSH is of importance in the sheep fetus.

The placenta allows the transfer of gammaglobulin antibodies in several species including the human. Long-acting thyroid stimulator (LATS) and LATS-protector are both gammaglobulins. In thyrotoxic patients in whom either or both of these antibodies may cross the placenta, the possible role of the placenta in the reported differences in T4 deiodination must also be investigated, in spite of the negative observations of Yamazaki, Noguchi and Slingerland (1960).

CONCLUSIONS

In conclusion we may ask two questions. First, how are the changes in the levels of activity in the various positions of the thyroid axis of the fetus brought about? Many of the answers to this question have been discussed above and there is now a fairly clear picture of the changes in the various thyroid hormones in the sheep fetus over the last third of gestation. The second question—how do the thyroid hormones influence growth and development?—still remains poorly understood.

ACKNOWLEDGEMENTS

My thanks are due over the years for stimulating discussion on the problems of fetal endocrinology in general and the thyroid in particular with several colleagues, especially Dr A. L. Thomas, Dr D. A. Fisher and Dr G. D. Thorburn. I am also grateful to Dr A. L. C. Wallace and Dr R. D. Hesch for generous gifts of antisera, without which much of this work would be very deficient. Our work reported here has been made possible by grants from the MRC, ARC and The Wellcome Trust.

REFERENCES

Alexander, D. P., Bashore, R. A., Britton, H. G. & Forsling, M. L. (1974) Maternal and fetal arginine vasopressin in the chronically catheterised sheep. *Biology of the Neonate,* **25,** 242–248.
Avery, M. E. (1975) Pharmacological approaches to the acceleration of fetal lung maturation. *British Medical Bulletin,* **31,** 13–17.
Azizi, F., Vagenakis, A. G., Bollinger, J., Reichlin, S., Braverman, L. E. & Ingbar, S. M. (1974) Persistent abnormalities in pituitary function following neonatal thyrotoxicosis in the rat. *Endocrinology,* **94,** 1681–1688.

Bakke, J. L. & Lawrence, N. (1966) Persistent thyrotrophin insufficiency following neonatal thyroxine administration. *Journal of Laboratory and Clinical Medicine,* **76,** 25–33.

Bakke, J. L., Gellert, R. J. & Lawrence, N. (1970) The persistent effects of perinatal hypothyroidism on pituitary, thyroid and gonadal functions. *Journal of Laboratory and Clinical Medicine,* **76,** 25–33.

Bassett, J. M. & Thorburn, G. D. (1969) Foetal plasma corticosteroids and the initiation of parturition in sheep. *Journal of Endocrinology,* **44,** 285–286.

Becks, H., Scow, R. O., Simpson, M. E., Asling, C. W., Li, C. H. & Evans, H. M. (1950) Response by the rat thyro-parathyroidectomised at birth to growth hormone and to thyroxine given separately or in combination. *Anatomical Record,* **107,** 299–317.

Bellabarba, D., Benard, B. & Langlois, M. (1972) Pattern of serum thyroxine, triiodothyronine and thyrotrophin after treatment of thyrotoxicosis. *Clinical Endocrinology,* **1,** 345–353.

Best, M. M., Duncan, C. H. & Best, M. M. (1969) Accelerated maturation and persistent growth impairment in the rat resulting from thyroxine administration in the neonatal period. *Journal of Laboratory and Clinical Medicine,* **73,** 135–143.

Brown-Grant, K. (1973) Recent studies on the sexual differentiation of the brain. In *Foetal and Neonatal Physiology. Proceedings of the Sir Joseph Barcroft Centenary Symposium* (Ed.) Comline, R. S., Cross, K. W., Dawes, G. D. & Nathanielsz, P. W. pp. 527–545. London: Cambridge University Press.

Chopra, I. J., Sack, J. & Fisher, D. A. (1976a) 3,3′,5′ Triiodothyronine (reverse T3) and 3,3′,5 triiodothyronine (T3) in fetal and adult sheep: studies of metabolic clearance rate, production rate, serum binding and thyroidal content relative to thyroxine. *Endocrinology,* **97,** 1080–1088.

Chopra, I. J., Sack, J. & Fisher, D. A. (1976b) Circulating 3,3′,5′ triiodothyronine (reverse T3) in the human newborn. *Journal of Clinical Investigation,* **55,** 1137–1141.

Comline, R. S., Hall, L. W., Lavelle, R. B., Nathanielsz, P. W. & Silver, M. (1974) Parturition in the cow: endocrine changes in animals with chronically implanted catheters in the foetal and maternal circulations. *Journal of Endocrinology,* **63,** 451–472.

Comline, R. S., Nathanielsz, P. W., Paisey, R. B. & Silver, M. (1970) Cortisol turnover in the sheep foetus immediately prior to parturition. *Journal of Physiology,* **210,** 141–142P.

Dawes, G. S. (1973) Breathing and rapid eye movement sleep before birth. In *Foetal and Neonatal Physiology. Proceedings of the Sir Joseph Barcroft Centenary Symposium on Foetal and Neonatal Physiology* (Ed.) Comline, R. S., Cross, K. W., Dawes, G. S. & Nathanielsz, P. W. pp. 49–62. London: Cambridge University Press.

Dussault, J., Row, Vas V., Lickrish, G. & Volpé, R. (1969) Studies of serum triiodothyronine concentration in maternal and cord blood: transfer of T3 across the human placenta. *Journal of Clinical Endocrinology and Metabolism,* **29,** 595–603.

Eayrs, J. T. (1954) The vascularity of the cerebral cortex in normal and cretinous rats. *Journal of Anatomy,* **88,** 164–173.

Eayrs, J. T. (1961) Age as a factor determining the severity and reversibility of the effects of thyroid deprivation in the rat. *Journal of Endocrinology,* **22,** 409–419.

Erenberg, A. & Fisher, D. A. (1973) Thyroid hormone metabolism in the foetus. In *Foetal and Neonatal Physiology. Proceedings of the Sir Joseph Barcroft Centenary Symposium* (Ed.) Comline, R. S., Cross, K. W., Dawes, G. D. & Nathanielsz, P. W. pp. 508–526. London: Cambridge University Press.

Escobar del Rey, F. & Morreale de Escobar, G. (1961) The effect of propylthiouracil, methylthiouracil and thiouracil on the peripheral metabolism of L-thyroxine in thyroidectomised, L-thyroxine maintained rats. *Endocrinology,* **69,** 456–465.

Fisher, D. A. & Dussault, J. H. (1971) Contribution of methodological artifacts to the measurement of T3 concentration in serum. *Journal of Clinical Endocrinology,* **32,** 675–679.

Fisher, D. A. & Dussault, J. H. (1974) Development of the mammalian thyroid gland. In *Handbook of Physiology* Section 7, *Endocrinology,* Vol. III *Thyroid,* pp. 21–38. American Physiological Society.

Fisher, D. A. & Odell, W. D. (1969) Acute release of thyrotrophin in the newborn. *Journal of Clinical Investigation,* **48,** 1670–1677.

Fisher, D. A., Lehman, H. & Lackey, C. (1964) Placental transport of thyroxine. *Journal of Clinical Endocrinology and Metabolism,* **24,** 393–405.

Fisher, D. A., Dussault, J. H., Hobel, C. J. & Lam, R. (1973) Serum and thyroid gland triiodothyronine in the human fetus. *Journal of Clinical Endocrinology and Metabolism,* **36,** 397–400.

Fisher, D. A., Hobel, C. J., Garza, R. & Pierce, C. A. (1970) Thyroid function in the preterm fetus. *Pediatrics,* **46,** 208–215.

Fisher, D. A., Odell, W. D., Hobel, C. J. & Garza, R. (1969) Thyroid function in the term fetus. *Pediatrics,* **44,** 526–535.

Hamburgh, M., Lynn, E. & Weiss, E. P. (1964) Analysis of the influence of thyroid hormone on prenatal and postnatal maturation of the rat. *Anatomical Record,* **150,** 147–162.

Hennen, G., Pierce, J. G. & Freychet, P. (1969) Human chorionic thyrotrophin: further characterisation and study of its secretion during pregnancy. *Journal of Clinical Endocrinology,* **29,** 581–594.

Hopkins, P. S. & Thorburn, G. D. (1972) The effects of foetal thyroidectomy on the development of the ovine foetus. *Journal of Endocrinology*, **54**, 55–56.

Hopkins, P. S., Wallace, A. L. C. & Thorburn, G. D. (1975) Thyrotrophin concentrations in the plasma of cattle, sheep and foetal lambs as measured by radioimmunoassay. *Journal of Endocrinology*, **64**, 371–387.

Hüfner, M., Hesch, R. D., Lüders, D. & Heinrich, U. (1973) Plasma T3 at the end of pregnancy in cord blood and during the first days of life. *Acta Endocrinologica*, Supplement, **173**, 16.

Jost, A. (1959) Action du propylthiouracile sur la thyroide du foetus de lapin intact, decapité ou injecté de thyroxine. *Compte Rendu de la Société de Biologie*, **153**, 1900–1902.

Kaiser, W. & Bygrave, F. G. (1969) Stimulation of phospholipid synthesis in isolated rat liver mitochondria after treatment *in vivo* with triiodothyronine. *European Journal of Biochemistry*, **11**, 93–96.

Kajihara, A., Kojima, A., Onaya, T., Takemura, Y. & Yamada, T. (1972) Placental transport of thyrotrophin releasing factor in the rat. *Endocrinology*, **90**, 592–594.

Koch, H. C., Reighert, W., Stolte, L., van Kesses, H. & Seelen, J. (1966) Placental thyroxine transfer and fetal thyroxine utilisation. *Acta Physiologica et Pharmacologica Neerlandica*, **13**, 363–365.

Mellor, D. J. & Slater, J. S. (1971) Daily changes in amniotic and allantoic fluid during the last three months of pregnancy in conscious, unstressed ewes with catheters in their foetal fluid sacs. *Journal of Physiology*, **217**, 573–604.

Meschia, G., Cotter, J. R., Breathnach, C. S. & Barron, D. H. (1965) The haemoglobin, oxygen, carbon dioxide and hydrogen ion concentrations in the umbilical bloods of sheep and goats as sampled via indwelling plastic catheters. *Quarterly Journal of Experimental Physiology*, **50**, 185–195.

Mott, J. C. (1975) The place of the renin–angiotensin system before and after birth. *British Medical Bulletin*, **31**, 44–49.

Nathanielsz, P. W. (1975) Thyroid function in the fetus and newborn mammal. *British Medical Bulletin*, **31**, 51–56.

Nathanielsz, P. W. (1976) *Fetal Endocrinology—An Experimental Approach*. Amsterdam: Elsevier, North Holland.

Nathanielsz, P. W., Silver, M. & Comline, R. S. (1973) Plasma triiodothyronine concentration in the foetal and newborn lamb. *Journal of Endocrinology*, **58**, 683–684.

Nathanielsz, P. W., Comline, R. S., Silver, M. & Paisley, R. B. (1972) Cortisol metabolism in the fetal and neonatal sheep. *Journal of Reproduction and Fertility*, Supplement **16**, 39–59.

Nathanielsz, P. W., Comline, R. S., Silver, M. & Thomas, A. L. (1973) Thyroid function in the foetal lamb during the last third of gestation and parturition. *Journal of Endocrinology*, **58**, 535–546.

Nathanielsz, P. W., Comline, R. S., Silver, M. & Thomas, A. L. (1974) Thyroid function in the foetal calf. *Journal of Endocrinology*, **61**, lxxi.

Nicholson, J. L. & Altman, J. (1972) The effects of early hypo- and hyperthyroidism on the development of rat cerebellar cortex. I. Cell proliferation and differentiation. *Brain Research*, **44**, 13–23.

Odell, W. D., Wilber, J. F. & Utiger, R. D. (1967) Studies of thyrotrophin physiology by means of radioimmunoassay. *Recent Progress in Hormone Research*, **23**, 47–78.

Pennel, M. T. & Kukral, A. J. (1946) An unusual case of holoacephalus. *American Journal of Obstetrics and Gynecology*, **52**, 669–671.

Rac, R., Hill, G. N. & Pain, R. W. (1968) Congenital goitre in Merino sheep due to an inherited defect in the biosynthesis of thyroid hormone. *Research in Veterinary Science*, **9**, 209–223.

Raiti, S., Holzman, G. B., Scott, R. L. & Blizzard, R. M. (1967) Evidence for the placental transfer of triiodothyronine in human beings. *New England Journal of Medicine*, **277**, 456–459.

Shelley, H. J. (1973) The use of chronically catheterised foetal lambs for the study of foetal metabolism. In *Foetal and Neonatal Physiology* (Ed.) Comline, R. S., Cross, K. W., Dawes, G. S. & Nathanielsz, P. W. pp. 360–381. London: Cambridge University Press.

Smith, D. W., Blizzard, R. M. & Wilkins, L. (1957) The mental prognosis in hypothyroidism of infancy and childhood: A review of 128 cases. *Pediatrics*, **19**, 1011–1022.

Tata, J. R. (1964) Biological action of thyroid hormones at the cellular and molecular levels. In *Actions of Hormones on Molecular Processes* (Ed.) Litwack, G. & Kritchevsky, D. pp. 58–131. New York: Wiley.

Tata, J. R. (1967a) The formation and distribution of ribosomes during hormone-induced growth and development. *Biochemical Journal*, **104**, 1–16.

Tata, J. R. (1967b) The formation, distribution and function of ribosomes and microsomal membranes during induced amphibian metamorphosis. *Biochemical Journal*, **105**, 783–801.

Tata, J. R. (1974) Growth and developmental action of thyroid hormones at the cellular level. In *Handbook of Physiology, Endocrinology*, Vol. III *Thyroid*. pp. 469–478. American Physiological Society.

Thomas, A. L., Abel, M. A. & Nathanielsz, P. W. (1974) The effect of cortisol on thyrotrophin secretion in the thyroidectomised calf. *Journal of Endocrinology*, **63**, 20P.

Thomas, A. L., Jack, P. M. B., Manns, J. G. & Nathanielsz, P. W. (1975) Effect of synthetic thyrotrophin releasing hormone on thyrotrophin and prolactin concentration in the peripheral plasma of the pregnant ewe, lamb fetus and neonatal lamb. *Biology of the Neonate,* **26,** 109–116.

Thorburn, G. D. (1974) The role of the thyroid gland and kidneys in fetal growth. In *Size at Birth. CIBA Foundation Symposium,* **27,** 185–214.

Thorburn, G. D. & Hopkins, P. S. (1973) Thyroid function in the foetal lamb. In *Foetal and Neonatal Physiology. Proceedings of the Sir Joseph Barcroft Centenary Symposium* (Ed.) Comline, R. S., Cross, K. W., Dawes, G. S. & Nathanielsz, P. W. pp. 488–507. London: Cambridge University Press.

Thorburn, G. D., Nicol, D. H., Bassett, J. M., Shutt, D. A. & Cox, R. I. (1972) Parturition in the goat and sheep: changes in corticosteroids, progesterone, oestrogens and prostaglandin F. *Journal of Reproduction and Fertility,* Supplement **16,** 61–84.

van Wynsberghe, D. M. & Klitgaard, H. M. (1973) The effects of thyroxine and triiodothyroacetic acid on neonatal development in the rat. *Biology of the Neonate,* **22,** 444–450.

Widnell, C. C. & Tata, J. R. (1966) Additive effects of thyroid hormone, growth hormone and testosterone on deoxyribonucleic acid-dependent ribonucleic acid polymerase in rat liver nuclei. *Biochemical Journal,* **98,** 621–628.

Wu, B., Kikkawa, Y., Orzalesi, M. M., Motoyama, E. K., Kaibara, M., Zigas, C. J. & Cook, C. D. (1973) The effect of thyroxine on the maturation of fetal rabbit lungs. *Biology of the Neonate,* **22,** 161–168.

Yamazati, E., Noguchi, A. & Slingerland, D. W. (1960) The *in vitro* metabolism of iodide, iodotyrosine and thyroxine by human placenta. *Journal of Clinical Endocrinology,* **20,** 794–797.

13

THE FETAL PITUITARY–ADRENAL AXIS AND ITS FUNCTIONAL INTERACTIONS WITH THE NEUROHYPOPHYSIS

John R. G. Challis and Geoffrey D. Thorburn

In this chapter two aspects of fetal endocrinology, which at first glance might appear to be completely independent, will be dealt with, namely the development and functional activity of the neurohypophysis and of the pituitary–adrenal axis. The areas of interaction and interdependence between the neurohypophysis and the adrenal will be indicated, and it will be seen that both glands secrete hormones which may interact directly or indirectly at a target organ, e.g. in the endocrine mechanisms controlling parturition, and presumably also in the regulation of sodium and water transport among various fluid compartments of the fetus. It will be shown that neurohypophyseal hormones may also have central actions which affect pituitary–adrenal function. The secretory activity of the neurohypophysis of the adult may be influenced considerably by circulating steroid levels and by prostaglandins. In the fetus these are uncharted areas which warrant future exploration.

Initially, the separate activities of the neurohypophysis and of the fetal adrenal will be discussed with respect to the roles of the latter in both oestrogen and cortisol biosynthesis. This leads to a consideration of those factors responsible for the regulation of cortisol production, particularly by the term fetus, and particularly in relation to the possible role of arginine vasopressin (AVP). Finally the importance of cortisol to the fetus, with special reference to the maturation of the fetal lungs and the initiation of parturition, will be considered.

THE FETAL NEUROHYPOPHYSIS

Development of the neurohypophysis occurs in parallel with the embryogenesis of the

232

adenohypophysis and the maturation of the hypothalamus. In the human, Rathke's pouch, which eventually forms the anterior pituitary (adenohypophysis), appears as an evagination of the stomadeum at about three weeks of gestation and by four to five weeks has grown dorsally to closely adjoin the floor of the diencephalon (Falin, 1961). By the sixth week, a hollow outgrowth has formed from the floor of the diencephalon and by eight weeks a prominent infundibulum is present. Also at about this time, differentiation of the supraoptic and paraventricular nuclei occurs, but it is not until 16 weeks that axons from the nuclei reach the neurohypophysis (Papez, 1940).

Stainable neurosecretory material first appears in the human fetal neurohypophysis at about 16 weeks, the material being observed initially in the cell bodies of the supraoptic and paraventricular nuclei (Benirschke and McKay, 1953). In parallel with this increase in stainable neurosecretory material, the biological activities of both oxytocin and vasopressin first appear in the human fetal pituitary at a relatively early stage in gestation and show a progressive increase throughout pregnancy. Vasopressin is present in greater amounts than oxytocin, giving a vasopressor to oxytocic (V:O) ratio greater than unity. As pregnancy proceeds this ratio gradually falls and by term has reached the adult value of one. High V:O ratios in fetal life are characteristic of all species studied to date and may represent an earlier maturation of the supraoptic nuclei as compared to the paraventricular nuclei (Perks and Vizsoyli, 1973). The physiological significance of the higher vasopressin levels is not clear.

A further feature of the fetal neurohypophysis in some species is the presence of a third principle during a portion of fetal life. Vizsoyli and Perks (1969) and Perks and Vizsoyli (1973), using pharmacological and chemical methods, have identified arginine vasotocin (AVT) in the pituitary of the fetal sheep and fur seal. Skowsky and Fisher (1973), employing a radioimmunoassay technique, have recently confirmed these observations in the sheep. These workers have also demonstrated the presence of AVT in pituitaries from human fetuses of 12 to 18 weeks of age, the ratio of AVT:AVP decreasing in the older fetuses. In both the fetal lamb and seal, AVT persists for only a portion of gestation and is absent or at very low levels by term. The hormone was formerly thought to be restricted to lower vertebrates, and its significance in the mammalian fetus remains to be determined.

Although the histological and pharmacological evidence suggests that the neurohypophysis functions early in the life of the human fetus, measurements of the circulating levels of oxytocin and vasopressin are largely confined to the perinatal period. The concentrations of both oxytocin and AVP increase markedly in the cord blood of patients in active labour in comparison with the levels in patients delivered by caesarean section (Hoppenstein, Miltenberger and Moran, 1968; Chard et al, 1971). In addition, the latter workers showed that the concentrations of both peptides were higher in the umbilical artery than in the vein, thereby providing evidence for their secretion by the fetus. The high circulating levels found during labour do not persist into postnatal life, and Hoppenstein, Miltenberger and Moran (1968) found very low plasma concentrations of AVP during the first few days of life, the levels gradually increasing during the first three months.

Studies carried out on exteriorised fetal lambs have demonstrated that the concentration of oxytocin and neurophysin in the pituitary at any stage of gestation was similar to that of the adult, although the level of AVP was somewhat less, and AVT was undetectable (Alexander et al, 1974b). Vasopressin may be released in response to hypoxia or haemorrhage as early as 90 days of gestation (Alexander et al, 1973). Oxytocin, on the other hand, was detected only in fetuses near term, and then only in trace amounts. Studies carried out on chronically catheterised fetal lambs in utero indicate that hypoxia, asphyxia and haemorrhage all result in a release of vasopressin at least during the last third of gestation (Rurak, unpublished observations, 1975). Indeed, fetuses as young as 60 days (0.43 of pregnancy) released vasopressin in response to haemorrhage. Resting plasma levels of the hormone appear lower than those observed in exteriorised fetuses, in most cases being below the sensitivity of the assay (2 to 5 μu/ml), except in cases of obvious fetal distress such as infection, chronic hypoxaemia or acidaemia. Similar low levels of vasopressin in the plasma of fetal lambs have been reported by Alexander et al (1974a).

In both fetal lambs and rhesus monkeys ^{125}I-labelled AVP is cleared from the circulation at a greater rate than in the adults (Skowsky et al, 1973; Rurak, unpublished observations, 1975). In the human, Chard's (1973) data indicate that the placenta may be a major site of metabolism, and a similar situation may exist in the sheep fetus. Although the liver and kidneys are major sites for inactivation of oxytocin and vasopressin in adults, little is known of their significance in the fetus. In the human fetus, immunoreactive oxytocin has been found in fetal urine (Seppala et al, 1972), which suggests a role for the fetal kidneys, although in view of the relatively low renal blood flow in utero, the importance of this mechanism may be questioned.

The neurohypophyseal hormones have a number of important functions in the fetus. Their roles in parturition and their interaction with the pituitary–adrenal axis will be considered later. In addition, they may have important influences on the fetal cardiovascular system; they may influence water and sodium transport between the fluid compartments of the conceptus; and AVP may play a role in controlling the tonicity of fetal urine. These subjects have been reviewed in detail by Challis et al (1975b).

THE FETAL ADRENAL

Developmental aspects

The human fetal adrenal is one of the largest fetal organs, and by the fourth month of gestation it is larger in size than the fetal kidney. Most of this increase in size is attributable to the fetal zone of the cortex, the cells of which assume the characteristics of a steroid-producing tissue during the first trimester, and by the second half of gestation comprise over 80 per cent of the gland. Many investigators have sought to understand the trophic factors responsible for the morphological and biochemical differentiation of the fetal zone, especially since its activities appear to represent a specialised aspect of intra-uterine life. In normal infants, the fetal zone regresses soon after birth. In anencephalic fetuses, however, the adrenal glands differentiate normally during the first trimester, but after the 20th week the fetal zone involutes prematurely (Benirschke, 1956). Both hCG and ACTH stimulate steroid secretion by the cells of the fetal zone (Johannisson, 1968), and it has been proposed that these hormones may exert a trophic influence on the fetal adrenal in utero. In the second half of pregnancy, when hCG production has declined, a functional hypothalamic–hypophyseal–adrenal axis and sustained ACTH secretion may assume increased importance in maintaining the fetal zone of the adrenal. Evidence for this concept is derived from experiments on the rhesus monkey (*Macaca mulatta*), in which it has been shown that fetal hypophysectomy (Chez et al, 1970) or suppression of fetal ACTH secretion following the maternal administration of dexamethasone (Challis et al, 1974b) causes atrophy of the fetal adrenals and a premature regression of the fetal zone. However, the normal regression of the fetal zone after birth in the human and monkey newborn implies a readjustment of the hypothalamic–pituitary–adrenal feedback system at this time and/or the loss of trophic support as that supplied by the placenta. The recent demonstration by immunoassay and bioassay that the human placenta contains a peptide resembling pituitary ACTH adds a further component to an already complicated area (Genazzani et al, 1975; Rees et al, 1975a). Genazzani et al (1975) obtained evidence using bioassay for the release of a corticotrophin-like molecule from human placental cultures in vitro, although with immunoassay, non-parellelism to α^{1-39} ACTH was observed. Clearly, further studies are warranted to characterise the placental corticotrophin and to elucidate the mechanisms controlling its production.

Fetal adrenal steroidogenesis

It is now well established that the fetal adrenal gland is a highly active endocrine organ, possessing the enzymes necessary to synthesise a considerable range of steroid hormones. This capacity, which appears to be related particularly to the fetal zone of the cortex, has been the subject of many detailed reviews (Solomon, 1966; Mitchell, 1967; Villee, 1969, 1972), and the general aspects will be described here only in outline.

General aspects

Much of our current thinking concerning steroidogenesis in the fetus has been derived from experiments on human material, generally obtained at mid-trimester abortion at 16 to 20 weeks. Extrapolation of this information to the full-term human fetus and to domestic animals is a dangerous, yet widely adopted practice. It is hoped to illustrate some of the pitfalls.

At mid-pregnancy, the human fetal adrenal is able to utilise acetate to synthesise the steroid nucleus, and to cleave the cholesterol side-chain to form pregnenolone. However, due to a relative deficiency of the Δ^5-3β-hydroxysteroid dehydrogenase (3β-HSD) there is a poor conversion of $C_{21}\Delta_5$ steroids like pregnenolone to $C_{21}\Delta_4$ steroids such as progesterone, which is an essential intermediate in the biosynthesis of another group of $C_{21}\Delta_4$ steroids, the corticosteroids. Nevertheless, the fetal adrenal does possess 17α-hydroxylase, C_{17-20} desmolase and sulphokinase activities, and therefore metabolises pregnenolone through the Δ_5 pathway to C_{19} steroids such as dehydroepiandrosterone (DHEA) and dehydroepiandrosterone sulphate (DHEAS) (for details see Diczfalusy and Mancuso, 1969; Ryan, 1969; Villee, 1969; Oakey, 1970; Davies and Ryan, 1972; Ryan and Hopper, 1974). The DHEAS produced by the fetal adrenal is then available for aromatisation by the placenta or 16α-hydroxylation in the fetal liver (see below and Figure 13.1).

The 3β-HSD deficiency, however, does not prevent glucocorticoid production, since the human fetal adrenal is able to utilise as substrate for cortisol biosynthesis, progesterone, secreted from the placenta into the fetal compartment. There is an increase in the activities of the 11β-hydroxylase and 21-hydroxylase systems of the fetal adrenal during pregnancy (perhaps under the influence of progesterone; Villee, 1966), which may influence the amount of cortisol that is secreted. It should be noted, by way of contrast, that in the fetal lamb, there is a highly potent 20α-hydroxysteroid dehydrogenase enzyme associated with fetal erythrocytes (Nancarrow and Seamark, 1968). This enzyme effectively reduces placental progesterone secreted into the umbilical vein to 20α-dihydroprogesterone, whilst the steroid is still in the vascular compartment, thereby presumably rendering it unavailable for corticosteroid biosynthesis. However, the sheep fetal adrenal, without the distinctive fetal zone of the primate, does possess 3β-HSD and Δ^5 isomerase activities (Anderson et al, 1973) and may not require a placental source of progesterone for cortisol biosynthesis. In species in

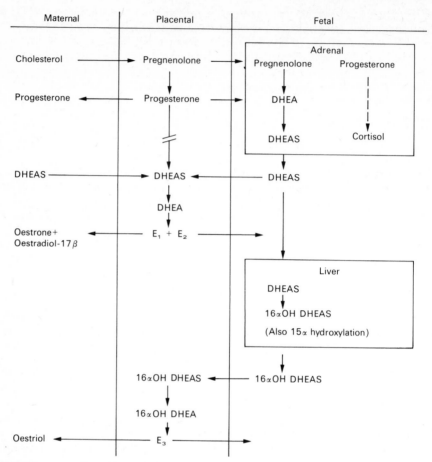

Figure 13.1. Summary of steroidogenesis in the human feto-placental unit (modified from Ryan and Hopper, 1974). The fetal zone of the fetal adrenal cortex has a relative deficiency of the 3β-HSD, and pregnenolone is metabolised through the Δ5 pathway to DHEAS. In the sheep, there is some evidence for 17α-hydroxylase and C_{17-20} lyase activities in the placenta, and a similar concept of a 'feto-placental unit' may not be applicable.

which the progesterone requirements of pregnancy are met by a sustained ovarian contribution (Davies and Ryan, 1972; Heap, Perry and Challis, 1973) such a source of substrate would be unavailable anyway.

The fetal adrenals in oestrogen biosynthesis

An increase in oestrogen production throughout pregnancy appears to occur in most of the animal species that have been studied, with the possible exception of those animals in which placental aromatase activity has not been demonstrated (Heap, Perry and Challis, 1973). Nevertheless, the primates, especially the higher primates, are peculiar in their production of large amounts of a 16α-hydroxylated oestrogen, oestriol, during pregnancy, the function and advantages of which are unclear (Ryan and Hopper, 1974).

It is now well established that the urinary excretion of oestrogens, and particularly oestriol, in human pregnancy continues in the absence of the maternal ovary, adrenal or adenohypophysis, but declines in the absence of a viable fetus (see Diczfalusy and Mancuso, 1969). Such findings have given rise to the concept of the feto-placental unit of human pregnancy, in which it is considered that whilst the fetus and placenta are anatomically distinct, they are biochemically complementary with respect of oestrogen, and particularly oestriol production (Diczfalusy and Mancuso, 1969; Ryan, 1969). Experiments carried out both in vitro and in vivo have demonstrated that the human placenta lacks the enzymes necessary to metabolise C_{21} neutral steroids such as progesterone and 17α-hydroxyprogesterone to C_{19} neutral steroids, but it is able to utilise exogenous C_{19} steroids as substrate for aromatisation. In addition, the placenta lacks the 16α-hydroxylase necessary for oestriol production, although this enzyme and the C_{17-20} lyase are found in the fetus, predominantly in the liver and adrenal respectively. Thus in the human, the major pathway of oestrogen biosynthesis in the feto-placental unit appears to be secretion of DHEAS by the fetal adrenal, and in particular by the fetal zone, followed by 16α-hydroxylation in the fetal liver. Some aromatisation may occur in the fetal liver (Diczfalusy and Mancuso, 1969), although most of the 16α-OH-DHEAS appears to be secreted into the blood by the liver, and can be measured in high amounts in fetal plasma (Magendantz and Ryan, 1964). This steroid then reaches the placenta, which normally contains both sulphatase and aromatase activities, where it is aromatised to oestriol. It should be noted that DHEAS from the fetal adrenal may reach the placenta directly, where it is aromatised to oestrone (E_1) and oestradiol-17β ($E_2\beta$). The maternal adrenal also secretes DHEAS, which is present in larger quantities in the maternal circulation and is available for oestrogen production. MacDonald and Siiteri (1965), and Siiteri and MacDonald (1963) have carried out extensive isotope kinetics studies in women during normal pregnancy, in molar pregnancies and in the presence of an anencephalic fetus. They have demonstrated that in normal pregnancy, about 50 per cent of the oestradiol-17β production rate is derived from maternal DHEAS, thus implying a 50 per cent contribution from the fetus. Diczfalusy and Mancuso (1969) have provided the complementary data, having shown that the oestradiol production rate in a pregnant adrenalectomised woman was about 50 per cent that of normal pregnant women (Siiteri and MacDonald, 1966). The high concentrations of oestradiol in molar pregnancies are due in part to trophoblastic aromatisation of maternally derived DHEAS (MacDonald and Siiteri, 1965) and in part to secretion from the hyperstimulated ovaries. In women pregnant with an anencephalic fetus, the oestradiol production rate was 25 to 50 per cent of normal and was derived almost entirely from maternal DHEAS (see Siiteri, 1973). Thus whilst oestriol production is largely a feto-placental function, oestradiol and oestrone production results from the combined activities of the placenta and both fetal and maternal adrenals.

These observations help to explain the relative usefulness of various steroid measurements as indices of fetal and placental function during pregnancy (see also Chapter 19). Maternal levels of oestriol are intimately related to the biosynthetic activity of the fetal hypothalamic–pituitary–adrenal pathway and the fetal liver, and are likely therefore to provide a reasonable index of 'fetal well-being'. Evidence has been presented elsewhere that variations in the placental aromatase or sulphatase activities are unlikely to provide a general mechanism controlling oestrogen biosynthesis (Townsley, Rubin and Crystle, 1973). The fetus specifically forms additional 15α-hydroxylated metabolites, and the measurement of a 15α-hydroxylated oestrogen such as oestetrol during pregnancy potentially offers a more useful indicator of fetal viability. It will be apparent on a theoretical basis that measurements of increments in oestradiol-17β following a loading injection of DHEA or DHEAS into the maternal compartment provide little hope of indicating more than an active placental aromatase system. Indeed patients with intra-uterine fetal death may respond with a similar increment in oestradiol to that seen in normal patients (Fraser et al, 1976). Similarly, measurements of progesterone or pregnanediol which essentially reflect a function of the placenta are unlikely to reveal useful information concerning fetal viability. In Cassmer's (1959) now classical experiment of ligating the umbilical cord, there was only a slight decrease in pregnanediol excretion, despite the occurrence of fetal death.

During normal human pregnancy, there is a gradual increase in the plasma levels of un-conjugated oestradiol-17β between the 8th and 30th weeks. This is followed by a more rapid increase from levels of about 8 ng/ml to concentrations of 20 to 30 ng/ml at 40 weeks, with a subsequent plateau or fall during the days immediately preceding parturition (Dawood and Ratnam, 1974; Turnbull et al, 1974). It has been suggested (Oakey, 1970) that the increase in plasma oestrogens seen during human pregnancy is closely related to the secretory activity of the fetal adrenal gland and its regulation by the levels of ACTH and cortisol in fetal plasma. Fetal cortisol is removed from the fetal circulation by hepatic metabolism and transferred to the mother, the latter process being facilitated by the greater number of corticosteroid-binding globulin (CBG) binding sites in maternal than in fetal plasma. As cortisol is cleared from the fetal compartment, this will tend to lower feedback inhibition, and to enhance the secretion of ACTH from the fetal pituitary. ACTH promotes growth of the fetal adrenal, and stimulates steroidogenesis. However, because of the 3β-HSD deficiency, the major secretory product of the fetal adrenal in response to ACTH is DHEAS rather than cortisol. The supply of C_{19} precursors for placental aromatisation to oestrogens is thereby increased.

The mechanism of oestrogen production by the materno-feto-placental system of lower primates appears to be essentially similar to that of man, although the amounts of oestriol produced are much less than in the human. The general aspects of this subject have been reviewed by Ryan and Hopper (1974). In the pregnant rhesus monkey (*Macaca mulatta*) the maternal plasma concentrations of unconjugated oestrogens (oestrone, oestradiol-17β) are much lower than in the human during pregnancy, but show a marked increase during the last seven to ten days before parturition (Bosu, Johansson and Gemzell, 1973; Challis et al. 1974a). This is unassociated with concomitant changes in maternal plasma C_{19} steroid (Challis et al, 1975a), thereby implicating an increase in fetal adrenal activity in providing the appropriate precursors. In other species of *Macaca* both the maternal and fetal adrenals can provide the appropriate precursors for placental aromatisation (Davies, Ryan and Petro. 1970). A reduction in maternal oestrogen levels is seen in *M. mulatta* following ligation of the umbilical cord in utero (Bosu, Johansson and Gemzell, 1974) or following suppression of the fetal adrenals with dexamethasone (Challis et al, 1974b).

A similar concept of the feto-placental unit and its relative importance in oestrogen production during pregnancy has hitherto been assumed to pertain to domestic animals. It is now apparent that not all aspects of the primate model are directly applicable to other species and with the disappearance of the capacity to secrete oestriol, the role of the maternal adrenals may have assumed greater importance. In pregnant sheep, for example, the mater-nal plasma concentrations of unconjugated oestrogens (oestrone and oestradiol-17β) are low throughout pregnancy, becoming elevated only during the last 24 hours before parturition (Challis, 1971; Thorburn et al, 1972). Although the placenta is the major site of aromatisa-tion (Ainsworth and Ryan, 1966; Findlay, 1970), and is able to utilise C_{19} steroids of both maternal and fetal adrenal origin as substrate for oestrogen biosynthesis (Davies, Ryan and Petro, 1970; Pierrepoint et al, 1973; Thompson and Wagner, 1974), some discrepancies have been noted. Potential precursors for oestrogen biosynthesis have been sought in vain in the fetal plasma; in fact, the fetal plasma levels of testosterone decrease before spontaneous or ACTH-induced delivery (Strott, Sundel and Stahlman, 1974). However, this change could presumably be related to either a decrease in secretion or an increase in metabolism.

Similarly, no consistent change is seen during late pregnancy in the fetal plasma levels of DHEAS (Seamark, personal communication, 1970), although more recently two steroids reactive to 17β-hydroxysteroid binding protein have been found in the solvolysable fraction from fetal lamb plasma during late pregnancy (Cox, Thorburn, Wong and Currie, unpublished observations, 1975). The identity of these steroids and their availability as substrate for aromatisation remain to be established. Unfortunately, the work is complicated by the extensive steroid metabolising activities of enzymes associated with the fetal erythrocytes.

In the sheep, a supply of fetal adrenal androgens may not be rate-limiting in oestrogen biosynthesis, because when parturition is induced by administration of dexamethasone to the fetus—a treatment which presumably suppresses fetal adrenal steroidogenesis—delivery is preceded by an increase in the maternal oestrogen concentrations similar to that seen at normal term (Liggins et al, 1972; Thorburn et al, 1972). Recently, evidence has been provided for the existence of a potent C_{17-20} lyase activity in sheep placentas during the latter part of gestation. Thus, the conversion of 17α-hydroxylated C_{21} steroids to C_{19} and conjugated C_{18} steroids was clearly demonstrated (John and Pierrepoint, 1975). Previous work had indicated the presence of a 17α-hydroxylase system in the placenta, the activity of which appeared to be influenced by fetal glucocorticoids (Anderson, Flint and Turnbull, 1974). It is conceivable therefore that the sheep placenta may, in apparent contrast to the human, possess all the enzyme systems necessary to metabolise cholesterol through progesterone and on to oestrogens. Alternatively, the fetus could provide some 17-hydroxylated precursors. In the sheep these placental reactions appear to be stimulated by exogenous dexamethasone. This is again in marked contrast to the primate, where exogenous glucocorticoids result in a suppression of maternal oestrogens, through their action in reducing the secretion of ACTH and C_{19} neutral steroids in the fetus (Simmer et al, 1974). Whether these differences between the sheep and the primate model result from divergent actions of dexamethasone at the level of the placenta or on the activity of the fetal pituitary–adrenal axis, are intriguing questions, answers to which seem fundamental to our understanding of the comparative aspects of the endocrine control of parturition.

A final point concerns the relative activities of the placental sulphatase and sulphotransferase systems. Under normal circumstances it appears that in the primate placenta, the former enzyme(s) predominates. In patients with placental sulphatase deficiency (France, Seddon and Liggins, 1973), who are unable to aromatise conjugated C_{19} neutral steroids from the fetus, very low maternal oestrogen concentrations have been found. In the sheep, sulphotransferase clearly predominates, and this is in part responsible for the low levels of unconjugated oestrogens normally seen in this species throughout all but the last few hours of pregnancy.

THE REGULATION OF CORTISOL CONCENTRATIONS IN THE FETUS

A consistent finding in a number of animal species has been a significant increase in the concentration of cortisol in fetal plasma during the final stages of pregnancy. The evidence that by 22 to 24 weeks of human gestation the fetal adrenal can synthesise cortisol either from progesterone derived from the placenta or from acetate synthesised in the fetal adrenal cortex has been discussed previously. Because of the relative deficiency of the 3β-HSD enzyme activity, however, most of the fetal cortisol synthesised during the second trimester is derived from placental progesterone rather than from acetate. However, since cortisol biosynthesis independent of placental progesterone is necessary for extra-uterine life, it is apparent that this capacity must develop in utero and be possible by 24 to 25 weeks of gestation. Nevertheless, the enzymatic activity of the neonatal adrenal cortex in general resembles that of the mid-trimester fetus, and is characterised by the relatively low 3β-HSD activity of the permanent zone and the predominance in excretion of Δ^5-3β-hydroxysteroids. Reynolds and Mirkin (1973) have examined the steroids excreted by newborns with intra-uterine growth retardation, whose adrenals are reduced in size due to a premature regression of the fetal zone. In these newborns the excretion of Δ^5-3β-hydroxysteroids is markedly reduced, although the quantitative excretion of cortisol metabolites resembles that of normally grown newborns and points to the relative importance of the permanent and fetal zones of the adrenal cortex. It should be noted that in subhuman primates such as the rhesus monkey, cortisol production by fetal adrenal tissue can be demonstrated by 75 days of gestation, and that ACTH administration increases the rate of cortisol production (Kittinger, 1973).

In the fetal lamb, a clearly distinct fetal zone of the adrenal is absent. The incubation of adrenals from fetal lambs at 100 days gestation with ^{3}H-pregnenolone resulted in the production of cortisol and corticosterone in reasonable yields, and demonstrated that in this species there is a substantial enzymatic capacity, including 3β-HSD, for corticosteroid biosynthesis throughout at least the last third of gestation (Anderson et al, 1973; Davies and Ryan, 1973).

The concentration of cortisol in fetal plasma is influenced by a number of important factors, including the rates of cortisol secretion into the maternal and fetal compartments, the extent of high affinity protein binding in plasma, the rates of metabolism in the fetal and maternal liver and in the placenta, and the extent to which cortisol traverses the placenta between the two compartments. The immediate discussion is concerned with the rates of binding and metabolism of cortisol and with the transplacental transfer of this steroid, since these factors largely determine the extent to which the fetal pituitary–adrenal axis may be regarded as autonomous.

By the application of continuous isotope infusion techniques, it has been possible to measure some aspects of fetal and maternal cortisol metabolism in the sheep, rhesus monkey and the human. Some of the results that have been obtained are summarised in Table 13.1. It can be seen that in spite of the marked differences in the absolute concentrations of total unconjugated cortisol in maternal and fetal plasma during late pregnancy, the ratio of the maternal:fetal levels in all three species is about 3:1. However, whilst in the human, a similar ratio pertains to the CBG binding capacity of maternal and fetal plasmas, in the monkey the corresponding ratio is 1:1 and in the sheep, where the transcortin concentration in both compartments is appreciably less than in the primate, the ratio has fallen to 0.4:1. The CBG concentration ratio might itself be adequate to maintain the transplacental cortisol differential in the human (Sandberg and Slaunwhite, 1959), but in the rhesus monkey and, to a greater extent, the sheep, the same cortisol concentration ratio can be maintained only by some additional mechanism, such as the rate of cortisol metabolism in the fetal liver or placenta. Kittinger's (1974) extensive studies in the rhesus monkey support the view that the rates of transfer of cortisol are not significantly different in either direction across the placenta, a major determinant of the fetal cortisol level being the extent of placental cortisol metabolism. Approximately 58 per cent of fetal cortisol is derived from transfer from the maternal circulation (Table 13.1). In addition, the monkey placenta metabolises cortisol to cortisone, which is biologically less active. The significantly greater concentration of cortisone in fetal plasma than in maternal plasma is consistent with placental metabolism being a major regulatory influence of the fetal cortisol concentration. It should be noted that more recent studies in the human reveal somewhat similar information. An appreciable fraction (20 to 50 per cent) of fetal cortisol may result from transplacental transfer (Beitins et al 1973). In addition, maternal cortisol is actively metabolised to cortisone by the placenta, and

Table 13.1. *Cortisol distribution between mother and fetus in the sheep, rhesus monkey and human.*

Species	Gestational age	Endogenous plasma cortisol (ng/ml)		Cortisol ratio M:F	CBG binding capacity (ng/ml cortisol)		CBG ratio M:F	Fractional source (percentage)	
		Mother	Fetus		Mother	Fetus		Δ^{MF}	Δ^{FM}
Sheep	135/145[a]	10–20[b]	2–10[b]	3:1	24[c]	40–70[b]	0.4:1	30–60[b,d]	0.2–2.0[b,d]
	143/145	10–20[b]	70–100[b]	0.2:1	24[c]	90–100[b]	0.25:1	3–20[b]	2.0–3.0[b]
Rhesus monkey	155/165	315[e]	121[e]	3:1	180[f]	210[f]	1:1	58[e]	4.4[e]
Human	Term (caesarian section)	200–250[g]	60–70[g,h]	3:1	330[f]	100[f]	3:1	20–50	–

[a] Gestational age/length of pregnancy.
[b] Liggins et al, 1973.
[c] Paterson and Hills, 1967.
[d] Dixon et al, 1970.
[e] Kittinger, 1974.
[f] Beamer, Hagemenas and Kittinger, 1972.
[g] Beitins et al, 1973.
[h] Murphy, 1973.

Δ^{MF} Fraction of fetal cortisol derived from the maternal compartment.
Δ^{FM} Fraction of maternal cortisol derived from the fetal compartment.

the proportion of fetal cortisone derived from maternal cortisol is of similar magnitude in the human at mid-trimester and at term, in the monkey (Beitins et al, 1973; Murphy et al, 1974 Pakravan et al, 1974). The recent report from Pakravan et al (1974) of a male newborn with familial congenital absence of the adrenal glands is of particular interest in this context The cord cortisol concentration (13 ng/ml) was much lower than the normal range and would correspond to the 20 to 25 per cent of fetal cortisol derived from maternal cortisol as calculated by Beitins et al (1973) (see Table 13.1). The cord cortisone concentration (96 ng/ml) was only one standard deviation below the mean of normal infants (136 $\pm$ 37 ng/ml mean $\pm$ s.d.), clearly illustrating the conclusions of other investigators that cortisone in the fetal plasma is derived from the placental metabolism of maternal cortisol. Of further interest was the finding of undetectable aldosterone and markedly suppressed levels of oestrone and oestradiol-17β in the umbilical cord plasma.

Similar kinetics studies in the sheep have also indicated the potential contribution of maternal cortisol to the cortisol pool of the fetus. However, more experiments on long-term chronically catheterised fetuses are necessary to provide more extensive and precise information. Transcortin binding in both compartments is much less than in the primate, despite the similar maternal:fetal cortisol concentration ratio of 3:1 at 10 days before term. By extrapolation from the monkey, one might suggest that the ovine placenta should be very active in metabolising cortisol and, in fact, a significant proportion of radioactive cortisol administered to the mother appears in the fetus as cortisol sulphate and cortisone (Anderson et al, 1973). The data of Liggins et al (1973) (Table 13.1) from two sheep suggest that the Δ^{MF} decreases at term. This could be due to the increase in the fetal contribution of secreted cortisol to the fetal production rate, but it could also reflect a change in placental utilisation or metabolism of maternal cortisol. It is of interest that the maternal:fetal cortisol concentration and CBG binding capacity ratios both appear to decrease near term and reach similar values. In part this is a function of the increase in fetal cortisol secretion, and in part it is attributable to the increase in CBG in the fetal compartment, the stimulus to which is unknown.

Whilst the above data indicate the contribution of maternal cortisol and placental metabolism to the fetal corticosteroid pool, they should not be taken to imply that the pituitary–adrenal system is poorly operative in the fetus. Fetal ACTH is necessary for both steroidogenesis and adrenal growth and differentiation; the anencephalic human fetus, with a presumed reduction or lack of ACTH secretion, shows premature regression of the fetal zone of the adrenal cortex in utero (Benirschke, 1956), and fetal adrenal steroidogenesis, as reflected in the maternal oestrogen levels, is markedly suppressed. In the human, ACTH has been measured in the fetal pituitary by the tenth week of gestation (Taylor, Loraine and Robertson, 1953) and in cord plasma at 12 to 19 weeks (Winters et al, 1974). Paired samples of fetal and maternal plasma from normal subjects and from patients in whom pregnancy was complicated by anencephaly showed no relationship in their ACTH concentrations suggesting that the ACTH in fetal plasma was probably derived from secretion by the fetus (Allen et al, 1973; Winters et al, 1974).

In the rhesus monkey it has been suggested that corticoids, but not ACTH, cross the placenta, and to a considerable extent the fetus may be autonomous with respect to controlling its ACTH secretion. Furthermore, it has been demonstrated that the constant infusion of ACTH into the maternal circulation of the pregnant rhesus monkey, at amounts which stimulated maximal cortisol secretion in the mother, had no effect on the fetal plasma cortisol. However, injection of ACTH directly into the fetal compartment provoked a marked increase in the fetal adrenal secretion of cortisol (Kittinger et al, 1972). In the human, similar conclusions have been derived from measurements showing a lack of correlation between ACTH levels in the plasma of normal pregnant women and their fetuses, and in

atients in which there was pathological evidence of a high maternal (Nelson's syndrome) or
ow fetal (anencephaly) plasma ACTH concentration (Allen et al, 1973). Experimental
tudies in the sheep (Nathanielsz et al, 1972; Bassett and Thorburn, 1973) have demonstrated
similar independence of maternal and fetal ACTH. Infusion of Synacthen (10 µg/hour) for
wo hours into the fetal lamb at 116 and 132 days of gestation produced no short-term change
i either fetal or maternal corticosteroid levels, whereas a similar infusion into the ewe
roduced a very rapid increase in the maternal corticosteroid levels (Bassett and Thorburn,
973).

ETAL CORTISOL AND PARTURITION

he experimental studies of Liggins and his various collaborators have established un-
quivocally in the sheep that the fetal lamb, and more specifically the fetal pituitary–adrenal
xis, plays a primary role in determining the length of gestation and the timing of parturition
ee Liggins et al, 1973). It has been shown that ablation of the pituitary of the fetal lamb in
tero led to an indefinite prolongation of pregnancy, whereas the infusion of ACTH or
lucocorticoids into the fetus resulted in premature delivery. Further evidence that activation
f the fetal pituitary–adrenal axis might be involved in parturition was provided by the fin-
ing that during the seven to ten days before birth there is a marked increase in the fetal
lasma corticosteroid concentration which is unrelated to the corticosteroid concentration in
ie maternal plasma (Bassett and Thorburn, 1969) and reflects an increase in the secretory
ctivity of the fetal adrenal gland (Nathanielsz et al, 1972; Liggins et al, 1973).

The evidence that the primate fetal pituitary–adrenal axis plays a similar role is still in-
omplete. However, measurements of cortisol in the amniotic fluid and in the umbilical cord
lasma of groups of patients during pregnancy and in active labour show a marked increase
i levels in association with labour and indicate that the primate fetus may play a role similar
o that of the sheep (Murphy, 1973; Challis and Thorburn, 1975; Fencl and Tulchinsky, 1975;
Murphy, Patrick and Denton, 1975).

A fundamental question therefore is whether the increase in fetal cortisol production
uring late pregnancy reflects a progressive maturation (sensitivity) of the fetal adrenal to
re-existing levels of ACTH, or whether the increased activity of the adrenal is a response to
n increase in the trophic stimulus (ACTH) applied to it? Although the evidence is still in-
omplete, the ultimate answer may lie with both the fetal pituitary and the adrenal. Since fetal
ypophysectomy prolongs the length of gestation and prevents normal adrenal hypertrophy,
ι pituitary factor, presumably ACTH, is of importance. However, providing a tonic level of
ACTH is sustained, it is suggested that the key then rests with the fetal adrenal and its ability
o respond.

The necessity for at least a basal secretion of ACTH is evidenced from the finding that
ypophysectomised fetal lambs, which do not deliver spontaneously at term, have very low
lasma cortisol concentrations and exhibit atrophy of their adrenal glands (Comline,
Nathanielsz and Silver, 1973). It is of interest that in the anencephalic human fetus, whilst the
etal plasma ACTH concentrations may be very low ($\leqslant$20 pg/ml), there is an appreciable
mount of ACTH in the pituitary which is readily dischargeable in response to an exogenous
njection of AVP (see below). However, the adrenal of the anencephalic was unable to res-
ond to an increment in plasma ACTH, presumably due to functional atrophy (Allen et al,
974). This observation may be of importance in relation to the different effects of ACTH or

dexamethasone administered to the sheep at varying time intervals after fetal hypophysectomy.

Infusion of synthetic ACTH (Synacthen) for three to five days into the fetal lamb results in premature parturition and in changes in the fetal plasma corticosteroid levels similar to those seen at normal term (Liggins et al, 1972; Thorburn et al, 1972). However, the fetal plasma levels of Synacthen (measured as ACTH by radioimmunoassay; Johnson et al, 1975) are elevated to values similar to those found during hypoxia or haemorrhage (Alexander et al 1972; Alexander et al, 1974b; Boddy et al, 1974). Measurement of ACTH in the plasma of fetal lambs is complicated by the possibility of diurnal or more subtle changes in hormon secretion during a 24-hour period, together with the relative insensitivity of most of the available assay technology.

Rees et al (1975b) reported a longitudinal study of plasma ACTH in samples taken daily in five fetuses. Values for individual animals were relatively constant until the last 24 hours of fetal life, when they rose to 1 ng/ml or greater. In no fetus did ACTH increase significantly before the elevation of plasma cortisol. Boddy, Jones, Mantell and Robinson (personal communication, 1975) have reported that fetal plasma corticosteroid concentrations of greater than 100 ng/ml may be achieved with ACTH concentrations of less than 200 pg/ml, which are not markedly elevated from basal values. Increases in ACTH to values in excess of 500 pg/ml were seen, however, during the final 9 to 12 hours of labour.

During the last ten days of gestation there is a marked increase in the size of the fetal adrenal gland, brought about by both cellular hypertrophy and hyperplasia (Comline and Silver, 1961). This growth appears to be a function of ACTH, since fetal hypophysectomy results in fetal adrenal atrophy, whereas the continuous infusion of ACTH into fetal lambs at amounts sufficient to precipitate premature parturition provokes an increase in the development of cortical tissue such that at delivery the fetal adrenal weighs as much as in normal full term lambs.

In conjunction with the increase in fetal adrenal weight, the gland's responsiveness to ACTH and secretion of glucocorticoids increases. Bassett and Thorburn (1973) demonstrated that the short-term intravenous infusion of Synacthen (10 µg/hour for two hours) into fetal lambs before 140 days did not induce a rapid increase in fetal corticosteroids, despite the effects of more prolonged infusions. As term approaches the response to exogenous Synacthen increases, such that the term newborn lamb responds with an elevation in plasma corticosteroids similar to that of the adult. In the goat, another species in which parturition may be induced prematurely by the fetal intravenous infusion of Synacthen, the response of the adrenal is poor during the first few hours of infusion, except in those fetuses in which the 'basal' level of corticosteroid is already raised (Bassett and Thorburn, 1973). It would appear therefore that the fetal adrenal requires exposure to a priming dose of ACTH before a secretory response is seen. Whether the secretory response requires a further elevation in ACTH is uncertain, although such an increase in ACTH might potentiate cortisol secretion. A puzzling aspect of this story is the failure or apparent absence of negative feedback between ACTH and cortisol at term. In part this could be related to the increase in CBG in the fetal plasma in late pregnancy (Liggins et al, 1973), which accounts for some of the 13-fold increase in total plasma cortisol in the fetus. However, the possibility exists that catecholaminergic or other stimuli potentiate the activities of corticotrophin releasing factor (CRF) through independent mechanisms (see below), and this area needs further exploration.

The priming action of ACTH on the fetal adrenal probably involves maturation of the steroid synthetic and secretory processes, and may include enzyme induction (11β hydroxylase, 17α-hydroxylase) by the ACTH. Madill and Bassett (1973) have demonstrated in an in vitro perifusion system that the mean secretion of corticosteroids by fetal adrenal issue in response to a fixed amount of ACTH increases with gestational age, and, in- erestingly, the ratio of cortisol to corticosterone that is produced increases between days 135 and 140 of pregnancy. The increase in the response of the fetal adrenal to ACTH timulation paralleled the increases in adrenal weight and plasma corticosteroid concen- rations which are seen in the fetal lamb in utero. These findings are consistent with stimula- ion of both 11β- and 17α-hydroxylating activities. However, quantitative interpretation of in *itro experiments is fraught with problems of different cofactor requirements, and it should be noted that Davies and Ryan (1973) were able to demonstrate significant 11β- and 17α- hydroxylating activity in fetal lamb adrenals as early as day 100 of gestation.

A final question concerns the molecular nature of ACTH in fetal plasma and the possibili- y that components are present with different immunological and biological activities. Coslovsky and Yalow (1974) have shown that cortisol is the principal glucocorticoid in a number of species in which the predominant component of immunoreactive ACTH is the usual α1–39 peptide (little ACTH). Other species in which corticosterone is the principal glucocorticoid have intermediate-sized ACTH in their pituitaries. Whether variations in hese molecular components occur in the fetus during gestation and the ways in which such modifications might relate to adrenal receptor activities for ACTH are intriguing questions or the future.

FACTORS AFFECTING ACTH RELEASE IN THE FETUS

The foregoing discussion does not preclude a role for an increase in ACTH as part of the nor- nal parturient endocrine mechanism. Furthermore, an increase in fetal ACTH may well be a contributory factor to premature labour, although some safeguard is provided, at least in the sheep, by the relative insensitivity of the fetal adrenal to acute changes in ACTH early in gestation.

In the sheep evidence has yet to be obtained for an elevation in fetal ACTH prior to the in- crease in fetal cortisol levels, although ACTH does increase during active labour. In the human there is additional evidence that an increase in ACTH may not be a prerequisite to the ncrease in fetal cortisol seen during late pregnancy. Since ACTH also stimulates DHEAS production, a concomitant increase in maternal oestrogens during the last week of gestation would be expected in parallel to such changes in cortisol (and ACTH); this has not been observed in the human (Turnbull et al, 1974). Winters et al (1974) have reported a decrease n umbilical cord ACTH levels of fetuses at term compared to the concentrations seen earlier n gestation at 20 to 34 weeks. However, in view of the rapid and dramatic increase in ACTH seen in response to hypoxia, at least in the fetal sheep (Boddy et al, 1974), the question of whether the appropriate fetal samples can ever be taken under ideal conditions in human experimentation is an important one.

It is now recognised that a variety of factors—haemorrhage, hypoxia, arginine vasopressin (AVP) and catecholamines—may influence the secretion of ACTH by the fetal lamb. Of the factors which are of potential physiological importance in normal or premature parturition, AVP has been studied most extensively. In the human, the evidence has been dis- cussed previously that the high levels of AVP seen in umbilical plasma reflect secretion of the hormone (Chard et al, 1971). In the sheep, the finding of an increase in the osmolality of fetal urine during the week before birth suggested the possibility that the secretion of AVP by the fetus might be increased during this time (Mellor and Slater, 1972). Recently Alexander et al (1974a) have demonstrated such an increase in AVP in the plasma of the fetal lamb during the last five days of intra-uterine life. Elevated levels of AVP in the plasma of fetal lambs may be stimulated by hypoxia, asphyxia or haemorrhage, at least during the last third of gestation (Alexander et al, 1973, 1974a; Rurak, unpublished observations, 1975).

The importance of AVP in relation to cortisol is that the peptide may augment the CRF-induced release of ACTH (Yates et al, 1971) and may cause the release of CRF from the median eminence, ACTH from the pituitary and, in high doses, glucocorticoids from the adrenals (Saffran, Matthews and Pearlmutter, 1971; Yates et al, 1971). In chronically catheterised fetal lambs, the intravenous infusion of AVP results in an increase in the plasma ACTH concentration (Jones and Rurak, unpublished observations, 1975). In adult monkeys, the levels of AVP and neurophysin in hypophyseal portal blood are far higher than in the systemic circulation, suggesting the specific delivery of AVP to the adenohypophysis (Zimmerman et al, 1974). In the adult sheep, the appropriate pathway from the paraventricular nucleus to the portal system has been described by Parry and Livett (1973). Stimulation of these nuclei may therefore provide an effective means of stimulating ACTH release. Recently it has been suggested that in rats genetically deficient in AVP, the basal plasma corticosterone concentrations and the corticosterone levels achieved during 'stress' or in response to exogenous ACTH were significantly lower than in normal animals (Wiley, Pearlmutter and Miller, 1974). This difference was attributed not to a corticotrophin-releasing action of AVP, but to a reduction in the adrenal sensitivity to ACTH in the deficient animals.

THE IMPORTANCE OF CORTISOL TO THE FETUS IN LATE PREGNANCY

Elevated levels of cortisol in the fetal plasma during late pregnancy are recognised as being important in at least two major respects. First, cortisol has been implicated in fetal lung maturation and the production of pulmonary surfactant (see review by Avery, 1975), and second, an increase in fetal cortisol is now recognised as an early link in a chain of endocrine events leading to parturition (see reviews by Klopper and Gardner, 1973; Liggins et al, 1973; Robinson and Thorburn, 1974; Challis and Thorburn, 1975).

A role for cortisol in promoting lung maturity was indicated by studies in the sheep in which premature delivery before 130 days was induced in fetal lambs by the administration of ACTH or cortisol. Such lambs were viable, although untreated animals delivered by caesarean section at the same time were unable to establish satisfactory respiration. Evidence has now been obtained in the rabbit for the presence of specific cytosol and nuclear receptors for cortisol in fetal lung tissue. The numbers of receptors increase with gestational age, reaching a peak at 28 days (Giannopoulos, Mulay and Solomon, 1972), which is also the time of high levels of unbound cortisol in fetal rabbit plasma. In the fetal lamb, pulmonary surfactant can be detected before the preparturition surge in cortisol, its production being due perhaps to basal levels of plasma cortisol. Nevertheless, lung maturation and differentiation of the alveolar type II cells is accelerated as the cortisol concentration increases. The role of cortisol appears to be as a timer in lung maturation; its continued presence is not required.

Avery (1975) points out that situations in which the fetus is 'stressed' in utero (such as infection and perhaps intra-uterine growth retardation) may give rise to precocious cortisol secretion and an enhancement of lung maturation. Liggins and Howie (1972) were the first to use exogenous glucocorticoids in an antepartum attempt to prevent respiratory distress in the human. In their series of premature infants, labour was delayed with either alcohol or salbutamol, since it is apparent that exposure to the glucocorticoid for greater than 24 hours in utero is required. Finally, it should be noted that other substances may also be involved in pulmonary surfactant production. In the fetal rabbit, both thyroxine and heroin were shown to stimulate lung maturation (surfactant production and increased numbers of osmiophilic inclusions in the alveolar type II cells). Whether the action of these compounds is a direct one or is mediated through cortisol release has not been established.

Surfactant production is one of many events surrounding the onset of labour. The role of cortisol in the complex sequence of events leading to delivery has not been entirely resolved, although a considerable body of evidence has accumulated, at least in the sheep, to suggest that it might be implicated as responsible for some of the changing aspects of placental steroidogenesis, viz. a decline in progesterone, and an increase in unconjugated oestrogen production. Evidence has been presented suggesting that cortisol is responsible for stimulating a placental 17α-hydroxylase enzyme which accelerates the metabolism of progesterone (Anderson, Flint and Turnbull, 1974). 17-hydroxy C_{21} steroids may be acted upon by the C_{17-20} lyase and the resultant C_{19} steroids are then available for aromatisation to unconjugated oestrogen. In the sheep and goat there is now persuasive evidence that increasing levels of unconjugated oestrogens stimulate prostaglandin $F_{2\alpha}$ ($PGF_{2\alpha}$) release by the maternal cotyledons and by the myometrium, and that elevated levels of $PGF_{2\alpha}$ may represent a final common intramyometrial pathway leading to membrane depolarisation and expulsion of the fetus (see Figure 13.2).

In the primate one can recognise a sequence of endocrine events which resembles in outline that of the sheep. $PGF_{2\alpha}$ is certainly a central component in the physiology of primate parturition, although the detailed mechanisms by which prostaglandin production is stimulated remain unknown. A clear understanding of the role of the primate fetus has been hampered by conflicting results in animal models (*Macaca mulatta*), and the need to rely, in the human, on abnormal fetuses (anencephalics, adrenal hypoplasia or aplasia) in which the necessary endocrine and pathological information has seldom been available. In contrast to the sheep, injection of large doses of long-acting glucocorticoids into abnormal human fetuses was ineffective in precipitating premature delivery (Liggins et al, 1973), as was the administration of dexamethasone to normal women (Anderson and Turnbull, 1973). However, the administration of large doses of betamethasone to women classified as past term does appear to reduce the mean interval to labour (Mati, Horrobin and Bramley, 1973; Liggins, personal communication, 1975). These studies need to be extended to include larger groups of patients. They do, however, indicate some similarities to the sheep model and provide some evidence for a similar role of the pituitary–adrenal system of the primate fetus in the initiation of term labour.

It has already been shown that the fetal neurohypophysis may interact with the fetal anterior pituitary during late pregnancy. Other possible sites of action for fetal oxytocin and AVP are the myometrium and the umbilical circulation.

The high levels of oxytocin found in human cord blood during delivery (Chard et al, 1971) suggest that fetal oxytocin may have a function in parturition, but this would require transfer of the peptide to the maternal side of the placenta and myometrium. There are clear umbilical arteriovenous concentration differences for both oxytocin and AVP in the human (Chard et al, 1971), indicating that placental transfer or uptake of these hormones may occur. Noddle (1969) reported that the sheep placenta was permeable to oxytocin, and intravenous injections of oxytocin (100 mu) to mature fetal lambs have been shown in some cases to result in an increase in uterine pressure (Nathanielsz, Comline and Silver, 1973). Thus, in the sheep, oxytocin released by the fetus may be capable of affecting the uterus. The guinea-pig placenta is also permeable to oxytocin (Burton, 1974), but in this species fetal oxytocin may be of

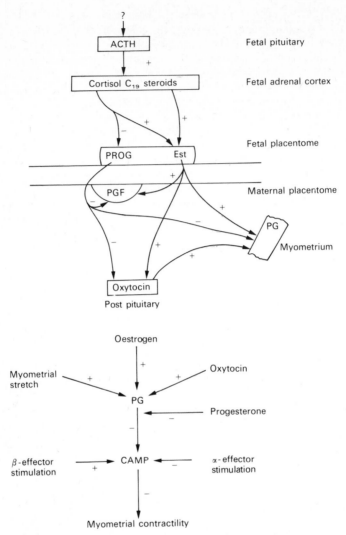

Figure 13.2. Schematic representation of the endocrine events at parturition in the sheep. Activation of the fet hypothalamic–hypophyseal–adrenal pathway results in an increase in fetal cortisol reaching the placenta. Place tal progesterone production falls, and oestrogen production increases dramatically. The change in the levels these steroids, particularly oestrogen, stimulates $PGF_{2\alpha}$ synthesis and release from the maternal cotyledons an from the myometrium. Placental $PGF_{2\alpha}$ may also affect the myometrium. An elevation in myometrial PGF_2 lowers the uterine threshold to oxytocin, and oxytocin and/or $PGF_{2\alpha}$ may interact with the smooth muscle aden cyclase system to lower cAMP levels and elevate cGMP levels. This results in the evolution of the myometrial co tractile response.

limited importance during labour, since maternal concentrations of the hormone are muc higher than the levels found in the fetus (Burton et al, 1974).

Chard (1973) has commented on the sensitivity of the umbilical circulation to vasoactiv compounds, and has suggested that enough oxytocin is normally present in the umbilica artery at the time of delivery to cause about 30 per cent of maximum constriction (Altura e

1, 1972). Whether this is a direct action, or whether it is the result of prostaglandin synthesis in these vessels (Karim, Hillier and Devlin, 1968) has not been investigated. A far higher dose of AVP was required to elicit a similar response, and the physiological significance of this effect is not clear.

In this chapter some of the dependent and independent activities of the fetal adrenal and neurohypophysis have been commented on. It is clear that physiological processes in the fetus represent a cumulative effect resulting from the complex interaction of a number of endocrine systems. Important clinical advances have already been made on the basis of some of the observations and experimental studies described. Clearly, there are many fundamental questions still to be answered, and the potential clinical benefit from future basic research is enormous.

ACKNOWLEDGEMENTS

We are indebted to our colleagues Drs J. S. Robinson, I. S. Fraser and D. W. Rurak for their advice, criticism and discussion. We thank Mrs Jane Hunter and Mrs Gay Harris for typing the manuscript. This work was supported in part by a grant from the MRC. G.D.T. is a member of the external scientific staff of the MRC.

REFERENCES

Ainsworth, L. & Ryan, K. J. (1966) Steroid hormone transformation by endocrine organs from pregnant mammals. 1. Estrogen biosynthesis by mammalian placental preparations *in vitro*. *Endocrinology*, **79,** 875–883.

Alexander, D. P., Bashore, R. A., Britton, H. G. & Forsling, M. L. (1974a) Maternal and fetal arginine vasopressin in the chronically catheterised sheep. *Biology of the Neonate*, **25,** 242–248.

Alexander, D. P., Britton, H. G., Forsling, M. L., Nixon, D. A. & Ratcliffe, J. G. (1973) Adrenocorticotrophin and vasopressin in foetal sheep and the response to stress. In *The Endocrinology of Pregnancy and Parturition* (Ed.) Pierrepoint, C. G. pp. 112–125. Cardiff: Alpha Omega Publishing Co.

Alexander, D. P., Britton, H. G., Forsling, M. L., Nixon, D. A. & Ratcliffe, J. G. (1974b) Pituitary and plasma concentrations of adrenocorticotrophin, growth hormone, vasopressin and oxytocin in fetal and maternal sheep during the latter half of gestation and the response to haemorrhage. *Biology of the Neonate*, **24,** 206–219.

Alexander, D. P., Forsling, M. L., Martin, M. J., Nixon, D. A., Ratcliffe, J. G., Redstone, D. & Tunbridge, D. (1972) The effect of maternal hypoxia on fetal pituitary hormone release in the sheep. *Biology of the Neonate*, **21,** 219–228.

Allen, J. P., Cook, D. M., Kendall, J. W. & McGilvra, R. (1973) Maternal–fetal ACTH relationship in man. *Journal of Clinical Endocrinology and Metabolism*, **37,** 230–234.

Allen, J. P., Greer, M. A., McGilvra, R., Castro, A. & Fisher, D. A. (1974) Endocrine function in an anencephalic infant. *Journal of Clinical Endocrinology and Metabolism*, **38,** 94–98.

Altura, B. M., Malaviya, D., Reich, C. F. & Orkin, L. R. (1972) Effects of vasoactive agents on isolated human umbilical arteries and veins. *American Journal of Physiology*, **222,** 345–355.

Anderson, A. B. M. & Turnbull, A. C. (1973) Comparative aspects of factors involved in the onset of labour in ovine and human pregnancy. *Memoirs of the Society for Endocrinology*, **20,** 141–162.

Anderson, A. B. M., Flint, A. P. F. & Turnbull, A. C. (1974) Mechanism of action of glucocorticoids in induction of ovine parturition; effect on placental steroid metabolism. *Journal of Endocrinology*, **61,** 36–37.

Anderson, A. B. M., Pierrepoint, C. G., Turnbull, A. C. & Griffiths, K. (1973) Steroid investigations in the developing sheep foetus. In *The Endocrinology of Pregnancy and Parturition* (Ed.) Pierrepoint, C. G. pp. 23–39. Cardiff: Alpha Omega Publishing Co.

Avery, M. E. (1975) Pharmacological approaches to the acceleration of fetal lung maturation. *British Medical Bulletin*, **31,** 13–17.

Bassett, J. M. & Thorburn, G. D. (1969) Foetal plasma corticosteroids and the initiation of parturition in the sheep. *Journal of Endocrinology*, **44,** 285–286.

Bassett, J. M. & Thorburn, G. D. (1973) Circulating levels of progesterone and corticosteroids in the pregnant ewe and its foetus. In *The Endocrinology of Pregnancy and Parturition* (Ed.) Pierrepoint, C. G. pp. 126–140. Cardiff: Alpha Omega Publishing Co.

Beamer, N., Hagemenas, F. C. & Kittinger, G. W. (1973) Development of cortisol binding in the rhesus monkey. *Endocrinology*, **93**, 363–368.

Beitins, I. Z., Bayard, F., Ances, I. G., Kowarski, A. & Migeon, C. J. (1973) Metabolic clearance rate, blood production, interconversion and transplacental passage of cortisol and cortisone in pregnancy near term. *Journal of Pediatric Research*, **7**, 509–519.

Benirschke, K. (1956) Adrenals in anencephaly and hydrocephaly. *Obstetrics and Gynecology*, **8**, 412–425.

Benirschke, K. & McKay, D. B. (1953) The antidiuretic hormone in fetus and infant. *Obstetrics and Gynecology*, **1**, 638–649.

Boddy, K., Jones, C. T., Mantell, C., Ratcliffe, J. G. & Robinson, J. S. (1974) Changes in plasma ACTH and corticosteroid of the maternal and fetal sheep during hypoxia. *Endocrinology*, **94**, 588–591.

Bosu, W. T. K., Johansson, E. D. B. & Gemzell, C. (1973) Peripheral plasma levels of oestrogens, progesterone and 17α-hydroxyprogesterone during gestation in the rhesus monkey. *Acta Endocrinologica*, **74**, 348–360.

Bosu, W. T. K., Johansson, E. D. B. & Gemzell, C. (1974) Influence of oophorectomy, luteectomy, foetal death and dexamethazone on the peripheral plasma levels of oestrogens and progesterone in the pregnant *Macaca mulatta*. *Acta Endocrinologica*, **75**, 601–616.

Burton, A. M., Illingworth, D. V., Challis, J. R. G. & McNeilly, A. S. (1974) Placental transfer of oxytocin in the guinea pig and its release during parturition. *Journal of Endocrinology*, **60**, 499–506.

Cassmer, O. (1959) Hormone production of the isolated human placenta. *Acta Endocrinologica*, Supplement **45**.

Challis, J. R. G. (1971) Sharp increase in free circulating oestrogens immediately before parturition in sheep. *Nature*, **229**, 208.

Challis, J. R. G. & Thorburn, G. D. (1975) Pre-natal endocrine function and the initiation of parturition. *British Medical Bulletin*, **31**, 57–62.

Challis, J. R. G., Davies, I. J., Benirschke, K., Hendrickx, A. G. & Ryan, K. J. (1947a) The concentrations of progesterone, estrone, and estradiol-17β in the peripheral plasma of the rhesus monkey during the final third of gestation and after the induction of abortion with PGF$_{2\alpha}$. *Endocrinology*, **95**, 547–553.

Challis, J. R. G., Davies, I. J., Benirschke, K., Hendrickx, A. G. & Ryan, K. J. (1974b) The effects of dexamethasone on plasma steroid levels and fetal adrenal histology in the pregnant rhesus monkey. *Endocrinology*, **95**, 1300–1305.

Challis, J. R. G., Davies, I. J., Benirschke, K., Hendrickx, A. G. & Ryan, K. J. (1975a) The effects of dexamethasone on the peripheral plasma concentrations of androstenedione, testosterone and cortisol in the pregnant rhesus monkey. *Endocrinology*, **96**, 185–192.

Challis, J. R. G., Robinson, J. S., Rurak, D. W. & Thorburn, G. D. (1975b) The development of endocrine function in the human fetus. In *Biology of Human Fetal Growth* (Ed.) Roberts, D. F. & Thompson, A. M. pp. 149–194. London: Taylor and Francis.

Chard, T. (1973) The posterior pituitary and the induction of labour. *Memoirs of the Society for Endocrinology*, **20**, 61–76.

Chard, T., Hudson, C. N., Edwards, C. R. W. & Boyd, N. R. H. (1971) Release of oxytocin and vasopressin by the human foetus during labour. *Nature*, **234**, 352–354.

Chez, R. A., Hutchinson, D. L., Salazar, H. & Mintz, D. H. (1970) Some effects of fetal and maternal hypophysectomy in pregnancy. *American Journal of Obstetrics and Gynecology*, **108**, 643–650.

Comline, R. S. & Silver, M. (1961) The release of adrenaline and noradrenaline from the adrenal glands of the foetal sheep. *Journal of Physiology*, **156**, 424–444.

Comline, R. S., Nathanielsz, P. W. & Silver, M. (1973) Foetal cortisol production and parturition in the sheep. In *The Endocrinology of Pregnancy and Parturition* (Ed.) Pierrepoint, C. G. pp. 141–152. Cardiff: Alpha Omega Publishing Co.

Coslovsky, R. & Yalow, R. S. (1974) Influence of the hormonal forms of ACTH on the pattern of corticosteroid secretion. *Biochemical and Biophysical Research Communications*, **60**, 1351–1356.

Davies, I. J. & Ryan, K. J. (1972) Comparative endocrinology of gestation. *Vitamins and Hormones*, **30**, 223–278.

Davies, I. J. & Ryan, K. J. (1973) Glucocorticoid synthesis from pregnenolone by sheep foetal adrenals *in vitro*. *Journal of Endocrinology*, **58**, 485–491.

Davies, I. J., Ryan, K. J. & Petro, Z. (1970) Estrogen synthesis by adrenal–placental tissues of the sheep and the Iris monkey *in vitro*. *Endocrinology*, **86**, 1457–1459.

Dawood, M. Y. & Ratnam, S. S. (1974) Serum unconjugated estradiol-17β in normal pregnancy measured by radioimmunoassay. *Obstetrics and Gynecology*, **44**, 194–199.

Diczfalusy, E. & Mancuso, S. (1969) Oestrogen metabolism in pregnancy. In *Foetus and Placenta* (Ed.) Klopper, A. & Diczfalusy, E. pp. 191–248. Oxford: Blackwell.

Dixon, R., Hyman, A., Gurpide, E., Dyrenfurth, I., Cohen, H., Bowe, E., Engel, T., Daniel, S., James, S. & Vande Wiele, R. (1970) Feto-maternal transfer and production of cortisol in the sheep. *Steroids*, **16**, 771–789.

Falin, L. (1961) The development of human hypophysis and differentiation of cells of its anterior lobe during embryonic life. *Acta Anatomica*, **44**, 188–205.

Fencl, M. & Tulchinsky, D. (1975) Concentrations of cortisol in amniotic fluid during pregnancy. *New England Journal of Medicine*, **292**, 133–136.

Findlay, J. K. (1970) *The Occurrence, Biosynthesis and Metabolism of Oestrogens in the Ovine Feto-Placental Unit*. PhD thesis, University of Adelaide.

France, J. T., Seddon, R. J. & Liggins, G. C. (1973) A study of a pregnancy with low estrogen production due to placental sulfatase deficiency. *Journal of Clinical Endocrinology and Metabolism*, **36**, 1–9.

Fraser, I. S., Leask, R., Drife, J., Bacon, L. & Michie, E. A. (1976) Plasma oestrogen response to dehydroepiandrosterone sulphate injection in normal and complicated late pregnancy. *Obstetrics and Gynecology*, **47**, 152.

Genazzani, A. R., Fraioli, F., Hurlimann, J., Fioretti, P. & Felber, J. P. (1975) Immunoreactive ACTH and cortisol plasma levels during pregnancy. Detection and partial purification of corticotrophin-like placental hormone: the human chorionic corticotrophin (HCC). *Clinical Endocrinology*, **4**, 1–14.

Giannopoulos, G., Mulay, S. & Solomon, S. (1972) Cortisol receptors in rabbit fetal lung. *Biochemical and Biophysical Research Communications*, **47**, 411–418.

Heap, R. B., Perry, J. S. & Challis, J. R. G. (1973) Hormonal maintenance of pregnancy. In *American Physiological Society Handbook of Physiology*, Section 7, *Endocrinology*, Vol. II, Part 2 (Ed.) Greep, R. O. & Astwood, E. B. pp. 217–260. Baltimore: Williams and Wilkins.

Hoppenstein, J. M., Miltenberger, F. W. & Moran, W. H. Jr (1968) The increase in blood levels of vasopressin in infants during birth and surgical procedures. *Surgery, Gynecology and Obstetrics*, **127**, 966–974.

Johannisson, E. (1968) Foetal adrenal cortex in human: its ultrastructure at different stages of development and in different functional states, *Acta Endocrinologica*, **58**, Supplement 130, 7–107.

John, B. M. & Pierrepoint, C. G. (1975) Demonstration of an active C_{17-20} lyase in the normal sheep placenta. *Journal of Reproduction and Fertility*, **43**, 559–562.

Johnson, P., Jones, C. T., Kendall, J. Z., Ritchie, J. W. K. & Thorburn, G. D. (1975) ACTH and the induction of parturition in sheep. *Journal of Physiology*, **252**, 64P.

Karim, S. M. M., Hillier, K. & Devlin, J. (1968) Distribution of prostaglandins E_1, E_2, $F_{1\alpha}$ and $F_{2\alpha}$ in some animal tissues. *Journal of Pharmacy and Pharmacology*, **20**, 749–753.

Kittinger, G. W. (1973) The regulation of cortisol levels in fetal plasma. *Primate News*, **11**, 2–5.

Kittinger, G. W. (1974) Feto-maternal production and transfer of cortisol in the rhesus (*Macaca mulatta*). *Steroids*, **23**, 229–243.

Kittinger, G. W., Beamer, N. B., Hagemenas, F., Hill, J. D., Baughman, W. L. & Ochsner, A. J. (1972) Evidence for autonomous pituitary–adrenal function in the near-term fetal rhesus (*Macaca mulatta*). *Endocrinology*, **91**, 1037–1044.

Klopper, A. & Gardner, J. (1973) Endocrine factors in labour. *Memoirs of the Society for Endocrinology*, **20**.

Liggins, G. C. & Howie, R. N. (1972) A controlled trial of antepartum glucocorticoid treatment for prevention of the respiratory distress syndrome in premature infants. *Pediatrics*, **50**, 515–525.

Liggins, G. C., Grieves, S. A., Kendall, J. Z. & Knox, B. S. (1972) The physiological roles of progesterone, oestradiol-17β and prostaglandin $F_{2\alpha}$ in the control of ovine parturition. *Journal of Reproduction and Fertility* Supplement **16**, 85–103.

Liggins, G. C., Fairclough, R. J., Grieves, S. A., Kendall, J. Z. & Knox, B. S. (1973) The mechanism of initiation of parturition in the ewe. *Recent Progress in Hormone Research*, **29**, 111–150.

MacDonald, P. C. & Siiteri, P. K. (1965) Origin of estrogen in women pregnant with an anencephalic fetus. *Journal of Clinical Investigation*, **44**, 465–474.

Madill, D. & Bassett, J. M. (1973) Corticosteroid release by adrenal tissue from foetal and newborn lambs in response to corticotrophin stimulation in a perifusion system *in vitro*. *Journal of Endocrinology*, **58**, 75–87.

Magendantz, H. G. & Ryan, K. J. (1964) Isolation of an estriol precursor, 16α-hydroxydehydroepiandrosterone, from human umbilical sera. *Journal of Clinical Endocrinology and Metabolism*, **24**, 1155.

Mati, J. K. G., Horrobin, D. F. & Bramley, P. S. (1973) Induction of labour in sheep and humans with single doses of corticosteroids. *British Medical Journal*, **ii**, 149–151.

Mellor, D. J. & Slater, J. S. (1972) Daily changes in foetal urine and relationships with amniotic and allantoic fluid and maternal plasma during the last two months of pregnancy in conscious, unstressed ewes with chronically implanted catheters. *Journal of Physiology*, **227**, 503–525.

Mitchell, F. L. (1967) Steroid metabolism in feto-placental unit and in early childhood. *Vitamins and Hormones*, **25**, 191–269.

Murphy, B. E. P. (1973) Does the human fetal adrenal play a role in parturition? *American Journal of Obstetrics and Gynecology*, **115**, 521–525.

Murphy, B. E. P., Patrick, J. & Denton, R. L. (1975) Cortisol in amniotic fluid during human gestation. *Journal of Clinical Endocrinology and Metabolism*, **40**, 164–167.

Murphy, B. E. P., Clark, S. J., Donald, I. R., Pinsky, M. & Vedady, D. (1974) Conversion of maternal cortisol to cortisone during placental transfer to the human fetus. *American Journal of Obstetrics and Gynecology*, **118**, 538–541.

Nancarrow, C. D. & Seamark, R. F. (1968) Progesterone metabolism in fetal blood. *Steroids*, **12**, 367–379.

Nathanielsz, P. W., Comline, R. S. & Silver, M. (1973) Uterine activity following intravenous administration of oxytocin to the foetal sheep. *Nature*, **243**, 471–473.

Nathanielsz, P. W., Comline, R. S., Silver, M. & Paisey, R. B. (1972) Cortisol metabolism in the foetal and neonatal sheep. *Journal of Reproduction and Fertility*, Supplement **16**, 39–59.

Noddle, B. A. (1969) Transfer of oxytocin from the maternal to the foetal circulation in the ewe. *Nature*, **203**, 414.

Oakey, R. E. (1970) The progressive increase in estrogen production in human pregnancy. An appraisal of the factors responsible. *Vitamins and Hormones*, **28**, 1–36.

Pakravan, P., Kenny, F. M., Depp, R. & Allen, A. C. (1974) Familial congenital absence of adrenal glands, evaluation of glucocorticoid, mineralocorticoid and estrogen metabolism in the perinatal period. *Journal of Pediatrics*, **84**, 74–78.

Papez, J. W. (1940) The embryological development of the hypothalamic area in mammals. *Research Publications of the Association for Nervous and Mental Disease*, **20**, 31–51.

Parry, H. B. & Livett, B. G. (1973) A neurohypothalamic pathway to the median eminence containing neurophysin and its hypertrophy in sheep with natural scrapie. *Nature*, **242**, 63–65.

Paterson, J. Y. F. & Hills, F. (1967) The binding of cortisol by ovine plasma proteins. *Journal of Endocrinology*, **37**, 261–268.

Perks, A. M. & Vizsoyli, E. (1973) Studies of the neurohypophysis in foetal mammals. In *Foetal and Neonatal Physiology* (Ed.) Comline, R. S., Cross, K. W., Dawes, G. S. & Nathanielsz, P. W. pp. 430–438. Cambridge: Cambridge University Press.

Pierrepoint, C. G., Anderson, A. B. M., Turnbull, A. C. & Griffiths, K. (1973) In vivo and in vitro studies of steroid metabolism by the sheep placenta. In *The Endocrinology of Pregnancy and Parturition* (Ed.) Pierrepoint, C. G. pp. 40–53. Cardiff: Alpha Omega Publishing Co.

Rees, L. H., Burke, C. W., Chard, T., Evans, S. W. & Letchworth, A. T. (1975a) Placental origin of ACTH in normal human pregnancy. *Nature*, **254**, 620–632.

Rees, L. H., Jack, P. M. B., Thomas, A. L. & Nathanielsz, P. W. (1975b) The role of foetal adrenocorticotrophin during parturition in the sheep. *Nature*, **253**, 274–275.

Reynolds, J. W. & Mirkin, B. L. (1973) Urinary steroid levels in newborn infants with intrauterine growth retardation. *Journal of Clinical Endocrinology and Metabolism*, **36**, 576–581.

Robinson, J. S. & Thorburn, G. D. (1974) The initiation of labour. *British Journal of Hospital Medicine*, **12**, 15–22.

Ryan, K. J. (1969) Theoretical basis for endocrine control of gestation—a comparative approach. In *Feto-placental Unit* (Ed.) Pecile, A. & Finzi, C. pp. 120–131. Amsterdam: Excerpta Medica Foundation.

Ryan, K. J. & Hopper, B. R. (1974) Placental biosynthesis and metabolism of steroid hormones in primates. *Contributions in Primatology*, **3**, 258–283.

Saffran, M., Matthews, E. K. & Pearlmutter, F. (1971) Analysis of the response to ACTH by rat adrenal in a flowing system. *Recent Progress in Hormone Research*, **27**, 607–647.

Sandberg, A. A. & Slaunwhite, W. R. Jr (1959) Transcortin: a corticosteroid binding protein of plasma. II. Levels in various conditions and the effects of estrogens. *Journal of Clinical Investigation*, **38**, 1290–1297.

Seppala, M., Aho, I., Tissari, A. & Ruoslahti, E. (1972) Radioimmunoassay of oxytocin in the amniotic fluid, fetal urine and meconium during late pregnancy and delivery. *American Journal of Obstetrics and Gynecology*, **114**, 788–795.

Siiteri, P. K. (1973) Overview of steroid hormone formation in pregnancy. In *The Endocrine Milieu of Pregnancy, Puerperium and Childhood*. Third Ross Conference on Obstetric Research (Ed.) Jaffe, R. B. pp. 51–54. Columbus: Ross Laboratories.

Siiteri, P. K. & MacDonald, P. C. (1963) The utilisation of circulating dehydroisoandrosterone sulfate for estrogen synthesis during human pregnancy. *Steroids*, **2**, 713.

Siiteri, P. K. & MacDonald, P. C. (1966) Placental estrogen biosynthesis during human pregnancy. *Journal of Clinical Endocrinology and Metabolism*, **26**, 751.

Simmer, H. H., Tulchinsky, D., Gold, E. M. & Frankland, M. (1974) On the regulation of estrogen production by cortisol and ACTH in human pregnancy at term. *American Journal of Obstetrics and Gynecology*, **119**, 283–296.

Skowky, R. & Fisher, D. A. (1973) Immunoreactive arginine vasopressin (AVP) and arginine vasotocin (AVT) in the fetal pituitary of man and sheep. *Journal of Clinical Investigation*, **52**, 77–78a.

Skowsky, W. R., Bashore, R. A., Smith, F. G. & Fisher, D. A. (1973) Vasopressin metabolism in the foetus and newborn. In *Foetal and Neonatal Physiology* (Ed.) Comline, R. S., Cross, K. W., Dawes, G. S. & Nathanielsz, P. W. pp. 439–447. Cambridge: Cambridge University Press.

Solomon, S. (1966) Formation and metabolism of neutral steroids in human placenta and fetus. *Journal of Clinical Endocrinology and Metabolism*, **26**, 762–772.

Strott, C. A., Sundel, H. & Stahlman, M. T. (1974) Maternal fetal plasma progesterone, cortisol, testosterone and 17β-estradiol in preparturient sheep: response to fetal ACTH infusion. *Endocrinology*, **95**, 1327–1339.

Taylor, N. R. W., Loraine, J. A. & Robertson, H. A. (1953) The estimation of ACTH in human pituitary tissue. *Journal of Endocrinology*, **9**, 334–341.

Thompson, F. N. & Wagner, W. C. (1974) Plasma progesterone and oestrogens in sheep during late pregnancy: contribution of the maternal adrenal and ovary. *Journal of Reproduction and Fertility*, **41**, 57–66.

Thorburn, G. D., Nicol, D. H., Bassett, J. M., Shutt, D. A. & Cox, R. I. (1972) Parturition in the goat and sheep: changes in corticosteroids, progesterone, oestrogens and prostaglandin F. *Journal of Reproduction and Fertility*, Supplement, **16**, 61–84.

Townsley, J. D., Rubin, E. J. & Crystle, C. D. (1973) Evaluation of placental steroid 3-sulfatase and aromatase activities as regulators of estrogen production in human pregnancy. *American Journal of Obstetrics and Gynecology*, **17**, 345–350.

Turnbull, A. C., Patten, P. T., Flint, A. P. F., Keirse, M. J. N. C., Jeremy, J. Y. & Anderson, A. B. M. (1974) Significant fall in progesterone and rise in oestradiol levels in human peripheral plasma before onset of labour. *Lancet*, **i**, 101–104.

Villee, D. B. (1966) Effects of progesterone on enzyme activity of adrenals in organ culture. *Advances in Enzyme Regulation*, **4**, 269–280.

Villee, D. B. (1969) Development of endocrine function in the human placenta and fetus (first of two parts). *New England Journal of Medicine*, **281**, 473–484.

Villee, D. B. (1972) The development of steroidogenesis. *American Journal of Medicine*, **53**, 533–544.

Vizsoyli, E. & Perks, A. M. (1969) New neurohypophysial principle in foetal mammals. *Nature*, **223**, 1169.

Wiley, M. K., Pearlmutter, A. F. & Miller, R. E. (1974) Decreased adrenal sensitivity to ACTH in the vasopressin-deficient (Brattleboro) rat. *Neuroendocrinology*, **14**, 257–270.

Winters, A. J., Oliver, C., Colston, C., MacDonald, P. C. & Porter, J. C. (1974) Plasma ACTH levels in the human fetus and neonate as related to age and parturition. *Journal of Clinical Endocrinology and Metabolism*, **39**, 269–273.

Yates, F. E., Russell, S. M., Dallman, M. F., Hedge, G. A., McCann, S. M. & Dhariwal, A. P. S. (1971) Potentiation by vasopressin of corticotrophin release induced by corticotrophin releasing factor. *Endocrinology*, **88**, 3–15.

Zimmerman, E. A., Carmell, P. W., Husain, M. K., Ferin, M., Tannenbaum, M., Frantz, A. & Robinson, A. G. (1974) Vasopressin and neurophysin: high concentrations in monkey hypophyseal portal blood. *Science*, **182**, 925–927.

14

THE DRIVE TO FETAL GROWTH

G. C. Liggins

The rate of growth and differentiation of the human fetus is determined in the main by genetic information contained within the dividing and growing cells themselves. Superimposed upon this genetic control of growth are two opposing influences. On the one hand there are various sorts of constraints, in particular that due to an inevitable limitation on the availability to the cell of nutrients. On the other hand, there are factors such as hormones that act on the cell from without and further stimulate the genetically determined drive to growth. The slope of the growth velocity curve and the birthweight are the outcome of the interaction with the fetal genotype of constraining and stimulating factors. In the first half of pregnancy, genetic control is dominant and gives rise to relatively narrow limits of variability of patterns of fetal growth; in the second half of pregnancy, constraints and stimuli become increasingly important and give rise to greater variability of growth and of maturational milestones.

This chapter is concerned with the factors that collectively determine the growth and development of the normal fetus. Abnormalities of growth will be considered only as far as they illustrate physiological mechanisms. Frequent recourse will be made to animal studies to help fill the many gaps in our knowledge of growth of the human fetus.

GENETIC CONTROL OF GROWTH

The way that the genetic information contained in the fertilised egg guides its multiplication and differentiation to eventual attainment of the perfect form of a human being is often taken for granted or is attributed to nebulous 'organisers' that mysteriously appear in the right place at the right time and direct the modelling of their particular pieces of anatomy. The description of growth in biochemical terms has lagged behind most areas of cell biology and is still poorly understood. Only recently has a hypothesis been developed that offers a satisfactory basis for answering such questions as how, in a differentiated cell, one set of genes can be active while the remainder are totally inactive; or how the genetic 'clocks' operate to determine that a particular developmental event will occur at a gestational age that is accurate almost to the hour. What is clear is that the programme is written in base sequences in the DNA; what is unclear is how the programme is translated into biochemical events on a precise time course.

The total number of cells in a term fetus lies within fairly narrow limits and is the result of 42 successive divisions of the fertilised ovum. Obviously the number of divisions must be precisely controlled if the fetus is to be of normal proportions. The consequences of inaccurate 'counting' will be appreciated from the fact that only five further divisions are required for the fetus to attain adult size. Thus, one of the fundamental genetic controls of growth depends on the ability of cells to 'count' the number of divisions it has gone through. There must be a mechanism whereby cell differentiation can be programmed to occur after a specified number of divisions of a cell-line.

Holliday and Pugh (1975) have postulated a developmental clock that depends on modification enzymes. Their hypothesis is necessarily speculative since modification enzymes, although known to occur in bacteria, have yet to be identified in higher organisms, but it will illustrate the sort of mechanism that could permit accurate division counting.

Modification enzymes have highly specific actions that result in modification of bases at particular positions in short, defined sequences of DNA; in the example to be described here, the modification consists of conversion of one base to another (adenine → guanine; A → G) and occurs during replication.

Figure 14.1 shows a hypothetical repeating sequence in a single strand of DNA. At the right hand end there is a sequence to which the modification enzyme binds. This sequence is first modified by an A–G transition. When this has occurred, the site of action for the enzyme has moved eight bases to the left. This process will be repeated during successive replications as many times as there are repeats of the sequence. At the end of the precisely determined number of divisions, the operator or promoter site is altered and the developmental switch

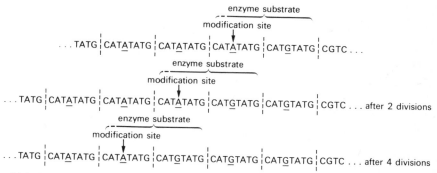

Figure 14.1. A mechanism for counting cell divisions based on an adenine–thymine → guanine–cystosine (AT → GC) transition. The modification enzyme recognises the first sequence of eight bases because it contains G at the 5-position together with the sequence to its left. The A at the 5-position of the second sequence is changed to G to give a new recognition sequence 8 bases to the left. When all the sequences have been modified during successive divisions a structural gene (not shown here) at the extreme left of the repeated controlling sequences is activated. Redrawn from Holliday and Pugh (1975) with kind permission of the authors and the editor of *Science*.

comes into operation. A similar system could work equally well on both strands of DNA, thus ensuring that all the progeny of a stem cell will possess synchronous switches.

A second issue of fundamental importance to development is the genetic stability of the differentiated state. Differentiated cells do not readily transform either to other types of differentiated cells or to undifferentiated cells. Although the switching on of a single gene may commit the cell to differentiation, it is unlikely to be sufficient to bring about all the changes required for differentiation. It is possible that the first activated gene codes for a modifying enzyme that is active at several sites in the genome which have the same controlling sequence. In this way, the cells of a particular line, when differentiated, contain altered DNA that distinguishes them from all other cells in the body and stability of the line is ensured.

Experiments on the development of the chick wing (Summerball, Lewis and Wolpert, 1973) provide convincing evidence of a developmental clock. The tip of the limb bud, the progress zone, contains dividing cells which form in strict sequence the various structures of the limb from its base to the extremity. If the progress zone from a limb in which the basic structures are nearly fully formed is transplanted to a very young limb from which the progress zone has been removed, none of the structures is formed. On the other hand, if a young progress zone replaces one on the end of a wing that has already laid down all the basic structures, another wing is formed at the end of the first. These results show that there is a temporal order in the laying down of successive structures and this order could well be related to the number of cell divisions that have elapsed in the cells of the progress zone.

Genetically controlled growth rates of normal human fetuses show some variability due to inherited characteristics. Approximately 15 per cent of total birthweight variation is attributable to fetal genotype. Of this, two per cent depends upon the sex chromosomes (Polani, 1974), males weighing 150 to 200 g more than females at term. The way in which the Y chromosome accelerates growth is not known and has been variously ascribed to the greater antigenic dissimilarity between the male fetus and his mother (Ounsted and Ounsted, 1970), or to effects of testicular hormones. Important genetic influences on growth may exist on a population basis. At one extreme, the American Indians of the Cheyenne tribe have a mean birthweight of 3800 g, while at the other extreme the Luni tribe of New Guinea have a mean birthweight of 2400 g (Meredith, 1970). Within ethnic groups a marked intrafamily similarity of birthweights can be demonstrated (Donald, 1939), while at an individual level, a correlation exists between birthweight and both height and weight of the parents. In the mother, weight is the more important and when this is corrected for, maternal height has little effect on the size of the fetus (Love and Kinch, 1965). Paternal height correlates positively with birthweight to the extent that birthweight increases by 9 g for each centimetre of the father's height above baseline (Abdul-Karim and Beydoun, 1974). The paternal contribution to birthweight can be mediated only through his contribution to the fetus's autosomal genes and sex. The maternal contribution is more profound and complex, being expressed not only through the genes of the fetus but also through the effect of her own genotype on the environment of the fetus; the latter is probably as important as the genotype of the fetus itself (Penrose, 1961).

CONSTRAINTS TO GROWTH

It is likely that the fetus rarely expresses fully its genetically determined potential for growth. Under normal conditions growth is constrained to a greater or lesser degree by unknown factors in the fetal environment. The classic demonstration of maternal constraint of fetal growth was made by Walton and Hammond (1938) who crossed Shire horses with Shetland ponies. The birthweights of foals born to Shetland dams were similar to those of pure Shetlands, while foals born to Shire dams were of similar birthweight to purebred Shires. This experiment showed that maternal factors in the horse override that part of the fetal genetic make-up acquired from the sire, but did not clearly distinguish between those maternal influences expressed through the genes of the fetus and those expressed through the fetal environment. In more recent experiments, the genetic component has been eliminated by transplantation of fertilised eggs. Smidt, Steinbach and Scheven (1967) transferred eggs from normal-sized pigs into dwarf sows and found that the piglets were about half the size of normal piglets. When the experiment was reversed by transferring eggs from dwarf sows into normal-sized sows, the piglets were about twice the size of usual dwarf piglets. Similar results of egg transfer experiments have been observed in sheep (Hunter, 1956) and rabbits (Venge, 1950).

In man, the evidence for maternal constraint of fetal growth must necessarily be more indirect. Nevertheless, it appears probable that maternal influences are no less important in man than in domestic animals. For example, it has been shown by Morton (1955) that the intraclass correlations of birthweight are high (0.581) for half-sibs related through a common mother but low (0.102) for half-sibs related through a common father. Maternal weight correlates with birthweight, as already noted. Ounsted (1971) found that the mean maternal weight in a group of infants of normal birthweight was 66.3 kg; in a growth-retarded group and a growth-accelerated group it was 62.9 kg and 74.7 kg respectively. She pointed out that both maternal stature and body weight have a larger effect at the upper than at the lower extremes of growth rate. Mothers of growth-retarded infants and normally-grown controls were of the same mean height, whereas mothers of growth-accelerated infants were 3.8 cm taller. Ounsted postulated that the effects of maternal height are apparent only when maternal constraint is relaxed.

The nature of maternal constraint is unknown. It could operate in many ways including such things as the factors determining placental weight, maternal placental perfusion and availability of nutrient materials. Ounsted and Ounsted (1966) proposed that constraint was exercised by the setting of a predetermined maternal regulator. They showed not only that the birthweights of the siblings of growth-retarded babies were significantly lower than those of siblings of babies of normal birthweight, but also that the mothers of growth-retarded babies were themselves of low birthweight. This suggests that the setting of the hypothetical regulator depends in part on the maternal genotype and in part on the extent to which the mother's growth was constrained during her own fetal development. Thus, it is possible for low birthweight to be transmitted through successive generations without being a part of the genotype.

The size that the human fetus could attain if maternal constraint was removed is a matter for speculation. Birthweights of 6 kg and more can be attained occasionally by normal babies in the absence of maternal disease such as diabetes. It is conceivable that the mean birthweight could double as it did in the piglets referred to above. A clearer understanding of the nature of maternal constraint has obvious implications in relation to the treatment of fetal growth retardation.

In this age when obesity in adults has become a major health problem there is reason to believe that maternal constraint of fetal growth has benefits extending beyond those of the mechanical problems of parturition. McCance and Widdowson (1947) have suggested that the subsequent rate of growth of an animal or child is predetermined by its rate of growth, or its size, during the critical period of development early in life when the regulating centres of the hypothalamus are being coordinated with the rate of growth. The appetite centres may be organised before birth in man and 'appetite control' may be ready to come into action immediately after birth. A small size at this time, arising from slow intra-uterine growth, might lead to an appetite geared to the small body size and hence to a smaller size at maturity. Conversely, the fetus who has enjoyed a gluttonous intra-uterine existence may retain the habit and suffer accordingly.

HORMONAL STIMULI OF FETAL SOMATIC GROWTH

Maternal hormones

None of the peptide or protein hormones can traverse the placenta from the maternal to the fetal circulation.

Of the remaining hormones, thyroxine and cortisol have metabolic functions and can pass the human placental barrier. In theory then, maternal thyroxine or cortisol could influence fetal growth, but in practice the transplacental passage of both hormones is impeded to the extent that even elevated maternal levels do not significantly raise fetal levels. In the case of thyroxine, passage is limited by restricted transport in the placenta, but with cortisol a unique mechanism exists to ensure a large gradient for cortisol while at the same time allowing free passage of other steroid hormones. The human placenta is rich in an enzyme, 11β-hydroxy-dehydrogenase, that converts cortisol to its inactive form, cortisone (Osinski, 1960). The fetus, unlike the adult, has little ability to reconvert cortisone to cortisol.

The elaborate precautions to limit transfer of hormones from mother to fetus are of importance to the orderly development of the fetus, for upon them depends his endocrine autonomy. If maternal hormones could freely enter the fetus, hormone levels in the fetus would be determined by the vagaries of maternal endocrine behaviour rather than by the needs of growth and development. Unfortunately for the fetus, these protective mechanisms cannot withstand the disturbances associated with certain maternal diseases. The fetus of the thyrotoxic mother may be thyrotoxic, not because of excessive passage of thyroxine from the maternal circulation but because of passage of immunoglobulins such as long-acting thyroid stimulator (LATS). Similarly, fetal pancreatic function is altered in maternal diabetes, not by any change in insulin transport but by fetal hyperglycaemia secondary to maternal hyperglycaemia. Fetal overgrowth associated with maternal acromegaly is more difficult to explain. In a recent case report, diabetes secondary to acromegaly was excluded and, in addition, the fetal macrosomia was not characteristic of diabetes (Fisch et al, 1974). It is possible that somatomedins, a group of small growth-promoting proteins which mediate the effects of growth hormone and which are elevated in acromegaly, can pass through the placenta. Erythropoietin, a protein related closely to somatomedins, may penetrate the human placenta (Finne, 1967).

Of course, failure of maternal hormones to enter the fetus does not exclude a function for them in fetal growth. Indirectly, by maintaining blood levels of glucose and other nutrients in the maternal circulation, they contribute to the drive to fetal growth. Hormones such as catecholamines, angiotensin II, aldosterone and prostaglandins maintain maternal cardiovascular homeostasis upon which adequate perfusion of the placenta depends. Indeed, Speroff (1973) has proposed that uterine blood flow is autoregulated by renin–angiotensin and prostaglandins generated within the uterus in a manner analogous to that of the kidney. From a clinical point of view, a future ability to promote fetal growth by pharmacological means is likely to depend on enhancement of placental perfusion rather than on stimulation of fetal hormones. Only in this way can *all* the ingredients of fetal growth be delivered in increased quantities to the fetus. Stimulation of fetal growth and, consequently, oxygen demand could create a potentially dangerous relative placental insufficiency unless at the same time efforts were made to increase placental blood flow.

Fetal hormones

Understanding the role of fetal hormones in growth cannot be obtained simply by extrapolating backward from a knowledge of growth in the postnatal period. While it is true that birth represents only a milestone in a continuing process of growth and development, there are certain peculiarities of the intra-uterine existence that call for controlling mechanisms that differ, at least in emphasis, from those of the growing child. Reference has been made already to the likelihood that fetal growth, even in optimal circumstances, is constrained to a considerable degree. The healthy, well-nourished child, on the other hand, probably achieves his full potential for growth. In a subsequent section it will be pointed out that intra-uterine existence is a period of life characterised by the beginnings of developmental events, and activation of a variety of 'time-clocks' forms an important component of ordered growth. By contrast, growth of the child is based on physiological systems already active at birth; with the important exception of puberty, activation of new systems is not needed. The diet before and after birth differs in ways that would be expected to be associated with an altered profile of hormones; apart from a requirement of essential fatty acids for the synthesis of lipids the fetus obtains little lipid in its diet; calories available to the child from dietary fat are replaced by a greater utilisation of glucose in the fetus (Battaglia and Meschia, 1973).

Growth hormone

The prominent place of growth hormone in postnatal growth is not apparent in the fetus. Indeed, the human fetus appears to have the capacity to grow at a near normal velocity in the total absence of growth hormone (Liggins, 1974). A number of disorders are known in which levels of human pituitary growth hormone (hGH) are low, but in none is growth markedly impaired. Anencephaly is associated with mean cord blood hGH levels only about 20 per cent of those of normal babies (Grumbach and Kaplan, 1973), yet growth occurs at a rate that allows the anencephalic fetus to attain a normal birthweight during prolonged pregnancy. The fetus that has suffered spontaneous decapitation in early pregnancy may reach a birthweight of 2600 g (Swinburne, 1967). Even more striking is the lack of effect on birthweight of two disorders of hGH secretion reported by Laron and Pertzelan (1969). They described birth measurements in a group of three children with familial isolated hGH deficiency and another group of 11 children with the familial syndrome of pituitary dwarfism with high levels of inactive hGH. All but two of the children (both in the growth hormone (GH) deficiency group) were of normal birthweight, but eight were significantly short. The authors suggest that hGH influences skeletal growth but not the mass of soft tissues.

The relatively small effect of hGH deficiency is surprising in view of the high levels of hormone present in the blood of normal fetuses (Figure 14.2). Even at term when maximal levels are past (Grumbach and Kaplan, 1973), the concentration of hGH corresponds to basal adult values found only in acromegalics. Both the lack of dependence of growth on GH and the high levels of hormone in fetal blood are not peculiar to man. In none of the mammals such as rats and rabbits with short gestation periods has fetal decapitation been found to

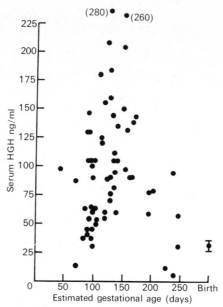

Figure 14.2. The concentration of hGH in umbilical cord serum of human fetuses. Note that peak values are attained at 100 to 150 days of pregnancy. Redrawn from Grumbach and Kaplan (1973) with kind permission of the authors and the publisher (London: Churchill).

cause growth retardation (Jost, 1966). Hypophysectomised fetal rhesus monkeys also grow at normal rates (Chez et al, 1970). On the other hand, fetuses that attain greater degrees of maturity at birth may show considerably retarded growth in the absence of pituitary function. Notable amongst these are fetal calves with pituitary hypoplasia (Kennedy, Kendrick and Stormont, 1957) and hypophysectomised fetal lambs (Liggins and Kennedy, 1968). In neither species, however, can the defective growth be attributed to growth hormone deficiency. Indeed, the fetuses have appearances more in keeping with thyroxine deficiency (see below).

Hoet (1969) considers that hGH may have the permissive role of increasing the glucose sensitivity of the pancreatic β-cell. In anencephalics born to normal mothers, the number of β-cells and the levels of insulin in cord blood are the same as those of controls. But anencephalics born to diabetic mothers fail to show the same increase in numbers of β-cells and in insulin levels found in normally formed fetuses of diabetic mothers. This relationship between hGH and insulin secretion could give hGH a minor share of the important place that insulin is thought to occupy in the hormonal control of growth.

Consideration of available evidence leads to the conclusion that hGH is not aptly named in the fetus—other hormones are better qualified for the title.

Thyroxine

The major role of thyroxine in cell metabolism would lead one to suspect that the fetal thyroid might make an important contribution to the regulation of fetal growth. At least in man, such seems not to be the case. Hypothyroid fetuses are usually of above average birthweight (Anderson, 1961), although they may show clear evidence of thyroxine deficien-

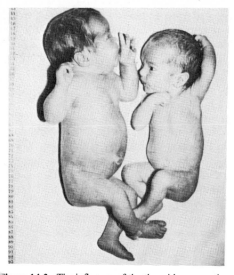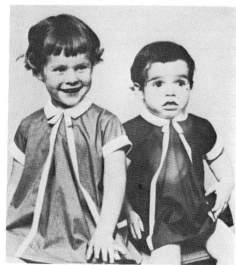

Figure 14.3. The influence of the thyroid on growth and development is illustrated in these two pairs of twins. In the photograph of the seven-day-old neonates, the large girl to the left had a birthweight of 4500 g, a birth length of 54 cm and prenatally retarded bone development. The thyroid gland was not palpable and radioiodine uptake was nil. Her sister had a birthweight of 2550 g, birth length of 49 cm and normal bone development and thyroid function. The photograph of the three-year-old twins shows a euthyroid girl on the left. Her untreated hypothyroid twin had a bone age of one year and the radioiodine uptake was five per cent. From Andersen (1961) with kind permission of the author and the editor of *Acta Paediatrica*.

y in the form of delayed maturation of the skeleton and nervous system (Figure 14.3). The thyroidectomised fetuses of rats and rabbits fail to show growth retardation, but this can be attributed to the short period of time from thyroidectomy to birth on the one hand and the long-lived biological effects of thyroxine on the other. Sheep fetuses thyroidectomised about seven weeks before birth show marked stunting of growth (Hopkins and Thorburn, 1972). This sharp discrepancy between the effects of absence of the fetal thyroid gland in man and in sheep is unlikely to result from a fundamental species difference in the functions of thyroxine, and another explanation must be sought. The difference is more likely to lie in the extent to which maternal thyroxine enters the fetus. The ovine placenta is almost completely impermeable to both thyroxine and triiodothyronine (Erenberg and Fisher, 1973; Thorburn and Hopkins, 1973). Thus the athyroid lamb is totally deprived of thyroxine. The human placenta is slightly permeable to thyroid hormones and it is for this reason that the classical signs of cretinism are seen in the newborn only when the function of the maternal thyroid, as well as the fetal, is deficient (Dussault et al, 1969). These observations suggest that small amounts of thyroxine are sufficient to maintain normal growth rates and that growth retardation is caused only by virtual absence of thyroxine. Excess thyroxine does not accelerate growth; indeed, the thyrotoxic fetus is likely to be small-for-dates (Samsamy, Jethwa and Ferriman, 1970).

The minimal effects of hypothyroidism on somatic growth of the human fetus should not be allowed to obscure the role of thyroxine in brain development. Ablation of the maternal and fetal thyroid gland by radioactive iodine administered to pregnant rhesus monkeys in mid-pregnancy reduces protein synthesis in the brain (Holt, Cheek and Kerr, 1973). Although the ratio of brain weight to body weight and the number of cells in the brain were found to be unaltered by thyroxine deficiency, there was depression of total RNA, total protein and of the activities of two enzymes concerned with protein synthesis (magnesium-dependent ATPase and carbonic anhydrase). The pattern of normal development of the fetal rhesus monkey brain is similar to that of the human in terms both of weight and composition. It is likely that the above observations apply equally well to the human (Cheek, 1975).

Insulin

Of the many factors causing birthweight to deviate from the mean, fetal insulin secretion appears to have the potential for inducing a wider range of variation than any other. On the one hand, birthweights of more than 6 kg can be associated with poorly controlled maternal diabetes, a state in which fetal hyperinsulinaemia is known to be present (Thomas, de Gasparo and Hoet, 1967). On the other hand, birthweights at term of 1250 g and 1800 g have been reported by Sherwood, Chance and Hill (1974) and Liggins (1974) respectively in diabetic neonates requiring insulin treatment who were presumably insulin-deficient during fetal life. Clinical evidence of this nature strongly suggests that insulin is the most important 'growth hormone' of the fetus.

Experimental evidence in animals supports the major role of insulin. Fetal injections of insulin in the rat cause an increase in both birthweight and total lipid content of the carcass (Picon, 1967). In sheep, the level of maternal nutrition has a positive correlation not only with birthweight but also with fetal insulin levels (Shelley, 1973; Bassett and Madill, 1974). Fetal rhesus monkeys made insulin-deficient by treatment with streptozotocin are growth retarded (Hill et al, 1972).

The function of insulin during fetal life differs from that after birth. The flow of glucose into the fetus is relatively constant because maternal blood levels are maintained within a narrow range by insulin secreted from the maternal pancreas. Thus the fetus has little need for the β-cells to be acutely responsive to glucose. In mid-pregnancy, glucose does not stimulate insulin release (Adam et al, 1969) and even at term the response is sluggish, resembling that of a diabetic (Oakley, Beard and Turner, 1972). Amino acids stimulate insulin secretion more vigorously than glucose, an observation which is consistent with insulin having an anabolic function in the fetus (Milner, Ashworth and Barson, 1972).

Although relatively unresponsive to short-term rises in glucose levels, the fetal pancreas is sensitive to more sustained hyperglycaemia and responds both by secretion and by β-cell hyperplasia. Increased responsiveness of the β-cell to glucose in fetal rats was observed after daily two-hour infusions of glucose to pregnant animals in the last five days of pregnancy (Asplund, 1970). β-cell hyperplasia is found in stillborn infants of women with mild gestational diabetes in whom hyperglycaemia is present for only short periods each day.

A prerequisite for enhanced growth in response to hyperinsulinaemia is the supply of additional substrate. Usually, the fact that elevated levels of substrate in the form of glucose is the cause of fetal hyperinsulinaemia ensures that the prerequisite will be met. Sometimes, however, the development of heightened responsiveness and hyperplasia of the β-cells in gestational diabetics is followed by progressive failure of placental perfusion as diabetic microangiopathy occludes the spiral arterioles of the decidua. The fetus may then become hypoglycaemic and be of low weight for gestational age. In such circumstances, there is a risk of intra-uterine death (Farquhar, 1959).

The action of insulin on cells is dependent on the presence of receptor sites for insulin and the degree of response to insulin is influenced by the concentration of receptor sites. Very little is known about insulin receptors in the fetus. It seems likely that the absence of response to insulin in early fetal life (Bocek and Beatty, 1969) is due to absence of receptors, but how their subsequent concentration varies with gestational age has not been investigated. The question is further complicated by the finding that insulin receptors are not specific to insulin but respond also to somatomedins (Hintz et al, 1972). The concentration of somatomedin in the blood of the overgrown fetus of the diabetic mother is unknown.

The fetal hyperglycaemia–hyperinsulinaemia theory of fetal obesity and hypersomia first proposed by Pedersen (1954) is not universally accepted. Attempts have been made to explain the occurrence of large babies born to women many years before the onset of diabetes by invoking mechanisms such as the passage into the fetus either of a synalbumin insulin antagonist (Vallance-Owen, McMaster and Bejaj, 1973) or of increased amounts of free fatty acids (Szabo and Szabo, 1974). Although it is unlikely that fetal overgrowth can be explained solely in terms of glucose and insulin, the evidence is overwhelming that they play the major roles.

Beckwith's syndrome

In case the impression has been gained that our knowledge of the major determinants of fetal growth is reasonably complete, it is salutary at this point to refer to Beckwith's syndrome, a bizarre syndrome of fetal overgrowth of which the cause is completely unknown (Beckwith, 1969). The most obvious features of the disorder are macroglossia, omphalocele and nephromegaly, but other evidences of cellular overgrowth are widespread. The birthweight is usually increased and somatic gigantism is the rule postnatally. With the exception of the thyroid, all of the endocrine organs, including the placenta, may show hyperplasia and cytomegaly. Siblings can be affected, the syndrome being transmitted as a genetic trait, probably of an autosomal recessive type.

The more severely affected fetuses abort in mid-pregnancy. Endocrine investigations of the less severely affected infants born near term have not been rewarding. It may well be that the abnormal drive to growth will be found by molecular biologists to be within the cells themselves.

Fetal kidney

Babies with renal agenesis (Potter's syndrome) are of low birthweight (Potter, 1965). The reason for this is unknown, but it does not seem to be due to the loss of the excretory function of the kidney. Electrolyte and urea concentrations in the plasma of fetal lambs are undisturbed by nephrectomy (Thorburn, 1974), presumably because the placenta is able to maintain electrolyte balance. However, growth of the lamb is considerably impaired (Table 4.1) and there is delay in bone development and in accumulation of liver glycogen. Thorburn considers that impaired growth could be due to interference with renal conversion of GH to a smaller active molecule. However, other possibilities exist. Fetal nephrectomy removes the source of renin, so that plasma renin activity in fetal lambs rapidly disappears after nephrectomy (Oakes, Catt and Chez, 1975). The effect of abnormally low levels of angiotensin II in the fetus is unknown, but it is possible that cardiovascular homeostasis is disturbed sufficiently to cause growth retardation. Another possibility needing investigation is that the absence of amniotic fluid, which invariably accompanies loss of renal function, could impair growth, perhaps by preventing fetal ingestion of amniotic fluid. The birthweight of fetuses unable to ingest amniotic fluid because of oesophageal atresia is reduced (Abbas and Tovey, 1960), but the mechanism is unknown; it could be due either to loss of calories usually acquired from amniotic fluid or to lack of stimulation of insulin secretion by gut hormones.

Table 14.1. *The effect of bilateral nephrectomy of the fetal lamb on body weight, estimated age and gestational age.*

Ewe No.	Treatment and sex of fetus		Gestational age		Body weight (g)	Estimated age (days)	Bone age (days)
			At operation	At delivery			
1	Nx	F	84	135	1380	107	127
	C	M			2700	120	132
2	Nx	F	85	134	1270	112	119
	C	F			2610	128	127
3	Nx	F	86	135	1700	113	122
	C	F			3130	134	132
4	Nx	M	87	135	2182	125	127
	C	F			2720	131	137
5	Nx	F	88	138	1750	114	131
	C	F			2530	128	140

The results are from five ewes carrying twin fetuses, one twin being nephrectomized (Nx), the other acting as control (C). From Thorburn (1974) with kind permission of the author and the publishers (Amsterdam Associated Scientific Publishers).

ENDOCRINE DEVELOPMENTAL CLOCKS

A distinction can be drawn between those developmental clocks in which the timing mechanism is activated by the genome itself and those in which the genome responds to a stimulus from hormones secreted by organs distant from the cells containing the activated enzymes. The former type of clock has already been considered in the earlier section on genetic control of growth and development; the latter type deserves separate consideration because it is potentially amenable to pharmacological modification, unlike the genetic clock which is relatively immutable.

A good example to illustrate the fundamental difference between the two varieties of developmental clock is afforded by hypothalamic imprinting of an androgen effect in male fetuses (see Chapter 1). In general, hypothalamic maturation is controlled by genetic information contained within the nerve cells. At a certain point in its development, the hypothalamus becomes susceptible to the effects of circulating androgen. If at that time the testis is programmed to secrete androgen, a permanent 'imprint' is left on the genomes of the hypothalamus such that a male, rather than a female, pattern of gonadotrophin secretion from the pituitary is ensured thereafter. The developing hypothalamus of the female fetus has precisely the same genetically determined susceptibility to androgen, but the endocrine clock is absent.

An endocrine clock of considerable clinical importance has been recognised in recent years. The fetal adrenal cortex has been shown to activate near term biochemical processes in various organs, both fetal and maternal, that are necessary for survival after birth.

Adrenocortical controlled preparations for birth

At birth, a critical situation develops that is usually, but not always, successfully resolved. On the one hand, the requirements of oxygen and calories increase abruptly to meet the demands for maintenance of body temperature and for the muscular exertion of respiratory effort, while on the other hand the accustomed source of oxygen and calories (the placenta) is suddenly lost. Functional maturation of the lungs and adequate stores of rapidly mobilisable calories are necessary if the newborn is to survive unharmed. There is evidence that cortisol plays an important part in ensuring that these needs are met.

Premature maturation of the embryonic intestine can be induced by treatment with cortisol. Moog and Kirsch (1955) noted this effect on alkaline phosphatase and other enzymes in explants of duodenum from chick embryos. Hayes (1965) observed accelerated morphological development of both the villus and the striated border in similarly treated cultures of duodenum. Intestinal invertase is also induced prematurely by cortisol (Doell and Kretchmer, 1964). Buckingham et al (1968) postulated that cortisol might have the same inductive effect on the developing lung because of the latter's embryological origin from foregut. Such proved to be the case and, as we shall see, other derivatives of the foregut are also responsive to cortisol.

Interest in the possibilities of the pharmacological use of glucocorticoids to induce precocious lung maturation in the human fetus (Liggins and Howie, 1973) has stimulated much basic investigation into the mode of action of corticosteroids on the developing lung. Cortisol has been found to enhance cell differentiation, which is manifested both morphologically and by specialisation of cell function. As is usual in developing tissues, differentiation occurs at the expense of cell division. The main target for the action of cortisol is the type II pneumocyte, which responds by a rapid accumulation of osmiophilic lamellar bodies containing surfactant material. Biochemical studies have shown that glucocorticoids act on the biosynthetic pathway of the phospholipid component of surfactant, dipalmitoyl

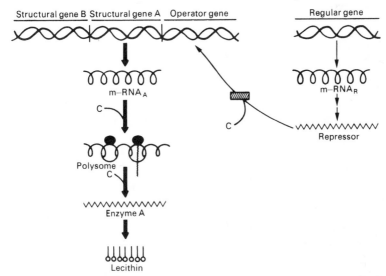

Figure 14.4. Possible molecular mechanisms for corticosteroid-mediated induction of enzymes in lung. Cortisol (C) is shown as interacting with a repressor protein, with some part of the ribosomal-mRNA-binding process and with the mechanism promoting release of newly synthesised enzyme from the polysome. Redrawn from Farrell (1973) with kind permission of the author and the publisher (New York: Academic Press).

lecithin, by inducing choline phosphotransferase (Farrell and Zachman, 1973), the enzyme controlling the final step in the synthesis of lecithin by the choline pathway. This property of glucocorticoids is not just a pharmacological curiosity, but probably has considerable physiological significance in the preparation of the lungs for breathing. Not only is cytodifferentiation of the type II pneumocyte delayed by fetal decapitation (Blackburn, 1973), but also there is a close relationship between the time-courses of the prepartum elevation of fetal corticosteroid levels and cytodifferentiation. Furthermore, developing lung contains a higher concentration of cytosol glucocorticoid receptors than any other fetal tissue (Ballard and Ballard, 1972). The manner in which cortisol transferred to the cell nucleus by cytosol receptor protein is thought to influence gene expression is shown in Figure 14.4.

Foregut derivatives include, in addition to the lungs, the liver and pancreas. In both of these organs, glucocorticoids can induce functional maturation. One of the earliest experiments in fetal endocrinology was described by Jost and Jacquot (1954) who showed that the rapid accumulation of liver glycogen normally preceding birth in fetal rats was prevented by fetal decapitation. Administration of a glucocorticoid after hypophysectomy restored glycogen accumulation. The concentration of glycogen in the liver of human fetuses also increases rapidly in the last month of pregnancy (Shelley and Neligan, 1966) and it is likely that it is related to the two or three-fold increase in the levels of corticosteroids in fetal blood occurring at the same time (Smith and Shearman, 1974). Certain liver enzymes, particularly tyrosine aminotransferase, are cortisol-inducible and become more active before birth. The relationship between liver glycogen content, the production of lecithin in the lung and fetal plasma cortisol concentration is shown in Figure 14.5.

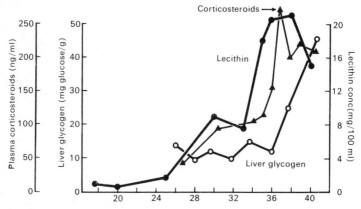

Figure 14.5. The time courses in human pregnancy of the concentrations of corticosteroids in umbilical cord plasma (data from Smith and Shearman, 1974), of lecithin in amniotic fluid (data from Gluck and Kulovich, 1973) and of glycogen in the fetal liver (data from Shelley and Neligan, 1966).

Reference has already been made to the lack of acute responsiveness of the human fetal pancreas to glucose. Although still sluggish in the newborn compared to the adult, the response does increase with advancing gestational age. In newborn lambs, the response is comparable to that of the adult, although shortly before term glucose elicits only a small release of insulin (Bassett and Thorburn, 1971). Stimulation of the immature fetal lamb adrenal with ACTH for three to four days converts the fetal type of pancreatic response to the adult type (Liggins and Rees, 1975). It seems likely that the surge of cortisol preceding the birth of the lamb is responsible for rapid maturation of the β-cells in anticipation of the need to regulate blood glucose levels soon after birth.

Mammalian preparations for birth would be incomplete without ensuring an ample supply of colostrum and milk. Many species depend for their survival not only on the food content of milk but also on passive immunity acquired from ingested antibodies. In such species, lactogenesis is initiated in advance of parturition through mechanisms controlled by cortisol secreted by the fetal adrenal. Elevated levels of cortisol cause a fall in the secretion of progesterone and a sharp rise in oestrogen. The maternal pituitary responds to these changes in levels of oestrogen and progesterone by secreting prolactin which, in turn, stimulates lactogenesis (Burd et al, 1975). In man, the fetal adrenal plays an important part in initiation of lactogenesis, but the mechanism is rather different from that of other species, being mediated by adrenal production of oestrogen precursors rather than of cortisol. In addition, absence of a prepartum fall in progesterone levels in women delays lactogenesis until progesterone secretion ceases with delivery of the placenta.

Finally, cortisol is the cornerstone of the mechanism by which the fetus initiates parturition and determines the timing of its birth. Although the evidence supporting this concept in the human fetus is largely circumstantial at present, it is firmly established in several experimental animals and there is detailed knowledge of the means by which fetal cortisol stimulates labour. In sheep, elevated levels of fetal cortisol cause an increase in placental secretion of oestrogen (Liggins and Howe, 1973). This action of cortisol probably depends on induction of two placental enzymes: one is a 17α-hydroxylase that acts on progesterone, the other is a 17–20 lyase that converts 17α-hydroxyprogesterone to a C 19 precursor of oestrogen (Anderson, Flint and Turnbull, 1975; Steele, Flint and Turnbull, 1975). Thus cortisol not only helps to prepare the fetus for birth but also causes birth when the preparations are complete.

CONCLUSION

Disorders of fetal growth and development form an important segment of the problems of obstetrics and neonatology. Accurate diagnosis and rational treatment (or preferably prevention) depend on a detailed understanding of normal fetal growth. This chapter has shown our knowledge to be superficial and fragmentary with little prospect that a sound basis for the treatment of fetal growth retardation is near at hand. The best that can be said is that those areas most deserving of research effort are becoming more clearly defined.

REFERENCES

Abbas, T. M. & Tovey, J. E. (1960) Proteins of the liquor amnii. *British Medical Journal*, i, 476–479.
Abdul-Karim, R. W. & Beydoun, S. N. (1974) Growth of the human fetus. *Clinical Obstetrics and Gynecology*, 17, 37–52.
Adam, P. A. J., Teramo, K., Raiha, N., Gitlin, D. & Schwartz, R. (1969) Human fetal insulin metabolism early in gestation: response to acute elevation of the fetal glucose concentration and placental transfer of human insulin—I-131. *Diabetes*, 18, 409–413.
Andersen, H. J. (1961) Studies of hypothyroidism in children. *Acta Paediatrica*, 50, Supplement 125, 1–150.
Anderson, A. B. M., Flint, A. P. F. & Turnbull, A. C. (1974) The mechanism of action of glucocorticoids on induction of ovine parturition: effect on placental steroid metabolism. *Journal of Endocrinology*, 66, 61–70.
Asplund, K. (1970) In *The Structure and Metabolism of the Pancreatic Islets* (Ed.) Falkmer, S., Hellman, B. & Taljedal, J. Oxford: Pergamon Press.

Ballard, P. K. & Ballard, R. A. (1972) Glucocorticoid receptors and the role of glucocorticoids in fetal lung development. *Proceedings of the National Academy of Sciences*, **69**, 2668–2672.

Bassett, J. M. & Madill, D. (1974) The influence of maternal nutrition on plasma hormone and metabolite concentrations of foetal lambs. *Journal of Endocrinology*, **61**, 465–477.

Bassett, J. M. & Thorburn, G. D. (1971) The regulation of insulin secretion by the ovine foetus in utero. *Journal of Endocrinology*, **50**, 59–74.

Battaglia, F. C. & Meschia, G. (1973) Foetal metabolism and substrate utilization. In *Foetal and Neonatal Physiology* (Ed.) Comline, R. S., Cross, K. W., Dawes, G. S. & Nathanielsz, P. W. pp. 382–397. London: Cambridge University Press.

Beckwith, J. B. (1969) Macroglossia, omphalocele, adrenal cytomegaly, gigantism and hyperplastic visceromegaly. *Birth Defects: Original Article Series*, **5**, 188–196.

Blackburn, W. R. (1973) Hormonal influences in fetal lung development. In *Respiratory Distress Syndrome* (Ed.) Villee, C. A., Villee, D. B. & Zuckerman, J. p. 271. New York: Academic Press.

Bocek, R. M. & Beatty, C. H. (1969) Effect of insulin on the carbohydrate metabolism of fetal rhesus monkey muscle. *Endocrinology*, **85**, 615–618.

Buckingham, S., McNary, W. F., Sommers, S. C. & Rothschild, J. (1968) Is lung an analog of Moog's developing intestine? I. Phosphatases and pulmonary alveolar differentiation in fetal rabbits. *Federation Proceedings*, **27**, 328.

Burd, L. I., Niswender, G. D., Lemons, J. A., Makowski, E. L. & Meschia, G. (1975) Relationship of mammary blood flow to parturition in the ewe. *Gynecologic Investigation*, **6**, 43.

Cheek, D. B. (1975) The growth of the brain. In *Fetal and Postnatal Cellular Growth* (Ed.) Cheek, D. B. pp. 3–22. New York: John Wiley.

Chez, R. A., Hutchinson, D. L., Salazar, H. & Mintz, D. H. (1970) Some effects of fetal and maternal hypophysectomy in pregnancy. *American Journal of Obstetrics and Gynecology*, **108**, 643–650.

Doell, R. C. & Kretchmer, N. (1964) Intestinal invertase: precocious development of activity after injection of hydrocortisone. *Science*, **143**, 42–44.

Donald, H. P. (1939) Sources of variation in human birth weights. *Proceedings of the Royal Society of Edinburgh*, **54B**, 91–108.

Dussault, J. H., Row, V. V., Lickrish, G. & Volpe, R. (1969) Studies of serum triiodothyronine concentration in maternal and cord blood transfer of triiodothyronine across the human placenta. *Journal of Clinical Endocrinology*, **29**, 595–603.

Erenberg, A. & Fisher, D. A. (1973) Thyrid hormone metabolism in the foetus. In *Foetal and Neonatal Physiology* (Ed.) Comline, R. S., Cross, K. W., Dawes, G. S. & Nathanielsz, P. W. pp. 508–526. London: Cambridge University Press.

Farquhar, J. W. (1959) The child of the diabetic woman. *Archives of Diseases in Childhood*, **34**, 76–96.

Farrell, P. M. (1973) Regulation of pulmonary lecithin synthesis. In *Respiratory Distress Syndrome* (Ed.) Villee, C. A., Villee, D. B. & Zuckerman, J. pp. 311–341. New York: Academic Press.

Farrell, P. M. & Zachman, R. D. (1973) Induction of choline phosphotransferase and lecithin synthesis in the fetal lung by corticosteroids. *Science*, **179**, 297–298.

Finne, P. H. (1967) On placental transfer of erythropoietin. *Acta Paediatrica Scandinavica*, **56**, 233–242.

Fisch, R. O., Prem, K. A., Feinberg, S. B. & Gehrz, R. C. (1974) Acromegaly in a gravida and her infant. *Obstetrics and Gynecology*, **43**, 861–866.

Gluck, L. & Kulovich, M. V. (1973) Lecithin/sphingomyelin ratios in amniotic fluid in normal and abnormal pregnancy. *American Journal of Obstetrics and Gynecology*, **115**, 539–546.

Grumbach, M. M. & Kaplan, S. L. (1973) Ontogenesis of growth hormone, insulin, prolactin and gonadotropin secretion in the human fetus. In *Foetal and Neonatal Physiology* (Ed.) Comline, R. S., Cross, K. W., Dawes, G. S. & Nathanielsz, P. W. pp. 462–487. London: Cambridge University Press.

Hayes, R. L. (1965) The maturation of cortisone-treated embryonic duodenum in vitro. *Journal of Embryology and Experimental Morphology*, **14**, 169–179.

Hill, D. E., Holt, A. B., Reba, R. & Cheek, D. B. (1972) Alterations in the growth pattern of fetal rhesus monkeys following the *in utero* injection of streptozotocin. *Pediatric Research*, **6**, 336 (abstract).

Hintz, R. L., Clemmons, D. R., Underwood, L. E. & Van Wyk, J. J. (1972) Competitive binding of somatomedin to the insulin receptors of adipocytes, chondrocytes and liver membranes. *Proceedings of the National Academy of Sciences*, **69**, 2351–2353.

Hoet, J. J. (1969) Normal and abnormal fetal weight gain. In *Foetal Autonomy* (Ed.) Wolstenholme, G. E. W. & O'Connor, M. pp. 186–213. London: Churchill.

Holliday, R. & Pugh, J. E. (1975) DNA modification mechanisms and gene activity during development. *Science*, **187**, 226–232.

Holt, A. B., Cheek, D. B. & Kerr, G. R. (1973) Prenatal hypothyroidism and brain composition in a primate. *Nature*, **243**, 413–415.

Hopkins, P. S. & Thorburn, G. D. (1972) The effects of foetal thyroidectomy on the development of the ovine foetus. *Journal of Endocrinology*, **54**, 55–56.

Hunter, G. L. (1956) Maternal influence on size in sheep. *Journal of Agricultural Science*, **48**, 36–60.

Jost, A. (1966) In *The Pituitary Gland* (Ed.) Harris, G. W. & Donovan, B. T. pp. 299–323. London: Butterworth.

Jost, A. & Jacquot, R. (1954) Recherches sur le contrôle hormonal de la charge en glycogène du foie foetal du lapin et du rat. *Comptes Rendu Hebdomadaire des Séances de l'Academie des Sciences*, **239**, 98–100.

Kennedy, P. C., Kendrick, J. W. & Stormont, C. (1957) Adenohypophyseal aplasia, an inherited defect associated with abnormal gestation in Guernsey cattle. *Cornell Veterinarian*, **47**, 160–178.

Laron, Z. & Pertzelan, A. (1969) Somatotrophin in antenatal and perinatal growth and development. *Lancet*, **i**, 680–681.

Liggins, G. C. (1974) The influence of the fetal hypothalamus and pituitary on growth. In *Size at Birth* (Ed.) Elliott, K. & Knight, J. pp. 165–183. Amsterdam: Associated Scientific Publishers.

Liggins, G. C. & Howie, R. N. (1973) A controlled trial of antepartum glucocorticoid treatment for prevention of the respiratory distress syndrome in premature infants. *Pediatrics*, **50**, 515–525.

Liggins, G. C. & Kennedy, P. C. (1968) Effects of electrocoagulation of the fetal lamb hypophysis on growth and development. *Journal of Endocrinology*, **40**, 371–381.

Liggins, G. C. & Rees, L. (1975) The effect of adrenal stimulation on the insulin response to glucose in the fetal lamb. Proceedings of the New Zealand Society of Endocrinology, 11th Annual Scientific Meeting, Massey, 1974. *New Zealand Medical Journal*, **81**, 486–490.

Liggins, G. C., Fairclough, R. J., Grieves, S. A., Kendall, J. Z. & Knox, B. S. (1972) The mechanisms of initiation of parturition in the ewe. *Recent Progress in Hormone Research*, **29**, 111–159.

Love, E. J. & Kinch, R. A. H. (1965) Factors affecting the birthweight in normal pregnancy. *American Journal of Obstetrics and Gynecology*, **91**, 342–349.

McCance, R. A. & Widdowson, E. M. (1974) The determinants of growth and form. *Proceedings of the Royal Society of London*, **185B**, 1–17.

Meredith, H. C. (1970) Body weights of viable human infants. A worldwide comparative treatise. *Human Biology*, **42**, 217–264.

Milner, R. D. G., Ashworth, M. A. & Barson, A. H. (1972) Insulin release from human fetal pancreas in response to glucose, lecithin and arginine. *Journal of Endocrinology*, **52**, 497–505.

Moog, F. & Kirsch, M. H. (1955) Quantitative determination of phosphatase activity in chick embryo duodenum culture fluid media with and without hydrocortisone. *Nature*, **175**, 722–723.

Morton, N. E. (1955) The inheritance of human birthweight. *Annals of Human Genetics*, **20**, 125–134.

Oakes, G. K., Catt, K. J. & Chez, R. A. (1975) Sheep plasma renin activity after fetal nephrectomy. *Gynaecologic Investigation*, **6**, 17.

Oakley, N. W., Beard, R. W. & Turner, R. C. (1972) Effect of sustained maternal hyperglycaemia on the fetus in normal and diabetic pregnancies. *British Medical Journal*, **i**, 466–469.

Osinski, P. A. (1960) Steroid 11β-oldehydrogenase in human placenta. *Nature*, **187**, 777–778.

Ounsted, C. & Ounsted, M. (1970) Effect of Y-chromosome on fetal growth rate. *Lancet*, **ii**, 857–858.

Ounsted, M. (1971) Fetal growth. In *Recent Advances in Paediatrics* (Ed.) Gairdner, D. & Hull, D. pp. 2–62. London: Churchill.

Ounsted, M. & Ounsted, C. (1966) Maternal regulation of intrauterine growth. *Nature*, **212**, 995–997.

Pedersen, J. (1954) Weight and length at birth of infants of diabetic mothers. *Acta Endocrinologica*, **16**, 330–341.

Penrose, L. S. (1961) In *Recent Advances in Human Genetics* (Ed.) Penrose, L. S. p. 56. London: Churchill.

Picon, L. (1967) Effect of insulin on growth and biochemical composition of the rat fetus. *Endocrinology*, **81**, 1419–1421.

Polani, P. E. (1974) Chromosomal and other genetic influences on birthweight variation. In *Size at Birth* (Ed.) Elliott, K. & Knight, J. pp. 127–164. Amsterdam: Associated Scientific Publishers.

Potter, E. L. (1965) Bilateral absence of the ureters and kidneys. *Obstetrics and Gynecology*, **25**, 3–12.

Ramsamy, B., Jethwa, A. K. N. & Ferriman, D. (1970) Congenital thyrotoxicosis. *Proceedings of the Royal Society of Medicine*, **63**, 577–578.

Shelley, H. J. (1973) The use of chronically catheterized foetal lambs for the study of foetal metabolism. In *Foetal and Neonatal Physiology. Barcroft Centenary Symposium* (Ed.) Comline, R. S., Cross, K. W., Dawes, G. S. & Nathanielsz, P. W. pp. 360–381. London: Cambridge University Press.

Shelley, H. J. & Neligan, G. A. (1966) Neonatal hypoglycaemia. *British Medical Bulletin*, **22**, 34–39.

Sherwood, W. G., Chance, G. W. & Hill, D. E. (1974) A new syndrome of pancreatic agenesis. *Pediatric Research*, **8**, 360.

Smidt, D., Steinbach, J. & Scheven, B. (1967) Die Beeinflussung der pra- und postnatalen Entwicklung durch Grosse und Korpergewicht der Mutter, largestellr an Ergebnissen reziproker Eitransplantatonen zwischen Zwergschweinen und grossen Hausschweinen. *Monatsschrift für Kinderheilkunde*, **115**, 533–545.

Smith, I. D. & Shearman, R. P. (1974) Fetal plasma steroids in relation to parturition. I. The effect of gestational age upon umbilical plasma corticosteroid levels following vaginal delivery. *Journal of Obstetrics and Gynaecology of the British Commonwealth*, **81**, 11–19.

Speroff, L. (1973) An essay: prostaglandins and toxemia of pregnancy. *Prostaglandins*, **3**, 721–728.

Steele, P. A., Flint, A. P. F. & Turnbull, A. C. (1975) Evidence of steroid $C_{17,20}$ lyase activity in ovine foeto placental tissue. *Journal of Endocrinology*, **64,** 41P.

Summerbell, D., Lewis, J. & Wolpert, L. (1973) Positional information in chick limb morphogenesis. *Nature* **244,** 492–496.

Sunshine, P., Kusumoto, H. & Kriss, J. P. (1965) Survival time of LATS in neonatal thyrotoxicosis: implication for diagnosis and therapy of the disorder. *Pediatrics*, **36,** 869–876.

Swinburne, L. M. (1967) Spontaneous intrauterine decapitation. *Archives of Disease in Childhood*, **42,** 636–641

Szabo, A. J. & Szabo, O. (1974) Placental free-fatty-acid transfer and fetal adipose-tissue development: a explanation of fetal adiposity in infants of diabetic mothers. *Lancet*, **ii,** 498–499.

Thomas, K., Gasparo, M. de & Hoet, J. J. (1967) Insulin levels in the umbilical vein and in the umbilical artery o normal and gestational diabetic mothers. *Diabetologia*, **3,** 299–304.

Thorburn, G. D. (1974) The role of the thyroid gland and kidneys in fetal growth. In *Size at Birth* (Ed.) Elliott, K & Knight, J. p. 185. Amsterdam: Associated Scientific Publishers.

Thorburn, G. D. & Hopkins, P. S. (1973) In *Foetal and Neonatal Physiology. Barcroft Centenary Symposiun* (Ed.) Comline, R. S., Cross, K. W., Dawes, G. S. & Nathanielsz, P. W. pp. 488–507. London: Cambridg University Press.

Vallance-Owen, J., McMaster, D. & Bajaj, J. S. (1973) Maternal synalbumin antagonism and large babies *Lancet*, **ii,** 358–359.

Venge, O. (1950) Maternal influence on birth weight in rabbits. *Acta Zoologica*, **31,** 1–8.

Walton, A. & Hammond, J. (1938) The maternal effects on growth and conformation in Shire horse–Shetlan pony crosses. *Proceedings of the Royal Society of London*, **125B,** 311–335.

15

FETAL GROWTH

Stuart Campbell

The factors which control normal fetal growth and development are not fully understood, but they certainly involve a complex interplay between genetic, immunological, endocrinological, nutritional and vascular influences. It is likely that a disturbance of any one of these controlling factors could cause abnormal fetal growth but the degree to which each of these elements contributes to this problem is at present difficult to evaluate. It is clearly important that the obstetrician should recognise abnormal fetal growth during the antenatal period, for both growth retardation and growth acceleration carry increased risks for the fetus. Growth-retarded babies in particular are associated with a significant increase in perinatal mortality (Gruenwald, 1969), intrapartum asphyxia (Low, Boston and Pancham, 1972) and are at increased risk in the neonatal period from pulmonary haemorrhage, hypoglycaemia, hypocalcaemia, hypothermia and fetal abnormality (Bard, 1970). In the long term there is evidence that a proportion of such babies continues to grow poorly after birth (Fitzhardinge and Stephen, 1972a; Bjerre, 1975), while a small number subsequently have educational difficulties (Fitzhardinge and Stephen, 1972b). Early and accurate recognition of fetal growth retardation will therefore reduce perinatal mortality and morbidity by permitting the delivery of the fetus at the optimal time to give the best chance of survival and the lowest risk of adverse sequelae. In the future it may also be possible to select those fetuses suitable for antenatal therapy to combat or counteract the effect of growth-retarding stimuli.

FETAL GROWTH

Definitions

A low-birthweight baby is defined as being 2.5 kg or less at birth and one-third of these are
due to growth retardation (Butler and Alberman, 1969). Recognition of the growth-retarded
baby at birth is vital so that the various associated complications can be anticipated and so
that mortality and morbidity data can be studied for this group of infants. Diagnostic
problems arise, however, because growth-retarded babies exhibit a wide spectrum of clinical
features reflecting the differing pathogenesis of the condition. Definition of this group is
therefore usually made on a basis of weight for menstrual age, hence the terms 'small-for
dates' and 'light-for-dates'. Babies whose birthweights fall on or below the 5th centile, or
alternatively two standard deviations of the mean (approximately 3rd centile), are usually
classified as light-for-dates. The 10th centile limit is also used by some workers but it is likely
that with this definition the growth-retarded population is being diluted by a large number of
babies of normal nutrition. It is essential in any study of light-for-dates babies to state the
centile limit being used and to classify every baby by using a chart whose data represent a
population of similar nutritional status and ethnic origin. Furthermore, classification should
include corrections for fetal sex, maternal parity and (where possible) maternal weight and
stature. Such an arbitrary classification must obviously include some babies that are not
growth-retarded; conversely, many growth-retarded babies will be excluded by the defini
tion. For example, a baby who by achieving its full growth potential would become 4 kg at
term may receive less than the optimal growth support from the mother and be only 3 kg.
This baby would fall outside the definition of light-for-dates but would be growth-retarded. It
is likely, however, that most severe cases of growth retardation will be included within the
light-for-dates definition and for practical purposes these terms should be regarded as
synonymous (see also Chapter 19).

Another system of classification frequently used in paediatric epidemiological surveys is
to take all low-birthweight babies and to arbitrarily divide them into preterm (36 weeks or
less) and mature (37 weeks or more) groupings; light-for-dates babies would fall into the se
cond group and preterm babies into the first. This system is simple to operate but does mis
classify the ten per cent of light-for-dates babies which are delivered before 37 weeks gesta
tion (Usher and McLean, 1974). It is, however, the only method of comparing the incidence
of fetal growth retardation in populations of different ethnic origin and socioeconomic status
For example, if the appropriate weight for gestation charts are used, the number of babies
below the 5th centile would be the same in the United Kingdom as in Guatemala (i.e. five pe
cent); the number of mature low-birthweight babies, however, would be at least four time
greater in the Guatemalan population.

A growth-accelerated baby is generally defined as being either above the 95th centile or
standard deviations (approximately 97th centile) above the mean weight for the menstrua
age of the fetus. This definition will include babies of excessive weight due to fluid retention
such as the hydrops of rhesus disease, and care should be taken to exclude these babies from
epidemiological studies of true growth acceleration.

Assessment of fetal growth

Information on fetal growth in the human can be obtained directly by ultrasonic measure ment during the antenatal period. Before discussing this technique, we will briefly review less direct ways of studying fetal growth and the information that has accrued from such studies. Intra-uterine growth of the human fetus can be charted by plotting birth dimensions and birthweight against the menstrual age of the fetus. Earlier in this century such data were obtained from postmortem specimens (Scammon and Calkins, 1929) but the information was misleading because it was largely obtained from pathologic material and because of artefactual errors (Campbell, 1970). There are now numerous published weight-for-gestation charts (Gruenwald, 1966; Thomson, Billewicz and Hytten, 1968; Freeman, Graves and Thomson, 1970; Sterky, 1970; Cheng, Chew and Ratnam, 1972) based on data obtained from liveborn infants which give the normal growth patterns for different ethnic and social groups. Criticisms can be made on two counts: first, that it is not valid to derive longitudinal growth patterns from cross-sectional data, and second, that babies delivered before 36 weeks cannot be representative of a 'normal' population. The first criticism can be discounted if large numbers of babies are used in the compilation of the graphs and care is taken to exclude those babies of uncertain menstrual age, but the second criticism would appear to be valid; weight for gestation charts show exponential growth up to 28 weeks (Lubchenco et al, 1963; Milner and Richards, 1974) which is refuted by all ultrasonic growth charts of all fetal dimensions (vide infra). After 34 weeks menstrual age, however, meaningful information on fetal growth can be derived from these charts.

Information on human fetal growth can also be obtained from animal studies but they have to be interpreted with care in view of wide species differences in the duration of pregnancy, in the timing of the growth spurts of the various organs and in the placental architecture. Animal studies have, however, contributed to our knowledge of growth at a cellular level. Cellular growth can occur as a result of an increase in cell number (hyperplasia), cell size (hypertrophy) or a simultaneous increase in both. Assuming that DNA resides exclusively in the nucleus and that the amount is constant within the diploid cell of a given species, it follows that total DNA content is an index of cell hyperplasia, while mean cell size (protein/DNA) is an index of hypertrophy, and DNA concentration (DNA/weight) is a function of both hyperplasia and hypertrophy. Bearing in mind the different time scales involved in animal studies, important information on fetal cellular response to maternal and placental 'insults' has been obtained. In the human, information on cellular growth can also be gathered from abortuses and stillbirths.

Normal fetal growth

Two basic factors govern the velocity of fetal growth: the intrinsic growth potential of the fetus, which is genetically determined, and the growth support it receives via mother and placenta (Gruenwald, 1966). From animal data the intra-uterine growth of the fetus describes a sigmoid curve (Widdowson, 1970) and it is likely that human fetal growth follows a similar pattern. The weight-for-gestation charts show that fetal growth is linear from 28 to about 38 weeks, after which there is a gradual reduction in growth rate to term, with only minimal growth thereafter. This is also true for other fetal dimensions (Usher and McLean, 1969). Gruenwald (1966) believes that if maternal growth support were unlimited, the growth rate of the fetus would proceed in a linear fashion past term and that one of the factors limiting growth potential is the diminution of supplies from the mother. In other words, there is a physiological utero-placental insufficiency from 38 weeks onwards. His view is supported by the fact that the immediate postnatal growth of the fetus quickly accelerates to the pre-38 weeks growth rate once it has been released from the constraints of the uterine environment, and that preterm babies do not follow the intra-uterine growth pattern. From this evidence it would seem that birthweight is determined by the slope of the growth potential line and the gestational age at which maternal growth support fails to maintain optimal fetal growth. Gruenwald (1966) demonstrated that in countries with the largest babies, such as Sweden, the deviation from the growth potential line occurs later in pregnancy than in countries with less well-nourished communities or social groupings.

Growth at a cellular level has been studied in the rat by Enesco and Leblond (1962) and Winick and Noble (1965). They described three stages of growth: first, a period when growth is entirely due to cell hyperplasia; second, a phase when growth is both by hyperplasia (now slower) and hypertrophy; and lastly, a phase when growth is entirely by hypertrophy. In the rat, hyperplastic growth occurs throughout the antenatal period and ceases postnatally, earliest in the brain and latest in muscle. In man less information is available, but the pattern is thought to be similar although over an extended time scale. Thus Dobbing and Sands (1970) found that cell hyperplasia ceased in the human brain during the second postnatal year while Cheek (1968) observed the continuing addition of muscle cells to 16 years of age. The importance of brain growth in determining the future intellectual status of the individual is obvious, but there is also evidence from animal studies that somatic stunting occurs if restriction is imposed during the brain growth spurt rather than during that of body growth (Dobbing, 1974). Brain growth would therefore appear to have an overriding influence on all aspects of human development. Dobbing and Sands (1973) from studies on abortuses obtained from legal termination of pregnancy, stillbirths and neonatal deaths, described two phases of accelerated brain growth: one from 12 to 18 weeks menstrual age, which is due to neuroblast proliferation, and the second from 25 weeks onwards which is the result of glial proliferation. Thus neuronal hyperplasia occurs during a highly protected phase of fetal growth. In addition to glial proliferation, many important changes are occurring in the late fetal brain such as myelination, dendritic arborisation and synapse formation which can have profound influence on intellectual development. The cerebellar growth spurt which begins in late pregnancy (30 weeks menstrual age) is more rapid than that of the forebrain, finishing by the end of the first postnatal year. In the placenta, growth by cell division ceases about four weeks before term, thereafter placental cellular growth being by hypertrophy (Winick and Noble, 1967).

Growth retardation

Light-for-dates babies can result from a reduction of the normal growth potential of the fetus or (more commonly) from inadequate maternal support for fetal growth. Reduced growth potential can result from chromosomal or genetic abnormality of the fetus or from viral infection such as rubella or cytomegalic inclusion disease during the process of organogenesis, resulting in a permanent loss of cells. The hypoplasia affects all organs equally but the placental size is usually unaffected (Winick, 1971).

Lack of maternal growth support can manifest itself in many ways but essentially all mechanisms cause (singly or in combination) a reduction in the supply to the fetus of amino acids for protein synthesis, glucose for energy requirements and oxygen for the various metabolic processes. The effect of growth retardation on the fetus is, however, very much determined by the particular aetiological mechanism and by its severity and duration.

On epidemiological grounds there is substantial evidence to support the theory of Ounsted and Ounsted (1966) who postulate that slow intra-uterine growth is due in part to constraint exercised by the maternal system operating through the predetermined setting of a maternal regulator (see Chapter 14). This hypothesis is supported by the epidemiological study of

Johnstone and Inglis (1974). The mechanism by which this growth restraint is imposed is obscure but it may involve some maternal limitation of trophoblastic invasion with a consequent reduction in the surface area available for placental transfer. This does not imply any vascular insufficiency, merely that a small placenta will result in a small baby.

Mechanisms of much more immediate practical import to the clinician can be conveniently allocated by virtue of their short and long-term effects to one of three groups, namely utero-placental vascular insufficiency, maternal undernutrition and chronic hypoxia.

Utero-placental vascular insufficiency is associated with such varied conditions as pre-eclampsia, essential hypertension, severe diabetes mellitus, chronic renal disease, multiple pregnancy and late recurrent bleeding from a normally situated placenta. In Western communities vascular insufficiency is the most commonly recognised cause of growth retardation because it often presents as an acute obstetrical problem with a high associated perinatal mortality rate. It is, however, important to realise that utero-placental vascular insufficiency in clinically recognisable form is not the major cause of inadequate maternal growth support. Low and Galbraith (1974) found that pre-eclampsia was a complicating factor in only ten per cent of their growth-retarded pregnancies while all forms of vascular insufficiency accounted for 31 per cent. These figures are supported by those of other workers (Dawes, 1974). Utero-placental vascular insufficiency results in a reduction of placental perfusion with a consequent decrease in the transfer rates of glucose, amino acids (Young, 1974) and oxygen (Longo, 1972). In this type of growth retardation the effects are to some extent mitigated by a redistribution of the fetal blood flow which results in a preferential perfusion of the fetal brain. This has been elegantly shown in the experiments on the pregnant ewe by Assali and Brinkman (1973) and Creasy et al (1974), the former by inducing maternal hypotension, the latter by injecting embolising microspheres. Both techniques resulted in a reduction in the utero-placental blood flow and oxygen transfer; this fall in fetal Po_2 is sensed by oxygen receptors in the ductus venosus and pulmonary vascular bed resulting in a diversion of blood from the pulmonary to the systemic circuits, and maintaining an effective cardiac output. The fall in Po_2 also resulted in the redistribution of blood to the fetal brain.

It has long been held that in developed countries, under-nutrition is an unlikely cause of fetal growth retardation. This appears to be supported by the classic studies of the 1944–1945 famine in Holland when the daily nutritional intake fell below 1000 calories and 40 g protein for a period of 27 weeks. Despite the severe insult, a reduction in the median birthweight only occurred when the nutritional deprivation occurred in the second half of pregnancy and then by a mere 240 g. Furthermore, there was no increase in neonatal mortality and long-term follow-up studies revealed no intellectual deficit in the undernourished group. On a world scale, however, maternal undernutrition is by far the commonest cause of fetal growth retardation. Lechtig et al (1975) in studies on a rural Guatemalan population with an incidence of low birthweight of 40 per cent have shown that women with the stigmata of severe undernutrition in childhood have a high incidence of low-birthweight babies and that there is a strong correlation between reduced maternal dietary intake and low birthweight. These low-birthweight infants had a four-fold increase in mortality during the first year of life. In this study dietary supplements resulted in a significant reduction in the number of low-birthweight infants. Thus maternal undernutrition appears to have a significant effect on fetal growth and perinatal mortality rates only if there is evidence of chronic undernutrition prior to pregnancy. Laga, Driscoll and Munro (1972) demonstrated that the principal effect of maternal undernutrition is to reduce placental size and showed a 24 per cent reduction in peripheral villous mass in a low social class urban Guatemalan population when compared with a middle class North American population. This deficit was attributed to a reduction in the number of villi rather than the dimension of the individual villi. Lechtig et al (1975) in their Guatemalan studies confirmed that these placental changes were due to maternal undernutrition and demonstrated that dietary supplements resulted in an increase in placental weight. Thus the mechanism whereby maternal undernutrition retards fetal growth would seem to involve a reduction in the placental surface area available for the exchange of nutrients. That this mechanism could be a factor in the aetiology of fetal growth retardation in Western communities is suggested by the fact that prepregnant maternal weight and pregnancy weight gain are the maternal factors which correlate most strongly with birthweight (Rush, Davis and Susser, 1972; Wehmer and Hafez, 1975). Naeye, Blanc and Paul (1973) performed autopsies on 467 stillborn babies having excluded those cases where there was a maternal or fetal disorder known to influence birthweight, such as fetal anomaly, diabetes or pregnancy hypertension. They found that mothers with the stigmata of chronic undernutrition (low prepregnancy weight) and undernutrition during pregnancy (low pregnancy weight gain) delivered babies of significantly lower weight than overweight mothers with a high pregnancy weight gain. The significance of these two factors was independent of social class, race, marital status, stature and other socioeconomic factors.

Chronic low-grade maternal hypoxia is probably a factor in limiting fetal growth. The median term birthweight in Lake County, Colorado in 1955 (10 000 feet) was 3.07 kg while at Denver (5000 feet) it was 3.29 kg and in Baltimore (sea level) 3.32 kg (Lichty et al, 1957). The low mean weight in the high altitude group was possibly related to hypoxia as the mothers in the study were matched for racial and nutritional factors. Babies born to women who smoke during pregnancy are significantly smaller than those born to non-smokers, which may be further evidence that hypoxia is a growth-retarding stimulus. Butler, Goldstein and Ross (1972) in a review of cases from the 1958 British Perinatal Mortality Survey found that the birthweight was reduced on average by 170 g (all other variables being equal) and that the reduction of birthweight was related to the number of cigarettes smoked and the duration of insult. The perinatal mortality was also raised but not as much as for light-for-dates babies in the same survey. Cole, Hawkins and Roberts (1972) demonstrated that the carbon monoxide in cigarette smoke caused not only significantly raised levels of carboxyhaemoglobin, which reduces the oxygen carrying capacity of fetal blood, but also a shift to the left in the haemoglobin dissociation curve, thus impairing the transfer of oxygen to the tissues. Although the fetal response to chronic hypoxia is an increase in haematocrit (Younoszai, Kacic and Haworth, 1968), this is unlikely to compensate for carboxyhaemoglobin levels as high as 20 per cent (Cole, Hawkins and Roberts, 1972) which can be even further aggravated in the presence of maternal anaemia (Dow, Rooney and Spence, 1975).

The effects of these mechanisms in limiting fetal growth can be better understood by studying their effect at a cellular level. Growth retardation during the hyperplastic phase limits cell division, leading to fewer cells and smaller organs than expected. The loss of cells is permanent, being proportional to the length of the period of undernutrition and the rate of cell division during this period. Undernutrition during the hypertrophic phase causes a reduction in cell size and again smaller organs, but the process is reversible. As human fetal growth is entirely hyperplastic, one would expect an insult during the antenatal period to result in a permanent loss of cells, especially if this occurs during a growth spurt. This hypothesis has been confirmed by Winick, Brasel and Velasco (1973) in rats and by Hill et al (1971) in Rhesus monkeys. Winick (1971) has contrasted the brain-sparing effect of vascular insufficiency with the symmetrical growth retardation pattern which results from maternal protein restriction. Extrapolation of this experimental data to the human situation must be made with extreme caution for two reasons. First, as the rate of cell division is slower in the human, the effects of maternal undernutrition will be less severe over the same time period (Payne and Wheeler, 1967). Second, unlike the rat, neuroblast proliferation occurs in the human at a time when growth-retarding stimuli do not usually operate (i.e. before 20 weeks menstrual age). On the other hand, retardation of cell division in late pregnancy in the human could have effects on cerebellar growth, dendritic arborisation and synapse formation which could be as important in the development of brain function as in neuronal cell number (Dobbing, 1974). Certainly there is definite evidence that the fetal brain in maternal undernutrition is less well protected than it is in utero-placental vascular insufficiency. In the previously mentioned study of Naeye, Blanc and Paul (1973) the brain weights of fetuses born after 33 weeks to the low maternal weight, low weight gain group were significantly lower than those of the high maternal weight, high weight gain patients. Dobbing (personal communication, 1975) reported a reduction in brain DNA content and brain weight in babies stillborn as a result of the 1974 famine in Ethiopia and that this deficit increased progressively after 32 weeks menstrual age. These data are particularly valuable in view of the reliable menstrual data provided by this community. Dobbing believes that the effects of prenatal undernutrition on brain growth could be reversed providing postnatal feeding was adequate; this however rarely occurs in underdeveloped countries. The educational handicap suffered by the children of heavy smokers (Davie, Butler and Goldstein, 1972) may indicate that chronic hypoxia does not provoke the same compensating fetal circulatory response as vascular insufficiency. Much work has to be done to elucidate the different effects that these mechanisms have on fetal growth and in particular brain growth. This subject is further discussed in the section on the measurement of fetal growth.

Growth acceleration

Growth acceleration causes few problems to the fetus as compared with growth retardation, although when associated with maternal diabetes mellitus it still carries a significantly raised perinatal loss (Brudenell and Beard, 1972). Most large babies are however unassociated with the diabetic state. Ounsted (1971) found that when the maternal growth-restraining factor was relaxed, other factors emerged to determine the fetal growth rate. In her growth-accelerated series she found that the mothers were older, of greater parity, taller and heavier than controls. Furthermore, the genetic influence of the father emerged as an important growth-determining factor; the mean birthweights of the fathers of growth-accelerated infants were even higher than those of the mothers. Maternal diabetes results in an increased intra-uterine growth rate of the fetus. This hyperplastic growth affects the whole fetus but in particular the fat (Osler, 1960) and body organs (Jackson, 1967). The placenta also shows evidence of hyperplasia (Winick, 1971). The role of insulin as a growth-accelerating factor has been mentioned in Chapter 8 by Beard and Oakley.

ANTENATAL MEASUREMENT OF FETAL GROWTH

Measuring the fetal growth rate involves the taking of accurate sequential fetal measurements. At present only x-ray and ultrasound are capable of providing readings sufficiently accurate for this purpose. As serial measurements by x-ray are clearly inadvisable on account of the radiation hazards to the fetus, ultrasound remains the only technique available for assessing the fetal growth rate. It is frequently observed that the various placental hormone and enzyme tests are means of assessing fetal growth but this is quite untrue; these tests reflect the integrity of the feto-placental unit and it would be most unwise to infer fetal growth rates from them. A crude assessment of the growth rate by abdominal palpation is of course practised daily in every obstetric unit in the country. Assessment of fetal size by this method is inexact and subjective because of variations in the amount of liquor amnii, in the length of the maternal abdomen, in the tone of the uterus, in the presentation and position of the fetus and in the thickness of the maternal soft tissues. The wide errors in predicting fetal size and maturity by abdominal examination both by measurement of the uterus and by simple palpation were explored by Beazley and Underhill (1970) and Loeffler (1967). In Queen Charlotte's Hospital during 1970 only 33 of 115 small-for-dates babies (i.e. below the 5th centile weight for gestation) were identified antenatally by abdominal palpation (i.e. the fundus was two or more weeks smaller than the expected size on two or more occasions). This is a serious cause for concern, casting considerable doubt on the value of the principal screening test for the growth-retarded fetus.

Ultrasound

Pulsed echo ultrasonic diagnosis was first introduced into obstetrics by Donald, MacVicar and Brown (1958) and reviews of its diverse applications in obstetrics were given by Donald (1968) and Campbell (1972). Comprehensive accounts of the basic physical principles of ultrasonic diagnosis have been given by Wells (1972) and Talbert and Campbell (1972). Only a brief and simplified account will be given here. Short pulses (2 µsec) of high frequency (2.5 mHz), low intensity sound are transmitted from a piezo-electric crystal (transducer) through the maternal abdomen. As the sound wave crosses the junction (interface) between different tissues it encounters an acoustic mismatch and a partial reflection of the wave occurs. The remainder of the ultrasonic beam passes on to the next interface where the process is repeated. The reflected sound waves are detected by the transducer which converts the acoustic signals into electric signals which are then amplified and processed by a cathode ray tube into visual signals. Strong echoes are obtained when the ultrasonic beam is at right angles (orthogonal) to the interface or when the acoustic mismatch between the tissues on each side of the interface is great. The transducer also receives weak signals from interfaces and tissue discontinuities that are not orthogonal to the ultrasonic beam. In the past these backscatter reflections were eliminated by signal processing in order to facilitate interpretation of the echograms but nowadays these echoes can be displayed by grey-scaling techniques (Kossoff, Garrett and Radovanovitch, 1974) aiding the visualisation of many organs which could previously not be detected.

There are two display systems commonly employed in antenatal measurement. In the first (A-scan) the echoes are displayed as vertical deflections (spikes) on a horizontal time base (Figures 15.2 and 15.3). The interval between any two spikes represents the difference in time taken by the sound wave to pass from the transducer to the relevant interface and back again; this difference is the time taken by the sound wave to pass from one interface to the other and if the sound velocity of this tissue is known, the distance between the two interfaces can be exactly determined. In the B-scan display, the echoes from each interface are shown on the time base as a bright spot. As the transducer travels over the maternal abdomen, the time base starting point and direction move in a corresponding manner so that the movements of the time base on the screen correspond with the movement of the ultrasonic beam in the body. To obtain optimal information the transducer is moved at different angles to the skin surface so the ultrasonic beam crosses all possible interfaces at right angles (compound scanning) and as the bright spots coalesce a two-dimensional outline of the abdominal structures is produced (Figures 15.1, 15.2 and 15.3).

All human and laboratory experimental data suggest that ultrasound at diagnostic power levels is a harmless technique (Taylor, 1974). Since it is also simple and rapid, causing no discomfort to the patient, it can be safely used for total population screening.

Ultrasonic apparatus

The ultrasonic machine most commonly used in obstetrics is the contact scanner (Donald and Brown, 1961) so called because the transducer is directly in contact with the skin of the maternal abdomen. As ultrasound waves are totally reflected at an air interface, it is necessary to put a thick layer of oil on the skin surface as a coupling medium. The alternative system is the water delay scanner (Kossoff, Robinson and Garrett, 1965) in which the patient presses her abdomen against the polythene window of a water tank in which the crystal is set. The contact scanner would seen to have considerable superiority in its mechanical versatility but the water delay scanner has one important advantage in that artefactual echoes due to the transmitter take place outside the region of interest; this does lead to improved definition of near structures in the abdomen and uterus. A large number of ultrasonic scanners is now being marketed; listed below are those features which are important in optimising measurements of the fetus:

1. The scanner must have both A-scan and B-scan facilities either displaying echoes simultaneously or at the turn of a switch. It is only by combining these displays that the most precise linear measurements are obtained.
2. The A-scan display should have an electronic caliper unit with two bright-up markers which when placed on the leading edges of the A-scan spikes will give the measurement to the nearest 0.1 mm. Measurements from the face of the tube using a graticule scale are imprecise.
3. The B-scan display must have a good dynamic range. In some machines as a result of signal processing some of the back scatter echoes are eliminated, which results in considerable loss of information. For example, backscatter reflections from the intracranial structures are vitally important in cephalometry for assessing the exact position of the fetal head.
4. The machine must be mechanically versatile and have a rigid scanning frame. This is especially important in cephalometry where the scanning arm must be adjusted quickly so that reproducible linear scans can be made at any angle and in any plane.
5. To facilitate cephalometry it is important to be able to follow fetal movements on the screen during B-scanning. This means that the scanner should have either a conventional long persistence oscilloscope or a variable persistence storage scope.
6. The apparatus should have a tilting scanning couch; by inclining the patient 20° 'head down' the deeply engaged head can be dislodged which greatly simplifies measurement.

The scan converter is a major advance in the imaging of ultrasonic echoes, for by conversion of the sector scan signal to a television raster display, computer techniques can be applied in processing the signal. Thus the scan converter is the most convenient method of obtaining grey-scale images in which the full range of echoes is displayed in various shades of grey according to echo strength. Furthermore the application of computer memory techniques enables the overwriting of echoes to be avoided thus lessening the need for scanning expertise. Once the signal has been processed into a television raster form it can be recorded on magnetic tape, printed on commercial hard copiers or used for any other television type of application. The scan converter will therefore permit life-size images (or larger) of the fetus in late pregnancy and these can then be transferred to paper for measuring. This greatly adds to the accuracy of predictions of fetal size. The difference between a conventional B-mode and a scan converter grey-scale echogram is shown in Figure 15.1, a and b.

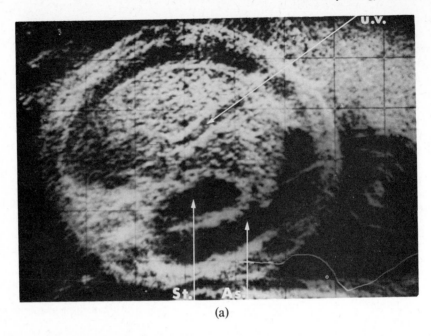

(a)

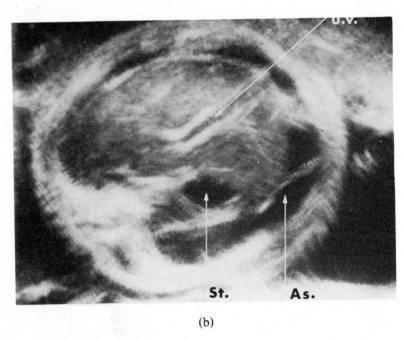

(b)

Figure 15.1. Echograms of: (a) conventional B mode, (b) grey-scale displays showing the same transverse section of the fetal abdomen. This fetus was affected by rhesus disease and the umbilical vein, fetal stomach and ascitic fluid can be observed on both echograms; the grey-scale picture, however, is easier to interpret and gives more information on minor variations in tissue density. u.v. = umbilical vein; As. = fetal ascites; St. = stomach.

Measuring techniques

Embryonic measurements

For examination of the pregnant uterus during the first 12 weeks of pregnancy, it is important that the maternal bladder should be moderately distended with urine (Donald, 1965). The cystic bladder improves the clarity of the intra-uterine echoes by pushing bowel away from the front of the uterus, reducing reverberation echoes and helping to raise the uterus out of the pelvis. An overfull bladder, however, distorts the anatomy and should be avoided.

The gestation sac can be reliably visualised from five weeks menstrual age and the increase in size monitored for the remainder of the first trimester. Various techniques for estimating size have been employed from simply measuring the largest diameter of the sac (Kohorn and Kaufman, 1974) to calculating sac volume from multiple longitudinal and transverse scans (Robinson, 1975). Gestation sac measurements, however, have been largely superseded by measurements of the embryonic crown–rump length.

Crown–rump length measurements have been facilitated by the newer machines which can give life-size images of the embryo. The technique is described by Robinson (1973). Several parallel longitudinal scans are first made to identify the long axis of the embryo. During this process, both poles of the embryo are observed and their respective positions marked on the patient's skin. As the embryo is usually lying transversely in the uterus, scanning between the marks to establish the crown–rump length usually involves a transverse scan. Measurement is then made directly from a polaroid photograph (Figure 15.2) with a ruler or when there is marked curvature of the embryo, a map measurer. Curvature of the embryo increases after 12 weeks and diminishes the accuracy of crown–rump length measurements as it is difficult to obtain the full length of the embryo on a single scan. Robinson found that the reproducibility of crown–rump length measurements was high; in a series of 30 experiments the average standard deviation of three readings was 1.2 mm.

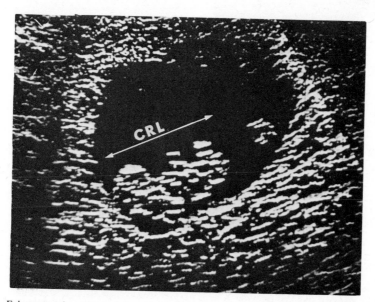

Figure 15.2. Echogram taken at ten weeks menstrual age illustrating crown–rump (CR) length measurement of the embryo. CRL = embryonic crown–rump length.

Fetal measurements

Biparietal diameter. Measurement of the fetal biparietal diameter is the most commonly made and the most precise measurement that can be obtained during the antenatal period. At least one cephalometry scan is performed on 60 per cent of patients attending Queen Charlotte's Hospital.

The technique is designed to ensure that the measurement is reproducible within acceptable limits. The midline echo of the fetal head makes this possible. The principal steps in the technique are listed below:

1. A longitudinal scan is made to determine the angulation of the fetal head to the vertical axis (angle of asynclitism). This is determined by placing the ultrasonic beam at right angles to the midline echo (Figures 15.3a and 15.4a) and reading the angle from a scale. The midline echo (which represents the medial aspect of each cerebral hemisphere) is strong when the head is occipito-transverse and becomes progressively less distinct the more the occiput is rotated anteriorly or posteriorly. Rotation means that the midline structures are being recognised by means of diffuse backscatter.

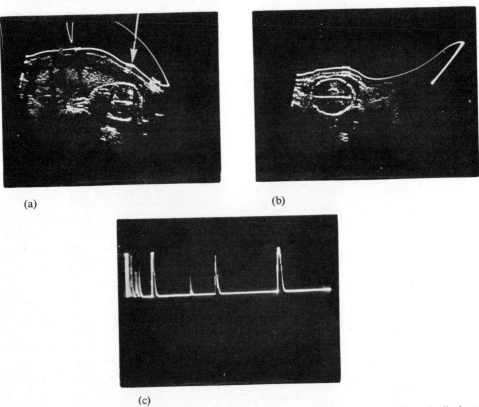

(a)   (b)

(c)

Figure 15.3. Illustration of the combined A and B-scan technique at 28 weeks gestation. (a) Longitudinal scan: the angulation of the ultrasonic beam (arrow) to the vertical axis is the angle of asynclitism (5° in this case). (b) Transverse scan with the transducer angled at 5° to the vertical to give a true transverse section of the fetal head with a strong continuous mid-line echo. (c) A-scan tracing showing cephalic echoes and mid-line echo; the measuring 'bright-up' markers are placed on the leading edges of the head echoes. The biparietal diameter is 76 mm.

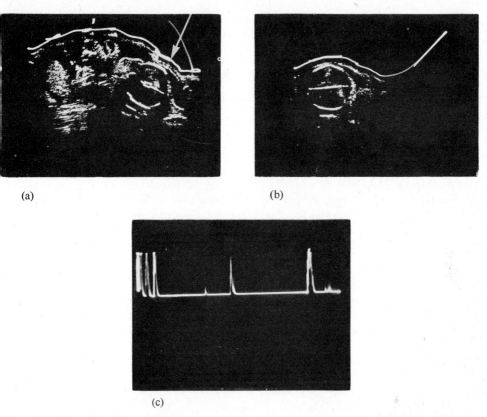

(a) (b)

(c)

Figure 15.4. Illustration of the combined A and B-scan technique at 36 weeks. (a) Longitudinal scan; angle of asynclitism is now 35°. At angles greater than this a tilting couch is helpful. (b) Transverse scan at 35° showing parietal bones and strong continuous mid-line echo. (c) A-scan display; the biparietal diameter is 95.6 mm.

2. A transverse scan is then made with the probe inclined to the angle of tilt of the head (asynclitism). This scan should give a true transverse section of the fetal head. The head is seen as an ovoid and a complete midline echo will bisect it in its longest axis (Figures 15.3b and 15.4b). The ultrasonic beam is then placed at right angles to the midline echo across the maximum convexity of the parietal bone and an A-scan measurement taken (Figures 15.3c and 15.4c). Further transverse scans are then made caudal and cephalad to this original transverse scan to establish the widest transcoronal diameter (which should be the biparietal diameter) with the proviso that the midline structures are still visible on both B and A-scan displays.

3. If the back of the head (occiput) is directly posterior or anterior then no midline structures can be visualised on the longitudinal scan and the angle of asynclitism cannot be measured. Gentle lateral pressure on the fetal head or body is then indicated in order to bring the midline structures into view. A transverse measuring scan at the appropriate angle with a similar degree of lateral pressure is then performed.

4. If the head is deeply engaged, cephalometry is difficult, due to the interposition of the symphysis pubis which physically limits the range of the scanning angles. Elevation of the foot of the scanning couch by 20 degrees will dislocate the head upwards and make cephalometry much more rapid and simple.

5. In cases of breech presentation the technique is no different from that described above but the movement of the head tends to be greater due to the respiratory excursion of the maternal diaphragm. It is then advisable to ask the patient to hold her breath intermittently while angles are measured and measurements taken. When the fetal lie is transverse the procedure is performed in reverse; the angle of asynclitism is assessed on the transverse scan and the measuring scan is performed longitudinally.

6. Measurement in early pregnancy can be difficult because of fetal movements. Violent movements rarely last longer than three or four minutes and the wisest course is to resume measurements only when the fetus is in a resting phase.

Good midline echoes can be obtained in 98 per cent of examinations. Assessment of the accuracy of cephalometry by the above technique was carried out on 35 babies delivered by elective caesarean section (Campbell, 1968) and 50 fetuses delivered by hysterotomy (Campbell, 1970). In 90 per cent of cases the discrepancy between the ultrasonic and postnatal caliper measurements was less than 2 mm and the mean error in both groups was less than 1 mm. In the later study three independent ultrasonic recordings were performed on each fetus and the average standard deviation was ±0.25 mm indicating a high degree of reproducibility.

Head circumference. To measure the circumference of the fetal head it is necessary to make a transverse scan to produce a horizontal section of the fetal head which will include both the biparietal diameter (coronal plane) and the occipital frontal diameter (saggital plane). Due to flexion of the fetal head, the straight transverse scan that is employed to measure the biparietal diameter usually displays the suboccipital bregmatic diameter (Figure 15.4b) and it is therefore necessary to rotate the scanning gantry until the fetal head appears as an ovoid

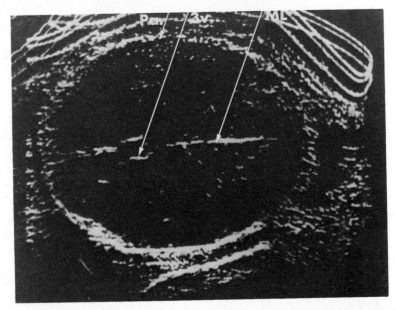

Figure 15.5. Echogram of a fetal head at 32 weeks menstrual age showing an optimal section for head circumference measurement; the mid-line echo is clearly shown and the third ventricle is observed approximately one-third of the distance from the sinciput. The measurement is made directly from the echogram by means of a map measurer. Pa. = parietal bone; ML = mid-line echo; 3v = third ventricle.

and the echoes from the third ventricle are detected in the midline, one-third of the distance from the sinciput (Figure 15.5). Measurement of the circumference is then made from a polaroid photograph (or hard copy) by means of a map measurer. Head circumference measurements are less reproducible than those of the biparietal diameter, the average standard deviation of three independent measurements on 20 fetuses being 1.8 mm.

Thoracic circumference. The fetal thorax is shaped like a cone with the base lying at the level of the diaphragm. One of the problems of thoracometry is to determine the level of the section for although heart pulsations are frequently used they can be observed throughout most of the thoracic length. Studies on circumference measurements of the fetal chest have been made by Hansmann, Voigt and Baeker (1973) and Levi and Erbsman (1975). Little detail about the measurement technique is described but the method involves making a transverse section at the base of the fetal heart at a point where the fetal heart pulsations disappear. Unfortunately, there is no positive reference point at this level and in view of its conical shape, measurements of the chest are less reproducible than abdominal circumference measurements.

Abdomen circumference. The fetal abdomen is shaped more like a cylinder than a cone and there are numerous structures which can act as reference points, including fetal vessels, stomach, kidneys and bladder. The author (1974) has found that the fetal umbilical vein is the optimal reference point for performing reproducible abdometry. Not only is it easily recognisable, but as the fetal liver is the most severely affected organ in cases of asymmetrical fetal growth retardation, this section is of most import in the assessment of fetal nutrition. The technique (Campbell and Wilkin, 1975) involves making scans at different angles to the

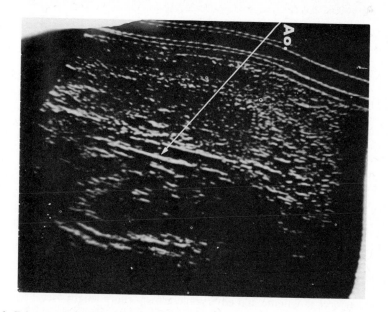

Figure 15.6. Echogram illustrating a significant length of fetal abdominal aorta; this is used to determine the long axis of the fetus. Ao. = fetal aorta.

midline of the maternal abdomen to identify the position of the long axis of the fetal body; where there is marked flexion of the fetal body it is essential to identify a significant length of fetal abdominal aorta (Figure 15.6) or fetal dorsal spine. Scans are then made orthogonal to the long axis of the fetal body and a section across the upper abdomen selected; this is recognised by the typical appearance of the umbilical vein as it passes under the fetal liver (Figure 15.7). Usually the umbilical vein can be easily recognised from 24 weeks onwards

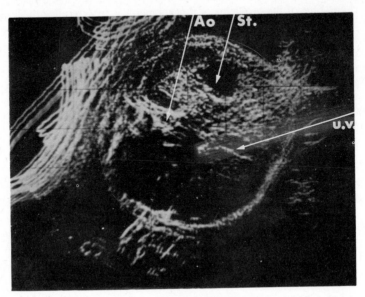

Figure 15.7. Echogram of the same fetus as on Figure 15.5 showing an optimal section for fetal abdomen circumference measurement; the umbilical vein and fetal stomach are the reference points and can be clearly identified. Abbreviations as in Figures 15.1 and 15.6.

except in about 10 per cent of cases when the fetal spine is directly anterior or posterior which means that the walls of the umbilical vein are not orthogonal to the ultrasonic beam. Under these circumstances, the fetal stomach is used as the reference point. It is not so precise a location as the umbilical vein for when distended it extends over a greater length of fetal abdomen but it does lie in the upper abdomen to the left of the fetal liver and both umbilical vein and fetal stomach can usually be visualised on the same section. Circumference measurements are made to the nearest millimeter on a polaroid photograph or hard copy by means of a map measurer. The abdomen can alter shape with different fetal positions and hence abdometry is less reproducible than either of the head measurements; the average standard deviation of three independent ultrasound readings (20 patients) was 2.95 mm.

Normal values

Graphs of gestation sac volume and embryonic crown–rump length measurements taken between 6 and 14 weeks menstrual age have been published by Robinson (1975) and Robinson and Fleming (1975). Both the sac and crown–rump length show exponential growth

om 6 to 12 weeks but after this growth appears to be linear. The 95 per cent confidence
mits of gestation sac measurements at each week of gestation are considerably wider than
ose for embryonic crown–rump length and the latter graph (Figure 15.8) is of greater value
making assessments of embryonic age and growth.

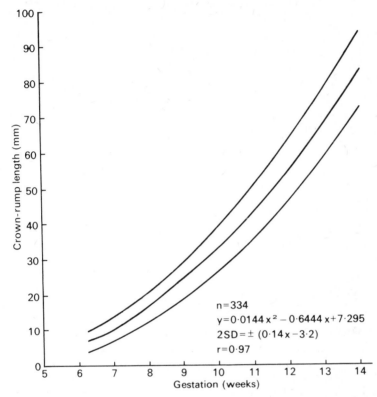

Figure 15.8. The mean growth of the embryonic CR length ± 2 s.d. from 6 to 14 weeks menstrual age as determined by a weighted non-linear regression analysis. From Robinson and Fleming (1975) with kind permission of
the authors and the editor of *British Journal of Obstetrics and Gynaecology.*

There are now several published graphs of biparietal diameter values taken during normal
pregnancy and plotted against the menstrual age of the fetus. Most of these graphs resemble
each other in the shape of the graph (an asymptotic curve) but there is a divergence in the ab-
olute size of the biparietal diameter for a particular week of gestation. For example the mean
alues of Campbell and Newman (1971) are about 5 mm larger for each week of gestation
when compared with those of Flamme (1972). The explanation is almost certainly due to the
act that various workers use different ultrasonic velocities for determining the distance
between the A-scan deflections, the higher ultrasonic velocities giving the larger readings.
For fetal growth measurements it is of little moment which ultrasonic velocity is used (as long
as an appropriate chart for the particular velocity chosen is used) for it is the relative increase
n head size that determines the growth rate. Where the absolute value is important, for
example in cases of suspected cephalo-pelvic disproportion, the velocity of 1600 m/sec determined by Willocks et al (1964) would seem to be the optimum figure for determining the true
unmoulded biparietal diameter. The growth curves of Campbell and Newman (1971) were

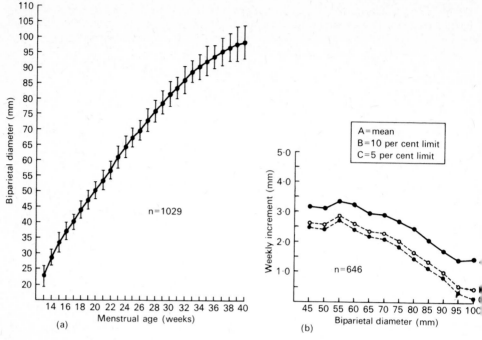

Figure 15.9. (a) Mean fetal biparietal diameter (mm) ± 2 s.d. for each week of pregnancy from 13 weeks to term (b) Mean growth rate of the fetal biparietal diameter with lower tolerance limits related to the size of the biparietal diameter.

made from measurements of a biparietal diameter using this velocity. These authors, who used strict criteria of normality (and included only those patients who went into spontaneous labour within one week of term), constructed two distinct types of graphs from their normal values; the first is used to assess size and maturity, while the second is used to assess growth. In the first graph a total of 1029 individual measurements of the biparietal diameter were plotted against the menstrual age of the fetus (Figure 15.9a). The mean weekly increase in the biparietal diameter is rapid and almost linear from 14 until 30 weeks menstrual age (3.. mm/week), slows significantly between 30 and 36 weeks (2.0 mm/week) and thereafter falls rapidly to term with a mean rate of increase of 1.2 mm/week. The range of values for a particular week of gestation is contained within narrow limits during the middle trimester and widens gradually after 30 weeks gestation. The second graph was based on longitudinal data and was compiled from 646 serial measurements. The mean weekly growth rate was related to the menstrual age of the fetus and also to the size of the biparietal diameter (Figure 15.9b). It was found that the latter graph was of more value when assessing the growth rate of the fetus. This is discussed more fully in the section on fetal growth.

Preliminary data illustrating the growth of the head and abdomen circumference in normal pregnancy are presented in Figures 15.10 and 15.11. Criteria of normality were strict as described for the biparietal diameter measurements. The head circumference chart has a similar shape to that of the biparietal diameter, i.e. rapid and linear growth from 14 to 30 weeks (11.5 mm/week), slowing from 30 to 36 weeks (7.2 mm/week) and a marked reduction to term (1.8 mm/week). Again confidence limits widen progressively after 30 weeks menstrual age. The abdomen circumference chart however shows almost linear growth from 14 to 30 weeks menstrual age (11.6 mm/week) with a moderate reduction thereafter (7.4 mm/week

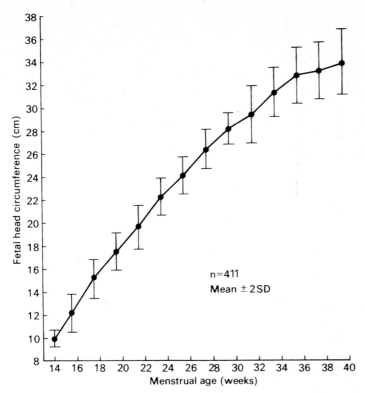

Figure 15.10. Mean head circumference values ± 2 s.d. taken during normal pregnancy from 14 to 40 weeks menstrual age (411 measurements). Values have been analysed in two weekly groupings to smooth out fluctuations due to small numbers.

nd no tendency to terminal flattening, although with the widening confidence limits towards he end of pregnancy there is obviously considerable variation of the growth rate in individual cases. Initially the mean abdomen circumference measurement is smaller than that f the head but by 36 weeks they are equal and thereafter the mean abdomen circumference xceeds that of the head. The ratio of the head to the abdomen circumference is of importance in antenatal monitoring and is discussed later.

Clinical applications

Estimation of fetal age, growth rate and size is dependent upon the capability of ultrasound o provide precise measurements of fetal dimensions. This in turn is dependent upon operator xperience and expertise which explains the disparity between the reliability of results eported by different centres (Davison et al, 1973; Varma, 1973).

Fetal age

The earlier in pregnancy the fetus is measured, the more accurate will be predictions of fetal ige. As growth is rapid, confidence limits are narrow and growth retardation is rare between

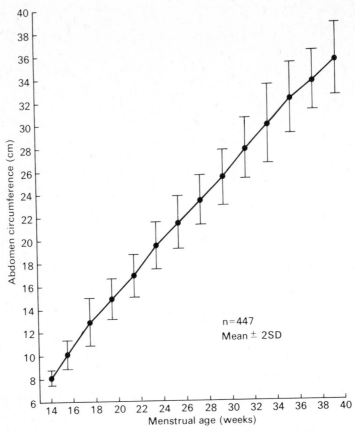

Figure 15.11. Mean abdomen circumference values ± 2 s.d. taken during normal pregnancy from 14 to 40 weeks menstrual age (447 measurements). Values have been analysed in two weekly groupings to smooth out fluctuations due to small numbers.

6 and 24 weeks, predictions of fetal menstrual age from single measurements can be made with great accuracy during this period of time. From Robinson's graph of CRL measurements, embryonic age predictions can be made to within five days with a 95 per cent probability. In a series of 34 patients who were certain of the date of their last menstrual period, he found that the ultrasonic prediction was within three days of the true menstrual age in 33 of these cases and within two days in 25. In our own laboratory, we have been able to estimate the menstrual age from a single CRL measurement to within one week in 95 per cent of cases.

Acceptable predictions of fetal age can be made between 13 and 24 weeks by measurement of the biparietal diameter. Campbell (1969) made menstrual age predictions during the middle trimester on 170 antenatal patients in whom menstrual age was in doubt; delivery occurred within nine days of the date predicted from the ultrasonic measurement in 84 per cent of patients in whom labour began spontaneously and who were delivered of mature babies. These predictions, however, were made in a small group of patients under optimal conditions and do not necessarily reflect the accuracy of fetal age predictions when made under the pressure of a total screening programme. For this reason, in Queen Charlotte's Hospital during 1972 alternate patients were screened routinely and predictions were made from

iparietal diameter measurements between 13 and 30 weeks menstrual age although the
najority of measurements were made between 13 and 20 weeks. The measurements were
nade by the author and a radiographer and no statistical difference in the accuracy of the
•redictions was found between these two workers; the results therefore are to some extent a
neasure of the degree of accuracy that can be expected under routine circumstances. Over
000 patients were studied and the first 332 patients to deliver spontaneously were analysed.
Ill patients at the first attendance at the antenatal clinic had an expected date of delivery
alculated from the last menstrual period by Naegle's calculation and also from clinical
ssessment of the uterine size. Following this visit, an ultrasonic examination was made, the
•iparietal diameter measured and an ultrasonic expected date of delivery calculated. Of the
32 babies, 19 were considered preterm on paediatric examination and were excluded from
he analysis. The relationship of the various predictions to the actual date of delivery is
hown in Table 15.1. Two cut-off points, i.e. 14 days and 10 days, were chosen to evaluate

Table 15.1. *Relative accuracy of the predicted dates of delivery made by ultrasonic cephalometry, Naegle's calculation and clinical examination, as
determined by the onset of spontaneous labour and the delivery of a mature
baby.*

Method of maturity prediction	Spontaneous labour		Total
	<14 days	<10 days	
Ultrasound EDD	292 (93%)	251 (80%)	313
Dates EDD[a]	261 (86%)	222 (73%)	304
Clinical EDD	216 (74%)	175 (60%)	291

[a]Nine patients (3 per cent) were totally unsure of the date of the last
menstrual period.

he relative accuracy of the three techniques. There was a seven per cent improvement at
•oth points in the ultrasonic predictions over those made from the patient's last menstrual
•eriod and a 20 per cent improvement over assessments made from the clinical examination.
The 304 patients with a last menstrual period were then divided into those with certain dates
ind those with suspect dates. Patients with suspect dates amounted to 39 per cent of the pop-
llation and were defined as those having been on oral contraceptives within two months of
he last menstrual period, having had bleeding during the first two months of pregnancy or
;iving a history of an irregular menstrual cycle. Table 15.2 shows that the ultrasonic fetal age
•redictions were 11 per cent better than those made from suspect dates and even in patients
vith certain dates the ultrasonic assessment showed a four per cent improvement at both cut-
•ff points.

Table 15.2. *Relative accuracy of the predicted dates of delivery from ultrasonic cephalometry and Naegle's calculation in patients with certain and
suspect dates.*

Method of maturity prediction	Spontaneous labour		Total
	<14 days	<10 days	
Ultrasound EDD	292 (93%)	251 (80%)	313
Impeccable dates EDD	163 (89%)	140 (76%)	184
Suspect dates EDD	98 (82%)	82 (68%)	120

Thus we now have a technique of routinely screening the obstetric population which will give more accurate predictions of fetal age than the last menstrual period. A case for routinely screening the whole obstetric population can be made, but even if this is disputed on grounds of cost effectiveness, it would be difficult to deny the advantage of screening all patients with suspect dates (i.e. approximately 40 per cent of the population) by ultrasonic examination in early pregnancy.

Fetal growth

Growth during the first trimester can be assessed by measurement of the fetal crown–rump length. Failure of growth at this stage inevitably results in embryonic death which can be quickly established from seven weeks onwards by failure to observe the fetal heart movements on the A-scan display as shown by Robinson (1973). In many cases of 'threatened abortion', death and shrinkage of the embryonic echo can be detected in the presence of an enlarging gestation sac and a positive pregnancy test.

Table 15.3. *Reproducibility of biparietal, head circumference and abdomen circumference measurements and the confidence limits for growth rate assessment according to the period of gestation.*

	No. of cases	Reproducibility s.d. (mm) (3 measurements)	95 per cent confidence limits weekly growth (mm)[a]	Mean growth rate (mm)		
				14–30	30–36	36–40
BPD	50	0.25	0.71	3.3	2.0	1.2
Head circumference	20	1.80	5.09	11.5	7.2	1.8
Abdomen circumference	20	2.95	8.35	11.6	10.1	7.4

[a] To determine the confidence limits for longer intervals, divide by the number of weeks between measurements.

In Table 15.3 the 95 per cent confidence limits for weekly growth measurements have been determined for biparietal diameter, head circumference and abdominal circumference measurements. It can be seen that weekly biparietal diameter measurements can be made with confidence throughout pregnancy. Head circumference measurements can be made every two weeks until 36 weeks, but thereafter the growth rate is too slow and the confidence limits too wide to give reliable information on growth. Despite the wider confidence limits for measurement of the fetal abdomen, its more rapid growth rate in late pregnancy makes fortnightly measurements clinically valuable from 14 weeks onwards.

Fetal growth has been principally studied by measurement of the biparietal diameter, partly because for many years it was the only fetal dimension to be measured, and partly because of its high precision and reproducibility. While in practice it is possible to make assessments of growth rate from two measurements separated by one week, there is no doubt that the more numerous the measurements and the earlier in pregnancy they are started, the more accurate and useful will be the diagnostic predictions. To measure the fetal growth rate, reference should be made to the two graphs of Campbell and Newman (1971). When the first measurement is taken it is compared with the graph of the biparietal diameter versus menstrual age (Figure 15.9a) to determine whether the reading is within the normal range for the particular week of gestation; subsequent growth is then assessed using the graph of the weekly growth rate versus biparietal diameter (Figure 15.9b). This method of assessment is best explained with an example; a fetus whose maturity is supposed to be 34 weeks is found to have a biparietal diameter measurement of 80 mm, i.e. equivalent to 30-week size. Excluding some cranial abnormality or dolichocephaly there are only two possible explanations for the small head size: either the assessment of fetal age is in error or fetal growth is retarded. A further measurement is then taken one week later. If the biparietal diameter measures 83 mm this indicates that growth is normal and that the calculated fetal age is in error. It is our practice to allow these patients to proceed past term provided fetal growth continues to be normal. On the other hand, if the biparietal diameter reading was only 81 mm then this would indicate growth retardation. It should be stressed that only by relating fetal growth rates to head size can rapid identification of growth retardation be achieved. This is because the smaller the fetal head the more rapid should be the growth rate. With severe degrees of growth retardation, however, the difference between the growth rate in a light-for-dates fetus and an immature fetus will be wide and separation becomes easy. This does not apply when growth rates are related to maturity; the difference in growth rate between a light-for-dates baby and a normal baby at 40 weeks is very small. A further advantage of using head size as the growth rate parameter is that it is not necessary to know the age of the fetus when assessing the significance of a fetal growth rate.

Campbell and Dewhurst (1971) studied 406 women with pregnancies carrying some risk to the fetus of whom 388 were believed on uterine palpation to be persistently smaller than normal for the gestational age: 149 were diagnosed as normal, 117 were diagnosed as having mistaken dates and 140 had retarded growth rates. In this latter group, 68 per cent of babies were below the 5th centile weight for gestation. The fetuses with retarded growth rates also had a significant increase in the incidence of low Apgar scores, perinatal death and fetal abnormality when compared with the other groups. Campbell and Kurjak (1972) compared the value of serial ultrasonic cephalometry and urinary oestrogen estimations in the assessment of a similar group of 284 'at risk' babies. All patients had at least three inpatient urinary oestrogen estimations which were continued to within one week of delivery. Ultrasonic cephalometry was found to be significantly better at diagnosing the light-for-dates fetus although no difference was demonstrated between the two techniques when predicting babies which would develop a low Apgar score at birth. Of the 11 light-for-dates perinatal deaths, 10 had a slow ultrasonic growth rate while there were nine in the abnormal oestrogen group. Varma (1973) in a similar study confirmed the superiority of ultrasound in the diagnosis of intra-uterine growth retardation but in addition showed that cephalometry was significantly superior to oestrogen assay in predicting perinatal asphyxia. Thus serial cephalometry compares favourably with steroid hormone assay of the feto-placental unit in the detection of a growth-retarded fetus.

Campbell (1974), from an analysis of cephalometry charts in cases of growth retardation, has described different patterns of intra-uterine growth which may be important in assessing the short and long-term risks to the fetus. These patterns generally fall into two main groups. In the first group there is an abrupt slowing and eventual cessation of the growth rate after a period of normal growth (Figure 15.12). This type is called a 'later-flattening' growth retardation pattern and is associated with maternal hypertension, intrapartum fetal asphyxia, postnatal hypoglycaemia, increased brain to liver ratio and a typically wasted appearance. The 'low-profile' growth retardation pattern demonstrates persistently low growth rate from early in the second trimester (Figure 15.13). There is usually no tendency to cessation of growth, no strong association with toxaemia or intrapartum asphyxia, and the brain to liver ratio is usually normal. These babies are more stunted than wasted in appearance and about 20 to 30 per cent of light-for-dates babies referred for ultrasonic examination conform to this growth pattern. A few of these babies have some genetic or chromosomal abnormality and are examples of reduced growth potential.

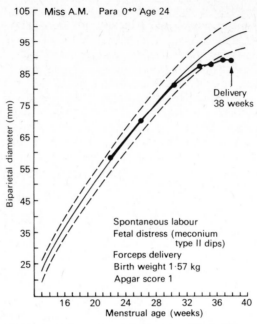

Figure 15.12. Example of 'late-flattening' growth retardation pattern. Typical history of pre-eclampsia, intrapartum fetal distress, low Apgar score and postnatal hypoglycaemia. Birthweight was below the 5th centile weight for gestation.

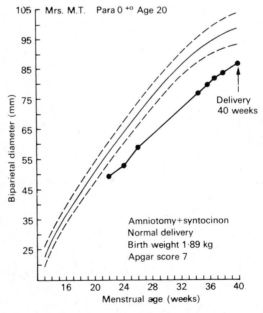

Figure 15.13. Example of 'low-profile' growth-retardation pattern. Uneventful pregnancy and labour. Baby cried at one minute and did not develop hypoglycaemia. Birthweight was below the 5th centile weight for gestation.

Our follow-up studies of these babies are still at an early stage but we have recently completed a study of 60 children who were light-for-dates at birth (below the 10th centile weight for gestation), who were born at term (more than 37 completed weeks), and whose antenatal growth had been followed by serial ultrasonic cephalometry (Fancourt et al, 1976). These children were examined at a mean age of four years by a paediatrician who had no knowledge of the ultrasonic growth pattern or birthweight. It was found that a height, weight and head circumference less than the 10th centile at follow-up occurred significantly more frequently in those children in whom the onset of growth failure of the biparietal diameter occurred before 34 weeks menstrual age (Figure 15.14). When the onset of growth failure occurred before 26 weeks there was a lower mean developmental quotient at follow-up using Ruth Griffiths extended scales. The longer the restriction of head growth in utero, the more serious the effects on subsequent somatic growth in childhood. All the 'low growth profile'

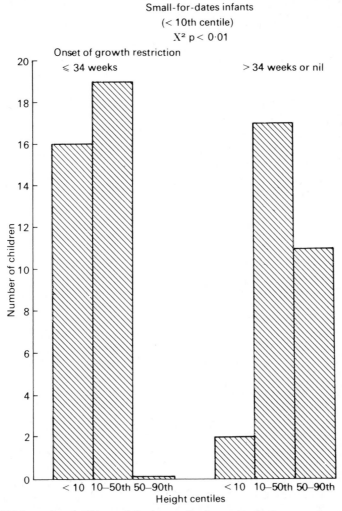

Figure 15.14. Height centiles of children at follow-up paediatric examination (mean age four years) according to whether the onset of growth failure of the biparietal diameter was before or after 34 weeks menstrual age. A similar distribution was demonstrated for weight and head circumference centiles.

fetuses were in the pre-34 weeks group, and the continued restriction of growth in childhood is predominantly a feature of this group. The reason for growth restraint in the 'low growth profile' group is not always apparent. Maternal undernutrition tends to cause slowing of brain growth after 30 weeks but in many of these fetuses brain growth was restricted before this time. What is clear however is that the intra-uterine growth pattern of the fetal head can indicate the subsequent somatic growth of the individual and in some cases the intellectual development.

Although serial cephalometry is an important means of detecting fetal growth retardation, it should be recognised that the technique, even when meticulously performed, has a significant incidence of false-positive results among growth-retarded fetuses; 21 per cent in the study of Campbell and Dewhurst had normal growth rates. This is due to the fact that the fetal brain and skull are usually preferentially protected from the effects of growth-retarding stimuli and that normal growth increments can occur when other parts of the fetal anatomy are failing to do so. It should be stressed, however, that when there is fetal growth retardation, the biparietal diameter will eventually show a significant slowing of growth before fetal demise occurs. Furthermore, the late slowing of the skull growth can be of advantage in that growth-retarded pregnancies can safely be prolonged to a time when the lecithin: sphingomyelin ratio indicates fetal pulmonary maturity provided that the biparietal diameter is showing normal weekly increments.

The principal disadvantage of serial cephalometry in the assessment of growth retardation is that it is time-consuming, making it impractical to screen a whole population by this technique. An undue reliance is thus placed on clinicians to refer cases at risk and as shown above the clinician recognises less than 30 per cent of growth-retarded fetuses during the antenatal period. For total screening of the obstetric population, an alternative technique is therefore required. In essence, this means accurate predictions of birthweight from single measurements of the fetus made during the third trimester of pregnancy.

Fetal weight and size

Despite the fact that the biparietal diameter is the most accurate linear measurement that can be obtained during the antenatal period, the prediction of birthweight from a single biparietal diameter measurement in late pregnancy is not particularly accurate. Campbell (1974) in a large series which included 211 babies below 2.5 kg found that the birthweight could be predicted to within 812 g with a 95 per cent probability. At the extremes of the birthweight range this may represent an improvement on predictions made from abdominal palpation, but in practical terms it still falls a long way short of acceptable accuracy.

Several workers have reported greater accuracy in predicting fetal weight from single measurements in late pregnancy by taking linear (Thomson and Makowski, 1971) or circumferential (Levi, 1972; Hansmann et al, 1973) measurements of the fetal thorax and 95 per cent confidence limits of between 400 and 600 g have been reported. Campbell and Wilkin (1975) made fetal weight predictions from a single fetal abdominal circumference measurement on 140 fetuses within 48 hours of birth; 36 had a birthweight below 2.6 kg and the birthweights ranged from 0.79 to 5.46 kg. The accuracy of predictions varied with the size of the fetus; at a predicted weight of 1 kg, 95 per cent of birthweights fell within 160 g, while at 2, 3 and 4 kg the corresponding values were 290, 450 and 590 g respectively (Figure 15.15). By computer analysis, extrapolation of this data to routine screening of the obstetric population was performed and this indicated that with a single measurement at 32 weeks menstrual age, 87 per cent of babies below the 5th centile could be detected by this method and that at 36 weeks the yield of small-for-dates babies would be 75 per cent. The false positive

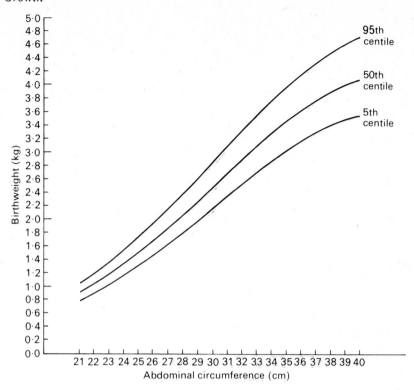

Figure 15.15. Relationship between the fetal abdomen circumference measurement and birthweight in 140 fetuses who were delivered within 48 hours of the ultrasound measurements; second degree polynomial regression, 95th and 5th centile confidence limits.

diagnosis rate would be very low at just over one per cent (Table 15.4). Thus by routinely screening all pregnancies with a single early measurement of CRL or biparietal diameter, combined with a late measurement of the fetal abdominal circumference, the majority of growth-retarded fetuses could be detected antenatally.

Table 15.4. *Correct classification of babies above and below the 5th centile weight at 32, 34, 36 and 38 weeks menstrual age, using the data in Figure 15.15*

Menstrual age (weeks)	5th centile limit[a] (kg)	Correct classification from fetal abdominal circumference measurements	
		>5th centile	≤5th centile
32	1.11	98.8%	86.7%
34	1.68	98.9%	81.8%
36	2.13	98.7%	74.9%
38	2.47	98.7%	63.2%

[a] From Table XI of Thomson, Billewicz and Hytten (1968).

Table from Campbell and Wilkin (1975) with kind permission of the editor of *British Journal of Obstetrics and Gynaecology*.

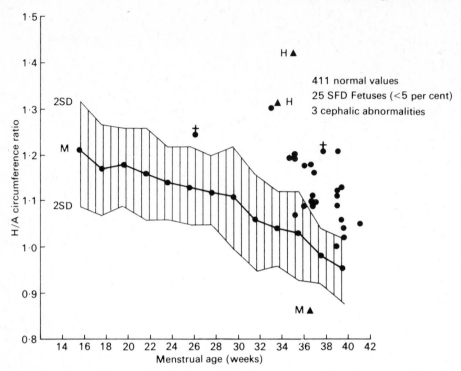

Figure 15.16. The head to abdomen circumference ratio (H/A ratio) in small-for-dates fetuses (i.e. below the 5th centile weight for gestation) and three fetuses with cephalic abnormalities; these are plotted on the normal H/A ratio graph showing the mean, 95th and 5th centile confidence limits. Twenty-two of the twenty-five small-for-dates fetuses had ratios above the 95th centile limit and the two fetuses who died (+) had high ratios. Hydrocephalus (H) is associated with very high and microcephaly (M) with very low H/A ratios.

Another parameter which may be of value in the assessment of fetal nutrition is the measurement of head to abdomen circumference ratio. During the second trimester the mean ratio is greater than 1 but after 36 weeks there is a reversal of the head to abdomen circumference ratio. In many cases of growth retardation, however, this reversal does not occur. Our preliminary results with this technique (Figure 15.16) suggest that the head to abdomen circumference ratio will prove to be a valuable means of assessing fetal nutrition in late pregnancy, and in addition it may provide a simple method of distinguishing between the stunted and wasted growth-retarded fetus.

REFERENCES

Assali, N. S. & Brinkman, E. R. (1973) The role of circulatory buffers in fetal tolerance to stress. *American Journal of Obstetrics and Gynecology*, **117**, 643–652.

Bard, H. (1970) Intrauterine growth retardation. *Clinical Obstetrics and Gynecology*, **13**, 511.

Beazley, J. M. & Underhill, R. A. (1970) Fallacy of the fundal height. *British Medical Journal*, **iv**, 404.

Bjerre, I. (1975) Physical growth of 5-year-old children with a low birth weight. *Acta Paediatrica Scandinavica*, **64**, 33.

Brudenell, M. & Beard, R. (1972) Diabetes in pregnancy. In *Clinics in Endocrinology and Metabolism* (Ed.) Pyke, D. A. Vol. 1, pp. 673–695. London: W. B. Saunders.

Butler, N. R. & Alberman, E. D. (1969) *The Second Report of the 1958 British Perinatal Mortality Survey: Perinatal Problems*. Edinburgh: Livingstone.

Butler, N. R., Goldstein, H. & Ross, E. M. (1972) Cigarette smoking in pregnancy: its influence on the birthweight and perinatal mortality. *British Medical Journal*, **ii**, 127.

Campbell, S. (1968) An improved method of fetal cephalometry by ultrasound. *Journal of Obstetrics and Gynaecology of the British Commonwealth*, **75**, 568.

Campbell, S. (1969) The prediction of fetal maturity by ultrasonic measurement of the biparietal diameter. *Journal of Obstetrics and Gynaecology of the British Commonwealth*, **76**, 603.

Campbell, S. (1970) Ultrasonic fetal cephalometry during the second trimester of pregnancy. *Journal of Obstetrics and Gynaecology of the British Commonwealth*, **77**, 1057.

Campbell, S. (1972) Ultrasound in obstetrics. *British Journal of Hospital Medicine*, **8**, 541.

Campbell, S. (1974a) Fetal growth. In *Clinics in Obstetrics and Gynaecology* (Ed.) Beard, R. W., Vol. 1, pp. 41–62. London: W. B. Saunders.

Campbell, S. (1974b) The assessment of fetal development by diagnostic ultrasound. *Clinics in Perinatology*, **1**, 507.

Campbell, S. & Dewhurst, C. J. (1971) Diagnosis of the small-for-dates fetus by serial ultrasonic cephalometry. *Lancet*, **ii**, 1002.

Campbell, S. & Kurjack, A. (1972) Comparison between urinary oestrogen assay and serial ultrasonic cephalometry in assessment of fetal growth retardation. *British Medical Journal*, **iv**, 336.

Campbell, S. & Newman, G. B. (1971) Growth of the fetal biparietal diameter during normal pregnancy. *Journal of Obstetrics and Gynaecology of the British Commonwealth*, **78**, 513.

Campbell, S. & Wilkin, D. (1975) Ultrasonic measurement of fetal abdominal circumference in the estimation of fetal weight. *British Journal of Obstetrics and Gynaecology*, **82**, 689.

Cheek, D. B. (1968) *Human Growth: Body Composition, Cell Growth, Energy and Intelligence*. Philadelphia: Lea and Febiger.

Cheng, M. C. E., Chew, P. C. T. & Ratnam, S. S. (1972) Birthweight distribution of Singapore, Chinese, Malay, and Indian infants from 34 weeks to 42 weeks gestation. *Journal of Obstetrics and Gynaecology of the British Commonwealth*, **79**, 149.

Cole, P. V., Hawkins, L. H. & Roberts, D. (1972) Smoking during pregnancy and its effects on the fetus. *Journal of Obstetrics and Gynaecology of the British Commonwealth*, **79**, 782.

Creasy, R. K., De Sweit, M., Kahanpaa, K. V., Young, W. P. & Rudolph, A. M. (1974) Pathophysiological changes in the foetal lamb with growth retardation. *Foetal and Neonatal Physiology. Proceedings of the Sir Joseph Barcroft Centenary Symposium*, pp. 398–402. Cambridge: Cambridge University Press.

Davie, R., Butler, N. R. & Goldstein, H. (1972) From birth to seven. *The Second Report of the National Child Development Study*. London: Longmans.

Davison, J. M., Lind, T., Farr, V. & Whittingham, T. A. (1973) Ultrasonic cephalometry. *Journal of Obstetrics and Gynaecology of the British Commonwealth*, **80**, 769.

Dawes, G. S. (1974) *Size at Birth. CIBA Foundation Symposium*, p. 393. Amsterdam: Excerpta Medica.

Dobbing, J. (1974) *Scientific Foundations of Paediatrics* (Ed.) Davis, J. A. & Dobbing, J. London: Heinemann.

Dobbing, J. & Sands, J. (1970) Timing of neuroblast multiplication in developing human brain. *Nature*, **226**, 639.

Dobbing, J. & Sands, T. (1973) Quantitative growth and development of human brain. *Archives of Disease in Childhood*, **48**, 757.

Donald, I. (1965) Ultrasonic echo sounding in obstetrical and gynaecological diagnosis. *American Journal of Obstetrics and Gynecology*, **93**, 935–41.

Donald, I. (1968) Ultrasonics in obstetrics. *British Medical Bulletin*, **24**, 71.

Donald, I. & Brown, T. G. (1961) Demonstration of tissue interfaces within the body by ultrasonic echo sounding. *British Journal of Radiology*, **34**, 539.

Donald, I., MacVicar, J. & Brown, T. G. (1958) Investigation of abdominal masses by pulsed ultrasound. *Lancet*, **i**, 1188.

Dow, T. G. B., Rooney, P. J. & Spence, M. (1975) Does anaemia increase the risks to the fetus caused by smoking in pregnancy? *British Medical Journal*, **iv**, 253.

Enesco, M. & Leblond, C. P. (1962) Increase in cell number as a factor in the growth of the organs and tissues of the young male rat. *Journal of Embryology and Experimental Morphology*, **10**, 530.

Fancourt, R., Campbell, S., Harvey, D. & Norman, A. P. (1976) A follow-up study of small-for-dates babies. *British Medical Journal*, **i**, 1435–1437.

Flamme, P. (1972) Ultrasonic fetal cephalometry; percentiles curve. *British Medical Journal*, **iii**, 384.

Fitzhardinge, P. M. & Steven, E. M. (1972a) The small-for-dates infant I. Later growth patterns. *Pediatrics*, **49**, 671.

Fitzhardinge, P. M. & Steven, E. M. (1972b) The small-for-dates infant II. Neurological and intellectual sequelae. *Pediatrics*, **50**, 50.

Freeman, M. G., Graves, W. L. & Thompson, R. (1970) Indigent Negro and Caucasian birthweight gestation tables. *Paediatrics*, **46**, 9.

Gruenwald, P. (1966) Growth of the human fetus. 1. Normal growth and its variation. *American Journal of Obstetrics and Gynecology*, **94**, 112.

Gruenwald, P. (1969) *The Second Report of the 1958 British Perinatal Mortality Survey. Perinatal Problems.* Edinburgh: Livingstone.

Hansmann, M., Voigt, U. & Baeker, H. (1973) Die Vertigkeit Intrauterine mit Ultra schall Messbarer Parameter für die Gewichtsklassen Schutzung Seten. *Archiv für Gynäkologie*, **214**, 194.

Hill, D. E., Myers, R. E., Holt, A. B., Scott, R. E. & Cheek, D. B. (1971) Fetal growth retardation produced by experimental placental insufficiency in the rhesus monkey. II. Chemical composition of the brain, liver, muscle, and carcass. *Biology of the Neonate*, **19**, 68.

Jackson, W. P. U. (1967) Diabetes and pregnancy. I–IV. *Acta Diabetologica Latina*, **4**, 317–347.

Johnstone, F. & Inglis, L. (1974) Familial trends in low birth weight. *British Medical Journal*, **iii**, 659–661.

Kohorn, E. I. & Kaufman, M. (1974) Sonar in the first trimester of pregnancy. *Obstetrics and Gynecology*, **44**, 473–483.

Kossoff, G., Garrett, W. J. & Radovanovitch, G. (1974) Grey scale echography in obstetrics and gynaecology. *Australasian Radiology*, **18**, 62–111.

Kossoff, G., Robinson, D. C. & Garrett, W. J. (1965) *The CAL Abdominal Ultrasonic Echoscope.* CAL report No. 31. Sydney: Commonwealth Acoustic Laboratories.

Laga, E. M., Driscoll, S. G. & Munro, N. H. (1972) Comparison of placentas from two socioeconomic groups, I. Morphometry. *Pediatrics*, **50**, 24–32.

Lechtig, A., Yarbrough, E., Delgado, H., Martorell, R., Klein, R. E. & Behar, M. (1975) Effect of moderate maternal malnutrition on the placenta. *American Journal of Obstetrics and Gynecology*, **123**, 191–201.

Levi, S. (1972) *Diagnostic par Ultrasons en Gynecologie Obstetrique*, p. 62. Paris: Masson et Cie.

Levi, S. & Erbsman, F. (1975) Antenatal fetal growth from the 19th week. *American Journal of Obstetrics and Gynecology*, **121**, 262–268.

Lichty, J. A., Ting, R. Y., Bruns, P. D. & Dyar, E. (1957) Studies of babies born at high altitude, I. Relation of altitude to birthweight. *American Journal of Diseases in Children*, **93**, 666.

Loeffler, F. E. (1967) Clinical foetal weight prediction. *Journal of Obstetrics and Gynaecology of the British Commonwealth*, **74**, 675.

Longo, L. D. (1972) Pathophysiology of gestation II. In *Disorders of Placental Transfer* (Ed.) Assali, N. S. & Brinkman, C. R. New York: Academic Press.

Low, J. A. & Galbraith, R. S. (1974) Pregnancy characteristics of intrauterine growth retardation. *Obstetrics and Gynecology*, **44**, 122–126.

Low, J. A., Boston, R. W. & Pancham, S. R. (1972) Fetal asphyxia during the intrapartum period in intrauterine growth retarded infants. *American Journal of Obstetrics and Gynecology*, **113**, 351.

Lubchenco, L. O., Hansman, C., Dressler, M. & Boyd, E. (1963) Intrauterine growth as estimated from liveborn birth weight data at 24–42 weeks of gestation. *Pediatrics*, **32**, 793–800.

Milner, R. D. G. & Richards, B. (1974) An analysis of birth weight by gestational age of infants born in England and Wales 1967 to 1971. *Journal of Obstetrics and Gynaecology of the British Commonwealth*, **81**, 966–967.

Naeye, R. L., Blanc, W. & Paul, C. (1973) Effects of maternal nutrition on the human fetus. *Pediatrics*, **52**, 494–502.

Osler, M. (1960) Body fat of newborn infants of diabetic mothers. *Acta Endocrinologica*, **34**, 277.

Ounsted, M. (1971) Fetal growth. In *Recent Advances in Pediatrics* (Ed.) Gairdner D. & Hull, D. London: Churchill.

Ounsted, M. & Ounsted, C. (1966) Maternal regulation of intrauterine growth. *Nature*, **212**, 995.

Payne, D. R. & Wheeler, E. F. (1967) Comparative nutrition in pregnancy. *Nature*, **215**, 1134–1136.

Robinson, H. P. (1973) Sonar measurement of fetal crown–rump length as a means of assessing maturity in the first trimester of pregnancy. *British Medical Journal*, **iv**, 28.

Robinson, H. P. (1975) Gestation "sac" volumes as determined by sonar at the first trimester of pregnancy. *British Journal of Obstetrics and Gynaecology*, **82**, 100–107.

Robinson, H. P. & Fleming, J. E. C. (1975) A critical evaluation of sonar "crown–rump length" measurements. *British Journal of Obstetrics and Gynaecology*, **82**, 702–710.

Rush, D., Davis, H. & Susser, M. (1972) Antecedents of low birth weight in Harlem, New York City. *International Journal of Epidemiology*, **1**, 375.

Scammon, R. E. & Calkins, L. A. (1929) *The Development and Growth of the External Dimensions of the Human Body in the Fetal Period.* Minneapolis: University of Minnesota Press.

Sterky, G. (1970) Swedish standard curves for intrauterine growth. *Pediatrics*, **46**, 7.

Talbert, D. G. & Campbell, S. (1972) Physical aspects of diagnostic ultrasound. *British Journal of Hospital Medicine*, **8**, 501.

Taylor, K. J. W. (1974) Current status of toxicity investigation. *Journal of Clinical Ultrasound*, **2**, 149.

Thomson, A. M., Billewicz, W. Z. & Hytten, F. E. (1968) The assessment of fetal growth. *Journal of Obstetrics and Gynaecology of the British Commonwealth*, **75,** 903.

Thompson, H. E. & Makowski, E. L. (1971) Estimation of birth weight and gestational age. *Obstetrics and Gynecology*, **37,** 44.

Usher, R. H. & McLean, F. (1969) Intrauterine growth of liveborn caucasian infants at sea level: standards obtained from measurements in seven dimensions of infants born between 25 and 44 weeks of gestation. *Journal of Pediatrics*, **74,** 901.

Usher, R. H. & McLean, F. (1974) *Scientific Foundations of Paediatrics* (Ed.) Davis, J. S. & Dobbing, J., p. 69. London: Heinemann.

Varma, Y. R. (1973) Prediction of delivery date by ultrasound cephalometry. *Journal of Obstetrics and Gynaecology of the British Commonwealth*, **80,** 316.

Wehmer, F. & Hafez, E. S. E. (1975) Maternal malnutrition, low birthweight and related phenomena in man; physiological and behavioural interactions. *European Journal of Obstetrics, Gynaecology and Reproductive Biology*, **5,** 177–187.

Wells, P. N. T. (1972) *Ultrasonics in Clinical Diagnosis*. Edinburgh, London: Churchill Livingstone.

Widdowson, E. M. (1970) Harmony of growth. *Lancet*, **i,** 901.

Willocks, J., Donald, I., Duggan, T. C. & Day, N. (1964) Fetal cephalometry by ultrasound. *Journal of Obstetrics and Gynaecology of the British Commonwealth*, **71,** 11.

Winick, M. (1971) Cellular changes during placental and fetal growth. *American Journal of Obstetrics and Gynecology*, **109,** 166.

Winick, M. & Noble, A. (1965) Quantitative changes in D.N.A. and R.N.A. and protein during prenatal and postnatal growth in the rat. *Developmental Biology*, **12,** 451.

Winick, M. & Noble, A. (1967) Cellular growth in the human placenta. 1. Normal placental growth. *Pediatrics*, **39,** 248.

Winick, M., Brasel, J. A. & Velasco, E. C. (1973) Effects of prenatal nutrition on pregnancy risk. *Clinical Obstetrics and Gynecology*, **16,** 184.

Young, M. (1974) *Size at Birth. CIBA Foundation Symposium*, pp. 21–22. Amsterdam: Excerpta Medica.

Younoszai, M. K., Kacic, A. & Haworth, J. C. (1968). Cigarette smoking during pregnancy: the effect upon the haematocrit and acid–base balance of the newborn infant. *Canadian Medical Association Journal*, **99,** 197.

16

FETAL CIRCULATION AND BREATHING MOVEMENTS

K. Boddy

INTRODUCTION: ANIMAL MODELS

Knowledge concerning fetal biological function has been derived mainly from studies involving the use of animal models. Inherent in such studies are the problems of species differences, the effects of surgical and other experimental interferences on the processes being examined, and the fact that controlled changes in individual variables do not normally occur in biological systems. The methods used for investigating the fetus have changed considerably as knowledge and expertise have increased, and as suitable techniques and equipment have become available.

Early observations of fetal cardiovascular function and breathing movements were made on exteriorised fetuses, usually of the ovine species. This species was the most extensively used since the fetus was large enough for the techniques available, and could survive when exteriorised for several hours before the umbilical–placental circulation failed. Apart from the effects of surgery and the short period available for study, such 'acute preparations' suffered from another disadvantage, that of the continuing effects of anaesthesia, usually chloralose or pentobarbitone. It is worth noting, however, that the main features of the fetal cardiovascular system including the pulmonary circulation were described using these techniques and are now well known.

The stimulus and information gained from these studies contributed significantly to our understanding of the fetus as well as many of the problems arising in the neonatal ward. Examples of such information include the changes taking place in the fetal circulation at birth, the effects of hypoxia on the redistribution of blood flow and particularly on the pulmonary circulation; the discovery of pulmonary surfactant and its clinical importance and the mechanism of temperature control in the newborn. Recently, however, observations have been made over many weeks of pregnancy with the fetus in a more natural environment, in utero. Catheters and flowmeters as well as electrophysiological leads are implanted into the fetus and several days' recovery allowed from the immediate effects of operation. In this way tactile and other environmental influences present in acute preparations and the continuance of general or local anaesthetic agents is avoided. To some extent the problems of a rapidly failing circulation are also overcome. Such 'chronic preparations' are not however without their own difficulties. The long-term effects of operation, usually related to placental damage as well as to the site and number of recording devices implanted in the fetus, may significantly alter fetal function and subsequently its growth and development. Postoperative infection and voluntary maternal starvation as well as the onset of premature labour, and repeated experimentation and withdrawal of blood samples, may all lead to a deteriorating fetal condition. Experience over the past five or six years has suggested that many of the so-called advantages of the chronic preparation for observing fetal physiology may be forfeited by attempting to sample and record simultaneously from multiple sites on frequently repeated occasions. Similarly fetal condition, and therefore the value of certain physiological information, may be influenced by not allowing sufficient recovery time after operation (at least seven days are probably necessary) (Mellor and Slater, 1971, 1973; Shelley, 1973) and by repeating experiments which are detrimental to the fetus such as those producing fetal hypoxaemia. It is not surprising that conflicting information has appeared in the literature and that some of the older observations, made with acute preparations, have been questioned.

INHERENT VARIATION AND INTEGRATION OF FETAL BIOLOGICAL SYSTEMS

As the limitations of animal models are increasingly appreciated and further experience is gained of the long-term behaviour of the fetus in utero, it might be expected that more critical assessments of such concepts as 'steady state' and 'fetal health' will be made. It is already clear that considerable variations occur in utero that were not previously recognised when the fetus was exteriorised and anaesthetised. Fetal heart rate and blood pressure are not steady but vary with fetal movements and sleep state as well as with breathing activity and swallowing. Diurnal rhythms are present in both the fetal electrocorticogram and in the incidence and minute volume of fluid breathing (Boddy, Dawes and Robinson, 1973). There is also increasing evidence from measurements of fetal arterial Po_2 and haematocrit that wide variations occur in fetal oxygenation. Partially compensated fetal hypoxaemia has been observed in chronic preparations, and such fetuses may appear healthy by the accepted criteria for experimental investigation. Their blood gas values, pH, heart rate and blood pressure may all be within normal limits. In such fetuses an episode of hypoxaemia may result in a rapid deterioration of fetal condition with acidaemia and subsequent death, whereas in a more stable preparation recovery would occur.

These observations show that the fetus exhibits as wide a range of normal variations as the adult. They also indicate that the changes and adaptations which occur in fetal physiological systems before safety margins are exhausted may not be readily appreciated. When observed they may provide more meaningful evaluations of fetal health than those at present in use.

The complexities and integration of fetal biological systems are only just beginning to be recognised and some of the so-called discrepancies between observations in acute and chronic animal preparations may be no more than a manifestation of the range of variation in different environmental circumstances. Two examples concerning the fetal circulation and breathing movements will serve to illustrate this:

1. Reports of fetal breathing movements, in both man and animal, have appeared from time to time over the past 80 years. Many were anecdotal; others were attributed to artefact or the conditions under which they were observed (see Windle, 1940). From observations made on exteriorised fetal lambs delivered under maternal spinal anaesthesia, Barcroft (1946) concluded that fetal respiratory movements were not normally present. They could be stimulated by application of tactile stimuli to the face at between 40 to 60 days gestation (term is 147 days), but after 60 days (0.4) the lambs were unresponsive and breathing movements only began after birth. (Figures in brackets after gestational ages refer to the proportion of gestation.) Fetal lambs, exteriorised from the uterus but with intact umbilical cords have been observed in apparently good condition and without the effects of general anaesthesia by many workers over the past 20 years. Such lambs, when placed either alongside the mother on a warm table or restrained in a warm saline bath, do not normally make breathing movements. More recently, when lambs were delivered into warm saline and were not restrained, and in chronic in-utero experiments when catheters and flowmeters were previously implanted, breathing movements were observed in all fetuses from 40 days gestation onwards (Dawes et al, 1970, 1972; Merlet et al, 1970).

Many centres have now confirmed these observations in several different species. Handling of the exteriorised fetus, or operating to implant catheters and other recording devices, reduces or abolishes breathing movements sometimes for many hours or days. Although several factors detrimental to the fetus may reduce or abolish breathing movements, the apparent differences observed between exteriorised restrained fetuses and those unrestrained in warm saline or replaced in utero cannot be explained by differences in blood gas values, heart rate or blood pressure. The most likely explanation lies in the responses of a complex physiological system to external environmental changes (temperature, light, touch, etc.). The range of results observed illustrates the spectrum of variation possible and the degree of integration present in fetal physiological systems.

2. The older work on exteriorised, anaesthetised fetuses in apparently good condition demonstrated that the two sides of the fetal heart worked in parallel and that their outputs were almost equal except during experimentally produced cardiac slowing or hypoxia (Dawes, 1968). More recently in chronic preparations the outputs of the two ventricles have been shown to be capable of altering differentially without evidence of bradycardia or blood gas values suggestive of hypoxaemia (Goodwin et al, 1973; Rudolph and Heymann, 1973). Also, estimates of the combined cardiac output and of the right ventricular component have been consistently higher than the values previously obtained in acute preparations (Table 16.1).

A range of results has therefore been observed in different experimental and environmental conditions. The spectrum of variation in the fetal cardiovascular system revealed in this way may have similar explanations to those seen in the investigations of fetal breathing movements. This conclusion is supported to some extent by the fact that high estimates of fetal cardiac output, similar to those found in chronic preparations, were obtained in acute experiments when the fetus was replaced into the uterus (Rudolph and Heymann, 1970.

Table 16.1. *Fetal cardiac output and right ventricular component in acute and chronic sheep preparations.*

	Combined ventricular output (ml/kg/min)	Right ventricular component (% of CVO)
Acute preparations		
Exteriorised fetal lamb		
Dawes, Mott and Widdicombe (1954)	315	45
Mahon, Goodwin and Paul (1966)	362	50
Assali, Morris and Beck (1965)	235 (excluding coronary flow)	58
In utero fetal lamb		
Rudolph and Heymann (1970)	525	
Chronic preparations		
Rudolph and Heymann (1972)	500	67

'able 16.1). Also there is no evidence in the literature that fetal condition in any way in-
1enced the results reported, or that the techniques used for measurement of cardiac output
ere significantly superior or inferior to one another. It is known however that the reflex con-
ol of the fetal cardiovascular system can be modified by anaesthesia and in the acute
eparations this may have resulted in reduced variability with equalisation of ventricular
tputs. It is equally possible that increased variability with redistribution of blood flow may
ave been present in the chronic preparations. Such changes might have resulted from both
e number and site of implanted recording devices as well as from the changes taking place
other systems with recovery from surgery. These factors do not however fully explain the
sults. The differences between the fetal environments warrants equal consideration and
ould accord with what is known about the complexity and integration of fetal physiological
stems.

These considerations raise several important issues. Investigation of the fetus and par-
cularly of the fetal circulation and breathing movements can no longer be considered in
olation from the influences of environmental factors including those operating in utero,
hether natural or produced by experimental interference. Results from transient methods
' investigation are difficult to interpret unless related to all the known variables. Even with
ntinuous recordings more critical evaluations of fetal condition are required, and in this
spect any single assessment and also some combinations will not suffice. The capacity for
laptation, and the complex nature and integration of the fetal physiological system need to
further appreciated before normal function can be properly assessed. For this purpose the
tus must be in utero. At the present time such extensive investigation can only be made by
e use of animal models and by a combination of physiological, biochemical and endocrine
udies. The following account attempts to review the available information on those factors
hich might normally control the fetal circulation and breathing movements.

HYSIOLOGICAL CONTROL OF THE FETAL CIRCULATION

he fetal heart rate and cardiac output

part from anatomical differences, the fetal cardiovascular system differs functionally
om the adult in several important respects. Throughout pregnancy the fetal heart rate and

Table 16.2. *Heart rate, blood pressure and cardiac output of the human fetus (at birth) compared to the adult.*

	Fetus	Adult
Resting heart rate (beats/min)	120–160	60–80
Systolic blood pressure (mm Hg)	50–60	100–120
Cardiac output (ml/kg/min)	200	80

cardiac output are high compared to the adult, and blood pressure is relatively low (Table 16.2). By inference the peripheral vascular resistance of fetal tissues must also normally be low, as is that of the umbilical vascular bed. Physiological control is however dependent on the same biological systems and is equally as complex as the adult. Changes occur as the fetus continues to grow and develop, but at no stage is there any evidence of an inadequate circulatory competence. This is true even in young fetuses when autonomic nervous control is poor and emphasises the importance of the high fetal heart rate. The effects of changes in fetal heart rate on cardiac output and ventricular stroke volume have been recently studied in utero, in late pregnancy, in sheep (Rudolph and Heymann, 1973). An initial increase in heart rate above resting values (150 to 180 beats/min) resulted in an increase in cardiac output since ventricular stroke volume was maintained. In the adult, stroke volume falls as the heart rate is increased above resting values, and in both the fetus and adult cardiac outputs fall when the heart rate is approximately doubled. The most significant changes however occurred with bradycardia and confirm what was previously known from acute experiments, that the fetal heart shows little ability to increase stroke volume and that cardiac output falls pari-passu with the heart rate. The explanation for these differences between the fetus and adult is not yet clearly defined but it would appear that the competence of the fetal cardiovascular system in terms of maintaining cardiac output is almost totally dependent on a high heart rate even in late pregnancy. It is interesting to recount the reasons given as to why this should be, and to speculate on the ability of the fetus to modify its own circulation. In order to provide a safety margin for gaseous exchange it might be expected that a large blood flow would be required to both the fetal tissues as well as the placenta. This may be necessary for several reasons. Unlike the lung, and contrary to what was previously thought, the structure of the placenta in terms of the organisation of its blood vessels is not especially designed for efficient gas exchange (Longo, Power and Foster, 1967). This is true of most species, including primates (Bartells and Moll, 1964; Meschia, Battaglia and Bruns, 1967). The diffusion rate for gases per unit weight of placenta is approximately one-fiftieth that of lung. For relatively efficient gas exchange blood flow on both the fetal and maternal sides must therefore be large. Since on the fetal side the resistance of the umbilical vascular bed is normally comparatively low and invariant and because it receives so large a proportion of fetal cardiac output (about 58 per cent of the combined output of both ventricles), normal changes in vascular resistance in the fetal tissues might be expected to have little effect on blood pressure and therefore on cardiac output and blood flow. In the presence of a comparatively low fetal blood pressure, blood flow to the placenta must be maintained by the high fetal heart rate. Again the structure of the fetal circulation is important since blood returning from the placenta is mixed in the heart and great vessels with poorly oxygenated blood returning from the fetal tissues. The oxygen concentration of fetal arterial blood is thus only about 80 per cent that of maternal, and the oxygen tension is reduced by 60 per cent. Also in younger fetuses the haemoglobin concentration, and therefore the oxygen carrying capacity of the blood, is much less than at term. Although this is adjusted during pregnancy and according to fetal needs, it may never reach maternal concentrations in some species nor in all human infants. Total carrying capacity can also be considerably reduced by haematological disrders such as rhesus incompatibility. The oxygen requirements of the fetus are nevertheless met during normal growth and development. There is also an adequate safety margin; many anaemic babies grow and survive in utero. In order to achieve this, cardiac output and blood flow rates to the tissues must normally be high, and are maintained by the relatively high fetal heart rate. This view of the importance of a high heart rate in maintaining a high cardiac output and so ensuring fetal oxygen needs throughout pregnancy is nevertheless an over-simplified one; other factors certainly operate.

Oxygen uptake is favoured in the fetus by the different interaction of 2,3-diphosphoglycerate with fetal and adult haemoglobin (Bauer, Ludwig and Ludwig, 1968). The efficiency of exchange both in the placenta and in the fetal tissues is influenced by the Haldane and Bohr effects, apart from the more obvious and perhaps more significant dependence on blood flow. Also blood flow to the fetal tissues and placenta will normally depend on the fetal arterial pressure and vascular resistance which may alter significantly, and more than was previously thought, to influence circulatory competence. Although fetal blood pressure is low compared to the adult, it is certainly not unchanging nor unrelated to other physiological systems. This is true not only as changes take place with fetal growth and development but also on a minute-by-minute basis. In chronic fetal lamb studies, relatively large changes in fetal blood pressure, cardiac output and flow in the descending aorta are seen in association with breathing movements. These changes occur particularly in older fetuses (after 0.75 of gestation) and when the movements are vigorous (Figure 16.1). They

140 DAYS GESTATION : 15 DAYS POSTOPERATIVE

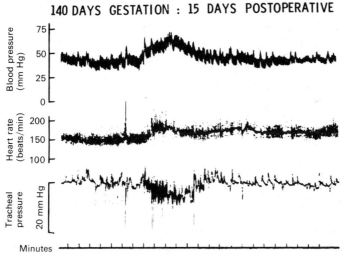

Figure 16.1. Fetal lamb in utero: short-lived changes in blood pressure and heart rate associated with breathing movements.

are sometimes clearly related to alterations in intrathoracic or abdominal pressures or volumes. Breathing movements have been observed from 40 days (0.2) of gestation in the sheep and from 11 weeks (0.27) of pregnancy in man (Boddy and Dawes, 1975). They may therefore influence the fetal circulation from a very early age. Independent of such mechanical factors, which have variable effects, the reflex control of the circulation may also alter, as in the adult, with those changes in the central nervous system that are associated with the state of sleep or arousal (Dawes, 1973). It is worth considering therefore the changes occurring with growth and development that might normally influence fetal vasomotor regulation.

The central nervous system

In the adult, cerebral cortical, hypothalamic and medullary activity are known to modif
cardiovascular function. In the fetus, systematic studies have not yet been made and th
evidence for central nervous system regulation of the circulation is scanty. Studies o
exteriorised, unanaesthetised fetal lambs have shown that before 60 days (0.4) the fetal cor
tex is electrically silent and that it is not electrically excitable before the 68th day (Bernhar
and Meyerson, 1973). After this time isolated bilaterally synchronised areas of the corte
show intermittent spontaneous activity, with bursts of spindles, not unlike the spindle activit
of the electroencephalogram (EEG) in the mature animal. These remain after transection c
the corpus callosum and are thus evidence of an afferent system driven from deep subcortica
structures such as the thalamus. The first evoked responses from the cortex to tactile stimula
tion of the trigeminal area occur at about 50 days (0.34) of gestation. From 70 to 75 day
(0.48 to 0.5) the electrocorticogram shows continuous activity but the electrocortica
characteristics associated with rapid-eye-movement (REM) sleep are not well develope
before 115 to 120 days (0.78 to 0.8). Cortical influences on the fetal cardiovascular systen
could not therefore arise much before 68 days (0.46) and probably not until some tim
later.

Spontaneous short-lived variations of heart rate and blood pressure have been observed i
fetal lambs in utero from as early as 85 days (0.55) of gestation. Studies before this time hav
not been made. These short-lived changes in the fetal cardiovascular system occur unrelate
to breathing movements (Figure 16.1) and even later, when seen in association with elec
trocortical activity (REM sleep), are not consistently related to it. Their presence suggest
normally occurring variations in fetal vasomotor tone, but their explanation is not yet cer
tain. Similar changes have been shown to result from electrical stimulation of the feta
hypothalamus as early as 115 days (0.75) gestation (Rudolph and Heymann, 1973). Othe
systems may however play a part. It is known for example that immature animal and huma
fetal tissues react vigorously in vitro to low concentrations of catecholamines o
acetylcholine (Boreus, 1973; Friedman, 1973; Owman et al, 1973). The renin–angiotensi
systems may also be active (Mott, 1973, 1975). The ability of the fetal cardiovascular systen
in late pregnancy to produce a pressor response to renin and angiotensin has been known fo
some time (Burlingame, Long and Ogden, 1942; Assali, Holm and Sehgal, 1962; Behrma
and Kittinger, 1968). Fetal hypophysial vasopressin release may similarly play a part i
regulating the responses of the fetal circulation, particularly in the last half of gestatio
(Skowky et al, 1973; Rurak, D., personal communication). The degree to which any of thes
complex systems normally affects fetal circulatory homeostasis in utero at various gestationa
ages is still however uncertain. Normally occurring changes in central nervous system activi
ty and stimulation of its various parts have complex effects which are difficult to evaluate, bu
recent evidence would suggest that physiological control of the fetal circulation may rely or
an integration of several systems, including the central nervous system, from an earlie
gestational age than was previously thought.

Development of autonomic and reflex control

The ability of the fetal cardiovascular system to respond by altering vasomotor tone, hear
rate and myocardial contractility, depends on several developments which result in a
progressive fall in heart rate and increase in blood pressure with increasing gestational age.

Autonomic nervous control of the fetal heart is known to be present late in gestation bu
may not be complete even at birth in some species. Although the pattern of innervation of the

heart is similar in all species so far studied, the rat (a relatively immature animal at birth) has no cardiac sympathetic nerves until about the end of the first week of life. The guinea-pig, on the other hand, which is relatively mature at birth has sympathetic nerves evident in the heart from just a little later than midway through pregnancy (0.66). In sheep, no sympathetic innervation is present up to 75 days (0.5). Prior to this time, however, dopamine-containing cells have been shown to exist throughout the myocardium and may influence cardiac regulation in early pregnancy (Rudolph and Heymann, 1973). Histological and histochemical studies on other fetal vascular structures have not yet been made in detail, but sympathetic nerve fibres and acetyl-cholinesterase have been demonstrated in the ductus arteriosus of fetal lambs in the last third of gestation (Silva and Ikeda, 1971). It is also known however that many immature fetal tissues, including the fetal heart, demonstrate a greater sensitivity to catecholamines than those of the adult. The same supersensitivity is present in adult tissues whose sympathetic nerve supply has been cut (Friedman, 1972).

These observations suggest that sympathetic innervation is incomplete in the fetus and therefore naturally occurring sympathetic amines may produce responses in the fetal circulation, of comparatively similar magnitude to those seen in adults, but at significantly lower concentrations. Some confirmation of this concept has been obtained using direct measurement or fluorescent microscopy to estimate the stores of catecholamines in many fetal tissues including the heart (Friedman, 1972; Boreus, 1973). These stores are less in several species before birth. There is no convincing evidence however that placental transfer of catecholamines occurs in sufficient quantities to increase fetal circulating levels, yet substantial increase in fetal plasma catecholamine concentration does occur in utero, particularly in such circumstances as fetal hypoxaemia, and is associated with major cardiovascular responses. Infusion of adrenaline and noradrenaline, in the same concentrations as those measured during hypoxia, also produces similar circulatory responses, in utero (Jones and Robinson, 1975). These considerations indicate an important role for naturally occurring fetal catecholamines in the regulation of the circulation throughout pregnancy but perhaps particularly so in early gestation when autonomic and central nervous system influences may be small. The exact timing of the earliest onset of sympathetic and parasympathetic influences is still in some doubt, but previous and recent observations in fetal lambs suggest that they might arise as early as 85 to 100 days (0.55 to 0.66) of pregnancy. In both the fetal heart and vascular smooth muscle, the development of beta- and alpha-adrenergic and parasympathetic receptor sites, as well as the ability to respond to autonomic and parasympathetic neurotransmitter substances, occurs about halfway through pregnancy (0.4 to 0.6) (Dawes, 1968; McMurphy and Boreus, 1971; McMurphy et al, 1972; Barrett, Heymann and Rudolph, 1972).

Some sympathetic influence is probably normally present from 100 days (0.66) gestation, since hexamethonium, a ganglion-blocking agent, produces a fall in both fetal blood pressure and heart rate in exteriorised fetal lambs. Small decreases in blood pressure were seen in utero before this time (at 85 days) when phenoxybenzamine or phentolamine (alpha-sympathetic blocking agents) were used, and after 100 days responses were similar in both fetal and newborn lambs. Propranolol or practolol (beta-sympathetic blocking agents) did not however produce significant changes till about 120 days (0.8) of gestation and there was always a greater effect in the newborn, increasing with age, suggesting continued development after birth. Experiments on fetal lambs in utero have shown that both alpha and beta-sympathetic stimulation and blockade can influence fetal heart rate, stroke volume and cardiac output in the last half of gestation (Rudolph and Heymann, 1973). These observations are in accord with a role for alpha-sympathetic influences on the fetal circulation from midway through pregnancy and beta-sympathetic influences in the last quarter of gestation. The results obtained with sympathetic blocking agents however may not be totally due to

autonomic blockade since these agents may interfere with the local effects of circulatory
catecholamines (van Petten and McCracken, 1973).

Reflex control

As pregnancy advances and fetal arterial pressure rises so the heart rate decreases (Figure
16.2). Observations in utero on fetal lambs have shown a fall in heart rate of 0.67

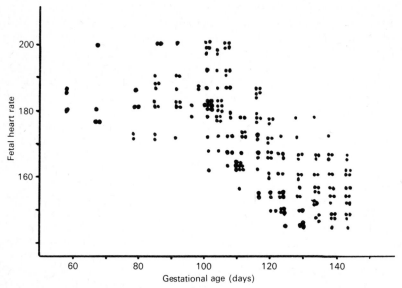

Figure 16.2. Fetal lamb heart rates in utero. Note the fall in heart rate after 100 days (0.66) gestation. Recordings
were made on unoperated ewes using Döppler ultrasound and gestational age was confirmed by x-ray.

beats/min/day from 100 days gestation (Boddy et al, 1974). In human pregnancy the fetal
heart rate falls from about 160 beats/min at 15 weeks gestation to about 140 beats/min at
term (Schifferli and Caldeyro-Barcia, 1973). This fall in heart rate from early in human
pregnancy suggests that parasympathetic vagal influences on the fetal circulation may be
present in the human fetus earlier than was previously thought. Parasympathetic blockade
using atropine produces a rise in fetal heart rate from as early as 85 days (0.55) gestation in
fetal lambs in utero (Rudolph and Heymann, 1973). Studies before this time have not been
made but the response is greater in older fetuses, increasing between 100 and 120 days (0.68
to 0.8) gestation. In human pregnancy atropine administered either to the mother or the fetus
results in a significant rise in fetal heart rate as early as the twentieth week (0.5) of pregnancy
and possibly from the 15th week (Schifferli and Caldeyro-Barcia, 1973). Again the response
is greater in older fetuses. These changes in fetal heart rate with gestational age and the
effects of parasympathetic blockade have been related to the development and function of the
aortic arch and carotid sinus pressure receptors (Dawes, 1968; Biscoe, Purves and Sampson,
1969). They suggest that the central cardiovascular centre together with the baroreceptors
and the efferent vagal fibres to the heart are active and capable of influencing the competency
of the fetal circulation throughout the whole of the last half of pregnancy, and possibly
earlier. Previously it has been suggested that the baroreceptor reflexes developed during the

st third of pregnancy from about 100 days (0.68) gestation. These earlier studies were ade on exteriorised and often anaesthetised fetal lambs and it is possible that reflex activity as modified by the different environment. Anaesthesia alone is unlikely to be a satisfactory xplanation since not all the experiments were performed under general anaesthesia and in cent acute experiments with unanaesthetised lambs in utero baroreflex activity was seen om 85 days (0.55) gestation (Rudolph and Heymann, 1973). An alternative explanation is at there may be a species difference between the sheep and human fetus. None of the recent vidence obtained from lambs in utero has however detracted significantly from the con- usions of the older work. Barcroft (1946) reported that in very young fetuses stimulation of e vagal nerves to the heart produced a small reduction in heart rate and it has long been nown that autonomic control of the fetal circulation is still incomplete even at birth. The ct that there is increasing tonic control of the fetal heart by an efferent cholinergic echanism due to the development of the baroreceptors was shown in animal experiments y recording aortic and carotid baroreceptor activity in time with the pulse in both late fetal d early neonatal life. Also, elevation of the fetal blood pressure, even halfway through station, caused a fall in heart rate which was abolished by section of the vagal pathways to e heart of the efferent baroreceptor nerves (Dawes, 1968; Rudolph and Heymann, 1973). he question as to whether before the last third of gestation sympathetic and parasym- athetic influences, in conjunction with other systems, normally modify fetal circulatory sponses in utero has not yet been studied in detail.

hemoreceptor reflex activity

part from baroreflex activity, the fetal circulation may also be regulated by the systemic terial chemoreceptors. Attempts to record chemoreceptor activity from the carotid nerves ave been unsuccessful in the exteriorised fetal lamb (Biscoe, Purves and Sampson, 1969). vidence in similar animal preparations has been obtained to show that both aortic and arotid chemoreceptor activity is capable of being stimulated from about 100 days (0.68) station (Dawes et al, 1969a, 1969b). In these experiments cardiovascular responses to ypoxaemia were abolished by section of the vagi or the aortic nerves but not by section of e carotid nerves. The carotid chemoreceptors were capable of responding to local injec- ons of cyanide which caused bradycardia, a fall in blood pressure, and fetal gasping, all of hich were abolished by section of the carotid nerves (Dawes, 1968). Such results led to the nclusion that the carotid chemoreceptor played only a small part, if any at all, in regulating e fetal circulation. The aortic chemoreceptors, on the other hand, were important in romoting the cardiovascular response to hypoxaemia and therefore influencing fetal sur- val under these conditions by redistribution of blood flow.

etal cardiovascular responses to hypoxaemia

he aortic chemoreceptors have been shown to operate over a range of fetal arterial Po_2 om 40 to <20 mm Hg (at a Pco_2 of 48 mm Hg). Their interaction with Pco_2 is important nce reduction by 10 mm Hg below the normal value of 48 mm Hg is sufficient to abolish or gnificantly reduce the cardiovascular responses to hypoxaemia (Baillie et al, 1971). The cir- ulatory responses to hypoxaemia however are too complex and variable to be explained urely by aortic chemoreceptor activity. They vary with gestational age as well as with the revious history and present condition of the fetus and are not readily predictable. The spec- um of different responses seen in fetal lambs in utero has been ascribed in part to central nervous system influences, baroflex responses and increases in circulatory plasma catecholamines (Boddy et al, 1974; Jones and Robinson, 1975). In exteriorised anaesthetised fetuses, the cardiovascular changes seen in response to hypoxia (and abolished by vagal or aortic nerve section) were those of a rise in fetal arterial pressure and vasoconstriction in the hind limbs, often, but not always, accompanied by tachycardia. The resultant redistribution of blood flow favoured the essential organs of the fetal brain and heart and maintained flow to the placenta, at the expense of the fetal body. Unlike the adult the fetal pulmonary circulation was found to be extremely sensitive to acute episodes of hypoxia and marked vasoconstriction occured due to both a direct effect of a fall in Pao_2 in the perfusing blood as well as the sympathetic reflex. The pulmonary circulation was also found to react vigorously to catecholamines as well as acetylcholine, bradykinin and histamine (vasodilator agents) (Dawes, 1968).

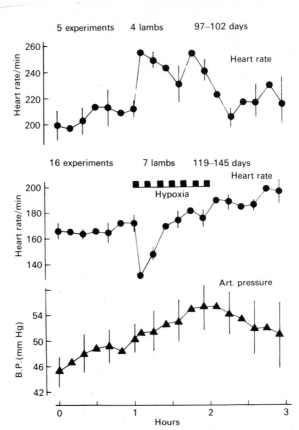

Figure 16.3. Fetal lambs in utero. Cardiovascular responses to hypoxia of one hour's duration (9 per cent O_2, per cent CO_2 in N_2 was administered to the ewe). There were no significant changes in blood pressure in the younger fetuses. Redrawn from Boddy et al (1974) with kind permission of the editor of the *Journal of Physiology*.

In recent investigations on fetal lambs in utero, the cardiovascular responses to hypoxia of one hour's duration were found to be age-dependent (Boddy et al, 1974). Resting heart rates were higher in younger fetuses (97 to 102 days) and the response to hypoxaemia was tachycardia (from 206 ± 13.4 beats/min to 256 ± 9.1 beats/min) with no significant change in blood pressure. Older fetuses (119 to 145 days) responded with an initial bradycardia

68 ± 6 beats/min to 131 ± 8 beats/min) and a rise in blood pressure (from 48 ± 2.3 mm
g to 55.3 ± 3.6 mm Hg) (Figure 16.3). The tachycardia seen in immature fetuses when the
rtic chemoreceptors are not yet fully functional, according to acute experiments, would
t indicate an earlier development of this system since there was no change in blood
essure. It could be due to a central effect or to an action of liberated catecholamines (which
ould cause cardio-acceleration). The fact that bradycardia did not occur in these young
uses or in older vagotomised fetuses does not rule out the presence of an active baroreflex
stem. In the absence of a rise in blood pressure no baroreflex stimulation would occur. The
pertension seen in older fetuses was abolished by vagal section and could therefore be at-
buted to excitation of the aortic bodies. It is known however that hypoxia is accompanied
some diminution of renin release and this may have limited the rise of blood pressure seen.
e hypertension was however maintained and the blood pressure only fell to resting values
the two hours following cessation of hypoxia. On the other hand, the bradycardia was not
aintained even in fetuses with intact vagal nerves and in spite of continuing hypoxaemia.
fter 20 minutes of continuous hypoxia the heart rate had returned to its original value and
ntinued to rise somewhat further, even though the fetus was by that stage becoming
idaemic. Continuous bradycardia throughout such periods of hypoxia has been observed
om time to time in fetal lambs in utero and is usually associated with a poor fetal condition
d an even greater rise in blood pressure than that seen in the above experiments.

These variable responses can be explained only by recognising both the complexity and in-
gration of the various physiological systems influencing fetal cardiovascular function as
ell as the capacity for adaptation and the changes taking place with increasing growth and
velopment. The variable nature and length of bradycardia may be attributed to differences
the degree of hypertension and baroreflex activity as well as the rise achieved in fetal
techolamines and other direct and second-order reflex effects of chemoreceptor stimula-
n. Large sustained falls in heart rate are usually only seen when the safety margins have
en exceeded. In severe hypoxia the bradycardia has two components, a primary reflex one
bolished by vagal section) and a secondary direct toxic effect upon the heart (Barcroft,
46). The fact that in acute exteriorised fetal lambs tachycardia was the usual initial
sponse to hypoxia even in the presence of hypertension does tend to suggest that baroreflex
tivity was modified in these preparations by the different environment or experimental con-
tions. The ability of the systemic arterial chemoreceptors to influence normally the fetal cir-
lation in utero is not yet known.

he renin–angiotensin system

he possible importance of the renin–angiotensin system in maintaining fetal circulatory
meostasis is suggested by evidence obtained principally from studies on animals that are
latively immature at birth (e.g. the rabbit and kitten) and from the fetal and newborn lamb
Mott, 1975). Systematic studies in utero have not yet been made. In the newborn of rabbits
d lambs as well as man, the plasma concentrations of angiotensin II are higher than in the
lult of the same species. Some of this difference has been explained in the rabbit by the
lative inability of an immature vasculature to inactivate as high a proportion of angiotensin
as the adult and in those species more mature at birth to those influences arising during
arturition that might stimulate the fetal renin–angiotensin system. In fetal lambs during the
st quarter of gestation the resting plasma concentrations of angiotensin II are similar to
ose of the mother, but plasma renin concentrations are higher and are also significantly
gher in fetuses above 130 (0.88) days gestation compared to those below 120 (0.86) days
Broughton Pipkin, Lumbers and Mott, 1974). It has been suggested that the low fetal levels of

circulating angiotensin II in the presence of high renin concentrations may be explained by th deficiency of converting enzyme in the immature fetus (Mott, 1975). The sensitivity of fet tissue to circulating angiotensin II may also alter with age. In new born rabbits at about the er of the second week of life when resting levels are maximal, the ability to obtain a pressc response is diminished (Broughton Pipkin, 1971). The same is true in various pathological co ditions where angiotensin II concentrations are high (Chinn and Dusterdieck, 1972).

These differences between the fetus and mother and the changes occurring with fetal ag have been linked with anatomical development of the kidney, which in species immature a birth shows a postnatal growth spurt, associated with increasing angiotensin II-like activit, Whilst fetal survival in most species does not depend on the presence of kidneys, rabbi nephrectomised at 25 to 29 (0.8 to 0.93) days gestation do not survive to term (Berton, 1970 In this species autonomic nervous development is demonstrably incomplete at birth (Friedma et al, 1968), yet fetal arterial blood pressure rises rapidly in the last quarter of gestation (Dawe Handler and Mott, 1957). There may therefore be a time in normal development when the fet: renin–angiotensin system is of importance to circulatory homeostasis. This is furthe suggested by the fetal response to a reduction of circulating blood volume. In terms of mai taining blood pressure, immature fetal rabbits have a superior ability to withstand removal of given fraction of blood volume, compared to the adult (Mott, 1975). This is greatly impaired the kidneys are removed, but is uninfluenced by section of the arterial baroreceptor nerves by sympathetic blockade using bethanidine. In the adult, bilateral nephrectomy has little effec on the response to haemorrhage (Mott, 1969). In fetal lambs plasma angiotensin II and reni concentrations fall to very low levels after bilateral nephrectomy in the last quarter of gestatio Similarly even small haemorrhages (producing a three per cent reduction in blood volume) ar sufficient to increase plasma renin concentrations in intact fetal lambs. The reduction of bloc pressure seen in newborn lambs after bilateral nephrectomy was however somewhat less tha that observed in rabbits and may be related to the lower concentration of angiotensin II seen i the young of more mature species (Mott, 1975). Apart from haemorrhage a reduction in fet: blood volume with increased renin release can be obtained by administration of a diuretic suc as frusemide (Trimper and Lumbers, 1972) and fetal renal concentrations have bee found to be higher in dogs when the uterus was made ischaemic (Hodgkinson, Hodari an Bumpus, 1967) or when the mother was nephrectomised (Hodari and Hodgkinson, 1968 These facts, together with the observation that expansion of the blood volume in fetal lamb results in a reduction of plasma renin and angiotensin II (Mott, 1975), suggest that the fet: renin–angiotensin system is functional and may be important in the maintenance and distribu tion of blood flow. The exact timing of when the system may normally influence the fetal ci culation is not however certain, but in both sheep and human pregnancy fetal nephrogenesis i usually complete by 0.7 of term and renal function is certainly present before this time in mar as judged by changes in amniotic fluid osmolability and concentration of creatinine and urea

CLINICAL IMPLICATIONS FROM ANIMAL STUDIES
OF THE FETAL CARDIOVASCULAR SYSTEM

Drugs influencing the fetal circulation

In both animal and human studies several drugs are known to affect the fetal circulation Two broad types of pharmacological agents will be discussed to illustrate the importance o

his subject; namely central nervous system depressants and drugs influencing the
utonomic nervous system. In assessing the clinical significance of pharmacological studies,
 must be remembered that drugs administered to the mother may or may not cross the
lacenta, and that this potential may be altered in various species and by changing maternal
lasma concentrations. Secondly drugs reaching the fetus may have different effects at
ifferent gestational age, and responses may be qualitatively and quantitatively different
rom the adult both because of the geometry of the fetal circulation and because of the func-
ional maturity of this and other fetal systems (e.g. liver and central nervous system).

So far as is known all general anaesthetic agents cross the placenta. Recent studies on fetal
ambs in utero showed that pentobarbitone administered to the ewe in a mild sedative dose (4
ng/kg) had complex age-related effects on the fetal circulation (Boddy and Dawes, 1976). In
ll fetuses the normal heart rate variations were abolished and a fall in blood pressure occurred
ttributable to systemic vasodilatation. This was prolonged in younger fetuses (87 to 97 days)
nd was associated with bradycardia. In older fetuses (116 to 137 days) the blood pressure was
estored in association with an increase in heart rate, a difference which can be attributed to the
evelopment of autonomic control. In human pregnancy, near term, maternal administration
f 0.2 mg/kg morphine results in significant fetal bradycardia (a fall of 12 to 20 beats/min)
Hon and Sze-Ya, 1969; Grimwade, Walker and Wood, 1971). Morphine, as well as
liazepam, also significantly reduces fetal heart rate variation (Hon and Sze-Ya, 1969;
Grimwade, Walker and Wood, 1970). The clinical use of central nervous system depressant
lrugs may therefore have important influences on the fetus. Although pethidine has shown no
onsistent effect (Boddy et al, 1976), further studies, with this and other drugs affecting the cen-
ral nervous system, are needed to asses the fetal responses, particularly during hypoxia. Pen-
obarbitone in anaesthetic doses has been reported to cause gross alterations in maternal utero-
lacental vasomotor reactivity (Assali, Brinkmann and Nuwayid, 1974). In both animal and
uman studies of the fetal cardiovascular system normal function should therefore be assessed
n the absence of this drug. The possible effects on the fetal and placental circulation of pen-
obarbitone and similar drugs need further investigation in both animals and man before they
an be regarded as entirely safe.

Drugs influencing the autonomic nervous system are the subject of renewed interest with
he use of such agents in the control of maternal hypertension during pregnancy and in the
reatment of premature labour. Parasympathetic blockade using atropine has been men-
ioned above but the question as to whether abolishing the fetal circulatory response to
ypoxia might be beneficial or otherwise has not been resolved. It is uncertain for example if
radycardia, apart from being a useful sign, may not also be physiologically useful in
educing cardiac work. Recently (van Petten, 1975) it has been suggested that beta-
drenoceptor agonists and antagonists may produce quantitatively different responses in the
etus compared to the adult. Propranolol (a beta-antagonist) administered in clinically rele-
ant doses to pregnant sheep produced full beta-blockade in the fetus, of three times longer
luration than that seen in the mother. The fetal plasma concentrations were only about five
er cent of those achieved in the maternal circulation (van Petten and Willes, 1970). By
locking the effects of circulating catecholamines on fetal tissues, propranolol may have
erious consequences to the fetus, particularly in the presence of hypoxaemia and at an early
estational age. Similarly isoxsuprine (a beta-agonist) has been seen to cause marked fetal
ardiac irregularities when administered either to the ewe or the fetus in clinically relevant
loses. The dysrhythmias were not attributable to fetal hypoxia and lasted one to two hours
fter drug injection (van Petten and McCracken, 1973). Both propranolol and isoxsuprine
re used in clinical practice and cross the human placenta. Other beta-adrenoceptor
gonists (e.g. bamethan) and antagonists (e.g. sotalol) produce little effect on the fetus in
tero when administered to the mother but produce similar responses to isoxsuprine and

propranolol when given directly to the fetus. These considerations are important when choosing drugs for use to control hypertension during pregnancy and to inhibit uterine activity. So far as is known no fetal deaths have been directly attributed to the use of adrenoceptor drugs in human pregnancy, but it is clear that more precise and additional information is required before such pharmacological agents become widely used in clinical practice. The not inconsiderable perinatal mortality and morbidity associated with maternal hypertension and premature labour should not be added to by the uninformed use of drugs which may be potentially dangerous to the fetus.

Fetal heart rate monitoring

The fetal heart beat can be continuously monitored in the human fetus both antenatally and in labour by several different methods. The most accurate of these, in terms of recording both the heart rate and the heart period (beat-to-beat interval), is that of obtaining the fetal electrocardiogram. As yet the wave form of the electrocardiogram has not been shown to be of great significance. Variation of the beat-to-beat interval between successive R-waves of the electrocardiogram has not been systematically analysed in fetal animals. Preliminary observations suggest that there is an inverse correlation with breathing movements and that a diurnal rhythm exists. The initial fetal response to hypoxia in utero would appear to be to increase beat-to-beat variation (Dalton, K., personal communication). The heart rate (measured in beats/min) and the beat-to-beat interval (measured in msec) have been used in human pregnancy to assess fetal well-being. That it is clinically useful to monitor continuously the fetal heart rate is widely accepted but the interpretation of such records remains a difficulty. In human labour there is good evidence to show that fetal bradycardias called 'delayed deceleration' (or Type II dips) are significantly associated with hypoxia (see Chapter 23) and the same is true in the sheep (Dawes, 1968, p. 121).

If the uterus is contracting, a variety of other responses may occur as the fetus becomes hypoxic. In the early stages, fetal heart rate decelerations which start at the onset of a contraction are often accompanied by tachycardia between contractions. As the condition of the fetus deteriorates, the decelerations are delayed relative to the contractions and the 'variability' of the fetal heart rate decreases, resulting in a flat trace. In contrast, in the absence of uterine activity, evidence of impending trouble may not be seen until the time of fetal death and even in labour warning signs can disappear only to return when the fetus is in extremis (Renou and Wood, 1974). These variable changes can be explained, by analogy with fetal lambs, on the basis that a high cardiac output and therefore a reasonable heart rate, are essential to maintain blood flow and hence fetal survival. Integration of central nervous system activity with chemoreflex and baroreflex responses and release of catecholamines, together with activation of the renin–angiotensin system, will all tend to result in redistribution of blood flow and maintenance of blood pressure and heart rate until the fetus can no longer adapt. A wide variation of responses would therefore be expected to changes which affect fetal blood gas and acid–base status, to uterine activity and to engagement and descent of the presenting fetal part. These responses will be difficult to predict and interpret; they will only appear simple when the physiological reserves have been exhausted. In fetuses which are growth-retarded or anaemic or subjected to repeated or prolonged hypoxaemia, a further adaptation may occur—that of a significant increase in fetal haemoglobin concentration adjusted by secretion of haemopoietin (Zanjani et al, 1973). In the event of glycogen stores being depleted such fetuses may rapidly succumb to mild hypoxia without warning signs (Shelley, 1969).

It should also be remembered that different cardiovascular responses to hypoxia may be expected from younger fetuses compared to the more mature fetus but the possible clinical significance of this has not yet been investigated (Boddy et al, 1974). It is for these reasons that other methods of assessing fetal well-being, such as the pH, are used. The fetal heart rate alone may be misleading and the various forms of 'stress-tests' at present in use may not only be detrimental to the fetus but would be expected to show similar variable responses. This is not to deny the practical clinical usefulness of fetal heart rate monitoring, particularly in labour, but to underline the complexity of fetal physiological systems and the need for further information before interpretation of responses can be made.

THE PHYSIOLOGICAL CONTROL OF FETAL BREATHING MOVEMENTS

Unlike the fetal heart rate, respiratory movements in utero do not appear to be necessary to maintain fetal health. Organised physiological control of these movements, and the development of the respiratory musculature, must be established in utero since both are essential to survival after birth. Observation of fetal respiratory movements and their responses to alterations in both the external and internal fetal environments, together with the changes taking place during growth and development, provide another opportunity of studying the range of variation present in fetal behaviour. The response to exteriorisation and handling of the fetus which has already been mentioned has led to the conclusion that breathing movements were not a normal accompaniment of fetal life. The ability to study the fetus with the use of sensitive pressure transducers, electromagnetic flowmeters and improved methods for measuring blood gas tensions, has now made it possible to describe more fully the nature and variability of fetal respiratory movements (Dawes, 1973; Boddy et al, 1974; Boddy and Dawes, 1975).

Initially, experiments similar to those of Barcroft (1946) were made on fetal lambs exteriorised from the uterus, with intact umbilical cords but unrestrained in warm saline. Episodic respiratory movements were observed in all fetuses studied. Tactile stimuli were seen to cause expiratory, not inspiratory efforts, and asphyxia abolished the normal movements and stimulated gasping. It is now a little over five years since these first observations were made, and the reasons appreciated why, previously, breathing movements had not normally been observed. Since that time breathing movements have been observed in utero in several other species, including the rabbit, guinea-pig and sub-human primates, as well as man. In sheep and man they are normally present from 0.27 of gestation (40 days, and 11 weeks respectively) and may even continue throughout labour to the time of birth. In man an A-scan ultrasound method has been used to record the heart beat and the movements of the fetal chest wall in utero (Boddy and Robinson, 1971) (Figure 16.4). The technique was validated using sheep with previously implanted fetal tracheal and carotid artery catheters.

Normal variation and diurnal rhythms

In fetal lambs in utero, '*episodic rapid irregular breathing movements*' occur at a frequency of 3 to 4 sec, are coincident with simultaneous activity in the diaphragm and intercostal muscles, and are associated with falls of tracheal pressure up to 5 to 15 mm Hg, occasionally up

Heart beat

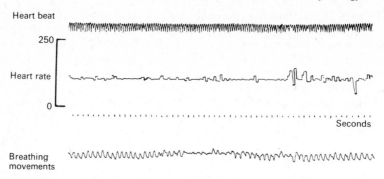

Figure 16.4. A-scan recording of human fetal heart beat, heart rate and breathing movements at term. Note the even depth and regular nature of the breathing movements. This pattern is first seen at the 34th week in clinically normal pregnancies.

to 30 mm Hg. The movements are usually of short duration (0.2 sec) and because of the viscosity and density of tracheal fluid, result in a fluid movement of only 1 to 5 ml which is insufficient to clear the dead-space. These observations are in accord with previous experiments where radio-opaque contrast medium was introduced into the amniotic cavity of both animals and man, and was not seen to enter the tracheobronchial tree (McCain, 1964; Carter et al, 1964). In previously catheterised lambs in utero a net outward flow of tracheal fluid has been observed to occur in association with short bursts of breathing movements accompanied by a rise in both carotid arterial and intrathoracic pressure. Net outward flow has been seen to increase with gestational age and is as much as 100 ml/kg/day near term. Outward gushes occur about 6 to 12 times per day and contribute more than half the total net outward tracheal flow (Dawes, 1973). Net inward tracheal flow is less common but occurs with the large falls in tracheal pressure seen from time to time during '*rapid irregular breathing movements*' and with gasping movements. Rapid irregular fetal breathing activity is present episodically about 40 to 50 per cent of the time and is seen in association with rapid-eye movement (REM) sleep. The onset and cessation of such episodes are unrelated to the fetal carotid blood gas tensions.

Another type of normally occurring breathing movement observed in utero is that of slow and relatively deep '*augmented breaths*', originally described as '*gasps or sighs*' (Dawes, 1973). They occur at a frequency of 1 to 4 min, cause falls in tracheal pressure of 20 mm Hg or more, and appear both independently and in association with '*rapid irregular breathing movements*'. Such '*augmented breaths*' are present about five per cent of the time and are not associated with either REM sleep or change in fetal blood gas tensions. A third variety of breathing activity seen in fetal lambs is that of '*panting*'. This can be brought about in exteriorised lambs, unrestrained and in warm saline, by increasing the bath temperature from 39.5°C by 1°C. '*Panting*' activity initiated in this way has been seen from 75 (0.5) days of gestation to term. It is characterised by strong expiration and protrusion of the fetal tongue but is not usually maintained for more than five to ten minutes. Similar episodes have been observed in utero associated with a rise in maternal temperature caused by disturbance (Robinson, J. S., unpublished observations). This activity is similar in character to portions of rapid irregular breathing movements and may be a variation of that activity.

Apart from this spectrum of normal variation seen in the character of fetal breathing activity, changes also take place with increasing gestational age and with the time of day. Early in pregnancy the movements are totally irregular and less frequent. They remain irregular for the most part but increase in rate and depth as pregnancy advances. Their incidence does not however alter with gestational age over the last third of fetal life until just before the onset of labour. The most vigorous periods of this fetal activity occur most often in the late evening and a diurnal variation is present from as early as 85 to 90 (0.58 to 0.6) days of gestation. This is persistent even when a 12-hour regulated light cycle is imposed in a temperature-controlled environment, and when disturbances associated with sound and feeding are reduced to a minimum (Boddy, Dawes and Robinson, 1973). The incidence of breathing movements approximately doubles between early morning and late evening. A quantitative estimate of breathing activity using an electromagnetic flowmeter (Clark and Wyatt, 1969) to record the rate and the minute volume of fluid breathing reveals a well-defined rhythm in both measurements from 110 days gestation. Fetal breathing movements thus vary with time of day in both their incidence and their activity (rate and depth). Before 110 days the alveoli are still solid and the lungs inexpansible so that tracheal fluid flow cannot be used as a measure of breathing activity. There is no evidence of a diurnal rhythm in net outward or inward tracheal flow. The fetal electrocorticogram shows a diurnal variation in the proportion of the low-voltage, rapid frequency activity which is present and is mainly associated with REM sleep. These rhythms all have their peak in the late evening (1900 to 2200 hours) and a broad trough in the early hours of the morning (0400 to 0900 hours). Their cause is not yet known. Preliminary observations suggest that a diurnal variation exists in fetal temperature (which passively follows that of the mother) but various endogenous fetal and maternal rhythms may also play a part. Variation might be expected with changes such as those occurring in light and sound, placental blood flow and concentrations of various blood constituents (e.g. fetal blood glucose and adrenocorticotrophic hormone (ACTH) concentrations). A reciprocal correlation between the incidence of fetal breathing movements in utero and the fetal plasma ACTH concentration has been described (Boddy, Jones and Robinson, 1974), and the proportion of time during which breathing movements are present in utero is significantly reduced in some apparently healthy fetuses two or three days prior to spontaneous delivery (Boddy and Dawes, 1975). These two observations may not be strictly 'normal' variations, although in both instances there was no correlation with fetal blood-gas value, pH, blood glucose concentration or fetal heart rate. They could be explained in part by changing conditions in utero that may be detrimental to the fetus (e.g. mild hypoxia and increasing uterine activity). If so then such changes are reflected earlier by alteration in fetal breathing movements than by responses in other systems used to assess fetal health. Similarly in otherwise healthy fetal lambs in utero, a fall in blood glucose concentration is accompanied by a reduction in both the amplitude and frequency of breathing movements, and with the appearance of abnormal 'gasping movements'. Normal movements do not disappear however until the fetal blood glucose concentration has fallen below 10 mg/100 ml (normal range 20 to 30 mg/100 ml). In such circumstances administration of glucose either to the fetus or the mother immediately restores the incidence and character of the breathing movements. There is also some evidence of a correlation with breathing movements and fetal blood glucose concentrations in the normal range but no diurnal variations in maternal or fetal blood glucose concentrations have been reported. These alterations which occur in fetal breathing movements with fetal age, electrocortical activity, time of day and other internal and external environmental changes all serve to emphasise the degree of integration and variability inherent in this fetal physiological function. Similar changes have been seen in recordings of human fetal chest wall movements in utero.

In clinically normal patients the proportion of time during which fetal breathing movements are present can vary from less than 10 per cent to above 90 per cent (Boddy and Wyn Pugh, unpublished observations). Usually apnoeic periods are short (< 1 min) and the incidence of breathing movements is above 50 per cent, altering little from one 15-min period to the next. A reduced incidence (below 50 per cent) has been seen in the early hours of the morning (0400 to 0700 hours); within 72 hours of the spontaneous onset of labour; immediately after cigarette smoking (Manning, Wyn Pugh and Boddy, 1975); and after maternal overnight starvation. Similarly maternal posture is important; supine hypotension can result in a marked reduction or abolition of fetal breathing movements and gasping may be seen. Previous maternal activity (e.g. walking upstairs) and palpation of the abdomen have also been seen to result in a reduced incidence of breathing movements in the fetus. Recovery to normal amounts may not occur for up to one hour.

In early human pregnancy breathing movements are less frequent and more irregular, as in the sheep. A periodic type of breathing movement is seen from 24 weeks of human pregnancy with rates varying from 30 to 90 breaths/min, and Figure 16.4 shows the more regular pattern which first appears at the 34th week and becomes an increasingly greater part of the breathing activity recorded between that time and term. These breathing movements are slower, vary less in frequency (40 to 60 breaths/min) and are usually of even depth. Initially it was felt that such changes with fetal age would not be clinically useful (Boddy and Dawes, 1975), but more recently the first appearance of a *regular pattern* has been seen to be a good index of gestational age (Boddy and Parboosingh, unpublished results). In diabetic pregnancies and some growth-retarded fetuses a *regular pattern* may be seen earlier than the 34th week. In such circumstances the incidence of breathing movements is reduced and periods of apnoea longer than one minute are also features of the records obtained. The variable nature of recordings obtained in patients with normal pregnancy makes detailed clinical knowledge and standardised techniques essential before results can be interpreted and compared with those of other centres. Experience from 1520 recordings made on 800 patients from 11 weeks (0.27) to 42 weeks gestation has shown that when normal fetal breathing movements are present for more than 50 per cent of the recording time (usually 15 minutes to 2 hours) and apnoeic periods are short (less than one minute), the fetus can be regarded as being in reasonably good health. Table 16.3 shows that intra-uterine fetal death and neonatal deaths did not occur in such fetuses and that fetal distress in labour was an uncommon finding.

Table 16.3. *Perinatal mortality and fetal distress in labour according to the incidence and type of human fetal breathing movements in utero (658 + 45 + 86 + 11 = 800 pregnancies).*

Fetal breathing Percentage	Type	Intra-uterine death	Neonatal death	Fetal distress in labour
> 50	Normal	0/658	0	5/658
5–50	Normal	0/45	0	5/41
5–50	Mixed	0/86	7	48/56
< 5	Apnoea + gasps	11/11	—	—

Data from Boddy and Wyn Pugh, unpublished observations.

Responses to changes in fetal blood gases and abnormal breathing movements

The effect of *hypercapnia* has been observed in fetal lambs in utero from 103 days (0.7) to term. The hypercapnia was achieved by exposing the pregnant ewe to a gas mixture containing four to six per cent CO_2 with 18 per cent O_2 in N_2 for one hour. A reduced oxygen content was used in order to limit the effect of maternal hyperventilation and hence the rise in both maternal and fetal oxygen tension (Po_2). In fact fetal Pao_2 increased by a mean value of only 3 mm Hg while the Pa_{CO_2} was increased from 44 to 57 mm Hg. The incidence of fetal breathing movements was approximately doubled during hypercapnia and the depth of these movements was also increased. The minute volume of fluid breathing increased three-fold but no increase was seen above the resting rate of breathing movements which was already high (> 3 Hz). The proportion of time spent in predominantly low voltage electrocortical activity was also significantly increased, as was the fraction of that time associated with breathing movements. These results indicate similar responses to hypercapnia as those seen after birth. It is known that an increase in carotid blood flow occurs when the EEG of fetal lambs in utero changes from predominantly high to low voltage activity (Jost, 1969). Hypercapnia is also known to cause cerebral vasodilatation (Campbell et al, 1967; Dunihoo and Quilligan, 1973). The increased incidence of fetal breathing movements and low voltage rapid frequency electrocortical activity seen with hypercapnia might therefore be attributable to an increase in blood supply of O_2 to the brain. Spontaneously occurring fetal *hypocapnia* associated with maternal hyperventilation has been observed occasionally in sheep. In such circumstances breathing movements are reduced (mean 15 per cent). Maternal administration of three per cent CO_2 in air is sufficient to increase the fetal Pa_{CO_2} from 30 to >40 mm Hg and restore a normal incidence of breathing activity.

Normal fetal breathing movements are reduced or arrested and gasping may be seen when the fetus is exposed to *hypoxia* sufficient to cause a fall in carotid arterial Pa_{O_2} from 25 to 17 mm Hg. There is no evidence of the hyperpnoea that occurs in the adult and newborn when exposed to low O_2 mixtures. This raises the question again as to whether the carotid bodies are normally active in the fetus. Direct recordings from carotid nerves in lambs (Biscoe and Purves, 1962) indicate that in the newborn the carotid bodies discharge more frequently in response to hypoxaemia. Also in newborn lambs and rabbits section of the carotid nerves abolishes the ventilatory response to hypoxia (Cross, Dawes and Mott, 1959; Dawes and Mott, 1959; Blotteis, 1964). The response to hypoxia of fetal lambs (Boddy et al, 1974) is therefore very like the behaviour of the newborn animal which lacks carotid body function. Nevertheless, in newborn lambs, rabbits and kittens, progressive hypoxaemia will ultimately lead to respiratory failure. Observation on unanaesthetised newborn lambs suggests that breathing is sustained until the Pa_{O_2} falls below 20 mm Hg (Johnson, P., personal communication) and that a reduction in respiratory minute volume, with incipient respiratory failure, occurs when the Pa_{O_2} falls below 25 mm Hg (Purves, 1966). The arrest of breathing movements seen in the fetus when the Pa_{O_2} falls below normal values, is therefore consistent with the progressive respiratory failure seen in the newborn when the Pa_{O_2} is reduced to similar values.

It is possible that carotid chemoreceptor activity may have been responsible for the 'gasping' activity seen during hypoxia. These deep slow inspiratory efforts however occur with asphyxia as early as 40 days (0.27) gestation in fetal lambs, and are present at term even after section of the vagi and carotid nerves (Dawes et al, 1972). They may therefore be due to a central action. Such observations, together with the fact that vagotomy does not influence normal fetal breathing activity in utero (or its abolition during hypoxia), would suggest that physiological control of breathing movements in utero has little dependence on the aortic chemoreceptor or the pulmonary stretch receptors or J-receptors. The present evidence indicates the importance of central control which may be influenced by a large number of variables. It is evident however from experiments attempting to raise the fetal Pa_{O_2} in utero (Boddy et al, 1974) that the normal incidence of breathing movements is not limited by oxygen lack. Increasing fetal Pa_{O_2} was not associated with more fetal breathing.

In man only limited observations have been made in circumstances where fetal blood gases could be measured (i.e. scalp pH; P_{O_2} and P_{CO_2} in labour). The results are not capable of statistical analysis because of the variability of the material, but they are consistent with those observed in fetal lambs. Evidence of fetal asphyxia, as judged by a reduction in fetal scalp pH and Po_2 with delayed deceleration of the fetal heart (Type II dips) has been seen to be associated with cessation of normal breathing movements and the appearance of *gasping* recorded by A-scan ultrasound. In normal labour of spontaneous onset, fetal breathing movements are usually reduced. In such circumstances maternal hyperventilation with consequent reduction of fetal scalp Pco_2 has been seen to be associated with the total absence of fetal chest wall movements. Also in some patients where labour has been induced and the fetal scalp Pco_2 was normal or raised (without evidence of hypoxia or acidaemia), the incidence of fetal breathing movements has remained high (60 to 90 per cent) (Boddy and Mantell, 1972). The absence of fetal breathing movements during labour may not therefore be of sinister significance, but the appearance of *gasping* has been associated with evidence of fetal asphyxia, acidaemia and low Apgar scores at delivery (Boddy and Mantell, 1973; Boddy and Dawes, 1976). By analogy, in the antenatal period a reduced incidence of fetal breathing with the appearance of *gasping* might be expected to be associated with fetal hypoxaemia, asphyxia or acidaemia. Table 16.3 shows that in 11 of 800 patients, the absence of normal fetal breathing movements and the appearance of gasping were followed by intra-uterine death. These fetuses were either growth-retarded or from pregnancies which were complicated by maternal hypertension, rhesus incompatibility or other factors. *Gasping* was noted 18 to 96 hours prior to fetal death. This abnormal pattern of fetal breathing is now used together with other clinical data as an indication for urgent delivery by caesarean section. It is not the only abnormal pattern that has been associated with imminent fetal demise. A diabetic pregnancy has been reported (Boddy and Dawes, 1976) where the incidence of fetal breathing movements was reduced and gasping was intermittently present. Within 48 hours of fetal death the nature of these movements changed to almost *continuous activity at unusually high rates* (100 to 200/min). Over the past three years observation on fetal lambs in utero has confirmed this suggestion that fetal death may be preceded by variable changes in breathing movements. Three preterminal types of abnormal breathing activity have been described. In all three types, prolonged periods of apnoea preceded the abnormality; in two, similar changes to those already described in human pregnancy were observed. Such observations indicate the need for further studies in human pregnancy before fetal breathing movements become widely used in clinical practice. Present evidence would indicate that in A-scan recordings of human fetal chest wall movements long periods of apnoea (30 min or more), and gasping in the absence of normal breathing activity, are indicative of impending fetal death. Immediate delivery (as has happened in two small-for-dates pregnancies so far)

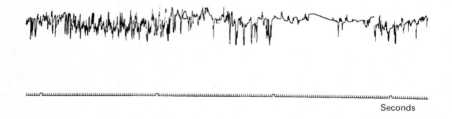

Seconds

Figure 16.5. A-scan recording of human fetal breathing in utero: a mixed pattern showing normal breathing movements, gasps and apnoea. (Periods of apnoea lasting longer than five minutes were seen in other parts of this recording.)

results in a living newborn which is acidaemic at birth but has few subsequent problems. The continued presence of normal fetal breathing activity (> 50 per cent incidence and with short apnoeic periods lasting less than two minutes) is a useful direct indication that the fetus is still in reasonably good health, even in the presence of low urinary oestriol excretion and intra-uterine growth retardation. By serial measurements a few important weeks may be gained before a deterioration in fetal condition is apparent. In such cases another pattern of breathing activity may be seen, with periods of apnoea greater than two to three minutes duration and a mixture of gasping and normal breathing movements (Figure 16.5). This *mixed pattern* has been observed in 86 of 800 pregnancies (Table 16.3) and has been seen to precede total apnoea and gasping, but may revert with the subsequent appearance of normal activity. The incidence of fetal distress in labour is high in pregnancies where a *mixed pattern* has been previously observed.

Drug actions

Like the responses seen in the fetal circulation, breathing movements can be used as an in-dicator of drug action in the fetus. From what has been said about the control and variability of these movements, drugs influencing central nervous system activity would be of special in-terest. In man few observations have been made, but recordings of fetal breathing movements, normal in incidence and character, have been obtained from mothers receiving long-term repeated doses of barbiturates, such as sodium amytal and phenobarbitone. The same is true of diazepam and the anticonvulsant phenytoin sodium (Epanutin). Such record-ings however did not take into account time-related responses, and measurements of drug concentrations were not made. Maternal administration of pethidine (100 mg i.m.) and diazepam (10 mg i.m.) has been seen to result in an arrest of fetal breathing activity. Obser-vations have been made in the last third of gestation on the effects of pentobarbitone and pethidine on fetal breathing movements in sheep (Boddy et al, 1976). Pethidine hydrochloride given to the ewe in doses of 100 to 200 mg and administered either in-tramuscularly, intravenously or retrograde via a carotid artery catheter into the maternal ascending aorta, showed no consistent effects on fetal breathing movements. Pethidine is known to cross the placenta and within 10 to 15 min of maternal injection gives fetal blood concentrations higher than those in the mother. A light sedative dose of pentobarbitone (4 mg/kg) administered intravenously to the ewe, caused an arrest of fetal breathing movements within one to five minutes, and a change in fetal electrocortical activity from low to high voltage. After a period of apnoea lasting from 8 to 31 min a series of single, in-spiratory breathing movements was seen, with a rate of 2 to 3/min. A further period of ap-noea was then followed by the return of '*rapid irregular breathing*'. Complex age and time-related responses are seen in both the fetal electrocortical and breathing activities over the two hours following pentobarbitone administration. Pentobarbitone crosses the sheep placenta rapidly and the concentration reaches a peak in the fetal arterial blood 20 to 30 min after maternal administration. Thereafter it exceeds the concentration achieved in the mother and subsequently declines over more than one hour. The arrest of fetal breathing movements seen after administration of pentobarbitone cannot be explained by alterations in fetal pH or blood gas values and the small doses used are insufficient to cause a significant change in blood glucose concentration. Small doses of pentobarbitone can cause excitement and catecholamine release but catecholamine infusion into fetal lambs has either no effect on fetal breathing movements or causes an increase. These results are important when considering fetal development and behaviour. They show that the episodic irregular breathing movements seen in utero are more susceptible to pentobarbitone than the more regular maintained breathing seen after birth. In the adult a small dose of pentobarbitone (4 mg/kg) causes a reduction in REM sleep activity. In the fetus the arrest and subsequent reduction of breathing activity seen after maternal pentobarbitone administration is most likely due to an effect on the state of sleep. The long-term effects of repeated doses of barbiturates on the fetal brain are not known, but there is evidence to suggest that, at certain periods in development, function is necessary for the proper development of structure (e.g. in the development of the visual cortex of kittens). Drugs used for maternal sedation and pain relief cannot therefore be assumed to be without significant consequences for the fetus.

Clinical implications and techniques

Recordings of fetal chest wall movements in human pregnancy provide a valuable direct measurement of fetal activity. At present the technique is still a research tool which is not sufficiently developed to be normally used in patient management. Experience and practice are required to obtain reasonable recordings and instrumental development is still necessary before the nature and character of breathing movements can be accurately described. In this regard the limitations and artefacts associated with the A-scan method need to be recognised. An ultrasound transducer placed on the maternal abdominal wall will be subject to displacements of that surface from various sources (e.g. material respiration, coughing, general movements and transmitted aortic pulsation; uterine contractions; transmitted fetal movements). Approximately one in every five recordings will need to be repeated because of artefacts produced in this way. Secondly, the A-scan method relies on identification of the fetal heart echoes prior to selection of echoes from the chest wall. The optimum transducer placement (at right-angles to the fetal chest wall) is obtained when the ultrasonic beam transects the mitral valve. Although fetal heart echoes are easily obtained, it is usually not possible to maintain mitral valve echoes for long periods of time. Changes in the angle of insonation of the narrow A-scan beam produce recordings which vary in amplitude and are not true reflections of the exact displacement of the fetal chest wall. This was clearly seen when the method was validated against tracheal pressure recordings from fetal lambs in utero (Boddy and Robinson, 1971). Also, the dependence on obtaining fetal heart echoes results in a further difficulty.

The fetal heart is in close proximity to the chest wall and it may not be possible to eliminate heart-echoes from recordings of anterior chest wall movements. Artefacts produced in this way can be reduced by integration of chest-wall echoes, by selection of posterior echoes or by recording from the fetal abdomen. The use of B-scan to select previously the site of recording will not eliminate these errors.

Apart from technical considerations, the physiology and pathophysiology concerned in the control of fetal breathing need extended investigation before any widespread clinical application is attempted. It is evident from the results already obtained in both animal and human studies that this control is multifactorial. Correct interpretation of recordings will therefore depend on appreciation of the factors which influence breathing movements in clinical practice (e.g. maternal smoking, drug use and food intake, as well as posture and abdominal palpation). It is because the importance of such factors was suggested by previous experience with animal models that initial human studies were made to assess their influence. Further animal and human studies together with improved recording techniques are needed before general clinical applications can be made.

In summary, the observations made in human pregnancy over the past three years have shown that it is possible to record and recognise the various patterns of normal and abnormal fetal chest wall movements referred to above. They have also indicated several clinical and esearch applications which may ultimately influence both patient management and regnancy outcome. Recordings of fetal breathing movements in utero can be used in the investigation of the effects and time course of action of drugs and other substances administered to the mother, including the inhalation of tobacco smoke. They are also useful as a uide to fetal health. The most sinister signs seen so far are those of *prolonged apnoea* and *pnoea and gasping* which have preceded fetal death on twelve occasions. In sheep *continuous fetal breathing movements* of almost constant frequency, duration and amplitude *picket-fence breathing*'), and *apnoea interrupted by brief episodes of rapid breathing accompanied by gasps* have also predicted fetal death. Such recordings have been seen to be econdary to a reduced incidence of normal fetal breathing activity. They may not be the only abnormal patterns to precede intra-uterine death. In human pregnancy apnoea and gasing give sufficient warning to obtain a living newborn but the long-term outcome of such abies remains to be seen. Similarly a '*mixed pattern*' of breathing movements which has een seen in both clinically normal and abnormal pregnancies may be a useful indicator of he fetus which later develops distress in labour. A screening programme in late pregnancy nay identify those patients for whom the costly facilities of continuous monitoring and lood-gas measurements in labour might be used most advantageously. The presence of normal breathing movements indicates good fetal health and sequential recordings may be useful to assess gestational age and the significance of low urinary oestriol values. Few observations have been made in labour but there is an association of reduced amounts of breathing movements and gasping with fetal bradycardia (delayed decelerations) and fetal acidaemia judged by scalp samples). Normal amounts, or the reappearance of normal breathing movements, have occasionally been observed even when early or late decelerations of the etal heart rate were present. In these and other circumstances they have provided direct vidence that the fetus was in good condition as also judged by scalp samples and Apgar cores at delivery. It is too early to say whether recordings in labour will be a useful addition o other monitoring methods.

These observations are all preliminary in nature and require verification in other centres ut they indicate a range of possible clinical usefulness as well as a prospect for learning more of the way that vital fetal functions are developed before birth. They provide information on he natural history of fetal breathing movements and their responses to changes in blood-gas alues as well as the correlations found with sleep state and the time of day. Then together vith new knowledge concerning the onset of labour and with blood glucose and adrenocorticotrophic hormone concentrations they all help in understanding the processes involved in growth and development. The so-called 'onset' of breathing at birth can now be seen as a continuation of what has gone before with the addition of the lungs acting for the first time as he organ of gas exchange.

REFERENCES

Assali, N. S., Brinkmann, C. R. III & Nuwayid, B. (1974) In *Modern Perinatal Medicine* (Ed.) Gluck, L. pp. 67–82. Chicago: Year Book Medical Publishers.
Assali, N. S., Holm, L. W. & Sehgal, N. (1962) Regional blood flow and vascular resistance of the fetus in utero. *American Journal of Obstetrics and Gynecology,* **83,** 809–817.
Baillie, P., Dawes, G. S., Merlet, C. L. & Richards, R. (1971) Maternal hyperventilation and foetal hypocapnia in sheep. *Journal of Physiology,* **218,** 635–650.
Barcoft, J. (1946) *Researches on Pre-Natal Life,* Vol. I. Oxford: Blackwell Scientific Publications.

Barrett, C. T., Heymann, M. A. & Rudolph, A. M. (1972) Alpha and beta adrenergic receptor activity in fetal sheep. *American Journal of Obstetrics and Gynecology,* **112,** 1114.

Bartells, H. & Moll, W. (1964) Passage of inert substances and oxygen in the human placenta. *Pflügers Archiv für die gesamte Physiologie des Menschen und der Tiere,* **280,** 165.

Bauer, C., Ludwig, I. & Ludwig, M. (1968) Different effects of 2,3-diphosphoglycerate and adenosine triphosphate on the oxygen affinity of adult and foetal human haemoglobin. *Life Science,* **7,** 1339.

Behrman, R. E. & Kittinger, G. W. (1968) Fetal and maternal responses to in utero angiotensin infusion in *Macaca mulatta. Proceedings of the Society for Experimental Biology and Medicine,* **129,** 305–308.

Bernhard, C. G. & Meyerson, B. A. (1973) Morphological and physiological aspects of the development of recipient function in the cerebral cortex. In *Foetal and Neonatal Physiology* (Ed.) Comline, R. S., Cross, K. W., Dawes, G. S. & Nathanielsz, P. W. pp. 1–19. London: Cambridge University Press.

Berton, J. P. (1970) Effects de la néphrectomie bilatérale chez le foetus de lapin (survie et metabolisme hydrique). *Compte Rendu Hebdomadaire des Séances de l'Acadamie des Sciences,* Series D, **271,** 219–222.

Biscoe, T. J., Purves, M. J. & Sampson, S. R. (1969) Types of nervous activity which may be recorded from the carotid sinus nerve in the sheep foetus. *Journal of Physiology,* **202,** 1–23.

Boddy, K. & Dawes, G. S. (1975) Fetal breathing. *British Medical Bulletin,* **31,** 3–7.

Boddy, K. & Dawes, G. S. (1976) Fetal well-being and fetal breathing. In *Prevention of Handicap through Antenatal Care.*

Boddy, K. & Mantell, C. D. (1972) Observations of fetal breathing movements transmitted through maternal abdominal walls. *Lancet,* **ii,** 1219–1220.

Boddy, K. & Mantell, C. D. (1973) Human foetal breathing in utero. *Journal of Physiology,* **231,** 105P–106P.

Boddy, K. & Robinson, J. S. (1971) External method for detection of fetal breathing in utero. *Lancet,* **ii,** 1231–1233.

Boddy, K., Dawes, G. S. & Robinson, J. S. (1973) A 24-hour rhythm in the foetus. In *Foetal and Neonatal Physiology* (Ed.) Comline, R. S., Cross, K. W., Dawes, G. S. & Nathanielsz, P. W. pp. 63–66. London: Cambridge University Press.

Boddy, K., Jones, C. T. & Robinson, J. S. (1974) Correlations between plasma ACTH concentrations and breathing movements in foetal sheep. *Nature,* **250,** 75–76.

Boddy, K., Dawes, G. S., Fisher, R., Pinter, S. & Robinson, J. S. (1974) Foetal respiratory movements, electrocortical and cardiovascular responses to hypoxaemia and hypercapnia in sheep. *Journal of Physiology,* **243,** 599–618.

Boddy, K., Dawes, G. S., Fisher, R. L., Pinter, S. & Robinson, J. S. (1976) The Effects of pentobarbitone and pethidine on fetal breathing movements in sheep. In press.

Boreus, L. O. (1973) Drug–receptor interations in the human fetus. In *Fetal Pharmacology* (Ed.) Boreus, L. A. pp. 111–126. New York: Raven Press.

Broughton Pipkin, F. (1971) Cardiovascular responses in rabbits of different ages to hypertensin and adrenalin. *Quarterly Journal of Experimental Physiology,* **56,** 210–220.

Broughton Pipkin, F., Lumbers, E. R. & Mott, J. C. (1974) Factors influencing plasma renin and angiotensin II in the conscious pregnant ewe and its foetus. *Journal of Physiology,* **243,** 619–636.

Burlingame, P., Long, J. A. & Ogden, E. (1942) The blood pressure of the fetal rat and its response to renin and angiotensin. *American Journal of Physiology,* **137,** 473–484.

Campbell, A. G. M., Dawes, G. S., Fishman, A. P. & Hyman, A. (1967) Regional redistribution of blood flow in the mature fetal lamb. *Circulation Research,* **21,** 229–235.

Carter, W. A., Becker, R. F., King, J. E. & Barry, W. F. (1964) Intrauterine respiration in the rat fetus. *American Journal of Obstetrics and Gynecology,* **90,** 247–256.

Chinn, R. H. & Dusterdieck, G. (1972) The response of blood pressure to infusion of angiotensin II. *Clinical Science,* **42,** 489–504.

Clark, D. M. & Wyatt, D. G. (1969) An improved peri-vascular flow meter. *Medical and Biological Engineering,* **7,** 185–190.

Cross, K. W., Dawes, G. S. & Mott, J. C. (1959) Anoxia, oxygen consumption and cardiac output in new-born lambs and adult sheep. *Journal of Physiology,* **146,** 316–343.

Dawes, G. S. (1968) *Foetal and Neonatal Physiology.* Chicago: Year Book Medical Publishers.

Dawes, G. S. (1973) Breathing and rapid-eye-movement sleep before birth. In *Foetal and Neonatal Physiology* (Ed.) Comline, R. S., Cross, K. W., Dawes, G. S. & Nathanielsz, P. W. pp. 49–62. London: Cambridge University Press.

Dawes, G. S. & Mott, J. C. (1959) The increase in oxygen consumption of the lamb after birth. *Journal of Physiology,* **146,** 295–315.

Dawes, G. S., Handler, J. J. & Mott, J. C. (1957) Some cardiovascular responses in foetal, new-born and adult rabbits. *Journal of Physiology,* **139,** 123–126.

Dawes, G. S., Mott, J. C. & Widdicombe, J. G. (1954) The foetal circulation in the lamb. *Journal of Physiology,* **126,** 563–587.

awes, G. S., Duncan, S. L., Lewis, B. V., Merlet, C. L., Owen-Thomas, J. B. & Reeves, J. T. (1969a) Hypoxaemia and aortic body chemoreceptor function in foetal lambs. *Journal of Physiology*, **201**, 105–116.

awes, G. S., Duncan, S. L., Lewis, B. V., Merlet, C. L., Owen-Thomas, J. B. & Reeves, J. T. (1969b) Cyanide stimulation of the systemic arterial chemoreceptors in foetal lambs. *Journal of Physiology*, **201**, 117–128.

awes, G. S., Fox, H. E., Leduc, B. M., Liggins, G. C. & Richards, R. T. (1970) Respiratory movements and paradoxical sleep in the foetal lamb. *Journal of Physiology*, **210**, 47P–48P.

awes, G. S., Fox, H. E., Leduc, B. M., Liggins, G. C. & Richards, R. T. (1972) Respiratory movements and rapid eye movement sleep in the foetal lamb. *Journal of Physiology*, **220**, 119–143.

unihoo, D. R. & Quilligan, E. J. (1973) Carotid blood flow distribution in the in utero sheep fetus. *American Journal of Obstetrics and Gynecology*, **116**, 648–656.

riedman, W. F. (1972) The intrinsic physiologic properties of the developing heart. In *Neonatal Heart Disease* (Ed.) Friedman, W. F., Lesch, M. & Sonnenblick, E. H. pp. 21–49. New York: Grune and Stratton.

riedman, W. F., Pool, P. E., Jacobowitz, D., Seagren, B. A. & Braunwald, E. (1968) Sympathetic innervation of the developing rabbit heart. *Circulation Research*, **23**, 25–32.

oodwin, J. W., Milligan, J. E., Thomas, B. & Taylor, J. R. (1973) The effect of aortic chemoreceptor stimulation on cardiac output and umbilical blood flow in the fetal lamb. *American Journal of Obstetrics and Gynecology*, **116**, 48–56.

rimwade, J., Walker, D. & Wood, C. (1970) Response of the human fetus to sensory stimulation. *Australian and New Zealand Journal of Obstetrics and Gynaecology*, **10**, 222.

rimwade, J., Walker, D. & Wood, C. (1971) Letter. Morphine and the fetal heart rate. *British Medical Journal*, **iii**, 373.

odari, A. A. & Hodgkinson, C. P. (1968) Fetal kidney as a source of renin in the pregnant dog. *American Journal of Obstetrics and Gynecology*, **102**, 691–699.

odgkinson, C. P., Hodari, A. A. & Bumpus, F. M. (1967) Experimental hypertensive disease of pregnancy. *Obstetrics and Gynecology*, **30**, 371–380.

on, E. H. & Sze-Ya, Y. (1969) Electronic evaluation of fetal heart rate, X. The fetal arrhythmia index. *Medical Research Engineering*, **8**, 14.

nes, C. T. & Rombinson, R. O. (1975) Plasma catecholamines in foetal and adult sheep. *Journal of Physiology*, **248**, 15.

st, R. G. (1969) *The Electroencephalogram of the Foetal Sheep*. PhD thesis, Yale University.

ongo, L. D., Power, G. G. & Foster, R. E. II (1967) Respiratory function of the placenta as determined with carbon monoxide in sheep and dogs. *Journal of Clinical Investigation*, **46**, 812.

ahon, W. A., Goodwin, J. W. & Paul, N. M. (1966) Measurement of individual ventricular outputs in the fetal lamb by a dye dilution technique. *Circulation Research*, **19**, 191–8.

cClain, C. R. Jr (1964) Amniography, a versatile diagnostic procedure in obstetrics. *Obstetrics and Gynecology*, **23**, 45–50.

cMurphy, D. M. & Boreus, L. O. (1971) Studies on the pharmacology of the perfused human fetal ductus arteriosus. *American Journal of Obstetrics and Gynecology*, **109**, 937–942.

cMurphy, D. M., Heymann, M. A., Rudolph, A. M. & Melmon, K. L. (1972) Developmental changes in constriction of the ductus arteriosus. *Pediatric Research*, **6**, 231.

anning, F., Wyn Pugh, E. & Boddy, K. (1975) Effect of cigarette smoking on fetal breathing movements in normal pregnancies. *British Medical Journal*, **i**, 552–553.

ellor, D. J. & Slater, J. S. (1971) Daily changes in amniotic and allantoic fluid during the last three months of pregnancy in conscious, unstressed ewes, with catheters in their foetal fluid sacs. *Journal of Physiology*, **217**, 573–604.

ellor, D. J. & Slater, J. S. (1973) The composition of maternal plasma and foetal urine after feeding and drinking in chronically catheterized ewes during the last two months of pregnancy. *Journal of Physiology*, **234**, 519–531.

erlet, C., Hoerter, J., Devilleneuve, C. & Tchobroutsky, C. (1970) Mise en evidence de mouvements respiratoires chez le foetus d'agneau in utero au cours du dernier mois de la gestation. *Compte Rendu Hebdomadaire des Séances de l'Academie des Sciences*, Series D, **270**, 2462–2464.

eschia, G., Battaglia, F. C. & Burns, P. D. (1967) Theoretical and experimental study of transplacental diffusion. *Journal of Applied Physiology*, **22**, 1171.

ott, J. C. (1969) The kidneys and arterial pressure in immature and adult rabbits. *Journal of Physiology*, **202**, 25–54.

ott, J. C. (1973) The renin–angiotensin system in foetal and newborn mammals. In *Foetal and Neonatal Physiology* (Ed) Comline, R. S., Cross, K. W., Dawes, G. S. & Nathanielsz, P. W. pp. 166–180. London: Cambridge University Press.

ott, J. C. (1975) The place of the renin–angiotensin system before and after birth. *British Medical Bulletin*, **31**, 44–50.

Owman, C., Aronson, S., Gennser, G. & Sjoberg, N. O. (1973) Histochemical and pharmacological evidence amine mechanism in human fetal vascular shunts. In *Fetal Pharmacology* (Ed) Boreus, L. O. pp. 179–192. Ne York: Raven Press.

Renou, P. & Wood, C. (1974) Interpretation of the continuous fetal heart rate record. In *Clinics in Obstetrics at Gynecology* (Ed.) Beard, R. W. Vol. I, pp. 191–215. London: W. B. Saunders.

Rudolph, A. M. & Heymann, M. A. (1970) Circulatory changes during growth in the fetal lamb. *Circulati Research*, **26**, 289–299.

Rudolph, A. M. & Heymann, M. A. (1972) Measurement of flow in perfused organs, using microsphere techniqu *Acta Endocrinologica* (Supplement), **158**, 112–127.

Rudolph, A. M. & Heymann, M. A. (1973) Control of the foetal circulation. In *Foetal and Neonatal Physiolo* (Ed.) Comline, R. S., Cross, K. W., Dawes, G. S. & Nathanielsz, P. W. pp. 89–111. London: Cambridge Univ sity Press.

Schifferli, P. Y. & Caldeyro-Barcia, R. (1973) Effects of atropine and beta-adrenergic drugs on the heart rate of t human fetus. In *Fetal Pharmacology* (Ed.) Boreus, L. O. pp. 259–279. New York: Raven Press.

Shelley, H. J. (1969) The metabolic response of the foetus to hypoxia. *Journal of Obstetrics and Gynaecology of t British Commonwealth*, **76**, 1–15.

Shelley, H. J. (1973) The use of chronically catheterized foetal lambs for the study of foetal metabolism. In *Foet and Neonatal Physiology* (Ed.) Comline, R. S., Cross, K. W., Dawes, G. S. & Nathanielsz, P. W. pp. 360–38 London: Cambridge University Press.

Silva, D. G. & Ikeda, M. (1971) Ultrastructural and acetyl cholinesterase studies in the innovation of the duct arteriosus, pulmonary trunk and aorta of the fetal lamb. *Journal of Ultrastructure Research*, **34**, 358–374.

Skowsky, W. R., Bashore, R. A., Smith, F. G. & Fisher, D. A. (1973) Vasopressin metabolism in the foetus and ne born. In *Foetal and Neonatal Physiology* (Ed.) Comline, R. S., Cross, K. W., Dawes, G. S. & Nathanielsz, P. V pp. 439–447. London: Cambridge University Press.

Trimper, C. E. & Lumbers, E. R. (1972) The renin–angiotensin in foetal lambs. *Pflügers Archiv für die gesam Physiologie des Menschen und der Tiere*, **336**, 1–10.

Van Petten, G. R. (1975) Pharmacology and the fetus. *British Medical Bulletin*, **31**, 75–79.

Van Petten, G. R. & McCracken, (1973) *Clinical Research*, **20**, 914 (abstract).

Van Petten, G. R. & Willes, R. F. (1970) β-Adrenoceptive responses in the unanesthetized ovine foetus. *Briti Journal of Pharmacology*, **38**, 572–582.

Windle, W. F. (1940) *Physiology of the Fetus: Origin and Extent of Function in Prenatal Life*. Philadelphia, Lo don: W. B. Saunders.

Zanjani, E. D., Gidan, A. S., Peterson, E. N., Gordon, A. S. & Wasserman, L. R. (1973) Human regulation erythropoiesis in the foetus. In *Foetal and Neonatal Physiology* (Ed.) Comline, R. S., Cross, K. W., Dawes, G. & Nathanielsz, P. W. pp. 448–455. London: Cambridge University Press.

7

AMNIOTIC FLUID ANALYSIS

C. R. Whitfield

AMNIOTIC FLUID FORMATION

In considering the turnover and volume of amniotic fluid (AF), molecular exchanges of water and electrolytes between the AF, the fetus and the maternal plasma must be distinguished from bulk inflows and outflows (mainly fetal micturition and swallowing). These molecular exchanges occur chiefly by diffusion across fetal skin, the membranes, the fetal surface of the placenta and the umbilical cord.

Direct measurements of the amount of AF in patients undergoing therapeutic abortion, and also ultrasonic estimations of 'gestational sac volumes' during the first trimester (Robinson, 1975) indicate that the AF volume is at first closely related to gestational age and fetal weight; it increases from less than 5 ml at six weeks to about 30 ml at ten weeks, and to about 350 ml when the fetus weighs about 300 g at 20 weeks. The permeability of the fetal skin during this stage allows free diffusion so that the early AF resembles fetal extracellular fluid, although the concentration of sodium is a little lower and that of urea slightly higher as a result of the voiding of very small amounts of fetal urine from as early as the 12th week.

As the fetal skin stratifies and becomes keratinised, diffusion across it is reduced and ceases at about 20 weeks. However, diffusion across the fetal placental surface remains unimpeded, and Abramovich (1973) has demonstrated in vivo that absorption of water from the AF to the fetus via the umbilical cord begins at 18 weeks. By these means all the AF water is replaced about every three hours.

From mid-pregnancy onwards the fetal kidney provides an increasing bulk inflow which reaches at least 500 ml/day by term. Normally the inflow is more or less balanced by increasing fetal swallowing, and in addition the tidal flow in the trachea results in a small net inflow of fluid from the fetal lungs. The composition and osmolality of the AF are now very similar to those of dilute fetal urine, while its volume is no longer closely related to fetal weight but shows an increasingly wide variation. As part of a joint Cornell–Belfast study of AF volume in normal pregnancies (Queenan et al, 1972), a large number of serial determinations were made showing that in many patients there are marked, but unpredictable and clinically undetectable, fluctuations in volume within the normal limits for the latter half of pregnancy. In addition, the diffusion rates of water into and out of the AF are not necessarily equal at all times.

As will be described, volume determinations may sometimes be of practical value when biochemical, hormonal or enzymatic measurements are being made on the AF; the total AF content of a particular constituent may be of more importance than its concentration when the amount of AF is grossly abnormal or has altered significantly between serial tests. For this purpose, a para-aminohippurate dilution technique using spectrophotometry rather than the diazo reaction has been established by Thompson, Lappin and Elder (1971) as a simple, rapid, accurate and reproducible test.

TECHNIQUE AND COMPLICATIONS OF AMNIOCENTESIS

Although careful palpation will usually locate collections of AF in the region of the fetal limbs or behind the fetal neck, preliminary ultrasonic B-scanning not only reveals the placental site but it should be used to locate pockets of AF when there is oligohydramnios. A point of practical value, which is often not recognised, is that when a suitable collection of AF has been located amniocentesis is best performed without moving the patient from the couch used for ultrasound scanning. As a general rule, a readily accessible collection of AF can be aspirated in the midline below the umbilicus where, due to separation of the rectus muscles, there is the least depth of maternal tissue to traverse. There is less likely to be a suitable pool of liquor at this site when the breech presents; in such cases, it is usually easy to tap an even larger collection of fluid beside the fetal head in the upper part of the uterus.

When an anterior placenta cannot be avoided, exact localisation by ultrasound of a collection of AF and measurement of its depth enables a transplacental tap to be made with deliberate precision, thereby reducing the likelihood of a heavily bloodstained sample or of feto-maternal bleeding. Thus, the introduction of routine preliminary ultrasonic scanning at a special amniocentesis clinic at the Royal Maternity Hospital, Belfast, reduced the incidence of feto-maternal bleeding (demonstrated in blood films by the Kleihauer technique) from 13.2 to 4.8 per cent and enabled most unavoidable transplacental taps to be made without detectable bleeds from fetus to mother (Robinson, personal communication, 1972). Rhesus negative women in whom a deliberate transplacental tap has been necessary, or in whom feto-maternal bleeding has been detected, should be protected from rhesus-sensitisation or from antibody boosting by injecting anti-D immunoglobulin.

When early amniocentesis is needed for genetic diagnosis, a placenta that is sited anteriorly cannot always be avoided and the midline subumbilical site is usually selected for these cases. Amniocentesis at an early stage of pregnancy should always be performed by xperienced operators. Thus, in an individual series of 105 such amniocenteses, Stewart has eported that abortion never occurred within one week of the procedure, that feto-maternal leeding could be detected in only eight women and that there was no instance of rhesus-ensitisation (Stewart, Ward and Lorber, 1975); he also failed to obtain AF (at two attempts) n seven patients, but it seems likely that this failure rate might well have been reduced had he lways used ultrasonic scanning for initial as well as second attempts.

Even when amniocentesis is not needed until late pregnancy, reference of patients to a mall team of obstetricians experienced in the procedure or perhaps the creation of a special mniocentesis clinic serving several hospitals is advantageous. In the aforementioned Belfast linic, Sproule (1974) noted only two serious complications attributable to the echnique—one already critically rhesus-affected fetus died two hours after puncture of its mbilical cord at amniocentesis (with resultant haematoma); another baby died from hyaline nembrane disease following premature delivery as a result of spontaneous labour on the day fter amniocentesis. In this large series, there was a 2.6 per cent incidence of spontaneous abour within one week of amniocentesis, but all these babies survived. In half of the cases abour occurred more than 48 hours after amniocentesis (perhaps not attributable), and there vere only eight instances of spontaneous labour before 36 weeks gestation (0.6 per cent).

AF samples should be protected from sunlight (ultraviolet light destroys bilirubin) and, xcept when cytological studies or cell cultures are required, they should immediately be cen-rifuged at low speed. Immediate use of a centrifuge kept nearby enables even heavily blood-ontaminated samples to be used for biochemical measurements. For culture, AF cells hould be allowed to settle in a transparent plastic container with a coned base, and it is best or someone from the cytogenetic laboratory to be present to receive the sample.

MANAGEMENT OF RHESUS DISEASE

t was in the management of the rhesus-immunised woman that amniocentesis was first es-ablished as a vital diagnostic procedure, the measured concentration of bilirubin in the AF iving some prediction of the likely eventual severity of haemolytic disease in the newborn. 3ecause bilirubin is also a normal constituent of AF which decreases during the third rimester, its level must be related to the stage of gestation. It has also become well es-ablished that predictive accuracy can be greatly improved by repeated amniocentesis, which nables the trend as well as the level of bilirubin to be considered. These principles remain the asis for assessing the severity and further trend of haemolysis in the fetus, and for predicting he optimal time for delivery or intra-uterine blood transfusion. Management along these ines has reduced attributable fetal and neonatal wastage to a rate of less than 10 per cent in everal centres where multidisciplinary teams provide a large and highly specialised (usually egional) reference service (Whitfield, 1970), compared with rates of 25 per cent without the se of amniocentesis and of almost 50 per cent before the introduction of neonatal exchange ransfusion.

The not uncommon practice of performing amniocentesis only when maternal serum an-ibody exceeds a critical titre is unwise because antibody titration is imprecise and because, ven in known first-affected pregnancies, sudden acute fetal haemolysis may necessitate im-nediate intervention to avoid intra-uterine death. When accurate automated measurement of ntibody protein (Fraser et al, 1972) is available, amniocentesis is unnecessary and term lelivery is safe if monthly testing shows persistently less than 1.0 μg/ml of antibody protein in he mother's serum, provided no previous baby was more than mildly affected by haemolytic lisease.

For adequate warning of dangerously severe haemolysis, amniocentesis should be timed according to the previous history. It is advisable to perform the first amniocentesis 10 weeks before the time of the earliest previous fetal death, fetal transfusion or birth of a very severely affected baby, but not before 20 weeks as intra-uterine transfusion is not really feasible until 22 weeks to 24 weeks. In the absence of such a history, an initial tap at 28 to 30 weeks is followed by another at 32 or 33 weeks. The interval of at least three weeks allows the bilirubin trend to be revealed clearly, and it also reduces spectrophotometric distortion in the second sample resulting from an initial bloody tap. Additional amniocenteses and/or shorter intervals may be needed when the AF bilirubin is very high or is rising sharply, or when an abrupt increase in antibody protein in the mother's blood suggests that a fetal haemolytic crisis is likely.

Interpretation and action, based on measurement of amniotic fluid bilirubin

The small amounts of bilirubin in the AF are best measured by spectrophotometry which, especially if a continuously recording instrument is used, is quick as well as sensitive. The methods of Liley (1961) for measuring the bilirubin peak (ΔOD at 450 nm) and for plotting such measurements in his three prediction zones (Figure 17.1), which slope in accordance with the physiological decline in AF bilirubin during the last trimester, are widely used. The expected downward trend between tests occurs with many affected fetuses (case A in Figure 17.1), but sometimes an abnormal trend results in the ΔOD at 450 nm approaching or reaching a different zone so that the prediction of severity must be revised (cases B, C and D).

Alternative similar prediction methods include that of Queenan and Goetschel (1968) who plot the ΔOD at 450 nm in an upper 'area of intra-uterine or neonatal deaths', a lower 'area of surviving infants', or in an intermediate 'area of overlap' which has no prognostic value but shows that repeat amniocentesis is needed to reveal the bilirubin trend. In Liley's and in most other prediction schemes, the forecast of severity has still to be translated into a decision on the time for delivery or fetal transfusion. Freda (1965) therefore grades ΔOD at 450 nm values to indicate the interval that can safely be left before a further tap or before either delivery or transfusion is called for: Grade 1+ (<0.20) signifies no fetal risk for at least two weeks, Grade 2+ (0.20 to 0.35) indicates some risk during the next two weeks, Grade 3+ (0.35 to 0.70) indicates that the fetus will die if not delivered or transfused within about 10 days, and Grade 4+ (> 0.70) calls for immediate action to avoid impending fetal death. These grades signify actual rather than predicted severity and their use seems to avoid some unnecessarily early fetal transfusions. On the other hand, a patient may require a very large number of amniocenteses, and no allowance is made for the physiological decline in AF bilirubin, so that fetal death may occur in the last six or seven weeks of pregnancy despite only Grade 2+ values. Robertson (1969) devised an effective practical scheme of management based on no less than 14 separate zones for the ΔOD at 450 nm, but this seems too complex for general use.

The curved action line, illustrated in Figure 17.2, was used to determine the time at which further conservative management carried a greater risk than delivery or fetal transfusion in 641 patients referred directly to the centralised rhesus service in Belfast during a three-year period, and the fetal and neonatal rhesus mortality rate was 8.9 per cent (Whitfield, 1970). Continued use of the action line has reduced rhesus wastage to less than two per cent in first-affected pregnancies and less than 40 per cent when there have been previous rhesus deaths. Before assessment of fetal lung development became possible, intra-uterine transfusion was always performed if the ΔOD at 450 nm or its extrapolated trend was related to the action line before 33 weeks (cases A, B and C in Figure 17.2). This part of the line corresponds

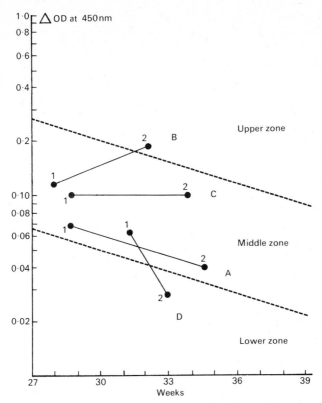

Figure 17.1. Liley's prediction zones in the third trimester, with the ΔOD at 450 nm plotted against gestational age. In each of the four examples shown the initial estimation was in the middle zone, giving a prediction of probably mild or moderately severe haemolytic disease. In case A the usual gradual reduction in amniotic fluid bilirubin occurred, with the ΔOD at 450 nm remaining low in the middle zone and with an unchanged prediction. The upward trend in case B resulted in a second estimation being in the upper zone, giving a revised prediction of probably severe haemolytic disease. In case C the static bilirubin trend approached (and could be extrapolated into) the upper zone, indicating that severe haemolysis would have become likely if the pregnancy had been continued to term. The steeply falling bilirubin trend in case D reached the lower zone, giving a revised prediction of an unaffected or only very mildly affected baby.

roughly with the transfusion zones of Liggins (1966) and of Robertson (1969), and with the lower borders of both Liley's upper zone and the upper danger area of Queenan and Goetschel; the use of less strict criteria results in the unnecessary transfusion of some less than severely affected fetuses. The action line is also effective in selecting 70 per cent of unaffected and mildly affected babies for term delivery (case G) and most of the remainder for delivery after 38 weeks.

Effect of amniotic fluid volume on prediction

Some serious errors of prediction are due to the effect of polyhydramnios or oligohydramnios on the concentration of bilirubin in the AF. Routine measurement of AF volume at 203 amniocenteses in 107 women with rhesus-affected fetuses confirmed a tendency to higher than average volumes when the fetus is severely affected, and showed that hydrops fetalis is

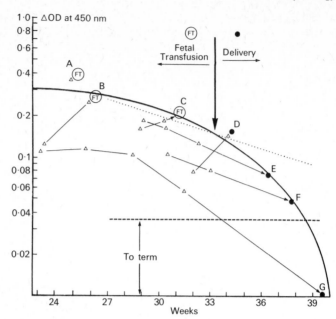

Figure 17.2. The action line, with the ΔOD at 450 nm plotted against gestational age. When the ΔOD at 450 nm is on or above the action line before 33 weeks (case A) or if its trend extrapolates to that part of the line (cases B and C), intra-uterine fetal transfusion is indicated. After 33 weeks, a ΔOD at 450 nm value beyond the line (case D) or extrapolation of the trend (cases E, F and G) indicate the optimal time for delivery without prior transfusion. The sloping dotted line represents the lower border of Liley's upper zone. The horizontal broken line represents a ΔOD at 450 nm value of 0.035. If the initial estimation is below this level, the pregnancy is continued to term without a further amniocentesis. Data from Whitfield (1970).

often present or about to develop if there is a gross excess of AF during the second trimester (Whitfield, 1971). It has not been possible to devise a formula to correct ΔOD at 450 nm values for variations in AF volume, but serial volume estimations enable the bilirubin trend to be related to significant changes in the amount of liquor. Intervention may be dangerously delayed if a rough allowance is not made for the diluting effect of polyhydramnios, and unnecessary transfusion or needlessly early delivery may be carried out if the concentrating effect of oligohydramnios is ignored. The alternative method of correcting for AF volume by determining the antibody: protein ratio (Morris, Murray and Ruthven, 1967) is not reliable, because the usual terminal fall in AF protein may not occur when fetal erythroblastosis is severe.

Amniotic fluid surfactant—very early delivery or transfusion?

Estimations of fetal pulmonary surfactant in the AF are of special value in the rhesus-immunised patient, because premature delivery is often required and some neonatal deaths are due to respiratory distress as well as haemolytic disease. As will be described, it seems that surfactant may be reduced in the critically anaemic fetus, although this may be preceded by an initial acceleration of its production, possibly occurring as a response to stress.

When intervention is required between 31 and 35 weeks, AF surfactant tests can distinguish between the baby who has functionally mature lungs and can be delivered safely and those that require intra-uterine transfusion because their lungs are still immature. This more flexible policy was introduced during a second three-year series of patients managed by the action line, in which only seven out of 706 infants, or 1.0 per cent, developed respiratory distress compared with a rate of 3.0 per cent in the reported first three-year series already referred to.

Other amniotic fluid measurements

A number of other constituents are measured at certain centres dealing with large numbers of rhesus-immunised women. It has been found that increased values for the ratio between diamine oxidase in the AF and in the mother's serum (Ward, Whyley and Millar, 1973) or high levels of either α-fetoprotein (Whyley, Ward and Hardy, 1974) or human placental lactogen (Niven, Ward and Chard, 1974) may provide useful additional evidence that a fetus is severely affected. Similarly, in Bristol, automated measurements of AF antibody protein have been found useful as an adjunct to bilirubin estimation (Fraser and Tovey, 1972).

Amniography and fetography before intra-uterine transfusion

Personal choice of technique for intra-uterine transfusion and the results that can be achieved by a small team experienced in it are described elsewhere (Whitfield et al, 1972) but it is relevant to emphasise the value of prior injection of radio-opaque contrast into the AF to improve visualisation of the fetus when the transfusion is performed. The author prefers to outline the fetal skin (vernix caseosa) with a lipo-soluble medium and also to mark the target area with water-soluble contrast (swallowed and concentrated in the fetal gut). Abnormal separation of the opacified scalp from the skull indicates a hopeless situation and the transfusion should not be carried out; such a grossly hydropic fetus may also fail to swallow any contrast up to one week before its demise.

ASSESSMENT OF FETAL MATURITY

Assessment of fetal maturity is a vital part of antenatal care, but it may be a difficult evaluation to make and, all too often, it seems not to be understood that ageing, growth and functional maturation are separate processes, that different tissues and systems mature at different rates, that these rates vary from fetus to fetus, and that functional development at birth is more important than weight or gestational age. Unlike clinical, radiological and ultrasonic methods of assessment, the AF tests used evaluate mainly functional maturation.

The maturing fetal skin sheds increasing numbers of cornified cells and anucleate squames into the AF. If 10 per cent of these cells contain lipid (sebum) that stains orange with Nile blue sulphate the fetus has almost certainly reached at least 38 weeks, but many patients have very few or no orange-staining cells even after term. Although Lind (1970), using haematoxylin and eosin stain, confirmed the predominance of cornified cells and anucleate cells from 38 weeks onwards, he pointed out that the cells are shed over an unknown period of time and they represent only very crudely the state of the fetal skin at the time of amniocentesis.

During the latter half of pregnancy the AF becomes increasingly hypotonic and contains increasing concentrations of creatinine and urea; these changes reflect the increasing contribution made by the maturing fetal kidneys to the formation of AF. Other normal changes include a falling bilirubin level that reflects maturation of the fetal liver, a rise and then fall in hydroxyproline which probably reflects alterations in fetal growth rate, and a terminal rise in surface-active lecithin from the developing fetal lungs. The concentrations of biochemical constituents show too gradual rates of change and too wide normal ranges to be precise guides to fetal age or growth; for example, although many laboratories use a creatinine concentration of about 1.8 mg/100 ml of AF as evidence that a fetus has probably reached 37 weeks, the gestational age range for that value extends from before 32 weeks to beyond 42 weeks.

Fetal pulmonary surfactant

The terminal rise in surface-active lecithin in the AF, beginning at about 32 weeks, provides a sensitive index of the functional development of the baby's lungs, and therefore of its ability to expand them and to survive ex utero.

Measurement of AF lecithin is a laborious process, even by the so-called 'quick' method of Bhagwanani, Fahmy and Turnbull (1972) and determination of its total content rather than its concentration, as advocated by Falconer, Hodge and Gadd (1973), necessitates an AF volume measurement as well. These methods hold no real advantages over the very much simpler determination of the lecithin : sphingomyelin ratio which is now widely established as a practical method of predicting, with remarkable accuracy, the likelihood (and likely severity) of neonatal respiratory distress and hyaline membrane disease if delivery is not delayed. The validity of the ratio rests upon the important observation by Gluck et al (1971) that the terminal rise in AF lecithin is not accompanied by a significant alteration in the level of sphingomyelin, a less important surface-active phospholipid. The ratio has the further obvious and important advantage that it is not affected by abnormal or changing AF volumes.

In their original method, Gluck and his colleagues used densitometry to measure the lecithin and sphingomyelin 'spots' on thin layer chromatograms made from AF extracts of the surface-active phospholipids. A technically much simpler, yet reliable method devised by the same research group is to measure the area of the spots after developing them with bromothymol blue and ammonia (Borer et al, 1971; described in detail by Wagstaff and Bromham, 1973). As reported by Whitfield and Sproule (1974), this method of colour-planimetry was used in a study of more than 1700 AF samples sent from many hospitals to a central laboratory in Belfast, the ratio so determined being referred to as the lecithin : sphingomyelin area ratio (LSAR). It was also shown that, although the concentration of each of the phospholipids is reduced if testing is delayed, the ratio between them remains virtually constant for about four days if the fluid is centrifuged (at 900 *g* for 5 min) immediately it is obtained and is then kept at room temperature. This and other methods for measuring AF surfactant are unreliable in the presence of meconium or certain antiseptic preparations including chlorhexidine. Heavy contamination with blood also gives rise to difficulties in the laboratory, but Hallman and Gluck (1974) are evaluating a two-dimensional thin-layer chromatography technique for overcoming this problem.

There is good correlation between the AF palmitic acid concentration and both the LSAR and neonatal respiratory function (Warren, Holton and Allen, 1974). The automated method for assaying palmitic acid merits further development and evaluation for both clinical and research purposes. Whatever basic laboratory method is used, so many modifications are in use that each centre must establish its own critical values.

The onset and rate of the terminal increase in AF surfactant shows much individual variation, with 'safe' values (3.5 mg lecithin/100 ml, or lecithin : sphingomyelin ratios of at least 2.0 in most laboratories) sometimes present as early as 32 weeks but not reached in other normal subjects until at least 38 weeks. Although initial abnormally high ratios are occasionally found in pregnancies complicated by very severe rhesus disease, the expected terminal surge does not occur, or does not persist, in about one-third of such cases; very abrupt falls in AF surfactant sometimes occur in association with evidence of an acute haemolytic crisis in the fetus. The well-known high risk of neonatal respiratory distress and hyaline membranes when the mother has diabetes is probably in part explained by the similar static or falling trends in surfactant that occur in some diabetics or latent diabetics; repeated amniocentesis is therefore advocated in such patients to identify the surfactant trend so that fetal lung maturation can be taken into account when timing delivery (Whitfield, Sproule and Brundenell, 1973). No other pregnancy complications associated with reduced levels of surfactant have been identified with certainty, but there is good evidence that there is some (as yet unrecognised) factor related to spontaneous premature rupture of the membranes that seems to bring about accelerated surfactant production and lung maturation (Richardson et al, 1974).

Table 17.1. *Incidence of respiratory distress in relation to 550 predelivery LSAR tests (i.e. on amniotic fluid obtained not more than 48 hours before delivery).*

Predelivery LSAR	No. of infants	Respiratory distress syndrome		
		No.	Percentage	Deaths
>2.0	466	3	0.6	—
1.5–2.0	65	13	20.0	1
<1.5	19	15	78.9	7
Total	550	31	5.6	8

The predictive accuracy of the LSAR is shown in Table 17.1 which summarises the results of 550 predelivery tests (i.e. in AF obtained not more than 48 hours before delivery) in the Belfast series. Of 466 such tests giving ratios above 2.0, only three were associated with neonatal respiratory distress, two of these babies being born to diabetic mothers and the third had haemolytic disease. It is of obvious practical importance that the LSAR exceeded 2.0 in 65 of 101 predelivery tests (64 per cent) at or before 36 weeks, including 6 of 11 made before 32 weeks, and, except for the rhesus-affected baby already referred to, these early 'safe' ratios all correctly predicted unimpaired respiration in the baby. In contrast, neonatal respiratory distress occurred in association with about four-fifths of predelivery ratios less than 1.5, and about half of the affected babies (7 out of 15) died as a result, whereas with intermediate predelivery ratios (1.5 to 2.0), one-fifth of the babies developed respiratory distress which was not usually severe (the only fatally affected baby in this group being associated with a value of 1.7). Very similar results have been reported from other centres, including Los Angeles where respiratory distress occurred in association with 13 out of 347 cases (3.7 per cent) in which the predelivery LSAR was more than 2.0 (Donald et al, 1973). It is noteworthy that in both the Belfast and Los Angeles studies, and in several other smaller series, unpredicted respiratory distress occurred only in association with maternal diabetes, severe birth asphyxia, rhesus disease or a combination of these factors.

Measurements of fetal lung surfactant in the AF (usually the lecithin: sphingomyelin ratio) have been widely adopted in the management of high risk pregnancies and to time delivery in women of uncertain gestational maturity. When placental insufficiency is suspected, even when (e.g. in severe pre-eclampsia) intervention is under consideration as early as 32 weeks, they enable the obstetrician to avoid the intra-uterine death of fetuses with sufficiently mature lungs for safe immediate delivery; in other cases he will postpone delivery to avoid the greater risk of neonatal death from respiratory immaturity. Similarly, when the membranes rupture prematurely it is now possible to identify (and expedite delivery of) the baby with adequate surfactant, whereas if this is still inadequate the risk of infection must be accepted and time allowed for the fetal lungs to mature. In such cases, lung maturation may occur very quickly (see above) and its occurrence can be confirmed by repeated sampling of the AF draining into the vagina. AF surfactant tests will also come to have an important role in monitoring the effects of treatment given in an attempt to accelerate pulmonary surface-activity in the fetus.

Accuracy depends on the receipt of enough AF samples for at least two technicians to perform these tests regularly. It will therefore often be best for a selected laboratory to provide the service on a group basis. In these circumstances, the other units could usefully adopt the bubble stability test ('shake test') of Clements et al (1972) as a simple screening procedure, either in their own laboratories or in a clinical side-room. Although as many as 20 per cent of bubble stability tests may give false-negative results, making it necessary to submit the AF sample to the central laboratory, false-positive tests (wrongly confirming adequate surface activity) are extremely rare (Sproule, Green and Whitfield, 1974).

Acceleration of the terminal rise in AF lecithin in mothers treated with steroids has been reported (Spellacy et al, 1973). A controlled trial in Auckland of glucocorticoid given to the mother in an attempt to accelerate pulmonary surfactant production in the fetus showed a significant reduction in hyaline membrane disease in babies born before 32 weeks (Liggins and Howie, 1972). The writer's experience so far of glucocorticoid therapy in 42 pregnancies, including 25 fetuses given hydrocortisone in the donor blood at intra-uterine transfusion for very severe rhesus disease, is inconclusive. Further evaluation is clearly needed. Meanwhile, until its efficacy is confirmed, over-enthusiastic adoption of this treatment is to be deplored, especially as there seemed to be an increased risk of fetal death in treated severe pre-eclamptics in the Auckland trial and also because of the possible deleterious effect of steroids in the presence of the infection that is so likely to follow membrane rupture. However, the apparent acceleration of fetal lung maturation when the mother is addicted to heroin (Glass, Rajegowda and Evans, 1971) and in a small number of patients treated with a derivative of bromhexine (Lorenz et al, 1974)—a drug used in the treatment of adult respiratory problems—and on the other hand, its apparent inhibition in methadone addicts (Hobbins, personal communication, 1974) encourage the belief that at least one of the mechanisms involved in the synthesis or release of lecithin in the fetal lung is a labile one that will eventually prove amenable to pharmacological stimulation.

ANTENATAL GENETIC DIAGNOSIS

For the early antenatal detection of genetic disorders and malformation causing serious handicap, amniocentesis should be performed during the 16th week when the experienced operator will almost always obtain a suitable sample. Before this time less than 150 ml of AF is usually present so that amniocentesis may be difficult, and the sample may not contain enough viable cells for satisfactory culture. Biochemical analysis of the supernatant fluid, determination of fetal sex (or blood type) from AF cells, and cytogenetic, biochemical and histochemical investigation of cultures of these cells will be considered in turn. For more detailed accounts the reader is referred to *Antenatal Diagnosis of Genetic Disease* by the

Department of Human Genetics at Edinburgh University (edited by Emery, 1973) or *The Prenatal Diagnosis of Hereditary Disorders* (Milunsky, 1973).

Amniotic fluid supernate

The first intra-uterine diagnosis of an inborn metabolic error was the identification of a fetus with the adrenogenital syndrome by demonstrating abnormally high pregnanetriol and 17-ketosteroid concentrations in the AF (Jeffcoate et al, 1965). This diagnosis has since been reported from several centres but it has always been made near full term. Reduction of the high pregnanetriol levels following injection of the fetus with hydrocortisone has also been reported (Nicholls, 1970) and it may well be useful to start treatment before birth in this way.

The probable exclusion of specific inherited disorders in the fetus by confirming normal concentrations of the relevant metabolites in the AF (e.g. normal phenylalanine levels when there is a family history of phenylketonuria) is reported with increasing frequency, but the positive diagnosis of an affected fetus from an abnormal value has so far been reported only very occasionally (e.g. Hurler's syndrome). Further, because there may be a normal acid mucopolysaccharide level when the fetus has Hurler's syndrome, the detection of this disorder (and probably also of others) cannot be relied on if only the AF supernate is tested.

Because it is likely that disorders associated with detectable abnormalities in the neonatal urine may be characterised by similar abnormalities in the composition of the AF, Emery et al (1970) determined the normal ranges and trends of 27 amino acids and related compounds in the AF. Other compounds have since been identified, but serial determinations in individual subjects (preferably with simultaneous measurements of AF volume) are needed, because, for the detection of some disorders and for the differentiation of a healthy carrier from an affected fetus, abnormal trends may have more value than single estimations and the total amount of a marker metabolite in the AF may sometimes be more significant than its concentration. Repeated measurements of phenylalanine in the AF might also be of value in monitoring the effect of dietary control of maternal phenylketonuria, with the aim of reducing the risk of malformation or subsequent mental retardation in the infant.

The same considerations probably apply to enzyme studies for the detection of such inborn metabolic errors as Pompe's disease (α-1-4-glucosidase deficiency) and Tay–Sachs disease (hexosaminidase-A-deficiency). The availability within two days of the results of such tests on the supernate minimises delay in aborting an affected fetus, but normal enzyme activity may be present when the fetus is abnormal (e.g. Pompe's disease) and cell cultures, which give clear separation between normal and abnormal enzyme activity, must be established.

α-Fetoprotein—neural tube defects

Since Brock and Sutcliffe (1972) reported that the AF α-fetoprotein concentration in cases of anencephaly at 25 to 35 weeks gestation was always several times greater than their highest normal control value, many further reports have confirmed this finding. For the purpose of terminating pregnancy, however, it is more important to identify the fetus with spina bifida as early as possible, because this malformation is compatible with life despite very severe handicap. Brock and Sutcliffe found a value four times as great as the highest control value in relation to a 13-week fetus with spina bifida and myelocoele, and subsequent similar reports include that of a grossly abnormal α-fetoprotein concentration in the AF of a fetus with open spina bifida as early as the second month of pregnancy (Nevin, Nesbitt and Thompson, 1973).

In a recently collected series of reports in the *British Medical Journal* (1975) of AF α-fetoprotein assays from 25 pregnancies in which the fetus had spina bifida, open defects were always associated with frankly abnormal values but some closed lesions were associated with values in the normal range. These findings have also been substantiated by Stewart, Ward and Lorber (1975) who, in a series of 400 pregnancies in which amniocentesis was performed, found clearly elevated values in 17 out of 18 cases with fetal neural tube defects, including four out of five cases of spina bifida without anencephaly (amniocentesis was between 13 and 20 weeks in these patients, and the false-negative result related to a closed defect). False-positive tests are very unusual but may result from fetal bleeding into the AF at the time of amniocentesis (Stewart, Ward and Lorber, 1975) (prompt centrifugation should avoid this problem) or perhaps in multiple pregnancy (Wald et al, 1975).

There may be other useful AF markers of neural tube defects in the fetus, although the claim that β-trace protein might serve to fulfil this role (Macri et al, 1974) has not been substantiated (Brock, 1976). Although fetoscopy, using a fibreoptic telescope, has not so far proved to be a practical method for inspecting the back of a fetus, ultrasonic scanning of its spine may detect spina bifida and its reliability for this purpose clearly requires thorough assessment. Fetographic outlining of a myelocoele (using lipo-soluble contrast) is not possible until about 24 weeks.

Unfortunately, more than 90 per cent of babies with spina bifida are born to mothers who have not previously given birth to babies with neural tube defects, indicating a need for a generally applicable screening method. The possibility that radioimmunoassay of α-fetoprotein in the mother's serum might provide such a mass screening test is under investigation at several centres, including Edinburgh and Oxford where one-third of fetuses with open or closed spinal defects were associated with maternal serum α-fetoprotein levels above the 98th percentile (Brock and Wald, 1975). Based on this statistic, some 15 000 amniocenteses would be needed to detect 800 of the 2400 babies born with spina bifida in Britain during one year, including about 400 that would survive beyond early infancy. However, if a one per cent risk of abortion resulting from early amniocentesis is assumed, the loss in this way of about 150 normal fetuses must be set against the possible identification and therapeutic abortion of 400 potential survivors with spina bifida (most, but not all of whom will have severe handicap). Formidable logistic and organisational problems would also be involved.

On balance, it would seem reasonable to suggest that such a two-tier screening and detection programme, using ultrasound as well as AF analysis in patients with elevated serum levels of α-fetoprotein (e.g. above the 98th percentile in two separate tests), should be established in areas with a high incidence of neural tube defects (e.g. Ireland, and parts of Scotland and Wales).

Uncultured amniotic fluid cells

The sex of the fetus can be determined, with almost 100 per cent accuracy, by examining uncultured AF cells for Barr bodies (indicating an XX constitution) or for F bodies (revealed by fluorescent staining, and confirming an XY constitution). In the case of X-linked recessive disorders causing serious handicap, and for which there is as yet no means of identifying the affected fetus with certainty (e.g. Duchenne's muscular dystrophy and haemophilia), known carrier mothers may be offered amniocentesis followed by selective abortion of male fetuses (one in two affected). If a specific diagnostic test is available (e.g. Hunter's and Lesch–Nyhan syndromes, and Fabry's disease) this should be carried out when a male fetus has been identified.

Genetic linkage analysis provides the most hopeful approach to the prenatal diagnosis of rare autosomal dominant diseases. Thus, there is an 80 per cent chance that an 'at risk' fetus is affected by dystrophia myotonica when the marker genes for lutheran blood group (determined in uncultured cells) and secretor status (diagnosed in the supernate) have both been shown to be present.

Amniotic fluid cell cultures

Cytogenetic studies

Improved culture techniques enable the chromosomal constitution of a fetus to be established within two or three weeks after amniocentesis. Down's syndrome (mongolism) is the only severely handicapping chromosomal disorder compatible with postnatal life, and most amniocenteses for genetic diagnosis are used to screen for this condition. If, because of a previous mongol child, a parent has been identified as a translocation carrier (D/G or G/G), or more rarely as a mosaic (having some trisomic cells), the risk of recurrent Down's syndrome is as high as 30 per cent. Amniocentesis is obviously indicated in such cases unless selective abortion is unacceptable to the couple. In 95 per cent of mongols, the underlying chromosomal abnormality results from non-disjunction during maternal gametogenesis (primary trisomy). As this is most likely to occur in older mothers, as are other less common chromosomal abnormalities, amniocentesis should be offered to mothers aged at least 40 years. In such women there is a one in 70 risk that the fetus has Down's syndrome, but the remaining mothers can continue their pregnancies with this fear allayed. In some centres amniocentesis is also offered to mothers of between 35 and 39 years, but the one in 200 risk of Down's syndrome in their babies is probably less than the risk of a serious complication of the amniocentesis.

Biochemical and histochemical studies

Some enzyme defects are expressed in the cells shed into the AF, making it possible to diagnose a growing list of rare autosomal and X-linked recessive disorders, which include galactosaemia, homocystinuria, glucose-6-phosphate dehydrogenase (G-6-PD) deficiency, Tay–Sachs and Pompe's diseases. A heterozygous fetus carrying Tay–Sachs disease has been detected by demonstrating intermediate hexosaminidase-A activity. The incorporation of radioactively labelled metabolites provides another useful method of study in cell cultures. Thus, the Lesch–Nyhan syndrome (a severe X-linked neurological disorder) has been diagnosed by the failure of cultured AF cells to utilise hypoxanthine, and a fetus carrying this disorder has been identified by the demonstration that some cells take up hypoxanthine while others do not. Similarly, heterozygosity for cystinosis has been detected during late pregnancy by measuring the incorporation of radioactive cystine.

In the storage disorders, intracellular accumulation of a mucopolysaccharide or other metabolite is revealed by histochemical staining, but metachromatic granules are not specific, both false-positive and false-negative results occur, and heterozygous carriers cannot be distinguished from homozygotes. Improved histochemical methods in conjunction with radioactive incorporation techniques and accelerated culture methods may soon enable the specific diagnosis of the various storage disorders (and perhaps also cystic fibrosis) to be made early enough for therapeutic abortion. Unlike chromosomal analysis, enzyme and radioactive investigations necessitate subculturing so that results are not available for at least a month. When cultures or subcultures fail, amniocentesis should be repeated unless the pregnancy will have proceeded too far for selective abortion by the time the fresh culture can be tested. It is vital, therefore, that known or probable carriers should be made aware of the need to report very early in pregnancy.

FUTURE DEVELOPMENTS

Banding techniques may reveal structural abnormalities of the chromosomes that are not visible with conventional cytogenetic techniques. Such structural variants in the chromosomes of amniotic cells must cause concern about the normality of the fetus, but in many such instances banding studies of the parents will reveal the same variant indicating that it is simply a normal polymorphic variant and that the pregnancy need not be terminated. On the other hand, banding techniques should make possible selective abortion of occasional fetuses with hitherto undetectable handicapping chromosomal disorders. In addition, a chromosomal basis may be recognised for some very rare syndromes of as yet uncertain aetiology. Urgent evaluation of these techniques is needed to establish their practical value in routine antenatal cytogenetic diagnosis.

There is need for the further development of sensitive methods to distinguish normal, heterozygous (carrier) and homozygous (affected) fetuses in relation to recessively inherited conditions, including cystic fibrosis, which is the commonest severe autosomal disease in Europeans. The basic biochemical defect in cystic fibrosis is still not recognised, but evidence that it is expressed in both skin and AF fibroblasts suggests that this disorder may soon prove amenable to intra-uterine diagnosis (Beratis et al, 1973).

Population screening methods are needed for the identification of carriers before the birth of an affected infant. This is already possible, using skin fibroblast cultures, in relation to Tay–Sachs disease in Ashkenazi Jewish communities (Kaback, Reynolds and Sonneborn, 1974). Linkage analysis may eventually prove helpful in screening for heterozygotes in certain communities or races, an example being the close relation between the loci for G-6-PD and haemophilia-A (factor VIII deficiency) on the X-chromosomes in black women.

In view of the rarity of most of these disorders and the sophisticated nature of many of the laboratory methods, expert genetic counselling and antenatal diagnostic services should be coordinated on a national basis. In this way, a particular expertise developed at one centre will be available to all the others. A case can be made for special antenatal reference clinics, but the vital early reference of at-risk patients to such clinics will depend not only on all obstetricians being aware of the scope of prenatal diagnosis, but also on adequate counselling of these women (and their husbands) by family doctors, paediatricians and community physicians.

REFERENCES

Abramovich, D. R. (1973) The volume of amniotic fluid and factors affecting or regulating this. In *Amniotic Fluid Research and Clinical Application* (Ed.) Fairweather, D. V. I. & Eskes, T. K. A. B. Ch. 3. Amsterdam: Excerpta Medica.

Beratis, N. G., Conover, J. H., Conod, E. J., Bonforte, R. J. & Hirschhorn, K. (1973) Studies on ciliary dyskinesia factor in cystic fibrosis III. *Pediatric Research,* **7,** 958.

Bhagwanani, S. G., Fahmy, D. & Turnbull, A. C. (1972) Quick determination of amniotic fluid lecithin concentration for prediction of neonatal distress. *Lancet,* **ii,** 66–67.

Borer, R. C., Gluck, L., Freeman, R. K. & Kulovich, M. V. (1971) Prenatal prediction of the respiratory distress syndrome. *Pediatric Research,* **5,** 655.

British Medical Journal (1975) Leading article: antenatal diagnosis of spina bifida. *British Medical Journal,* **i,** 414.

Brock, D. J. H. (1976) Prenatal diagnosis—chemical methods. *British Medical Bulletin,* **32,** 16–20.

Brock, D. J. H. & Sutcliffe, R. G. (1972) Alpha-fetoprotein in the antenatal diagnosis of anencephaly and spina bifida. *Lancet,* **ii,** 197–199.

Brock, D. J. H. & Wald, N. (1975) Previously unpublished data quoted in leading article. *British Medical Journal,* **i,** 414.

Clements, J. A., Platzker, A. C. G., Tierney, D. F., Hobel, C. J., Creasy, R. K., Margolis, A. J., Thibeault, D. W., Tooley, W. H. & Oh, W. (1972) Assessment of the risk of the respiratory distress syndrome by a rapid new test for surfactant in amniotic fluid. *New England Journal of Medicine,* **268,** 1077–1081.

Donald, I. R., Freeman, R. K., Goebelsmann, U., Chan, W. H. & Nakamura, R. M. (1973) Clinical experience with the amniotic fluid lecithin/sphingomyelin ratio. *American Journal of Obstetrics and Gynecology,* **115,** 547–552.

Emery, A. E. H. (Ed.) (1973) *Antenatal Diagnosis of Genetic Disease.* Edinburgh, London: Churchill Livingstone.

Emery, A. E. H., Burt, D., Nelson, M. M. & Scrimgeour, J. B. (1970) Antenatal diagnosis and amino acid composition of amniotic fluid. *Lancet,* **i,** 1307–1308.

Falconer, G. F., Hodge, J. S. & Gadd, R. L. (1973) Influence of amniotic fluid volume on lecithin estimation in prediction of respiratory distress. *British Medical Journal,* **ii,** 689–691.

Fraser, I. D. & Tovey, G. H. (1972) Estimation of antibody protein in amniotic fluid to predict severity in rhesus haemolytic disease. *Journal of Obstetrics and Gynaecology of the British Commonwealth,* **79,** 981–984.

Fraser, I. D., Tovey, G. H., Lockyear, W. J. & Sobey, D. F. (1972) Antibody protein levels in the maternal serum in rhesus isoimmunisation. *Journal of Obstetrics and Gynaecology of the British Commonwealth,* **79,** 1074–1079.

Freda, V. J. (1965) The Rh problem in obstetrics and a new concept of its management using amniocentesis and spectro-photometric scanning of amniotic fluid. *American Journal of Obstetrics and Gynecology,* **92,** 341–374.

Glass, L., Rajegowda, B. K. & Evans, H. E. (1971) Absence of respiratory distress syndrome in premature infants of heroin-addicted mothers. *Lancet,* **ii,** 685–686.

Gluck, L., Kulovich, M. V., Borer, R. C., Brenner, P. H., Anderson, G. G. & Spellacy, W. N. (1971) Diagnosis of the respiratory distress syndrome by amniocentesis. *American Journal of Obstetrics and Gynecology,* **109,** 440–445.

Hallman, M. & Gluck, L. (1974) Phosphatidyl glycerol in lung surfactant I. *Biochemical and Biophysical Research Communications,* **60,** 1–7.

Jeffcoate, T. N. A., Fliegner, J. R. H., Russell, S. H., Davis, J. C. & Wade, A. P. (1965) Diagnosis of the adrenogenital syndrome before birth. *Lancet,* **ii,** 553–555.

Kaback, M. M., Reynolds, L. W. & Sonneborn, M. (1974) Tay–Sachs disease: a model for the control of recessive genetic disorders. In *Birth Defects* (Ed.) Motulsky, A. G. & Lenz, W. Amsterdam: Excerpta Medica.

Liggins, G. C. (1966) Current indications for intrauterine transfusion. *Fifty-third Ross Conference: Intrauterine Transfusion and Erythroblastosis Fetalis* (Ed.) Lucey, J. & Butterfield, L. J. p. 28. Columbus, Ohio: Ross Laboratories.

Liggins, G. C. & Howie, R. N. (1972) A controlled trial of antepartum glucocorticoid treatment for prevention of the respiratory distress syndrome in premature infants. *Pediatrics,* **50,** 515–525.

Liley, A. W. (1961) Liquor amnii analysis in management of pregnancy complicated by rhesus sensitisation. *American Journal of Obstetrics and Gynecology,* **82,** 1359–1370.

Lind, T. (1970) The estimation of fetal growth and development. *British Journal of Hospital Medicine,* **3,** 501–507.

Lorenz, U., Ruttgers, H., Fux, G. & Kubli, F. (1974) Fetal pulmonary surfactant induction by bromhexine metabolite VIII. *American Journal of Obstetrics and Gynecology,* **119,** 1126–1128.

Macri, J. N., Weiss, R. R., Joshi, M. S. & Evans, M. I. (1974) Antenatal diagnosis of neural-tube defects using cerebrospinal-fluid proteins. *Lancet,* **i,** 14–15.

Milunsky, A. (1973) *The Prenatal Diagnosis of Hereditary Disorders.* Springfield: Charles C. Thomas.

Morris, E. D., Murray, J. & Ruthven, C. R. J. (1967) Liquor bilirubin levels in normal pregnancy: a basis for accurate prediction of haemolytic disease. *British Medical Journal,* **i,** 352–354.

Nevin, N. C., Nesbitt, S. & Thompson, W. (1973) Myelocele and alpha-fetoprotein in amniotic fluid. *Lancet*, **i**, 1383.

Nicholls, J. (1970) Antenatal diagnosis and treatment of the adrenogenital syndrome. *Lancet*, **i**, 83.

Niven, P. A. R., Ward, R. H. T. & Chard, T. (1974) Human placental lactogen in amniotic fluid in rhesus isoimmunisation. *Journal of Obstetrics and Gynaecology of the British Commonwealth*, **88**, 988–990.

Queenan, J. T. & Goetschel, E. (1968) Amniotic fluid analysis for erythroblastosis fetalis. *Obstetrics and Gynecology*, **32**, 120–133.

Queenan, J. T., Thompson, W., Whitfield, C. R. & Shah, S. J. (1972) Amniotic fluid volumes in normal pregnancies. *American Journal of Obstetrics and Gynecology*, **114**, 34–38.

Richardson, C. J., Pomerance, J. J., Cunningham, M. D. & Gluck, L. (1974) Acceleration of fetal lung maturation following prolonged rupture of the membranes. *American Journal of Obstetrics and Gynecology*, **118**, 1115–1118.

Robertson, J. G. (1969) Management of patients with Rh iso-immunisation based on amniotic fluid examination. *American Journal of Obstetrics and Gynecology*, **103**, 713–722.

Robinson, H. P. (1975) 'Gestation sac' volumes as determined by sonar in the first trimester of pregnancy. *British Journal of Obstetrics and Gynaecology*, **82**, 100–107.

Spellacy, W. N., Buhi, W. C., Riggall, F. C. & Holsinger, K. L. (1973) Human amniotic fluid lecithin/sphingomyelin ratio changes with oestrogen and glucocorticoid treatment. *American Journal of Obstetrics and Gynecology*, **115**, 216–218.

Sproule, W. B. (1974) Unpublished data for thesis submitted to Dublin University.

Sproule, W. B., Greene, E. & Whitfield, C. R. (1974) Amniotic fluid bubble stability test as a screening procedure for predicting the risk of neonatal respiratory distress. *American Journal of Obstetrics and Gynecology*, **119**, 653–656.

Stewart, C. R., Ward, A. M. & Lorber, J. (1975) Amniotic fluid α-fetoprotein in the diagnosis of neural tube malformations. *British Journal of Obstetrics and Gynaecology*, **82**, 257–261.

Thompson, W., Lappin, T. R. J. & Elder, G. E. (1971) Liquor volume by direct spectrophotometric determination of injected PAH. *Journal of Obstetrics and Gynaecology of the British Commonwealth*, **78**, 341–344.

Wagstaff, T. I. & Bromham, D. R. (1973) A comparison between the lecithin–sphingomyelin ratio and the 'shake test' for the estimation of surfactant in amniotic fluid. *Journal of Obstetrics and Gynaecology of the British Commonwealth*, **80**, 412–417.

Wald, N., Barker, S., Peto, R., Brock, D. J. H. & Bonnar, J. (1975) Maternal serum α-fetoprotein levels in multiple pregnancy. *British Medical Journal*, **i**, 651–652.

Ward, H., Whyley, G. A. & Millar, M. D. (1973) A comparative study of diamine oxidase in amniotic fluid and serum in normal pregnancy and in pregnancy complicated by rhesus iso-immunisation. *Journal of Obstetrics and Gynaecology of the British Commonwealth*, **80**, 525–530.

Warren, C., Holton, J. B. & Allen, J. T. (1974) Assessment of fetal lung maturity by estimation of amniotic fluid palmitic acid. *British Medical Journal*, **i**, 94–96.

Whitfield, C. R. (1970) A three-year assessment of an action line method of timing intervention in rhesus isoimmunization. *American Journal of Obstetrics and Gynecology*, **108**, 1239–1244.

Whitfield, C. R. (1971) Effect of amniotic fluid volume on prediction. *Clinical Obstetrics and Gynecology*, **14**, 537–547.

Whitfield, C. R. & Sproule, W. B. (1974) Fetal lung maturation. *British Journal of Hospital Medicine*, **12**, 678–690.

Whitfield, C. R., Sproule, W. B. & Brudenell, M. (1973) The amniotic fluid lecithin: sphingomyelin area ratio (LSAR) in pregnancies complicated by diabetes. *Journal of Obstetrics and Gynaecology of the British Commonwealth*, **80**, 918–922.

Whitfield, C. R., Thompson, W., Armstrong, M. J. & Reid, M. McC. (1972) Intrauterine fetal transfusion for severe rhesus haemolytic disease. *Journal of Obstetrics and Gynaecology of the British Commonwealth*, **79**, 931–940.

Whyley, G. A., Ward, H. & Hardy, N. R. (1974) Alpha-fetoprotein levels in amniotic fluid in pregnancies complicated by rhesus isoimmunisation. *Journal of Obstetrics and Gynaecology of the British Commonwealth*, **81**, 459–465.

18

MATERNAL AND FETAL INFECTION

Pamela Davies

The true extent to which maternal infection is transmitted to the fetus is unknown. There is ignorance too of the precise mechanisms—whether dependent on mother, fetus or placenta—which, when combined with variation in the virulence of infecting organisms, determine the fate of an individual offspring. For example, it is not always clear why, in apparently similar circumstances, one embryo or fetus escapes completely unscathed and another becomes infected; and, in the latter instance, why the result may range through abortion, stillbirth, a newborn infant severely or mildly damaged, to one apparently healthy and capable of entirely normal development. Timing of the maternal infection is clearly a most important variable, particularly with regard to the stage of fetal organ differentiation, and maturity of the fetal immune system. Important too are the numbers of invading organisms, and the route by which they enter. The occasional marked difference in degree of twin involvement suggests that other factors must also have a role.

The present state of knowledge is often insufficient to guide the obstetrician in the management of a pregnancy. Frequently maternal infective illness goes unsuspected and undiagnosed until the birth of an affected infant. In some cases, infection may be found in an apparently well woman in the course of some routine screening procedure, and only very rarely is there a clinically recognisable and proven illness. Even then, the risk to the fetus can be expressed for only a very few infecting organisms with any sort of precision. It must also be emphasised that what may be valid in one country for a population of a given social and economic standing may not be so for another. With these reservations in mind, this chapter will try to record what is known so far of the risk to the fetus, and to give details of diagnostic tests which may be helpful. Not all of the latter are available in the routine laboratory.

GENERAL ASPECTS

Defence mechanisms

It is now known from the work of several groups pursuing an explanation for the survival of the genetically incompatible 'fetal allograft' that pregnancy is accompanied by an altered immune state. The alteration is one of a reduced cell-mediated immunity (T-cell activity) as judged by the in vitro phytohaemagglutinin-induced lymphocyte transformation rate. This is thought to be due to a serum inhibitor rather than a reduction in the number of T-cells (St. Hill, Finn and Denye, 1973), and the possibility of its being hormonal has to be considered in view of a similar depression of cellular immunity in women on the contraceptive pill (Hagen and Frøland, 1972). Clearly any reduction of immunity due to pregnancy cannot be sufficiently severe as to jeopardise the future of the human race, and any evidence that gravidae are more susceptible to illness in general is difficult to collect, though local susceptibility of the genital tract may be altered. However, pregnant women are thought to have a more severe illness in the course of certain viral diseases than non-pregnant women of the same age (Frucht and Metcalfe, 1954; Hardy, 1965).

Mechanisms of immunity in the fetus develop steadily from early in gestation and are elaborated in detail in recent reviews (Gotoff, 1974; Stiehm, 1975). Stem cells in the liver and spleen form the basis of the cellular immune or T-cell system and are thought to enter the thymus at about eight weeks of gestation. After maturation they leave the thymus and go particularly to lymph nodes and spleen, and presumably have an important role to play in limiting intra-uterine infection. In vitro cell cultures from 10-week abortuses will produce interferon—important for its ability to prevent further multiplication inside infected cells when challenged with virus (Banatvala, Potter and Best, 1971). Interferon can also be produced by the placenta. Complement is being synthesised by the fetus from the eighth week, but is only 50 per cent of adult levels at birth. The production of the antibody or B-cell system starts at about 11 to 12 weeks with the synthesis of IgM, mainly in the spleen; IgG synthesis follows at 12 weeks, and IgA at 30 weeks. Antibody production is very limited unless challenged by infecting organisms (see below). The fetus receives maternal IgG by active placental transport largely in the last trimester. Granulocyte cells are synthesised by the bone marrow from about five months, and before that in the liver. The phagocytic white cells of the newborn are not as effective as those of adults in disposing of bacteria, and presumably this applies to fetal cells as well. There is growing evidence that fetal undernutrition, itself so often a product of maternal malnutrition, may impair fetal immune defence.

Geographical and socioeconomic factors

Variations in pregnancy infections are to be expected in different parts of the world, depending on the immune status of women of child-bearing age and differing strains of infecting organisms. Densely populated countries such as the United Kingdom may in general expect a high degree of immunity among their citizens. Vaccination and immunisation policies have now removed the fear of certain diseases in this country, though the scope of modern international travel suggests that we should not be too parochial in our outlook.

There seems to be increasing evidence that women in poor social and economic circumstances in this country, and the world over, are more likely to have certain pregnancy infections than are those who are more privileged. The fetuses of this group are then inevitably at greater risk also.

Mechanisms of fetal damage

Miscarriage, fetal death or preterm live birth may undoubtedly occur in the course of certain maternal infections, though actual serological or cultural evidence that the conceptus itself is infected or damaged may not be forthcoming. Neither the extent to which this happens, nor the underlying mechanisms for it, are fully known. When the pregnancy goes forward, the most important factors determining fetal damage are the timing of the maternal infection, the special properties of the infecting organisms themselves, and the routes by which they reach the fetus. There are several theoretical paths of entry, but two—the transplacental, and that ascending from the birth canal—are by far the most important, and may not always be easy to distinguish. In the former placental infection is thought to be invariably present first, and in some cases it may be quite extensive without inevitable fetal involvement.

If organ formation in the first trimester is disturbed by an infecting organism, congenital anomalies may follow. Such anomalies however are known to occur with certainty only with rubella and varicella-zoster infections, if the central nervous damage caused by cytomegalovirus (CMV) and toxoplasmosis for instance are excluded. The rubella virus inhibits or retards cell growth, and malformations may occur with this arrest of cell division, though the virus' predilection for infecting vascular endothelium, with resulting vessel thrombosis and tissue necrosis, as well as its chronic persistence, account for many of the effects seen (Menser and Reye, 1974). Reasons put forward to explain the persistence of rubella virus excretion after birth in the presence of high antibody titres are that the antibody forming cells (B-lymphocytes) are only partly damaged; that because mitotic division of infected thymic lymphocytes is impaired they are less capable of destroying infected cell clones; and that the rubella antibody produced by uninfected B-lymphocytes is stimulated in utero without the development of tolerance. As unaffected clones of T-lymphocytes become available they destroy infected cells, the B-lymphocytes then neutralising the released virus (Plotkin, 1975). The lesions following infection with the varicella-zoster virus, which is well known for its neurotropic properties, may result from damage to motor nerves (Savage, Moosa and Gordon, 1973). Such viruses as CMV and *herpesvirus hominis* (HVH) may exert their damaging effect by cell lysis; in the first trimester of pregnancy this will cause morphological disruption, most seriously of the brain, without evidence of inflammation.

It is not until the development of fetal antibody-producing cells in the second trimester that the inflammatory response to *Treponema pallidum* occurs and though spirochaetes may be present in the fetus in the earlier weeks, they are not themselves damaging during this time (Plotkin, 1975). That fetal damage of the order caused by certain viruses or protozoa early in pregnancy could also be caused by other bacteria remains a theoretical and so far largely un-investigated possibility.

Maternal infection and possible childhood malignancy

Very recently the suggestion has been made that there may be a link between viral disease in pregnancy and malignant disease in the child. Fedrick and Alberman (1972) found that children whose mothers had had 'influenza' during pregnancy had an unexpectedly high incidence of leukaemia, and neoplasms of lymphatic and haematopoietic tissue. (This was not serologically confirmed influenza, but the illness occurred at the time of a recognised pandemic.) Bithell, Draper and Gorbach (1973) and Hakulinen et al (1973) have produced data which are not as striking, but nevertheless suggest a significant similar association. On the other hand, Curnen et al (1974) in Connecticut, and Leck and Steward (1972) from the north-west of England, where registration of these diseases is known to be lower (together with Scotland) than other parts of the United Kingdom, have failed to confirm these findings, as have Donovan, Adelstein and Leighton (1974) in a preliminary report. Bithell, Draper and Gorbach (1973) postulate as well an association between chickenpox infection in pregnancy and later central nervous system tumour in the child, an association also apparent in the data of Donovan et al. Lack of laboratory confirmation of maternal infection must constitute a very large variable in these studies and, as several of the authors point out, even if these suspicions were to be confirmed on a larger scale, the number of cases of childhood cancer and leukaemia attributable to maternal infection is probably very small. Nevertheless, there is growing interest in the idea of an increased incidence of neoplasia with impairment of immunological function, and the latter is known to exist following at least some of the congenital intra-uterine infections.

Diagnostic tests

It may be helpful to mention briefly some of the more frequently used terms and diagnostic tests. The definitions for these are taken from *A Dictionary of Immunology* (Herbert and Wilkinson, 1972).

All antibodies so far described are immunoglobulins, and we are concerned with three of the major classes, IgA, IgG and IgM. The first is found in secretions, and is concerned with the protection of mucosal surfaces. IgG, the only one to be actively transported across the placenta, fixes complement. IgM is produced first in response to primary infection, also fixes complement, and can be manufactured by the fetus along with IgA, in response to intra-uterine infection. Specific IgM is that antibody reacting specifically with a given antigen (e.g. rubella-specific IgM). In primary postnatal infection, it is usually only present for a few weeks (see also page 357), but in congenital infection for considerably longer.

Immunofluorescent techniques are of considerable diagnostic help where the location of tissue antibodies or antigens is concerned, or even bacteria in smears, and viruses in cells. An antigen or antibody can be conjugated to a substance such as fluorescein (a yellow dye with an intense green fluorescence) and then allowed to react with the corresponding antibody or antigen in a tissue section or smear. With ultraviolet light as the source of microscope light the location of tissue antibodies or antigens on the slide can be seen by the pattern of fluorescence.

Haemagglutination inhibition (HI), complement fixation (CF) and neutralisation tests are in common use in the diagnosis of infection. In general, a four-fold rise in titre over a two to hree-week period would suggest a primary infection. In the first, antibody against certain iruses which agglutinate red blood cells is detected by its ability to inhibit such agglutina-ion. The second detects antibody, usually IgG and IgM, which, in reacting with antigen, inds complement. Neutralisation tests measure the capacity of antibody to neutralise the in-ectivity of a virus, or effects of a bacterial toxin.

VIRUSES

These will be considered first as there is more information on their effects on the fetus com-pared with many of the other organisms. Individual viruses are listed alphabetically in Table 8.1, rather than grouped under their genus, for the nomenclature of the latter still seems con-roversial. There is space to discuss only a few, and not all in detail. Brief information about he others is given in Table 18.2, and the maximum extent of fetal involvement is shown in Table 18.3.

Table 18.1. *Some infecting organisms which may involve the fetus during pregnancy, labour and delivery.*

Transmitted via placenta [a]		Acquired from birth canal and perineum
Bacterial [b]	Viral	Bacterial [c]
Borrelia	Coxsackie virus	*Listeria monocytogenes*
Brucella abortus	Cytomegalovirus	*Neisseria gonorrhoeae*
Leptospira	ECHO virus	*Salmonella* spp.
Listeria monocytogenes	Hepatitis B virus	*Shigellae* spp.
Mycobacterium tuberculosis	Herpesvirus hominis	Enteropathogenic
Pasteurella tularensis	Influenza virus	*Escherichia coli*
Salmonella typhi	Mumps virus	
Treponema pallidum	Polio virus	Viral
Vibrio fetus	Rubella virus	
	Rubeola virus	Cytomegalovirus
	Vaccinia virus	Herpesvirus hominis
	Varicella-zoster virus	
	Variola virus	Protozoal
	Western equine	
Protozoal	encephalitis virus	*Trichomonas vaginalis*
Plasmodia		
Toxoplasma gondii		Fungal
Trypanosoma spp.		
		Candida albicans
Fungal	Other	Other
Candida albicans	*Mycoplasma*	*Chlamydia*
		Mycoplasma

[a] Evidence conclusive or reasonable.
[b] Only unusual bacteria known to have caused fetal disease listed. Any others causing maternal infection could be involved.
[c] Only unusual bacteria listed. Any others colonising birth canal and perineum or causing local disease could be involved.

Table 18.2. *Possible effects of some viruses and other organisms* (not described in text).

Infecting organism	Fetal and/or neonatal involvement
Viruses	
ECHO	No consistent reports of fetal damage but overwhelming infection with severe hepatic necrosis has occurred.
Influenza (most studies related to A)	Possible risk increased abortion. No consistent pattern congenital anomalies in different parts of the world; evidence in favour increased teratogenic risk in conclusive. Increased infant mortality during recent epidemic year reported (DHSS, 1971). Possible association with later development leukaemia, and neoplasms of lymphatic and haematopoietic tissue (see text).
Mumps	Postulated association with endocardial fibroelastosis (Noren, Adams and Anderson, 1963), but subsequent reports conflicting, and neutralising antibody to mumps virus in children's sera frequently absent. Not yet proven.
Poliovirus	No increase of congenital defects, inconclusive evidence preterm birth, fetal death in 35 to 40 per cent first trimester infections, neonatal poliomyelitis most frequently seen with paralytic maternal illness occurring just before delivery (Siegel and Greenberg, 1956).
Rubeola	Increased risk abortion and premature labour. Congenital measles very rare usually severe.
Vaccinia	No harmful effect first trimester vaccination in prospective study involving 4172 women (Greenberg et al, 1949). Virus can involve placenta and fetus quite extensively; isolated case reports describe abortion, stillbirth, livebirth with generalised vaccinia. Vaccination should be avoided in pregnancy; if essential give specific anti-vaccinial gammaglobulin (central PHL) at same time.
Varicella-zoster	Risk small, but herpes zoster and varicella both reported in newborn when infection late in pregnancy. Teratogenic effects of infection in early pregnancy include reduction deformities of limbs with skin scarring, choroidoretinitis and meningoencephalitis (Savage, Moosa and Gordon, 1973).
Variola	High fetal loss.
Western equine encephalitis	Infection not invariable, risk unknown, central nervous system damage to infant may be severe.
Protozoa	
Plasmodia	Congenital malaria very rare among indigenous population of endemic areas who have substantial immunity, but not uncommonly found when mothers poorly immune, and inadequately treated or untreated. Placental involvement can be massive without fetal infection.
Trichomonas vaginalis	Reports of infection involving infant girls in this country rare, but more common elsewhere, probably in association with untreated maternal infection.
Trypanosomes	Transplacental infection shown to occur with African and South American trypanosomiasis, but precise risk unknown. Difficult to know to what extent chronic maternal infection itself may predispose to probable increase in abortion and stillbirth.
Fungi	
Candida albicans	Intra-uterine infection of fetus, placenta and membranes recorded in few isolated cases, and organism demonstrated on fetal surface placenta in 0.8 per cent cases (Maudsley et al, 1966). Pinkish-yellowish-white lesions may be seen on cord surface. Incidence oral and perineal moniliasis in offspring of women with inadequately or untreated monilial vulvovaginitis is high (Shrand, 1961). Possibility exists that transmission could be via hands after birth, rather than birth canal.
Other	
Chlamydia	Inclusion blenorrhoea may occur in infants colonised by maternal cervical infection.

Table 18.3. *Neonatal signs of prenatal infection* [a]

Possible clinical involvement	Infecting organisms
Central nervous system	
Meningitis, meningo-encephalitis (may lead to microcephaly, hydrocephalus, abnormal CNS signs, fits and in some cases to cerebral calcifications)	Bacteria, *Candida albicans*, Coxsackie virus, Cytomegalovirus (CMV), ECHO virus, Herpesvirus hominis (HVH), poliovirus, rubella virus, *Toxoplasma gondii*, *Treponema pallidum*, varicella-zoster virus, variola virus
Special sensory organs	
Eye: cataracts	Rubella virus, *Toxoplasma gondii*
choroidoretinitis	CMV, HVH, rubella virus, *Toxoplasma gondii*, varicella-zoster virus
microphthalmia	HVH, rubella virus, *Toxoplasma gondii*
keratitis and corneal opacity	HVH, rubella virus, *Treponema pallidum*
purulent ophthalmia	*Neisseria gonorrhoeae*, or other bacteria, *Mycoplasma hominis*, *Chlamydia*
Ear: eighth nerve damage (may not be detected even with special techniques)	CMV, rubella virus, *Treponema pallidum*
otitis media	Bacteria
Cardiovascular system	
Congenital heart disease (patent ductus arteriosus, pulmonary artery stenosis, pulmonary valve stenosis, ventricular septal defect, aberrant subclavian vessels)	Rubella virus
Peripheral arterial stenoses	Rubella virus
Myocarditis	Coxsackie B virus, poliovirus
Pericarditis	Bacteria
Respiratory system	
Pneumonia	Bacteria, *Candida albicans*, Coxsackie virus, CMV, HVH, *Mycobacterium tuberculosis, Mycoplasma hominis*, poliovirus, rubella virus, *Treponema pallidum*, vaccinia virus, varicella-zoster virus, variola virus
Skeletal system	
Periostitis and/or defective mineralisation and growth disturbance	CMV, HVH, rubella virus, *Toxoplasma gondii*, *Treponema pallidum*
Reduction deformities of limbs	Varicella-zoster virus
Osteomyelitis, septic arthritis	Bacteria
Gastrointestinal system	
Hepatosplenomegaly with or without jaundice	Coxsackie virus, CMV, ECHO virus, hepatitis B virus, HVH, *Mycobacterium tuberculosis, Plasmodium*, rubella virus, *Toxoplasma gondii*, *Treponema pallidum*, vaccinia virus, varicella-zoster virus, variola virus
Enteritis	Enteropathogenic *Escherichia coli*, *Shigellae*, *Salmonellae*
Genitourinary system	
Nephritis, nephrotic syndrome	*Treponema pallidum*
Vaginitis	*Trichomonas vaginitis*
Urinary infection	Bacteria

Table 18.3 *contd.*

Possible clinical involvement	Infecting organisms
Haematopoietic system	
Anaemia, sometimes haemolytic with jaundice	Bacteria, CMV, HVH, rubella virus, *Toxoplasma gondii*, *Treponema pallidum*
Purpura, with or without disseminated intravascular coagulation (some haemorrhagic skin nodules are erythropoietic in nature)	Coxsackie virus, CMV, ECHO, HVH, rubella virus, *Toxoplasma gondii*, *Treponema pallidum*
Skin and mucous membrane	
Vesicular lesions, single, grouped or scattered, sometimes unilateral	HVH, varicella-zoster virus, *Treponema pallidum*
Large umbilicated lesions	Vaccinia and variola viruses
Macular or maculo-papular lesions	*Treponema pallidum*
Mouth—'milk curd' lesions leaving raw area when removed	*Candida albicans*
Skin—papulo-vesicular and scaling	*Candida albicans*
Pustules, abscesses	Bacteria, *Mycoplasma hominis*
Intra-uterine growth retardation	CMV, *Plasmodium*, rubella virus, *Treponema pallidum*

Adapted from Davies et al (1972) with kind permission of the publishers (London: Heinemann).
ᵃMaximum involvement listed.

Coxsackie virus

The largest prospective survey available is that of Brown and Karunas (1972) who studied 22 935 pregnant women with serological testing in the first trimester and at delivery. Their results suggested a significant association between infection with certain Coxsackie types during the pregnancy and congenital malformations in their offspring compared with controls. First trimester Coxsackie B4 infection was associated with an excess of urogenital defects. Infection with Coxsackie B3 and B4 viruses throughout pregnancy was associated with cardiovascular defects, but of a wide variety; similarly Coxsackie A9 infection, again throughout pregnancy, showed a link with digestive tract anomalies. The wide range of anomalies, and the fact that the infections were not necessarily limited to the first trimester, make this study difficult to assess. Further data would have to be collected before a definite teratogenic effect could be ascribed to these viruses. Infection later in pregnancy is now well recognised as a cause of pneumonia, meningitis and myocarditis in the newborn, though a numerical risk cannot be given. Burch et al (1968) have suggested that intra-uterine infections of occult Coxsackie virus B might be responsible for some forms of heart disease in later life.

Cytomegalovirus (CMV)

Maternal involvement. The epidemiology of acquired as opposed to congenital CMV infection is not fully known. It is geographically widespread, but unlike rubella it appears to be more common in those of poorer socioeconomic status, and the incidence may vary between racial groups. In a study in the north-west of England, the infants of young unmarried mothers were found to be infected six times more frequently than those of married ones (Collaborative Study, 1970). Stern and Tucker (1973) found that two-thirds of 1040 London women in a prospective pregnancy survey possessed antibody to CMV, and they demonstrated its presence in 58 per cent of native white English women, and in 90 per cent of immigrant Asian women. Four per cent of women developed a primary infection during the course of their pregnancy. Although many fewer of the Asian women were without antibodies in the first trimester, and thus susceptible, the rate of primary infection among them was considerably higher than among the white women.

Virus has been recovered from the cervix more frequently than from the urine during pregnancy and in the third trimester of pregnancy more often than in the second or first. In a prospective pregnancy survey of Caucasian and Negro women from Pittsburgh, 58 per cent were found to have antibodies to CMV, but the virus was recovered from the cervix in only four per cent (Montgomery, Youngblood and Medearis, 1972). Women known to have antibodies to CMV before the onset of pregnancy may start to excrete CMV in pregnancy (urine and cervix), presumably because of their temporary alteration of immunity.

Risk to the fetus. Both placenta and fetus may be infected by the viraemia occurring with primary infection, though the fetus is not always infected when the placenta is. Stern and Tucker (1973) found the overall incidence of fetal infection to be almost 50 per cent following primary infection in the mother, and noted that it was higher in early pregnancy. They calculated that about 4000 CMV infected infants would be born yearly in England and Wales. Prospective American surveys have shown that CMV can be recovered from the urine of between 0.5 per cent and 3.0 per cent of newborn infants (Birnbaum et al, 1969; Feldman, 1969), but the majority of them appear normal at birth, and are thus presumably affected late in the second or third trimester, for clinical manifestations are primarily a reflection of the duration of intra-uterine infection (Monif et al, 1972). Weller (1970) has pointed out that positive cultures are higher by three to four months of age, and it is possible that this increase represents infections acquired at birth during passage through the birth canal.

It has been said that reactivation of latent infection in pregnancy does not appear to involve the fetus (Montgomery, Youngblood and Medearis, 1972; Stern and Tucker, 1973). However, there are now some well documented case reports which show that successive fetuses may be involved (Embil, Ozere and Haldane, 1970; Stagno et al, 1973). The extent of this mode of infection may have been underestimated, for it has never been studied on a prospective scale. It may happen when the interval between pregnancies is short. Despite the excretion of virus in breast milk (Hayes et al, 1972), it seems unlikely that this is a significant source of infection for the infant. No correlation has beeen found between breast feeding and CMV excretion in infants (Levinsohn et al, 1969). Intra-uterine transfusion of donor blood infected with CMV may be a hazard for erythroblastotic babies (King-Lewis and Gardner, 1969). The severe manifestations of CMV infection in the newborn, seen in only a tiny minority of infants, are shown in Table 18.3.

The realisation that apparently normal children excreting virus at birth greatly outnumber those with obvious central nervous system damage has been relatively recent, and the exact prognosis for fetal infection is not yet accurately known, conflicting findings having been reported. Hanshaw (1966) found CMV antibodies in 43.9 per cent of microcephalic children compared with 3.9 per cent in normocephalic controls; but showed that 16 of 22 children infected with CMV at birth were developing normally, while three of the remaining six were deaf. Cytomegalovirus was thought to account for 10 per cent of mental retardation in children under six living at home in the London area (Stern et al, 1969). On the other hand, Baron and colleagues (1969) could find no significant association between microcephaly and evidence of CMV infection; and a follow-up study of children congenitally infected yet normal at birth showed no difference in their mean I.Q. compared with controls (Kumar, Nankervis and Gold, 1973). Further sizeable follow-up studies of congenitally infected children with carefully matched controls will be necessary before the long-term significance of intra-uterine infection with CMV can be accurately assessed.

Diagnosis. The lack of an obvious clinical illness in most cases of primary CMV infection means that a rising antibody titre is unlikely to be detected during pregnancy unless a prospective survey is being made. Specific IgM antibody is normally present for 6 to 12 weeks after primary infection, and may be more useful. Tobin (1973) does not believe that routine cervical culture to identify maternal virus excretors is a helpful measure.

Newborn screening which is based only on raised cord blood IgM levels (>20 mg per cent), will miss a significant proportion of CMV urine excretors; and children severely damaged at birth with raised levels at birth may be seronegative after a few years. Viral excretion in the urine may persist for many months, and is probably the most useful means of diagnosing congenital infection, along with detection of CMV-specific IgM antibody. Infected cells with a greatly increased diameter (which gives the virus its name) may be found in freshly passed urine.

Hepatitis B

At present it is considered there are two types of viral hepatitis—infective (virus A) and serum (virus B)—the former with a short, the latter with a long incubation period. It has not proved possible so far to isolate the causative viruses, but the discovery of the hepatitis B surface antigen (HB_sAg), also variously known as the Australia or hepatitis-associated antigen, present in the blood late in the incubation period and in the acute phase of serum hepatitis, makes a valuable marker for the latter. It has allowed study of maternal–fetal transmission, for in addition a number of apparently healthy people are carriers. All blood donors and many pregnant women in this country are screened for its presence. It can be found in about 0.1 per cent of the population, though the incidence is higher, sometimes considerably, in certain racial groups.

Risk to the fetus. Two relatively large surveys (Skinhøj et al, 1972; Desmyter, Liu and Van den Berghe, 1973) have shown risk to the baby to be minimal, and no cord blood positive for HB_s Ag was found among a total of 723 tested from infants born to healthy carrier mothers in these two series. The infants can theoretically become infected at birth by swallowing maternal blood during the birth process, and some have become HB_sAg carriers later in the first year. Hepatitis B surface antigen-positive cord blood has, however, been reported (see Desmyter, Liu and Van den Berghe, 1973) from infants whose mothers had hepatitis at the end of pregnancy. Reviewing such cases, Skinhøj et al (1972) report that two out of eight such infants themselves developed hepatitis.

Diagnosis. More sensitive tests for detection of the antigen are continually being developed, and one or other of two commercial haemagglutination tests (Hepanosticon reagent, Organon Scientific Development Group; HAA test, Wellcome Reagents Ltd) have been recently recommended as suitable for routine screening, with the more expensive and laborious radioimmunoassay being kept for confirmatory testing (Vandervelde et al, 1974). These three tests are all much more sensitive than electrophoresis. Contamination of cord blood with maternal blood probably occurs on occasions for HB_s Ag detected in cord blood by the sensitive radioimmunoassay test has not always been confirmed in specimens drawn directly from the infant. Thus positive cord blood tests should always be confirmed in this way later. This is especially important if specific antibody is to be given to infants negative at irth in an effort to protect them from developing chronic antigenaemia (Kohler et al, 1974). rials of such immune globulin treatment are at present in progress in this country.

Management of HB$_s$Ag positive pregnancy. It has become customary in some hospitals to ake careful precautions against transmission of the antigen from pregnant women to ospital staff. The major risk appears to be from blood contamination, though theoretically rine, faeces and amniotic fluid are also possible sources. Particular precautions have to be aken with vaginal bleeding at any time throughout pregnancy, with venepuncture and with lisposal of excreta. The patients are usually admitted and delivered in areas designated solely or them. Experience suggests that breast feeding is not contraindicated, though it seems like-y that antigen may be present in breast milk.

Herpesvirus hominis (HVH)

Maternal involvement. These infections in man are due to two antigenic types, 1 and 2. Type isolates are those responsible for genital tract infections in 95 per cent of cases, whereas nost strains from non-genital sites such as mouth, eyes and central nervous system are type . The socioeconomic state of the population is an important influence on incidence, as with CMV infection, and antibodies at relatively young ages are found most commonly among he less privileged. The incidence of type 2 antibodies is greatest among the sexually promiscuous, for the virus is believed to be venereally transmitted. Primary and recurrent herpetic disease can involve the external genitalia in males and females, but in the latter the cervix and vagina may also be involved, the cervix usually being the principal site of infecion. Cervicitis and vaginitis frequently cause no symptoms (Kibrick, 1973). Female herpetic genital infection is found in about one per cent of pregnant women, the incidence being three imes that in the non-pregnant (Nahmias et al, 1971). Even this, however, may well be an unlerestimate, and the depressed cellular immunity of pregnancy again presumably accounts or this recurrence.

Risk to the fetus. Nahmias et al (1971), in a study of 283 women with genital herpes, found hat the abortion rate during the first 20 weeks in those with primary infection was five times ligher than in non-infected women and three times higher when all types of herpetic infecion—primary, recurrent and undetermined—were taken together. It should be noted that listological examination of the abortuses did not reveal evidence of viral invasion, but twohirds showed evidence of fetal death prior to abortion. Genital infections detected after 20 weeks of gestation were not associated with an increased rate of preterm birth compared with he uninfected group. When HVH was detected after 32 weeks, the fetus became infected in 0 per cent of cases, and the later in pregnancy the infection was found, the greater the risk to he infant. Primary infections were associated with a higher risk than recurrent infections, perhaps because of longer persistence of the virus. Genital infection at term appeared to offer he greatest risk, with at least 40 per cent of fetuses involved. However, as in so many other naternal infections, not all infected fetuses are damaged, and the overall risk of a dead or affected infant appears to be 20 per cent when maternal infection occurs at term. There are, o far, few large surveys of this problem, and as more figures are collected it may well be the isk will eventually prove lower still. We do not yet know with accuracy the long-term prognosis particularly where neurological handicap is concerned, for the brain along with iver and adrenals is frequently involved. Skin vesicles are another feature of congenital infecion and may become recurrent, and with the other lesions, may not develop until after birth. Although the common mode of infection is thought to be ascending, transplacental infection has been reported in the first trimester, leading to central nervous system damage such as microphthalmia, microcephaly and choroidoretinitis (Nahmias, Alford and Korones, 1970).

When Kibrick (1973) reviewed the evidence for and against abdominal as opposed to vaginal delivery, he concluded that results presented so far did not suggest that caesarean section prevented fetal infection. If, as has been suggested, maternal genital herpetic infection at term is associated with sufficiently prolonged viraemia, fetal infection could in some cases be transplacental even late in pregnancy, in which case abdominal delivery would have no role in prevention. Infection during passage through the birth canal however is probably much more common, and Amstey and Monif (1974) reviewing data on 43 mothers with virologically proved HVH infections believe that elective caesarean section before or less than four hours after ruptured membranes significantly reduces the likelihood of neonatal infection.

Males diagnosed as having active genital herpes should be warned of the risk to the fetus if intercourse occurs during pregnancy, particularly in the latter part of it.

Diagnosis. Detection of a four-fold rise in neutralising antibody titre in maternal serum, in paired specimens, would be considered significant of recent infection, as would the finding of HVH-specific IgM antibody. Characteristic cellular changes can be seen in Papanicolaou-stained cervicovaginal smears in a high proportion of virologically proven cases of genital HVH infection (Ng, Reagan and Yen, 1970). *Herpesvirus hominis* can be isolated from the maternal urine and cervix, and from skin lesions, throat swabs and urine in the infant. Immunofluorescent techniques have been used for rapid identifications of HVH in the infant's nasopharynx, but are not generally available.

Rubella

Maternal involvement. Gregg (1941) first drew attention to the association between fetal defect and maternal pregnancy rubella. The isolation of the virus in 1962, and the widespread epidemic of 1964, have made further advances in knowledge possible. It is a disease of low communicability, and approximately 20 per cent of women reach reproductive age having escaped it in childhood (Public Health Laboratory Service, 1967). When infection occurs in adult life it is more frequently subclinical, and may go undiagnosed without special serological tests. Substantial immunity exists after naturally occurring primary rubella infection, and reinfection, though reported, is rare. It is nearly always subclinical, and often diagnosed only by a boost in IgG antibody titre.

Risk to the fetus. Dudgeon (1972) has estimated that in non-epidemic years (and presumably in the prevaccination era) 200 children with congenital rubella would be born in the United Kingdom yearly. From a survey of the world literature he deduced that, following first trimester rubella, the overall risk of fetal damage resulting from spontaneous abortion, stillbirth, death in infancy, as well as major and minor defects, was between 30 and 40 per cent. Congenital malformations occurred in 20 per cent of infants, but between 0 to 4 weeks the risk was 33 per cent, between 5 to 8 weeks 25 per cent, between 9 and 12 weeks 9.0 per cent, between 13 and 16 weeks 4.0 per cent and between 17 and 30 weeks 1.0 per cent (Dudgeon, 1970). Rubella virus was isolated from 90 per cent of abortuses from pregnancies in which first trimester clinical maternal rubella had been proved or supported by laboratory investigation (Thompson and Tobin, 1970). Deafness may not be present (and not just undiagnosed) until towards the end of the first year or even later; diabetes mellitus has now been reported as an even later complication in a few patients, and learning difficulties may also be evident when schooling starts. Reinfection following natural infection and occurring in pregnancy has been considered unlikely to harm the fetus so long as viraemia and the development of rubella-specific IgM antibody do not occur (Boué, Nicholas and Montagnon, 1971; *Lancet*, 1973a); the extent to which they do occur in reinfection, if at all, is uncertain as yet (Banatvala and Best, 1973; Haukenes, Haram and Solberg, 1973; *Lancet*, 1973a).

Diagnosis. Theoretically the diagnosis of rubella could be established in a number of ways, but in practice, particularly when the patient is a pregnant woman, speed and reliability and reproducibility of results are essential. The HI antibody test is the most important, CF antibody and rubella-specific IgM determination sometimes being necessary in addition. Banatvala (1972) outlines clear rules, given below, for investigation during pregnancy, and stresses that close cooperation between patient, clinician and virologist is necessary for accurate interpretation of serological results. Clinical details should be as precise as possible.

Exposure to rubella. 1. Blood should be withdrawn for testing of serum HI antibodies to rubella as soon as possible after exposure. If antibodies are present in high titre well within the incubation period, the patient can be considered protected by previously acquired infection.

2. If the antibody titre is low, probably particularly important when contact is within the family, a second sample should be taken seven to ten days later, and if time allows also 21 to 25 days after first exposure, and HI and CF tests performed to ensure that there has been no rise in antibody titre. A significant rise in titre (say four-fold) confirms recent infection. Allowance should be made if the patient has been given gammaglobulin which may prolong the incubation period.

3. If the patient first presents at a stage when termination of pregnancy, if it is to be done at all, must be done immediately (say approaching 18 to 20 weeks gestation), determination of rubella-specific IgM antibody may be the most helpful, for if present it suggests recent infection (though see below).

Development of rubella-like illness. Confirmation of true rubella is most often required urgently. Blood should be taken as soon as possible after symptoms develop, and if time permits four to five days later. The serum samples should be tested in parallel for a rise in HI antibody titre. If the situation is as in (3) above, the sample should be tested for rubella-specific IgM antibody.

Interpretation of results. Banatvala (1972) has stressed that considerable care in conducting tests and interpreting their results is essential, and that the titres obtained by one laboratory may not be applicable to another. However in most laboratories antibody titres of the order $\leqslant$ 1:64 (HI) and $\leqslant$ 1:8 (CF) would be unlikely to be due to recent infection. Low levels of HI antibody may be due to the presence of nonspecific inhibitors which have not been removed by pretreatment of the serum, hence the necessity wherever possible for a second or even third sample to detect the significant rise (Banatvala, 1972). Rubella-specific IgM has not always been detected in the first week of illness. Conversely, while it has sometimes disappeared as soon as three to four weeks after the onset of the rash, it is now realised it can persist for a year or more after the acute illness (Pattison, Dane and Mace, 1975). Thus the finding of rubella-specific IgM cannot guarantee rubella virus infection in the current pregnancy as was at first thought, re-emphasising the need always to consider laboratory results in the light of history and clinical findings.

Rubella vaccination and the fetus. Trials of four different live attenuated rubella virus vaccines are in progress in several centres, and preliminary results are appearing. It is as yet uncertain whether the immunity conferred by a single dose of vaccine will be life-long, as in the natural infection. Locally produced rubella-specific IgA in the nasopharynx, which may be important in preventing viral multiplication at sites of entry, appears to be less efficient and long-lasting with at least three of four vaccines when compared with the natural infection (Al-Nakib, Best and Banatvala, 1975). The United Kingdom policy, started in 1970, of vaccinating 12 to 14-year-old girls will, it is hoped, safeguard women during their reproductive years. Booster doses may eventually be shown to be necessary. Immediate postpartum vaccination of seronegative women is also practised but cannot protect the firstborn who constitute 40 per cent of births (*British Medical Journal*, 1972). In such cases it may be important to check the seroconversion rate if large blood transfusions or anti-D-immunoglobulin have also had to be given, to ensure they have not influenced the serological response.

Reinfection may be more common in those with vaccine acquired rather than natural immunity. Rubella virus has been recovered from the placenta, decidua and various organs of therapeutically aborted conceptuses of seronegative women who had been vaccinated (*Lancet*, 1973b). Thus vaccination must be avoided during pregnancy, and similarly pregnancy avoided, probably for several months, after vaccination. An injectable 'depot' progestogen, given for contraceptive purposes at the same time as the vaccine in postpartum cases, is said to have proved effective in this respect (Sharp and MacDonald, 1973).

Use of gammaglobulin. Trials of passive protection of the mother and fetus against rubella with 700 to 1500 mg of immunoglobulin (Public Health Laboratory Service, 1970) did not suggest that the incidence of rubella was affected. Peckham (1974) was later able to examine the children of those women involved in this trial who subsequently showed serological evidence of the infection despite immunoglobulin prophylaxis. She found the incidence of congenital defects to be lower when the mother had subclinical rubella as opposed to clinical rubella. Although it was not possible to rule out reinfection in the subclinical cases, she nevertheless felt that immunoglobulin could be of limited usefulness, particularly in those who do not wish pregnancy terminated, since it may suppress the clinical manifestations of the disease. Although some controversy still surrounds its use, Dudgeon (1974) advocates the giving of 1500 mg of immunoglobulin as soon as possible after contact, and after a blood sample has been taken. If the latter does not show HI antibodies, a further similar dose is given three to four days later (about six days after contact) and presumptively just before the viraemic phase. As it may be possible for the incubation period to be prolonged a few days by immunoglobulin, a second sample is tested between 21 and 28 days later for seroconversion.

PROTOZOA

Toxoplasma gondii

Toxoplasma gondii, found in many parts of the world, and infecting a large number of warm-blooded animals including man, is the protozoan parasite responsible for toxoplasmosis. It exists in three forms—trophozoite, tissue cyst (containing many trophozoites) and oocyst. The mode of human infection, and the life cycle of the parasite—now known to involve the domestic cat—have been recently reviewed by Beverley (1973).

Maternal involvement. Congenital toxoplasmosis may occur if a woman acquires her primary infection in pregnancy, with temporary parasitaemia leading to placental involvement. Her infection is most likely to be subclinical, though occasionally it may present as an infectious mononucleosis-like illness. Parasitaemia has been demonstrated as long as 14 months after the onset of illness (Miller, Aronson and Remington, 1969). The risk of contracting the illness in this country is probably not high. In a recent British survey (Ruoss and Bourne, 1972), 3187 mothers were tested at the first antenatal visit, and again at the 20th and 30th week, and finally at delivery. Seven contracted toxoplasmosis during pregnancy, a further two developing it either shortly before or during early pregnancy. In an American series (Kimball, Kean and Fuchs, 1971) serological tests were made at the first antenatal visit and at delivery in 4048 women; 2765 were initially negative, of whom 6 converted to positive; 1283 had positive first tests, 17 showing a substantial rise in titre. On the other hand, in a recent French series, the rate of pregnancy infections was 6.3 per cent (Desmonts and Couvreur, 1974). The national penchant for eating undercooked meat is generally held to blame for this high risk in France. Equally, however, as Fleck (1973) has pointed out, the reputation of Britons 'for close and sentimental contact with cats' might have been expected to lead to a similar state of affairs here, but it has not! Nevertheless, until more is known about modes of spread, he believes pregnant women would be well advised to leave the mopping up of kitten faeces to others, and of course to avoid eating raw meat.

Risk to the fetus. The role *Toxoplasma gondii* plays in abortion has been much debated, and the large literature has been ably and critically reviewed by Remington (1973). His own studies in California where the prevalence of infection in the childbearing age group is low (30 per cent), and in El Salvador, Central America, where it is more than twice as high, led him to the following conclusions: the parasite can definitely cause abortion in chronically infected women (California study); it is not a significant cause of perinatal mortality in Central America; and serological surveys are inadequate to answer the question of whether or not *Toxoplasma* can be transmitted from a chronically infected woman to her fetus, for the parasite has been reported to have been isolated from an abortus and placenta in a woman with a negative dye test.

Fleck (1973) has estimated the incidence of congenital toxoplasmosis in England and Wales as 1 : 20 000 births. In France it is about 1 : 2000 births. In the prospective British survey already cited (Ruoss and Bourne, 1972), eight out of ten infants born to mothers with a primary pregnancy infection were followed for two years, and showed no evidence of infection; one was stillborn and one died in the neonatal period, but there was no definite evidence that *Toxoplasma* played a contributory role in either of these deaths. In the prospective American survey, only three of the 19 women involved transmitted the infection to their fetuses, and only one of the three showed any abnormality (Kimball, Kean and Fuchs, 1971). Desmonts and Couvreur (1974) reported 11 abortions and seven stillbirths or neonatal deaths from the 183 mothers who acquired toxoplasmosis in pregnancy; and the disease occurred in 59 of the non-aborted offspring. Among the latter, two died and seven had severe disease. Of the remaining 50, 11 had mild and 39 had subclinical illness, but severe disease was noted only when the maternal infection was acquired in the first or second trimesters. Third trimester infection appeared to give subclinical or no fetal involvement. A suggestion that intellectual deficits might occur following subclinical congenital toxoplasmosis has appeared (Saxon et al, 1973) but the number of children involved was small, and the observation will require confirmation. The offspring of successive and closely spaced pregnancies have, rarely, been reported involved (Langer, 1963; Garcia, 1968).

Treatment with spiramycin during pregnancy reduced the overall frequency of the fetal infections, but not of obvious disease (Desmonts and Couvreur, 1974). To identify the converters would entail testing pregnant women at three, six and nine months of pregnancy, and the low British incidence would seem to make this unjustifiable at present. Since the degree of fetal involvement is likely to be greatest the earlier in pregnancy infection occurs (see Table 18.3 for maximal involvement), there could be grounds for termination with serological conversion in the first trimester, but a numerical risk cannot be given. Choroidoretinitis and occasionally intracranial calcification may not develop for many months after birth in congenital infection.

Diagnosis

Serological. The diagnosis of primary toxoplasmosis is established by the demonstration of rising antibody titres. All too often a stable high titre, which may persist for several years after infection, may have been reached when the patient is first tested, and a conclusive diagnosis may not be possible (Remington, 1973). The most commonly used tests are the Sabin–Feldman dye test, the CF test, the HI test, and the toxoplasma-specific IgM fluorescent antibody test. If dye test or IgM fluorescent antibody titres are already high when first seen (>1:512), a negative CF test turning positive, or increasing CF titres, together with stable high dye test titres are indicative of active infection. The indirect fluorescent antibody test has occasionally given false positive results with some sera containing antinuclear antibodies. Thus, in patients with disorders such as lupus erythematosus, a dye test or HI test should be performed to confirm a positive indirect fluorescent antibody test (Remington, 1973).

In the newborn, the toxoplasma-specific IgM fluorescent antibody test will be positive in those infected but asymptomatic, as well as in those who have signs of disease. Remington (1973) demonstrated that several infants with false positive tests showed no serological evidence of congenital toxoplasmosis in later life. It must also be remembered that a majority of infants in whom congenital infection is later proved have *no* antibodies demonstrated by the IgM fluorescent antibody test at birth, so that their absence then, or even during the first months of life, does not rule out congenital infection, and suspect infants should be carefully followed clinically and serologically.

Histological. Trophozoites and tissue cysts can be demonstrated in tissues and body fluids such as CSF. If placental evidence is sought, the organ should be fresh and not formalin-fixed. Parasites were isolated from the placenta in 25 per cent of the French series (Desmonts and Couvreur, 1974).

BACTERIA

Bacteria can theoretically reach the fetus by several routes—transplacental, ascending from cervix and vagina, from the peritoneal cavity via the fallopian tubes, or from an infected uterine wall. In practice, the first two are presumed to be the most frequent, with the ascending route well in the lead. It seems unlikely that 'intact' membranes create a perfect safeguard for the fetus, for their biopsy near the os at term has not infrequently shown degeneration and necrosis (Bourne, 1962). There are conflicting views too about the ability of amniotic fluid to inhibit bacterial growth. In the presence of meconium it becomes a good culture medium (Galask and Snyder, 1968); and bacteria have been cultured from it following amniocentesis in 9.5 per cent of a very small series of women with intact memranes in early labour (Prevedourakis et al, 1972). It seems reasonable to assume that the majority of acute, symptomatic bacterial infections in pregnant women are now likely to be treated promptly with antimicrobial therapy, and that the risk of transplacental infection would be small. As with viral infection, however, factors governing transfer of bacterial infection to the fetus are imperfectly understood, and this assumption may not be valid. Chronic asymptomatic infection of the genitourinary tract nevertheless would appear to pose the greatest risk to the fetus, who is most likely to be infected by the ascending route in such cases.

Risk to fetus in systemic and genital tract infections

It is quite impossible to give a quantitative risk, particularly of transplacental infection. Ascending infection is frequently associated with chorioamnionitis. In unselected consecutive pregnancies, this is present in 11 per cent of cases, an incidence higher than that of all perinatal morbidity and mortality; this incidence increases further with an increasing interval between membrane rupture and delivery, and with decreasing birthweight (Benirschke and Driscoll, 1967). These authors have found evidence of chorioamnionitis in 50 per cent of pregnancies resulting in the birthweight of an infant less than 1000 g.

Three other related comprehensive studies of stillbirths and early neonatal deaths have shown that about one-third are associated with an infected intra-uterine environment, as judged by the presence of chorio-amnionitis. This proportion is substantially increased with low socioeconomic status, and a maternal history of previous unsuccessful pregnancies. Congenital pneumonia was the most frequent diagnosis among infected infants. Adrenal glands were found to be 19 per cent heavier in the infected than in the non-infected, and it was suggested that their 'hyperfunction' might have played a role in initiating premature labour (Naeye and Blanc, 1970, 1973; Naeye, Dellinger and Blanc, 1971).

There has been much recent emphasis in the American literature of the role of maternally derived beta-haemolytic streptococci (Lancefield Group B) in causing serious, often devastating, neonatal infection. This organism was isolated from the vagina of 5.3 per cent of 780 unselected pregnant women attending a London hospital's antenatal clinic for the first time (De Louvois et al, 1975). A very similar incidence is reported from the United States, though Baker and Barrett (1973) using a selective broth medium, were able to show an isolation rate of 25.4 per cent from women admitted in labour, and pointed out that 58.9 per cent of the isolates would have been missed if the selective medium had not been used, because of the overgrowth of gram-negative organisms. Thus they were able to show that the incidence of Group B streptococcal colonisation among mothers was 254 per 1000, among infants 262 per 1000, with an attack rate for proved neonatal infection with that organism of 2.9 per 1000. Neonatal mortality has been high—70 per cent or more—in many of the reported series. It is possible that infants who develop serious Group B streptococcal illness are born to mothers deficient in antibody, and thus have not received any protective transplacental transfer themselves (Klesius et al, 1973; Baker and Kasper, 1976).

As the beta-haemolytic streptococcus has reputedly been responsible for 25 per cent of neonatal infection in some centres, there has naturally been much discussion about the desirability of identifying and treating maternal carriers in the hope of eradicating the organism before delivery. Even if the numbers cited above are not generally applicable, this would be a very large task. The organism may be found in the male urethra and reinfection could presumably easily occur. There is also no guarantee as yet that treatment would eradicate the streptococcus, and even less desirable gram-negative organisms might flourish immoderately as a consequence of penicillin therapy. The tendency to 'planned delivery' and thus surgical induction does mean that organisms could be introduced into the amniotic sac of more women than previously. At present, at least in this country, although serious neonatal streptococcal infections occur, it does not seem justifiable to single out one organism in this way when many other similarly maternally transmitted perinatal infections occur. An appreciation of the need for the strictest aseptic precautions on the part of obstetricians, and a much greater awareness among paediatricians of the possibility of early neonatal infection are of paramount importance.

We have only an imperfect idea of the extent of permanent damage from intra-uterine bacterial infection in children who survive. Isolated reports suggest the need for prospective investigation. For instance Dungal (1961), reporting a case of congenital listeriosis, wondered whether three previous children in the family who were considered to have congenital cerebral malformation could all be victims of listeriosis of the central nervous system. After treatment with oxytetracycline in the fifth pregnancy, the mother was delivered of her first normal healthy child. Lang (1955) investigated a group of mentally retarded children; antilisteria titres were significantly higher in those children in whom the cause of retardation was uncertain compared with those in whom it was known. Although perinatal listeriosis has always been rare in this country, it is conceivable that other bacteria of the birth canal could cause similar defects. Certainly the prognosis for intact survival following serious bacterial infection acquired during pregnancy, labour and delivery has not been good, at least until relatively recently (see review by Davies, 1971).

Risk to fetus in pregnancy bacteriuria

Kass and Zinner (1973) state that bacteriuria occurs in the female at the rate of about one per cent for each decade of life from at least age five years onwards. It is present rather more commonly in pregnancy though and, depending on age, parity and social class, may be found in three to eight per cent of the population. Kass (1962) reported that an excess of low birthweight infants were born to bacteriuric women, and showed that this could be corrected if sterilisation of the urine was achieved with antimicrobial therapy. This has remained a controversial topic, for certain authors reproduced Kass's findings while others did not.

The reasons for these apparent contradictions may be multiple. First, strict criteria for the collection of urine specimens and diagnosis of bacteriuria laid down by Kass have not always been adhered to. He states that the labia should be spread, the introitus washed with green soap solution from before backwards four times, and the urine voided into a sterile receptacle. If not cultured immediately it should be refrigerated at 4 to 6°C until this is possible. Specimens yielding more than 10^5 colonies/ml are considered bacteriuric. Second, the terms prematurity and low birthweight may have been variously defined. 2500 g is usually taken as the dividing line between infants of low and normal weight. This weight has been used synonymously with prematurity in several of the studies, and small-for-dates infants (birthweight below the 10th percentile for gestational age) have not always been identified separately from those of preterm (<37 weeks) gestation. Since one sample may vary in the number of small-for-dates and preterm infants in a low birthweight group, mortality rates may vary. In addition there is an association between low social class and an increased incidence of bacteriuria, and between low social class and increased perinatal mortality. Thus these interlocking variables mean, as Kass and Zinner (1973) have pointed out, that very large numbers are needed in any trial of antibacterial therapy for pregnancy bacteriuria before clearcut results can be obtained.

Treponema pallidum

A pregnant woman with primary and secondary syphilis is likely to transmit the infection to her fetus at any stage in the pregnancy. Plasma cell infiltration in response to spirochaetal entry will not occur until a certain stage of immune competence is reached, and the recognised lesions of congenital syphilis are the result of this inflammation (Benirschke, 1974). Prompt treatment of the mother should effect a cure in the majority of infants.

Diagnostic tests. The scope of serological tests now available has recently been reviewed by Wilkinson (1972) and his recommendations are given below. The tests measure the presence of antibodies and are of two main kinds.

Antitreponemal antibody (reagin, the antibody is both IgG and IgM, the latter predominating in early infection) is regularly produced by syphilitic infection, but also by some other diseases, and may be measured by the Wasserman reaction, the Venereal Disease Research Laboratory (VDRL) slide test, the rapid plasma reagin (RPR) test, or the automated reagin test (ART). Biological false positives have been found in autoimmune diseases such as disseminated lupus erythematosus, thyroiditis and acquired haemolytic anaemia; following enterovirus infection; following vaccination; and in drug addicts.

Antitreponemal antibody tests can be further subdivided into (1) group and (2) specific tests.

1. *Treponema pallidum* has antigen in common with various commensals, particularly those in the mouth. The Reiter protein complement fixation test (RPCFT) detects *group antitreponemal antibody,* which appears about the same time as reagin.
2. These include the treponemal immobilisation (TPI) test, the absorbed fluorescent treponemal antibody (FTA–ABS) test (mainly IgG, also IgM and IgA), and the treponemal haemagglutination (TPHA) test. False positives with the FTA–ABS test have been reported.

Use and interpretation. The reagin tests have a high sensitivity in untreated, early latent, and in most cases of late syphilis. False positives occur in less than one per cent and are usually quite different from those (also less than one per cent) which occur for instance in RPCFT. The RPR and ART are particularly useful when sera are being examined in bulk. Reagin tests are essentially screening procedures and positive results require confirmation with antitreponemal antibody tests such as FTA–ABS. If this is negative a TPI should be done though discrepancies between them are rare. False positive reactions due to abnormal macroglobulins or antinuclear factor have very occasionally been reported with the FTA–ABS test. Both the TPI and FTA–ABS tests may be positive for many years unless treatment is first given during the primary or secondary stage, and thus cannot be used to assess progress after treatment. Positive TPI and FTA–ABS tests are an indication of past or present syphilitic infection, but the VDRL, particularly if reactive at a dilution of 16 or above, and with a rising titre, may be a better guide to activity. There are no tests yet available which differentiate syphilis from yaws (Wilkinson, 1972). Negative tests early in pregnancy may give a false sense of security. Congenital syphilis has been reported following primary infection acquired after such tests (Al-Salihi, Curran and Shteir, 1971) and it has been suggested that in high risk cases, serology should be repeated at the beginning of the third trimester, and even at the time of admission for delivery. In certain communities this may be sound advice, but in general, laboratories could not be asked to do this as a routine.

Finally *Treponema pallidum* may be demonstrated in material from early lesions by using conventional dark ground microscopy, and by indirect or direct immunofluorescence. They are sometimes difficult to find in the placenta, examination of which is now often neglected. However, focal villitis, endovascular and perivascular proliferation in villous vessels, and relative immaturity of villi may be found (Russell and Altshuler, 1974).

Neisseria gonorrhoeae

The risk of neonatal ophthalmia caused by the organism is well known. There are occasional case reports of systemic gonococcal infection in the infant following maternal infection.

Diagnosis. In the acute phase a positive smear from cervical and urethral discharge showing gram-negative intracellular diplococci, and a positive culture, are the most reliable. As the infection wanes, or in asymptomatic contacts, only cultures can be relied on, though false negatives will occur. Swabs of vaginal material alone yield a lower isolation rate, and it is essential to include urethral and cervical cultures for improved diagnosis. The sensitivity of cultures will be lessened by lubricant on speculum or surgical glove.

A direct fluorescent antibody test does not have any advantage over ordinary cultural methods, and gonococcal complement fixation tests have not been proved reliable.

OTHER INFECTING ORGANISMS

Mycoplasma

The mycoplasmas are neither bacteria, because they lack a rigid cell wall, nor viruses, because they contain both DNA and RNA.

Maternal involvement. Mycoplasma hominis and the T-mycoplasmas (so called because they form 'tiny' colonies) are to be found in the female genital tract, are sexually acquired, and like CMV and HVH are found more commonly in the less affluent sections of the community. They can be cultured more easily from the vagina and periurethral area than from the cervix (McCormack and Lee, 1973).

Risk to the fetus. There is controversy about their role in disease, because of difficulties in getting suitable controls for the sexually promiscuous and economically unfavoured (Chanock, 1965). There is however at least suggestive evidence that genital mycoplasmas in pregnancy are associated with spontaneous abortion, preterm birth, and low birthweight.

Mycoplasma hominis has been isolated from the blood stream in some cases of febrile abortion (Tully et al, 1965; Harwick et al, 1967, 1970). Significant levels of CF antibody in maternal sera in association with isolation of *Mycoplasma hominis* from the tissues of abortuses in two cases, and a rise in antibody titre of *Mycoplasma hominis* in paired sera in some patients in whom the vagina was colonised by the organism at the time of abortion have also been reported (Jones, 1967). *Mycoplasma hominis* has been recovered from the cervix three times more commonly in febrile abortion than in afebrile abortion and normal pregnancy (Harwick et al, 1970). In cell cultures, *Mycoplasma hominis* type 1 has been shown to increase abnormalities of chromosome structure (Allison and Paton, 1966) and these authors have suggested that the possible relationship of mycoplasmas to chromosomal aberrations in portuses should be studied further. The risk of stillbirth was significantly more common in women from whom *Mycoplasma hominis* was recovered on blood culture made within a few minutes of vaginal delivery (McCormack et al, 1975).

A highly significant association ($P = <0.003$) between isolation of T mycoplasmas, and a less significant association ($P = <0.05$) between isolation of *Mycoplasma hominis* from the cervix and/or urine at first antenatal visit and subsequent low birthweight of the infant has been reported (Braun et al, 1971). The genital mycoplasmas have been cultured from the nose and throats of newborns more commonly as birthweight decreases (Klein, Buckland and Finland, 1969). Apart from the obvious disadvantage of low birthweight and preterm birth, however, proved infection with mycoplasmas in the newborn has been rarely reported. *Mycoplasma hominis* was cultured from a supraclavicular abscess in a seven-day-old infant, and from her mother's vagina (Sacker, Walker and Brunell, 1970). The same organism has been isolated from some infants with neonatal ophthalmia (Jones and Tobin, 1968); whether it could be cultured from the conjunctival sac in the absence of eye infection however is not known.

Diagnostic tests. Serological evidence of *Mycoplasma* infections can be sought by CF and HI tests. The organisms need special culture media for their recovery.

PREVENTION OF INFECTION

Mothers are likely to continue transmitting infection to their fetuses for the forseeable future, although many diseases which killed or maimed their fetuses at the beginning of this century have now been successfully controlled. The risks both for a few viral and bacterial illnesses seem likely to be greatest in the poorest communities, and for instance where CMV is concerned, with its possibility of later intellectual deficit in the child, a vicious cycle may exist. The remedies are complex, and are social as much as medical. It is still too early to assess the results of rubella vaccination reliably, though a preliminary report from the United States suggests that it has been successful in reducing the morbidity of the congenital infection (Modlin et al, 1975). Nevertheless, the vagaries of case reporting would suggest that any such interpretation should be extremely cautious. The development of a vaccine for CMV is being debated, and a live tissue-culture-adapted strain of the virus has been tested in volunteers (Elek and Stern, 1974). Such strains may not be eliminated in the way that poliovirus, rubella and rubeola viruses are, raising problems of oncogenicity and attenuation.

Overseas travel is now common, and obstetricians may be faced with decisions regarding protection of their patients with vaccine and the safety of such protection for the fetus. Killed vaccines are probably not important, though live vaccines may pose a hazard. In a recent review of the available evidence it has been concluded that immunisation against poliomyelitis and yellow fever is indicated in women travelling to affected zones. As already stated, rubella vaccination is contraindicated in pregnancy, as are mumps and smallpox vaccination. If the patient cannot be dissuaded from travel to an endemic smallpox area, she should be vaccinated with specific immune globulin cover. Measles vaccination is not indicated (Levine, Edsall and Bruce-Chwatt, 1974). Malarial prophylaxis in the form of 50 mg pyrimethamine, given as a single dose once monthly to pregnant African women, has been considered safe and effective, and resulted in a greater fetal weight gain during pregnancy compared with untreated controls (Morley, Woodland and Cuthbertson, 1964).

CONCLUSIONS

It has to be reiterated that the true extent to which maternal infection is transmitted to the fetus is unknown. In addition, possible long-term effects, inapparent at birth, are only gradually being revealed. Rubella is probably one of the few infections for which a numerical risk to the fetus *at a given gestational age* can be hazarded, but even this varies in different parts of the world. The discrepancy between the very high rate of recovery of the virus from abortuses and the much lower incidence of clinically detected damage at birth and later underlines how little we still know of protective mechanisms. In general, the earlier in pregnancy an infection occurs the more serious may be the consequences for the fetus; infection with HVH, however, may be an exception, for serious damage, particularly to the central nervous system, can also occur when infection is acquired at birth.

Where bacterial infections are concerned, we have little factual knowledge. It is well known that many bacteria encountered by the fetus in sufficient numbers during passage through the birth canal can cause widespread and lethal disease. While the extent of spontaneous abortion is uncertain, it seems likely that infection with bacteria or *Mycoplasma* accompany such abortion in a proportion of cases. Damage in an infant when the pregnancy is retained in the face of bacterial infection may at present be underestimated.

Screening procedures undertaken in antenatal clinics come into two categories. First, they aim to detect illness in the mother, the persistence of which untreated would be detrimental to her, if not always to her fetus. Into this category come serological tests for syphilis, chest radiography for tuberculosis and urine culture for bacteriuria. In addition, early detection and treatment of local infection of the genital tract such as gonorrhoea, moniliasis and trichomoniasis will minimise any risk to the infant. Second, large prospective surveys aim to identify the incidence of one or more infections among a given population of pregnant women, and to establish the risk to the fetus. Although a formidable task, these surveys will be most productive of badly needed facts when accompanied by careful follow-up of the children involved.

REFERENCES

Allison, A. C. & Paton, G. R. (1966) Chromosomal abnormalities in human diploid cells infected with Mycoplasma and their possible relevance to the aetiology of Down's syndrome (mongolism). *Lancet,* **i**, 1229–1230.

Al-Nakib, W., Best, J. M. & Banatvala, J. E. (1975) Rubella-specific serum and nasopharyngeal immunoglobulin responses following naturally acquired and vaccine-induced infection. Prolonged persistence of virus-specific IgM. *Lancet,* **i**, 182–185.

Al-Salihi, F. L., Curran, J. P. & Shteir, O. A. (1971) Occurrence of fetal syphilis after a nonreactive early gestational serologic test. *Journal of Pediatrics,* **78**, 121–123.

Amstey, M. S. & Monif, G. R. G. (1974) Genital herpesvirus infection in pregnancy. *Obstetrics and Gynecology,* **44**, 394–397.

Baker, C. J. & Barrett, F. F. (1973) Transmission of Group B streptococci among parturient women and their neonates. *Journal of Pediatrics,* **83**, 919–925.

Baker, C. J. & Kasper, D. L. (1976) Correlation of maternal antibody deficiency with susceptibility to neonatal Group B streptococcal infection. *New England Journal of Medicine,* **294**, 753–756.

Banatvala, J. E. (1972) Maternal rubella and its virological diagnosis. *Postgraduate Medical Journal,* **4** (Supplement), 11–17.

Banatvala, J. E. & Best, J. M. (1973) Letter. Rubella reinfections. *Lancet,* **i**, 1452.

anatvala, J. E., Potter, J. E. & Best, J. M. (1971) Interferon response to Sendai and rubella virus in human foetal cultures, leucocytes and placental cultures. *Journal of General Virology*, **3**, 193–201.

aron, J., Youngblood, L., Siewers, C. M. F. & Medearis, D. N. (1969) The incidence of cytomegalovirus, herpes simplex, rubella, and toxoplasma antibodies in microcephalic, mentally retarded, and normocephalic children. *Pediatrics*, **44**, 932–939.

enirschke, K. (1974) Syphilis—the placenta and the fetus. *American Journal of Diseases of Children*, **128**, 142–143.

enirschke, K. & Driscoll, S. G. (1967) *The Pathology of the Human Placenta*. Berlin: Springer.

everley, J. K. A. (1973) Toxoplasmosis. *British Medical Journal*, **ii**, 475–478.

irnbaum, G., Lynch, J. I., Margileth, A. M., Lonergan, W. M. & Sever, J. L. (1969) Cytomegalovirus infections in newborn infants. *Journal of Pediatrics*, **75**, 789–795.

ithell, J. F., Draper, G. J. & Gorbach, P. D. (1973) Association between malignant disease in children and maternal virus infections. *British Medical Journal*, **i**, 706–708.

oué, A., Nicolas, A. & Montagnon, B. (1971) Reinfection with rubella in pregnant women. *Lancet*, **i**, 1251–1253.

ourne, G. L. (1962) *The Human Amnion and Chorion*. London: Lloyd-Luke.

raun, P., Lee, Y-H., Klein, J. O., Marcy, M., Klein, T. A., Charles, D., Levy, P. & Kass, E. H. (1971) Birth weight and genital mycoplasmas in pregnancy. *New England Journal of Medicine*, **284**, 167–171.

ritish Medical Journal (1972) Rubella vaccination. *British Medical Journal*, **iii**, 305–306.

rown, G. C. & Karunas, R. S. (1972) Relationship of congenital anomalies and maternal infection with selected enteroviruses. *American Journal of Epidemiology*, **95**, 207–217.

urch, G. E., Sun, S-C., Chu, K-C., Sohal, R. S. & Colcolough, H. L. (1968) Interstitial and Coxsackie virus B myocarditis in infants and children. A comparative histologic and immunofluorescent study of 50 autopsied hearts. *Journal of the American Medical Association*, **203**, 1–8.

hanock, R. M. (1965) Mycoplasma infections of man. *New England Journal of Medicine*, **273**, 1199–1206.

ollaborative Study (1970) Cytomegalovirus infection in the north west of England: A report on a two year study. *Archives of Disease in Childhood*, **45**, 513–522.

urnen, M. G. M., Varma, A. A. O., Christine, B. W. & Turgeon, L. R. (1974) Childhood leukemia and maternal infectious diseases during pregnancy. *Journal of the National Cancer Institute*, **53**, 943–947.

avies, P. A. (1971) Bacterial infection in the fetus and newborn. *Archives of Disease in Childhood*, **46**, 1–27.

avies, P. A., Robinson, R. J., Scopes, J. W., Tizard, J. P. M. & Wigglesworth, J. S. (1972) *Medical Care of Newborn Babies*. London: Heinemann.

e Louvois, J., Stanley, V. C., Leask, B. G. S. & Hurley, R. (1975) Ecological studies of the microbial flora of the female lower genital tract. *Proceedings of the Royal Society of Medicine*, **68**, 269–270.

epartment of Health and Social Security (1971) *On the State of the Public Health. Annual Report of the Chief Medical Officer, 1970*. London: HMSO.

esmonts, G. & Couvreur, J. (1974) Congenital toxoplasmosis. A prospective study of 378 pregnancies. *New England Journal of Medicine*, **290**, 1110–1116.

esmyter, J., Liu, W. T. & Van den Berghe, H. (1973) Viral hepatitis type B: studies of congenital transmission. In *Intrauterine Infections* (Ed.) Elliott, K. & Knight, J. (Ciba Foundation Symposium 10, New Series) London: Associated Scientific Publishers.

onovan, J., Adelstein, A. M. & Leighton, P. (1974) Sequelae of virus infections in pregnancy. *British Medical Journal*, **ii**, 5021.

udgeon, J. A. (1970) Recent advances in the study of rubella. *Scientific Basis of Medicine Annual Reviews*, pp. 61–88.

udgeon, J. A. (1972) Congenital rubella: A preventable disease. *Postgraduate Medical Journal*, Supplement **48**, 7–11.

udgeon, J. A. (1974) γ-globulin and congenital rubella. *British Medical Journal*, **ii**, 723–724.

ungal, N. (1961) Listeriosis in four siblings. *Lancet*, **ii**, 513–516.

lek, S. D. & Stern, H. (1974) Development of a vaccine against mental retardation caused by cytomegalovirus infection in utero. *Lancet*, **i**, 1–5.

mbil, J. A., Ozere, R. L. & Haldane, E. V. (1970) Congenital cytomegalovirus infection in two siblings from consecutive pregnancies. *Journal of Pediatrics*, **77**, 417–421.

edrick, J. & Alberman, E. D. (1972) Reported influenza in pregnancy and subsequent cancer in the child. *British Medical Journal*, **ii**, 485–488.

eldman, R. A. (1969) Cytomegalovirus infection during pregnancy. *American Journal of Diseases of Children*, **117**, 517–521.

leck, D. G. (1973) The problem of congenital toxoplasmosis. In *Intrauterine Infections* (Ed.) Elliott, K. & Knight, J. (Ciba Foundation Symposium 10, New Series). London: Associated Scientific Publishers.

rucht, H. L. & Metcalfe, J. (1954) Mortality and late results of infectious hepatitis in pregnant women. *New England Journal of Medicine*, **251**, 1094–1096.

Galask, R. P. & Snyder, I. S. (1968) Bacterial inhibition by amniotic fluid. *American Journal of Obstetrics and Gynecology*, **102**, 949–955.

Garcia, A. G. P. (1968) Congenital toxoplasmosis in two successive sibs. *Archives of Disease in Childhood*, **43**, 705–710.

Gotoff, S. P. (1974) Neonatal immunity. *Journal of Pediatrics*, **85**, 149–154.

Greenberg, M., Yankauer, A., Krugman, S., Osborn, J. J., Ward, R. S. & Dancis, J. (1949) The effect of smallpox vaccination during pregnancy on the incidence of congenital malformations. *Pediatrics*, **3**, 456–467.

Gregg, N. McA. (1941) Congenital cataract following German measles in the mother. *Transactions of the Ophthalmological Society of Australia*, **3**, 35–46.

Hagen, C. & Frøland, A. (1972) Depressed lymphocyte response to PHA in women taking oral contraceptives. *Lancet*, **i**, 1185.

Hakulinen, T., Hovi, L., Karkinen-Jääskeläinen, M., Penttinen, K. & Saxen, L. (1973) Association between influenza during pregnancy and childhood leukaemia. *British Medical Journal*, **iv**, 265–267.

Hanshaw, J. B. (1966) Congenital and acquired cytomegalovirus infection. *Pediatric Clinics of North America*, **13**, 279–293.

Hardy, J. B. (1965) Viral infection in pregnancy. A review. *American Journal of Obstetrics and Gynecology*, **93**, 1052–1056.

Harwick, H. J., Iuppa, J. B., Purcell, R. H. & Fekety, F. R. (1967) *Mycoplasma hominis* septicemia associated with abortion. *American Journal of Obstetrics and Gynecology*, **99**, 725–727.

Harwick, H. J., Purcell, R. H., Iuppa, J. B. & Fekety, F. R. (1970) *Mycoplasma hominis* and abortion. *Journal of Infectious Diseases*, **121**, 260–268.

Haukenes, G., Haram, K. & Solberg, C. O. (1973) Letter. Rubella reinfection and the fetus. *Lancet*, **i**, 1313.

Hayes, K., Danks, D. M., Gibas, H. & Jack, I. (1972) Cytomegalovirus in human milk. *New England Journal of Medicine*, **287**, 177–178.

Herbert, W. J. & Wilkinson, P. C. (1972) *A Dictionary of Immunology*. Oxford, London, Edinburgh, Melbourne: Blackwell Scientific Publications.

Jones, D. M. (1967) *Mycoplasma hominis* in abortion. *British Medical Journal*, **i**, 338–340.

Jones, D. M. & Tobin, B. (1968) Neonatal eye infections due to *Mycoplasma hominis*. *British Medical Journal*, **iii**, 467–468.

Kass, E. H. (1962) Pyelonephritis and bacteriuria. A major problem in preventive medicine. *Annals of Internal Medicine*, **56**, 46–53.

Kass, E. H. & Zinner, S. H. (1973) Bacteriuria and pyelonephritis in pregnancy. In *Obstetric and Perinatal Infections* (Ed.) Charles, D. & Finland, M. Ch. 21. Philadelphia: Lea & Febiger.

Kibrick, S. (1973) Herpes simplex. In *Obstetric and Perinatal Infections* (Ed.) Charles, D. & Finland, M. Ch. 4. Philadelphia: Lea & Febiger.

Kimball, A. C., Kean, B. H. & Fuchs, F. (1971) Congenital toxoplasmosis: a prospective study of 4048 obstetric patients. *American Journal of Obstetrics and Gynecology*, **111**, 211–218.

King-Lewis, P. A. & Gardner, S. D. (1969) Congenital cytomegalic inclusion disease following intrauterine transfusion. *British Medical Journal*, **ii**, 603–605.

Klein, J. O., Buckland, D. & Finland, M. (1969) Colonization of newborn infants by mycoplasmas. *New England Journal of Medicine*, **280**, 1025–1030.

Klesius, P. H., Zimmerman, R. A., Mathews, J. H. & Krushak, D. H. (1973) Cellular and humoral immune response to Group B streptococci. *Journal of Pediatrics*, **83**, 926–932.

Kohler, P. F., Dubois, R. S., Merrill, D. A. & Bowes, W. A. (1974) Prevention of chronic neonatal hepatitis B virus infection with antibody to the hepatitis B surface-antigen. *New England Journal of Medicine*, **291**, 1378–1380.

Kumar, M. L., Nankervis, G. A. & Gold, E. (1973) Inapparent congenital cytomegalovirus infection. A follow-up study. *New England Journal of Medicine*, **288**, 1370–1372.

Lancet (1973a) Rubella reinfection and the fetus, *Lancet*, **i**, 978.

Lancet (1973b) Rubella vaccination and pregnancy. *Lancet*, **ii**, 769–770.

Lang, K. (1955) Listeria-Infektion als mögliche Ursache früh erworbener Cerebralschaden. *Zeitschrift für Kinderheilkunde*, **76**, 328–339.

Langer, H. (1963) Repeated congenital infection with toxoplasma gondii. *Obstetrics and Gynecology*, **21**, 318–329.

Leck, I. & Steward, J. K. (1972) Incidence of neoplasms in children born after influenza epidemics. *British Medical Journal*, **iv**, 631–634.

Levine, M. M., Edsall, G. & Bruce-Chwatt, L. J. (1974) Live-virus vaccines in pregnancy. Risks and recommendations. *Lancet*, **ii**, 34–38.

Levinsohn, E. M., Foy, H. M., Kenny, G. E., Wentworth, B. B. & Grayston, J. T. (1969) Isolation of cytomegalovirus from a cohort of 100 infants throughout the first year of life. *Proceedings of the Society for Experimental Biology and Medicine*, **132**, 957–962.

audsley, R. F., Brix, G. A., Hinton, N. A., Robertson, E. M., Bryans, A. M. & Haust, M. D. (1966) Placental inflammation and infection. *American Journal of Obstetrics and Gynecology*, **95**, 648–659.

cCormack, W. M. & Lee, Y-H. (1973) Genital mycoplasmas. In *Obstetric and Perinatal Infections* (Ed.) Charles, D. & Finland, M. Ch. 5. Philadelphia: Lea & Febiger.

cCormack, W. M., Rosner, B., Lee, Y-H., Rankin, J. S. & Lin, J-S. (1975) Isolation of genital mycoplasmas from blood obtained shortly after vaginal delivery. *Lancet*, **i**, 596–599.

enser, M. A. & Reye, R. D. K. (1974) The pathology of congenital rubella: A review written by request. *Pathology*, **6**, 215–222.

iller, M. J., Aronson, W. J. & Remington, J. S. (1969) Late parasitemia in asymptomatic acquired toxoplasmosis. *Annals of Internal Medicine*, **71**, 139–145.

odlin, J. F., Brandling-Bennett, A. D., Witte, J. J., Campbell, C. C. & Meyers, J. D. (1975) A review of five years' experience with rubella vaccine in the United States. *Pediatrics*, **55**, 20–29.

onif, G. R. G., Egan, E. A., Held, B. & Eitzman, D. V. (1972) The correlation of maternal cytomegalovirus infection during varying stages in gestation with neonatal involvement. *Journal of Pediatrics*, **80**, 17–20.

ontgomery, R., Youngblood, L. & Medearis, D. N. (1972) Recovery of cytomegalovirus from the cervix in pregnancy. *Pediatrics*, **49**, 524–531.

orley, D., Woodland, M. & Cuthbertson, W. F. J. (1964) Controlled trial of pyrimethamine in pregnant women in an African village. *British Medical Journal*, **i**, 667–668.

aeye, R. L. & Blanc, W. A. (1970) Relation of poverty and race to antenatal infection. *New England Journal of Medicine*, **283**, 555–560.

aeye, R. L. & Blanc, W. A. (1973) Unfavourable outcome of pregnancy: repeated losses. *American Journal of Obstetrics and Gynecology*, **116**, 1133–1137.

aeye, R. L., Dellinger, W. S. & Blanc, W. A. (1971) Fetal and maternal features of antenatal bacterial infections. *Journal of Pediatrics*, **79**, 733–739.

ahmias, A. J., Alford, C. A. & Korones, S. B. (1970) Infection of the newborn with *Herpesvirus hominis*. *Advances in Pediatrics*, **17**, 185–226.

ahmias, A. J., Josey, W. E., Naib, Z. M., Freeman, M. G., Fernandez, R. J. & Wheeler, J. H. (1971) Perinatal risk associated with maternal genital Herpes simplex virus infection. *American Journal of Obstetrics and Gynecology*, **110**, 825–837.

g, A. B. P., Reagan, J. W. & Yen, S. S. C. (1970) Herpes genitalis. Clinical and cytopathologic experience with 256 patients. *Obstetrics and Gynecology*, **36**, 645–651.

oren, G. R., Adams, P. & Anderson, R. C. (1963) Positive skin reactivity to mumps virus antigen in endocardial fibroelastosis. *Journal of Pediatrics*, **62**, 604–606.

attison, J. R., Dane, D. S. & Mace, J. E. (1975) Persistence of specific IgM after natural infection with rubella virus. *Lancet*, **i**, 185–187.

eckham, C. S. (1974) Clinical and serological assessment of children exposed in utero to confirmed maternal rubella. *British Medical Journal*, **i**, 259–269.

otkin, S. A. (1975) Routes of fetal infection and mechanisms of fetal damage. *American Journal of Diseases of Children*, **129**, 444–449.

revedourakis, C. N., Strigou-Charalambis, E., Michalas, St. & Alvanouiakovakis, M. (1972) Intrauterine bacterial growth during labor. *American Journal of Obstetrics and Gynecology*, **113**, 33–36.

ublic Health Laboratory Service Rubella Working Party, Report to (1967) Incidence of rubella antibodies among pregnant women in six areas: prophylactic effect of two doses of gammaglobulin. *British Medical Journal*, **iii**, 638–640.

ublic Health Laboratory Service Working Party on Rubella, Report to (1970) Studies of the effect of immunoglobulin on rubella in pregnancy. *British Medical Journal*, **ii**, 497–500.

emington, J. S. (1973) Toxoplasmosis. In *Obstetrics and Perinatal Infections* (Ed.) Charles, D. & Finland, M. Ch. 3. Philadelphia: Lea & Febiger.

uoss, C. F. & Bourne, G. L. (1972) Toxoplasmosis in pregnancy. *Journal of Obstetrics and Gynaecology of the British Commonwealth*, **79**, 1115–1118.

ussell, P. & Altshuler, G. (1974) Placental abnormalities of congenital syphilis. A neglected aid to diagnosis. *American Journal of Diseases of Children*, **128**, 160–163.

acker, I., Walker, M. & Brunell, P. A. (1970) Abscess in a newborn infant caused by mycoplasma. *Pediatrics*, **46**, 303–304.

avage, M. O., Moosa, A. & Gordon, R. R. (1973) Maternal varicella infection as a cause of fetal malformations. *Lancet*, **i**, 352–354.

axon, S. A., Knight, W., Reynolds, D. W., Stagno, S. & Alfred, C. A. (1973) Intellectual deficits in children born with subclinical congenital toxoplasmosis: A preliminary report. *Journal of Pediatrics*, **82**, 792–797.

narp, D. S. & MacDonald, H. (1973) Use of medroxyprogesterone acetate as a contraceptive in conjunction with early postpartum rubella vaccination. *British Medical Journal*, **iv**, 443–446.

hrand, H. (1961) Thrush in the newborn. *British Medical Journal*, **ii**, 1530–1533.

Siegel, M. & Greenberg, M. (1956) Poliomyelitis in pregnancy: effect on fetus and newborn infant. *Journal Pediatrics,* **49,** 280–288.

Skinhøj, P., Olesen, H., Cohn, J. & Nikkelsen, M. (1972) Hepatitis-associated antigen in pregnant women. *Ac Pathologica et Microbiologica Scandinavica,* **80B,** 362–366.

St. Hill, C. A., Finn, R. & Denye, V. (1973) Depression of cellular immunity in pregnancy due to a serum fact *British Medical Journal,* **iii,** 513–514.

Stagno, S., Reynolds, D. W., Lakeman, A., Charamella, L. J. & Alford, C. A. (1973) Congenital cytomegalovir infection: consecutive occurrence due to viruses with similar antigenic compositions. *Pediatrics,* **52,** 788–79

Stern, H. & Tucker, S. M. (1973) Prospective study of cytomegalovirus infection in pregnancy. *British Medic Journal,* **ii,** 268–270.

Stern, H., Elek, S. D., Booth, J. C. & Fleck, D. G. (1969) Microbial causes of mental retardation. The role prenatal infections with cytomegalovirus, rubella virus, and toxoplasma. *Lancet,* **ii,** 443–448.

Stiehm, E. R. (1975) Fetal defense mechanisms. *American Journal of Diseases of Children,* **129,** 438–443.

Thompson, K. M. & Tobin, J. O'H. (1970) Isolation of rubella virus from abortion material. *British Medi Journal,* **ii,** 264–266.

Tobin, J. O'H. (1973) The virus laboratory in the diagnosis and prevention of congenital infection. In *Intrauteri Infections* (Ed.) Elliott, K. & Knight, J. (Ciba Foundation Symposium 10, New Series). London: Associa Scientific Publishers.

Tully, J. G., Brown, M. S., Sheagren, J. N., Young, V. M. & Wolff, S. M. (1965) Septicemia due to *Mycoplas hominis* Type 1. *New England Journal of Medicine,* **273,** 648–651.

Vandervelde, E. M., Mahmood, N., Goffin, C., Porter, A., Megson, B. & Cossart, Y. E. (1974) User's guide some new tests for hepatitis-B antigen. *Lancet,* **ii,** 1066–1071.

Weller, T. H. (1970) Cytomegaloviruses: the difficult years. *Journal of Infectious Diseases,* **122,** 532–539.

Wilkinson, A. E. (1972) Recent progress in venereal disease. Serology of syphilis. *British Medical Journal,* 573–575.

19

HORMONAL ASPECTS OF
FETO-PLACENTAL FUNCTION

M. G. R. Hull and T. Chard

Quantitative assessment of synthetic functions of the placenta provides an indirect means of assessing fetal health. The involvement of the fetus in many of these synthetic processes has given rise to the concept of the 'feto-placental unit', the products of which will provide a more accurate indication of fetal state than products of the placenta alone. These products which pass to the mother may be assayed in blood or urine in their original or metabolised form. The concentration of a substance in blood reflects the balance at a given moment between production and metabolism or excretion; the absolute amount in a timed urine collection reflects production rate, given normal renal excretion, though the substance as measured may be several steps removed from the original product.

Products of potential clinical value, as shown in Table 19.1, must be distinguishable from substances normally present in non-pregnant women because they occur either uniquely in pregnancy, as with proteins like cystine aminopeptidase (CAP) and human placental lactogen (hPL), or in much larger amounts, as with the steroids. Their measurement must meet certain criteria to be of clinical use. The values, or change in values, that occur with advancing gestation, must distinguish normal from abnormal conditions of the fetus. Any abnormal change in values must occur in time for therapeutic action to be taken. If the normal range is wide and early recognition of the abnormal depends on individual trends within this range, then a further requirement is that fluctuation of values in the individual must be within narrow limits.

Table 19.1. *Fetal and placental products used in assessing feto-placental function.*

Placental products independent of the fetus
    Progesterone
    Placental lactogen (hPL)
    Cystine aminopeptidase

Placental products partly from fetal precursors
    Oestrone   ⎫
    Oestradiol-17β ⎬   60% from fetal DHEAS
    Oestriol   90% from fetal DHEAS

Fetal products from placental precursors
    Oestetrol   ≥90% fetal, mainly from oestradiol-17β
    16α-OH-progesterone   ? 90% fetal, from progesterone

The placental hormones discussed in this chapter all originate in the trophoblast, which at term has a mass of about 60 g, representing about one-fifth of the placental parenchyma and being its largest nucleated component (Laga, Driscoll and Munro, 1974). Synthesis of hormones by the trophoblast depends on precursors reaching it from the maternal blood in the intervillous space and, in some cases, from fetal blood in the villous capillaries. Unlike other endocrine systems, placental hormones appear to have no feedback control and it seems likely that their synthesis is governed simply by the rate at which products are removed and nutrients supplied—in other words, primarily on materno-placental blood flow—and thus ultimately on the nutritional state of the mother. In addition, the synthetic capacity of the trophoblast depends on its total mass, which may be increased in maternal diabetes or rhesus isoimmunisation, or reduced by genetic factors or damage due to infection.

The fetal share in the synthesis of many steroids is variable, as shown in Table 19.1: the greater the share, as in the case of oestriol, the more closely would that steroid be expected to reflect fetal state. However, production of steroids does not appear to be influenced by the fetus through any endocrine-mediated control.

In order to interpret measurements of feto-placental hormones it is essential to understand the pathophysiology of the wide variety of disorders that can impair feto-placental function (Table 19.2). Many maternal disorders reduce nutrition of the fetus and placenta and so reduce hormone production; a similar constraint to production may be applied by disorders of the fetus itself. However, in maternal diabetes and rhesus isoimmunisation, hyperplasia of the trophoblast elevates hormone production regardless of the condition of the fetus; the latter is not subject to nutritional impairment unless some other complication is present. In rhesus isoimmunisation, hPL production is abnormally increased in proportion to the severity of the disease. Though the steroids remain within the normal range, those derived from the placenta alone are elevated relative to others derived from the fetus (see section on steroids below). In uncomplicated diabetes feto-placental hormones generally remain within the normal range and the disorder can be managed only on the basis of metabolic control in the mother (Gillmer and Beard, 1975).

Feto-placental function in multiple pregnancy must be judged by standards appropriate to the increased mass of the feto-placental unit. A serious problem in interpretation is that occasionally one twin may grow at the expense of the other; the effect on the deprived fetus would be poorly reflected by the combined hormone production.

Endocrine factors dependent on the fetus and/or the placenta may play a part in the initiation of premature labour (Klopper and Gardner, 1973). In those cases in which abnormal en

Table 19.2. *Causes of feto-placental impairment.*

Maternal

    Factors that impair nutrition of the fetus and placenta

        Maternal undernutrition
        Utero-placental vascular insufficiency
            Hypertensive disorders
            Prolonged pregnancy
            Infections (placental)
        Maternal hypoxia
            Cardiorespiratory diseases
            High altitude
        Tobacco smoking

        Diabetes mellitus
        Rhesus isoimmunisation

Fetal

        Malformations and genetic disorders
        Infections (transplacental)
        Multiple pregnancy
        ? Endocrine disorder leading to premature labour

Unidentified causes

ocrine production is responsible, premature labour may be predicted by measurement of the appropriate hormones (see section on steroids).

At present the greatest clinical value of feto-placental hormone measurements is in the recognition of nutritional deprivation of the fetus, the consequences of which are summarised in Table 19.3. Overt fetal nutritional deprivation occurs in only a minority of pregnancies complicated by clinical disorders such as pre-eclampsia. Feto-placental function tests should help to define the actual fetal risk in these conditions and not the condition itself. Emphasis should be placed on the value of these tests in predicting the outcome for the fetus rather than their correlation with clinically recognisable syndromes of pregnancy.

Table 19.3. *Consequences of fetal nutritional deprivation.*

Intra-uterine death
Intra-uterine growth retardation
Perinatal asphyxia
Neonatal metabolic disorders (hypoglycaemia, hypocalcaemia)
Intellectual and/or motor impairment

A major problem exists in the correlation of feto-placental hormone measurements with fetal outcome. Syndromes such as fetal growth retardation, fetal distress and neonatal asphyxia are often poorly defined and, furthermore, have a variety of causes often unrelated to feto-placental function. Fetal growth retardation is, in most cases, impossible to define from observations on the live newborn. 'Light-for-dates', arbitrarily defined by varying criteria (below the 3rd, 5th or 10th normal percentile), is not synonymous with 'fetal growth retardation'. The latter may not be the sole cause of light-for-dates babies, and is also likely to be present in some babies of apparently normal weight. Feto-placental hormone determinations should distinguish the fetus of poor functional capacity, irrespective of body size.

STEROID HORMONES

Steroids are substances chemically related to and biologically derived from cholesterol and have as their fundamental carbon skeleton the 17-carbon cyclopentanoperhydrophenanthrene ring (Figure 19.1). Steroid hormones can be classified according to their biologic effects and chemical configuration:

1. Progesterone (Figure 19.2) contains 21 carbon atoms (C_{21}) and is a Δ^4-3-oxo compound. 'Δ^4' implies a double bond between C4 and C5. The precursor of progesterone is pregnenolone (Figure 19.2), which differs from progesterone only by its Δ^5-3β-hydroxy configuration; 'Δ^5' implies a double bond between C5 and C6.

Figure 19.1. The cyclopentanoperhydrophenanthrene ring system on which the chemical structure of all steroids is based. Each numbered point represents a fully hydrogenated carbon atom.

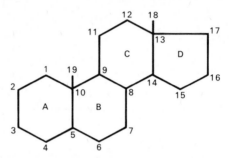

Pregnenolone (Δ^5P)   Progesterone (P)

Figure 19.2. The chemical structures of pregnenolone and progesterone. The abbreviations in brackets are as in Figure 19.4.

2. Glucocorticoid and mineralocorticoid hormones are C_{21} steroids with Δ^4-3-oxo configuration, like progesterone from which they are derived, and are characterised by a keto ($-CO-CH_2OH$) side-chain at C17.
3. Androgens are C_{19} steroids; dehydroepiandrosterone (DHEA) is the Δ^5 precursor of the Δ^4 compounds androstenedione and testosterone.
4. Oestrogens (Figure 19.3) are C_{18} steroids, C18 being attached to C13, having an aromatic A-ring and a phenolic hydroxyl group at C3.

The main function of placental progesterone in some mammals, and probably in women, is the maintenance of pregnancy by inhibition of myometrial contractility (Heap, 1972). The role of oestrogens in pregnancy is uncertain and deficiency due to placental enzyme defect (Oakey, Cawood and Macdonald, 1974) is not harmful to the fetus. The fetus may be protected from the effect of excess androgens by their conversion to oestrogens (Figure 19.4), although the effect of the resulting high concentrations of oestradiol-17β is not known. The biosynthesis of oestriol via the Δ^5 pathway may to this extent bypass the most potent androgens *and* oestrogens.

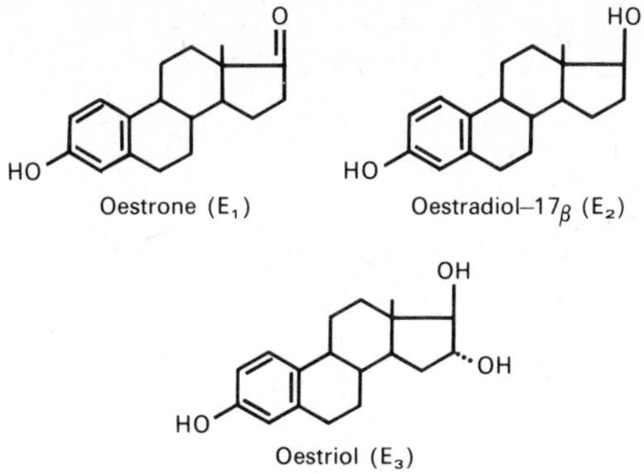

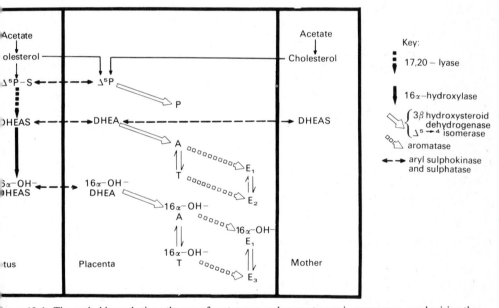

Figure 19.3. The chemical structures of the main oestrogens. The abbreviations in brackets are as in Figure 19.4. The orientation of the hydroxyl groups at C16 and C17 may be α (dotted line) or β (continuous line). Oestrone is an oxo (ketone) molecule at C17 and a single hydroxyl group at C3. Oestradiol-17β has two hydroxyl groups, at the 3- and 17-β positions, and oestriol has an additional 16α-hydroxyl group. Oestetrol is not shown but differs from oestriol only by a fourth hydroxyl group in the 15α-position.

Figure 19.4. The main biosynthetic pathways of oestrogens and progesterone in pregnancy, emphasising the roles of enzymes. The key to the enzymes is on the right. For explanation see text.

Oestrogens

Physiology

The study of steroid physiology in human pregnancy is complicated by the lack of any suitable animal model, due to major species differences (Heap, 1972). Abortions in mid-pregnancy have provided the classic human experimental models: the perfused, isolated fetus, the isolated placenta in situ, and the distribution of radioisotopes in mother and fetus

(Diczfalusy and Mancuso, 1969). Umbilical arterial and venous blood can easily be sample at delivery, but steroid levels are likely to be affected by the stress of labour. Howeve caesarean section at term gestation allows collection before labour of not only umbilic blood but also retroplacental (intervillous) and peripheral maternal blood (Tulchinsk 1973).

Biosynthesis. There are numerous detailed reviews of oestrogen synthesis in middle and la pregnancy (e.g. Beling, 1974). The adrenals, gonads and placenta all have a common potenti for synthesising most steroid hormones, but their characteristic products reflect tl predominance in each of particular enzymes. Any diagram of feto-placental steroid bi synthesis is likely to be incomplete or excessively confusing; Figure 19.4 is designed to sho only the major pathways of oestrogen and progesterone synthesis and to emphasise the roles the characteristic enzymes, some of which achieve different steroid interconversions via con mon pathways.

The fetus utilises progesterone (P, as in Figure 19.4) for conversion to glucocorticoid ho mones but cannot synthesise it. The fetus can synthesise cholesterol and pregnenolone (Δ^5F but it cannot convert pregnenolone (and other Δ^5 steroids) to progesterone (and other co responding Δ^4 steroids), because it lacks the necessary 3β-hydroxysteroid dehydrogena and $\Delta^{5\rightarrow4}$ isomerase enzyme system. Conversely, the placenta is deficient in the 17,20-lya enzyme system required to split off the side-chain from pregnenolone or progesterone, so cannot in this way make the oestrogen precursors dehydroepiandrosterone (DHEA) or a drostenedione (A). Thus placental synthesis of oestrone (E_1), oestradiol-17β (E_2) and oestri (E_3) is entirely dependent on the adrenal cortex of both the fetus and mother for the commc precursor DHEA-sulphate (DHEAS). On the other hand the fetus is unable to achieve tl $\Delta^{5\rightarrow4}$ conversion of DHEA to androstenedione or of 16α-hydroxy-DHEA to 16α-hydrox androstenedione, which are essential steps before aromatisation to oestrogens can occu The conversion of androstenedione to testosterone (T), E_1 to E_2, and of their 16 hydroxylated counterparts that give rise to E_3, is achieved by reduction at C17.

The main precursor of E_3 is 16α-hydroxy-DHEA derived by conversion of DHEA in tl fetal liver. The placenta lacks 16α-hydroxylase, while the maternal liver effects 16 hydroxylation mainly of oestrogens in preference to DHEA. Very little E_3 owes its origin fetal 16α-hydroxylation of E_1 and E_2, because the bulk of the oestrogens produced by tl placenta, particularly E_2, pass immediately into the maternal rather than the fetal circulatio Finally, due to the presence of aryl sulphokinase, Δ^5 steroids and oestrogens exist mainly a C3 sulphoconjugates in the fetus and mother, whereas in the placenta these conjugates a hydrolysed by aryl sulphatase. Hydrolysis of DHEAS and 16α-hydroxy-DHEAS is esse tial before $\Delta^{5\rightarrow4}$ isomerisation and aromatisation to oestrogens can occur.

Of the oestrogens synthesised by the trophoblast about 60 per cent of E_1 and E_2, and 9 per cent of E_3 originate from fetal precursors, the rest of the precursors coming from tl mother. Thus production of E_3 depends almost entirely on the fetus at precursor stages, b production of E_1 and E_2 partly reflects placental activity independent of the fetus. On tl other hand progesterone production is entirely dependent on the placenta. At term, dai production rates of oestrogens calculated from measured concentration gradients betwee maternal intervillous and peripheral blood and estimated intervillous blood flow are ap proximately: E_1 12 mg, E_2 15 mg and E_3 19 mg (Tulchinsky, 1973).

Of the numerous other oestrogens produced in much smaller quantity by the fet placental unit, oestetrol (15α-hydroxy-oestriol, or E_4) is of particular interest in the asses ment of fetal condition because it is at least 90 per cent dependent on 15α-hydroxylatio (and 16α-hydroxylation) in the fetal liver. The synthetic pathway is different from tl main oestrogens in that its precursors are oestrogens (especially E_2) rather than DHE.

able 19.1). Tracer studies have shown that the production rate of E_4 by the feto-placental unit about 1 mg/day (Fishman, 1973).

ntrol of placental oestrogen production. There is no evidence of any endocrine regulation feto-placental oestrogen production in normal circumstances (Hull, 1975). Though in tro studies on placental enzyme activity suggest that human chorionic gonadotrophin CG) stimulates, and unconjugated steroids inhibit oestrogen synthesis, in vivo studies tend discount any regulatory role for hCG and show that the supply of precursors is more im- ortant than enzyme capacity, except in the case of rare enzyme defects. Though impaired zymic conversion of oestrogen precursors has been demonstrated in various disorders of egnancy in vitro, there is no in vivo information to support this.

Fetal ACTH independently influences the production of DHEAS by the fetal adrenal cor- x, since ACTH from the mother does not cross the placenta (Simmer et al, 1974). Thus tal ACTH may regulate oestrogen production, though there is no evidence that it normally ays any important part. However, this is the mechanism by which oestrogen production is pressed by elevated maternal levels of cortisol or by administered glucocorticoids, which oss the placenta and suppress fetal ACTH.

The demonstration that precursor supply affects oestrogen production (Townsley, Rubin d Crystle, 1973) and that perfusion rate controls hCG and hPL (human placental lac- gen) production (McNeilly et al, in preparation) suggests that blood flow, presumably both llous and intervillous, is normally the major determinant of the synthetic activity of the ophoblast.

etabolism in the mother. Oestrogens are released by the trophoblast into maternal blood in nconjugated form but are excreted in urine almost entirely in conjugated form, redominantly as conjugated E_3. The unconjugated oestrogens are cleared from the plasma ith a half-life of about 15 min and subsequently in conjugated form are almost totally iminated in the urine: unconjugated E_3 is eliminated within 24 hours, while unconjugated E_2 is iminated over several days. The metabolic pathways of oestrogens in the mother have been eviewed by Hull (1975) and are illustrated diagrammatically in Figure 19.5; they are ualitatively the same as in non-pregnant women. Conjugation with sulphuric acid at C3 oc- urs widely, particularly in the liver. Conjugation with glucuronic acid at C16 occurs in the ver and to an undetermined extent in the kidneys, and at C3 in intestinal mucosa. The in- stinal reabsorption of oestrogens, excreted in bile as 3-sulphate, 16-glucuronides and 16- lucuronides, is largely dependent on hydrolysis by intestinal bacteria prior to 3- lucuronidation. About 25 per cent of E_3 passes through this hepato-intestinal circuit. About 0 per cent of E_1 and E_2 pass through after conversion, E_2 via E_1, to various conjugated estrogens, mainly E_3 and 16α-hydroxy-E_1; the latter is later partly reduced in intestinal ucosa to (conjugated) E_3. Thus conjugated E_3 which is present in relatively large amounts in lasma and urine (see below), is derived partly by metabolism of E_1 and E_2, and does not reflect roduction of only E_3 by the feto-placental unit.

Oestrogens *in maternal plasma* are partly conjugated (Figure 19.5) and are largely bound proteins. E_1, as in the non-pregnant state, is mainly sulphoconjugated and bound to lbumin. E_2 is 50 per cent conjugated; in both conjugated and unconjugated form more than 9 per cent is strongly bound to sex hormone binding globulin (SHBG). About 13 per cent of 3 is unconjugated, 25 to 43 per cent glucuronides, the remainder being sulphates including ulphoglucuronides. E_3 in any form is not significantly bound to SHBG but is weakly bound albumin. The sulphates of E_1 and E_3 are bound more than E_3-glucuronides, which may xplain why the E_3-glucuronides are more freely filtered by the renal glomeruli. In addition, 3-glucuronides are excreted by the renal tubules. The predominance of E_3-glucuronides in

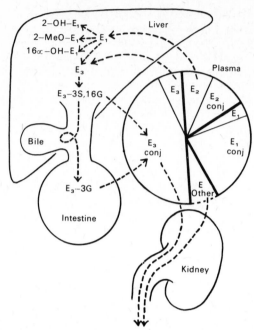

Figure 19.5. The main metabolic pathways of oestrogens in the mother. For explanation see text. 'Conj' = conjugated; 'Other E' = oestrogens other than E_1, E_2 and E_3.

urine reflects a production rate greater than that of E_3-sulphates, but the lower proportion in blood indicates the greater efficiency of excretion (Figure 19.6; see also Swapp, Masson and Klopper, 1975). Unconjugated oestrogens are poorly soluble in water and so are only found in small quantities in urine.

Disorders of maternal metabolism can alter oestrogen concentrations in plasma and excretion in urine:

1. Severe liver damage impairs the metabolism of unconjugated oestrogens but is rare.
2. Cholestasis, with or without jaundice, diminishes hepato-intestinal circulation of oestrogens and so reduces the production of conjugated E_3.

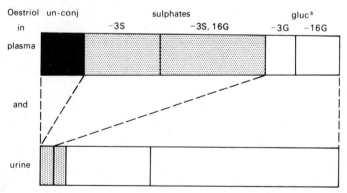

Figure 19.6. Oestriol in plasma and urine. Redrawn from Goebelsmann et al (1973) and Goebelsmann and Jaffe (1971).

3. A number of antibiotics have a similar effect which is much more marked, due to destruction of intestinal bacteria. After a course of ampicillin it has been found that the levels of plasma total E_3 (i.e. conjugated and unconjugated) and of urinary oestrogens (i.e. all conjugated oestrogens) are suppressed, but not plasma unconjugated E_2. From this, and from assumptions based on the normal derivation of conjugated E_3 and of unconjugated E_2 and E_3, it can be inferred that conjugated E_3 (particularly E_3-3-glucuronide) in plasma is reduced but not unconjugated E_3.

4. Impaired renal function associated with hypertensive disorders has been shown to elevate total (presumably conjugated) but not unconjugated E_3 levels in plasma, while urinary oestrogens are lowered (Figure 19.7).

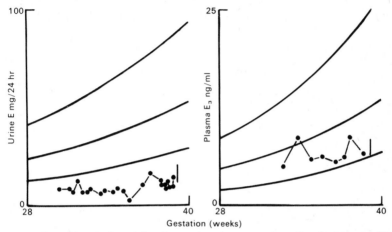

Gestation (weeks)

Figure 19.7. The effect of impaired renal function on the urinary excretion of total oestrogens (Urine E) in a hypertensive pregnant woman. She delivered a baby weighing only 2.2 kg at 39 weeks gestation, but it was otherwise healthy despite urinary oestrogen values that mostly suggested impending fetal death except on retrospective examination of their overall trend. Plasma unconjugated oestriol (E_3) values were normal. The day of delivery is indicated by the short vertical line. The continuous lines define the normal means $\pm$ 2 s.d. The normal ranges are skewed, the means geometric.

In addition to E_1, E_2 and E_3 there are small amounts of many other oestrogens in maternal plasma, derived both from the feto-placental unit and by maternal metabolism of the first three. Oestetrol (E_4) is probably mainly conjugated and derived from fetal E_4, while tracer studies have shown that the bulk is eliminated in the urine, mainly as E_4-glucuronides (Fishman, 1973).

In maternal urine oestrogens are present almost entirely as conjugates, mainly of E_3, while there are only minute quantities of E_1 and E_2. However, as other oestrogens have been identified and quantitated, they have been found to represent at least 33 per cent of the total (Adlercreutz and Luukkainen, 1970) and the list continues to grow. Thus E_3 accounts for only 60 to 67 per cent of the total oestrogen fraction. E_4 and 16α-hydroxy-E_1 are the major oestrogens after E_3, though they occur in only one-tenth the amount. Almost all oestrogens in maternal urine are derived from oestrogens produced by the feto-placental unit, after metabolic interconversion in the mother.

In fetal blood and *amniotic fluid* (reviewed by Scommegna, 1974) the major oestrogen is E_3 which is present in much higher concentrations than in maternal blood. In fetal blood E_3 is present mainly as the sulphoconjugate, whereas in amniotic fluid it occurs mainly as the glucuronide. This difference may be due to differences both in excretion of E_3 conjugates by the fetal kidneys and in removal from amniotic fluid after hydrolysis. No equilibrium exists between fetal, amniotic and maternal E_3. Because of the pooled nature of amniotic fluid and the very wide range of E_3 concentrations, and because of the problem of access, there is no clinical use for measurement of E_3 in amniotic fluid.

Summary. There is a strong case for measuring unconjugated oestrogens in maternal plasma because:

1. Conjugated E_3, both in maternal plasma and urine, is to a large extent the metabolic product of E_1 and E_2 and thus does not specifically reflect E_3 production by the feto-placental unit.
2. The individual production rates of E_1, E_2 and E_3, but perhaps not of E_4, by the feto-placental unit can only be specifically related each to the concentration of its own unconjugated form in maternal plasma, assuming constant metabolic clearance rates.
3. Maternal metabolic disorders are less likely to affect levels of unconjugated oestrogens in plasma than of conjugated E_3 in plasma or urine.

The case for measuring conjugated oestrogens, in maternal plasma or urine, will depend on questions such as: (1) whether oestrogens originating mainly in the placenta correlate as well with fetal condition as oestrogens dependent on fetal precursors; (2) the rate and degree of fluctuations in concentration; and (3) the ease of assay.

Measurement

In obstetric practice oestrogens have usually been measured in maternal 24-hour urine specimens. Increasing use is now made of plasma or serum, which allows immediate and error-free collection, easy handling and storage, and the possibility of measuring responses to dynamic tests. With the advent of radioimmunoassay rapid determinations in blood are now fully practical, and the numbers of samples which can be processed are already considerably greater than using classical methods.

Urinary oestrogen methodology has been reviewed by Wilde and Oakey (1975). Measurement of E_3 conjugates has generally given way to measurement of total oestrogen conjugates, because it is simpler and because of the biological advantages discussed earlier. The most recent development is based on the performance of Kober colour reaction directly on urine followed by Ittrich extraction and fluorimetry (Brombacher, Gijzen and Verheeson, 1968). This permits automation and continuous-flow systems which allow up to 70 samples to be assayed each day with a high degree of precision and clinical reliability (Hull, Braunsberg and Irving, 1975).

Plasma oestrogen assays in current use have been reviewed by Hull (1975). The earlier colorimetric, double-isotope derivative and gas–liquid chromatography methods are too time-consuming for clinical application and have generally given way to radioligand assays. However, fluorimetric methods are also in use for both conjugated and unconjugated oestrogens, but are often imprecise and may give overestimates due to nonspecific fluorescence. Radioligand assays employing natural receptor-proteins such as uterine cytosol or sex hormone binding globulin have been superseded by radioimmunoassays. The recent development of highly specific antisera to E_1, E_2 and E_3 permits assay of the unconjugated steroid after simple extraction of plasma, without any need for further purification. Measurement of total E_3 or total oestrogens requires prior hydrolysis of the conjugates. E_4 is less easily assayed because of its relatively low concentration, and with current antisera may be overestimated due to cross-reaction with E_3, though recently Tulchinsky et al (1975) have reported that this is not a problem in practice. Unconjugated E_2 and E_3 and total E_3 can now be assayed in small volumes of plasma with a throughput of 40 samples each day, or 100 using semi-automated techniques (Hull and Monro, 1975). Much further technical refinement is possible, and modifications that avoid organic solvents (Christner and Fetter, 1974) could permit full automation.

Clinical studies

The results of oestrogen determinations in normal and abnormal pregnancy have been extensively reviewed, both for urine (Beischer and Brown, 1972; Scommegna, 1973) and for plasma (Hull, 1975).

1. Normal pregnancy

Progression and fluctuation of values. Urinary excretion of conjugated total oestrogens or conjugated E_3 increases exponentially in late pregnancy and does not fall before labour. The plateau reported by some for late pregnancy may well be partly due to the overlapping of subjects with mistaken gestational maturity. In plasma, conjugated and unconjugated oestrogens rise exponentially, except unconjugated E_1 which slows down in the last few weeks. Unconjugated E_3 rises more rapidly than E_2 in late pregnancy, although after a later start, reflecting increasing activity of the fetal adrenal cortex and liver. Unconjugated E_4 rises even more steeply than E_3 towards term.

The mean urinary excretion of conjugated E_3 in women at term with normal pregnancies is about 28 mg/24 hours (see Scommegna, 1973); whereas for total oestrogens it is about 53 mg (Hull, Braunsberg and Irving, 1975). From the numerous reports on plasma oestrogens mean normal values at term are approximately: unconjugated E_1, 9 ng/ml, E_2 20 to 25 ng/ml, E_3 14 ng/ml and E_4 1 to 4 ng/ml; and total E_3 200 to 250 ng/ml, the higher values being obtained by fluorimetric methods. (It is of interest that the ratio of reported values of total to unconjugated E_3 is twice as high as that found in compartmental studies (Goebelsmann et al, 1973; Klopper et al, 1973) and is probably due to lack of methodological specificity in the former case.) The normal ranges for all oestrogens in urine and plasma are wide and their distributions are skewed, being greater above the geometric mean than below it (Figure 19.8).

The rate and degree of fluctuation of values are important determinants of the clinical usefulness of any oestrogen measurement. The coefficient of variation of 24-hour urinary E_3 excretion is about 20 per cent, but it is often greater in clinical practice due to errors in collection. To overcome this and also to shorten the collection interval, the concentration ratio of E_3 or total oestrogens to creatinine is used by some (Lockwood and Newman, 1974). This makes the assumption that the rates of production and excretion of creatinine are constant, and has not been widely accepted. In plasma no consistent diurnal pattern of unconjugated E_1, E_2 or E_3, or total E_3, has been demonstrated, nor any relationship to posture, exercise or food. The day-to-day and circadian coefficients of variation for the concentrations of plasma oestrogens are each about 15 per cent. This degree of fluctuation also occurs even from minute to minute for unconjugated E_2 and E_3 and may be partly due to changes in placental blood flow; this is inferred from the acute reductions in unconjugated E_3 levels that occur with uterine contractions.

Urinary and plasma oestrogen concentrations correlate, although poorly, with

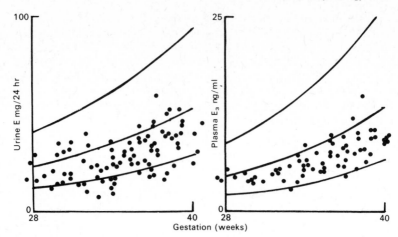

Figure 19.8. Urinary total oestrogen (Urine E) and plasma unconjugated oestriol (E₃) values in pregnant women, irrespective of any disorder of pregnancy, whose babies were light-for-dates (weighing less than the 10th percentile) but otherwise in good condition at birth. The continuous lines define the normal means ± 2 s.d. The values of the case illustrated in Figure 19.7 are not included.

birthweight—low mean values are consistently found with healthy light-for-dates babies (Figure 19.8)—but do not correlate with parity or fetal sex.

Dynamic studies. Dynamic responses of oestrogens in the mother have been measured after intravenous injection of 50 mg or more of the precursor DHEAS. The test response was first based on changes in urinary conjugated E_3 but these are not immediate or large enough to be useful (Lauritzen, 1974). These changes are now known to reflect increased production of E_1 and E_2 alone. There is no rise in unconjugated E_3 because the injected DHEAS is presumably taken up by the trophoblast and little reaches the fetus (Buster et al, 1974). Unconjugated E_2 levels increase about four-fold within 15 to 30 min of the injection and remain elevated for several hours. Compared with DHEAS the response to DHEA, taken orally because it is poorly soluble in water, is smaller and slightly delayed. The response to DHEAS or DHEA might be expected to be impaired in disorders that reduce its transfer to the placenta or its conversion by placental enzyme activity. However, the DHEAS test, at least with the dose used, is not sensitive enough to detect impairment of feto-placental function, though it is of value in the recognition of placental sulphatase deficiency.

The oestrogen response in the mother after an intra-amniotic injection of DHEAS is similar to that following intravenous injection, but a dose of 150 mg is needed to evoke a maximal response (Crystle et al, 1973). Since there is no rise in unconjugated E_3 it can be presumed that the DHEAS passes mainly into the maternal blood across the amnion rather than entering the fetal circulation.

2. Abnormal pregnancies

Abnormal oestrogen values. The recognition of abnormal oestrogen levels may be based on either single values or trends in serial values. The normality or otherwise of individual values are defined by the limits of the normal range (Figures 19.7, 19.8, 19.9). The normality or otherwise of a trend is more difficult to define. In general the greater the deviation of the trend in a specific patient from normal, which is parallel to the mean and limit lines of the normal range, the greater is the risk implied. From what is known about normal short-term fluctuation in levels it can be taken that any acute fall of 40 to 50 per cent is abnormal, provided that in the case of 24-hour urinary oestrogens the sample volumes have been consistent.

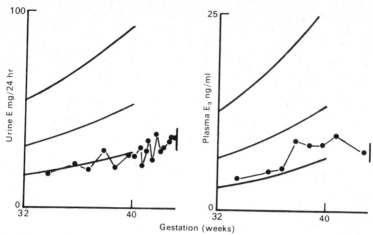

Figure 19.9. Urinary total oestrogen (Urine E) and plasma unconjugated oestriol (E_3) values in a woman who appeared to have a light-for-dates fetus and whose pregnancy later appeared to be prolonged to 43 weeks. The day of delivery is indicated by the short vertical line. The normal trend in oestrogen values allowed safe continuation of the pregnancy without interference; in retrospect gestational maturity was found to have been mistaken. The continuous lines define the normal means $\pm$ 2 s.d.

Low oestrogen values may be difficult to interpret if occurring as a single value in an individual, or if the gestational maturity is in doubt. However, a low value is more likely to be abnormal if it has been preceded by a significant fall or is followed by an abnormal trend. Low values that follow a normal upward trend, at least parallel to the lower limit of the normal range, provide evidence of continuing growth and well-being of the fetus, although the fetus and placenta are likely to be small. Some of the lowest oestrogen values occur in association with healthy fetuses, due to placental enzyme defects. In these cases the large disparity between the oestrogen values and the normal fetal growth is obvious enough not to be misleading.

Fetal complications. Intra-uterine death associated with fetal growth retardation, for instance as a result of hypertensive disorders, is invariably preceded by low or falling oestrogen values both in urine and blood. This is not the case with diabetes and rhesus isoimmunisation (see below). Intra-uterine deaths unheralded by any disorder of pregnancy, and presumably due to unrecognised nutritional or vascular impairment, are also often preceded by low urinary oestriol excretion (Beischer and Brown, 1972) and the same would be expected for plasma oestrogens.

Light-for-dates babies in general and perinatal asphyxia are frequently associated with low urinary oestrogen excretion in pregnancy (MacLeod, Mitton and Avery, 1971). Light-for-dates babies that are born in good condition, irrespective of any maternal disorder, are less likely to be suffering from intra-uterine starvation and their pregnancies are usually associated with normal oestrogen values. The values tend to fall within the lower part of the normal range (Figure 19.8), but continue to rise with advancing gestation.

Follow-up of children born to mothers with low urinary oestrogens in pregnancy was said to reveal a high incidence of neurological defects (Wallace and Michie, 1966), but this has not been confirmed (Greene et al, 1969).

Fetal abnormality is often associated with low urinary oestrogen excretion; this occurs, for instance, in more than half the cases of Down's syndrome (Jorgensen and Trolle, 1972) and is probably related to the generally reduced fetal size rather than any particular defect of the adrenal cortex or liver. Adrenal hypoplasia, by reduced production of DHEA, results in particularly low urinary oestrogen values (Fliegner, Schindler and Brown, 1972). Anencephaly causes adrenal hypoplasia as a result of ACTH deficiency, due to absence of the hypothalamus.

Specific disorders of pregnancy. Hypertensive disorders, including pre-eclampsia, are associated with low oestrogen values in urine and plasma, which correlate well with the severity of the disorder and risk to the fetus. In some cases plasma total E_3 concentration is elevated, unconjugated E_3 is normal (Mathur, Leaming and Williamson, 1973) and urinary oestrogen excretion is reduced (Figure 19.7), indicating impaired renal clearance of conjugated E_3.

Prolonged pregnancy beyond 42 weeks is not associated with low urinary oestrogen excretion. Since low oestrogen values can be expected in some cases due to mistaken gestational maturity, the trend rather than the absolute value provides the best index of fetal well-being (Figure 19.9). Doubt about gestational maturity frequently compounds the clinician's anxiety of the small but definite risk to the fetus from postmaturity. In these cases rising oestrogen values are a reliable indication that it is safe to allow the continuation of the pregnancy until the onset of spontaneous labour.

Antepartum haemorrhage from any cause has been reported by Beischer and Brown (1972) to be followed by low urinary oestrogen excretion in about half the cases in which the fetus survives the acute episode of bleeding. This suggests impaired placental function in many of these cases, even though fetal growth retardation is recognised in only a few and subsequent fetal death usually occurs in association with recurrent major bleeding.

Tobacco smoking in pregnancy is associated with reduced birthweight but there is no increase in the incidence of fetal death or low urinary oestrogen excretion (Targett et al, 1973).

Diabetes mellitus is generally associated with normal oestrogen values both in urine and blood except when vascular complications result in starvation of the fetus (Gillmer and Beard, 1975).

Rhesus isoimmunisation resulting in fetal death is often associated with normal oestrogen values both in urine and blood. However, fetal progress after intra-uterine blood transfusion appears to be reflected by the subsequent urinary oestrogen values, which fall and remain low when fetal death follows (Michie and Robertson, 1971). Excretion of E_4 in urine has been correlated with fetal haemoglobin concentration (Heikkila and Luukkainen, 1971), but no advantages over other oestrogens have been found for E_4 in plasma (Tulchinsky et al, 1975). The best correlation with fetal outcome appears to be the ratio between unconjugated E_2 and E_3 in plasma, which is high when fetal death occurs later (Lindberg, Johansson and Nilsson, 1974). A similar relationship between plasma progesterone and unconjugated E_3 has also been reported (Tulchinsky et al, 1972). These findings indicate the disparity between the placental and fetal conditions in this disorder. However, steroid values alone do not provide a clear guide to the timing of delivery in rhesus isoimmunisation.

Multiple pregnancy is associated with elevated oestrogen values both in urine and blood. An upward trend in values in the upper range of normal is usually observed but cannot be relied on as an index of well-being of *both* fetuses. A failure of oestrogen values to rise with advancing gestation is always a bad sign, as in singleton pregnancy.

Premature labour has been reported to be preceded by elevation of plasma unconjugated E_2 concentrations (Tamby Raja, Anderson and Turnbull, 1974) except when due to cervical incompetence (Csapo, Pohanka and Kaihola, 1974). The value of such measurements in the clinical management of patients at risk of premature labour has still to be determined.

Screening for the 'at risk' pregnancy. The incidence of low urinary oestrogen excretion occurring at some time in a complete population of women in late pregnancy is about 14 per cent (Targett et al, 1973). Amongst these cases the incidence of birthweight below the 10th percentile is increased seven-fold and fetal death 15-fold, and it has been suggested that many stillbirths might be prevented if the test were applied routinely (Beischer and Brown, 1972). However, there is an incidence of false-positive results which might entail an equal risk because of inappropriate clinical action. The balance of risks and advantages of screening all pregnant women has yet to be determined. The practical drawbacks of 24-hour urine collection for this purpose could now be overcome by the use of plasma oestrogen assays.

Progesterone

The synthesis, metabolism and functions of progesterone in pregnancy have been extensively reviewed (e.g. Goldman and Zarrow, 1973). Biosynthesis (Figure 19.4) of progesterone (P) from pregnenolone (Δ^5P) by the placenta is dependent mainly on maternal cholesterol. The fetus is unable to convert pregnenolone to progesterone and the corpus luteum produces comparatively negligible amounts from the 12th week of pregnancy. Thus progesterone production in late pregnancy reflects placental function alone. There appears to be no mechanism controlling production, which may depend primarily on intervillous blood flow. The average production rate at term is about 350 mg/day (Tulchinsky and Okada, 1975).

In maternal plasma 90 per cent of progesterone is bound to protein, half of this to corticosteroid-binding globulin. It is rapidly metabolised in the liver, kidneys, and other sites, the half-life being about 90 min. Negligible amounts are found in urine, but some 10 to 15 per cent is excreted in urine as pregnanediol.

In normal pregnancy maternal plasma progesterone levels rise linearly to a mean of about 150 ng/ml at term, with a wide range (Tulchinsky and Okada, 1975). There is no obvious circadian fluctuation of values and the day-to-day coefficient of variation is about 20 per cent.

Measurement of pregnanediol excretion was one of the first tests used for the assessment of placental function, but is now largely of historic interest. Plasma progesterone concentrations do not usually change before fetal death (Tulchinsky and Okada, 1975), but they may be of value in rhesus isoimmunisation: in this condition the ratio to plasma unconjugated E_3 is high prior to fetal death, reflecting the disparity between the condition of the placenta and of the fetus (Tulchinsky et al, 1972). Progesterone is now easily measured in plasma by rapid competitive protein binding radioassay or by radioimmunoassay.

A related steroid that might prove to be clinically valuable is 16α-hydroxyprogesterone, which is present in maternal plasma in concentrations similar to, and closely correlated with, unconjugated E_3 (Abraham and Samojlik, 1974). It is presumably synthesised in the fetal liver by 16α-hydroxylation of progesterone derived from the placenta. Thus it involves a very much simpler pathway than the oestrogens, while the immediate placental precursor, progesterone, is readily available for comparative measurement.

PROTEIN HORMONES

The best characterised of the protein hormones of the human feto-placental unit are human chorionic gonadotrophin (hCG) and human placental lactogen (hPL). There is also some evidence for the production of other hormones, including chorionic corticotrophin (hCCT), chorionic thyrotrophin (hCT), and peptides like those of the hypothalamus, thyrotrophin-releasing hormone (TRH) and gonadotrophin-releasing hormone (LH/FSH–RH). Only hCG and hPL will be considered in any detail here.

Human chorionic gonadotrophin (hCG)

Physiology

Chorionic gonadotrophin was the first of the hormones of the feto-placental unit to be clearly identified. Chemically it is very similar to pituitary luteinising hormone (LH), and like the pituitary glycoproteins consists of two non-identical subunits, α and β. The function is unknown, though as it is produced from a very early stage of pregnancy it has been suggested that it might form part of a luteotropic complex responsible for the maintenance of the corpus luteum. In common with the other specific protein hormones of the feto-placental unit it is produced by the syncytiotrophoblast. No specific control mechanisms have been identified, though the rate of release may be related to blood-flow in the intervillous space (McNeilly et al, in preparation). A notable feature of the production of hCG is the observation that the placenta releases substantial amounts of the free α-subunit, and that the latter can be identified in the maternal circulation by means of specific radioimmunoassays. Maternal metabolism occurs chiefly in the liver and kidneys.

Measurement

Bioassays are no longer used in clinical or research practice, and have been replaced by immunological assays. Methods of agglutination inhibition, using coated red cells or latex particles, are still widely used in the detection of early pregnancy; two weeks after the first missed period positive results are 97 per cent reliable, although a quarter of negative results are false (Stringer et al, 1975). However, if hCG determinations prove to be of any value for the detailed monitoring of fetal well-being in early pregnancy, these techniques are likely to be replaced by the more precise and sensitive radioimmunoassays, particularly of the free α-subunit which may prove to be superior to that of the intact hormone for practical clinical applications.

Clinical studies

Chorionic gonadotrophin levels reach a peak in maternal urine and blood between the seventh and eighth weeks of pregnancy. A small secondary peak occurs between 32 and 36 weeks, the levels in women at term being higher when the fetus is female rather than male (Broditsky et al, 1975). There is evidence for differential release of the intact hormone and the free α-subunit, but this needs further elucidation.

Other than in the diagnosis and management of trophoblastic tumours, there is surprisingly little recent information on the clinical significance of hCG levels in the mother in relation to fetal well-being. In principle, it might be expected that the significance would be similar to that of other specific placental products such as hPL. However, the very different pattern of production, and the fact that it is synthesised as two subunits, suggests the possibility that maternal levels may reflect a hitherto unexplored aspect of placental function.

Human placental lactogen (hPL)

Physiology

The term 'human placental lactogen' is now preferred to the less elegant 'human chorionic somatomammotrophin'. The physiology of hPL has been extensively reviewed (see

Josimovich, Reynolds and Cobo, 1947). It is a single-chain protein of molecular weight around 22 000 which is chemically and immunologically similar to pituitary growth hormone and prolactin. The function of hPL, like oestriol, is uncertain, although it may play an important part in mammary growth and development and in the altered carbohydrate and lipid metabolism of pregnancy. It is produced by the syncytiotrophoblast at rates which reach 1 g/day at term. No specific control mechanisms have been identified; the circulating levels in the mother fall after intravenous administration of glucose, but the extent of the reduction is small and unlikely to be of great physiological significance (Pavlou et al, 1973). In the mother hPL is metabolised in the liver and kidneys; relatively small quantities are excreted in maternal urine (about 5 mg/day).

Measurement

The relatively weak biological activities of hPL have vitiated attempts to develop a biological assay. For this reason most studies have been based on the use of radioimmunoassay, though other types of immunological systems have been described. Measurement of hPL by radioimmunoassay does not demand a system of high sensitivity, since the circulating levels in the second half of pregnancy are of the order of 4 to 10 μg/ml; it is therefore possible to use relatively high concentrations of reagents, yielding in turn high precision and rapid equilibration. One of the great advantages of the measurement of hPL in maternal blood samples is that a result can be available in one to two hours, and that highly skilled technicians are not essential.

Clinical studies

1. Normal pregnancy. Placental lactogen levels in the mother rise progressively throughout most of pregnancy and reach a plateau in the last four to five weeks of delivery (Figure 19.10). As with other hormonal tests of feto-placental function, the levels show a skewed distribution, the variation above the geometric mean being greater than below it. The rate and

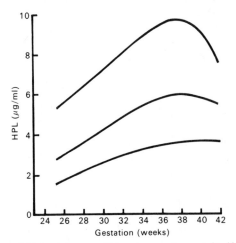

Figure 19.10. Maternal plasma hPL levels in normal late pregnancy (mean ± 2 s.d.). As for oestrogens, the range is skewed and the mean geometric.

degree of individual fluctuation is somewhat less than that reported for urinary oestrogen determinations in normal pregnancy, but comparable to that of plasma oestrogens. The coefficient of variation is approximately 15 per cent; there is some circadian variation but no obvious circadian rhythm, and posture, bedrest, exercise and smoking have no consistent effects on hPL levels.

Placental lactogen levels in the mother do not vary with parity or fetal sex, but correlate, although poorly, with the delivered weight of the fetus and placenta (Sciarra et al, 1968; Letchworth et al, 1971). Clinical tests based on a dynamic response of hPL levels have not been described.

2. Abnormal pregnancy

Fetal complications. Though maternal hPL levels reflect only the function of the placenta, they are often found to be reduced in many disorders prior to resulting *fetal death* (Ward et al, 1973). However, in the occasional patient the levels remain within the normal range until after death occurs.

Low levels of hPL have been described in association with the *light-for-dates* fetus (Lindberg and Nilsson, 1973). Except in those cases in which growth retardation is based solely on placental insufficiency, it may be anticipated that the oestrogens, being dependent on fetal precursors, would be a better index of this complication.

Several workers have shown a close relationship between maternal hPL levels and *perinatal asphyxia* (e.g. England et al, 1974). This association may hold in the absence of other obvious complications, even in babies of normal birthweight (Letchworth and Chard, 1972). There have been no studies involving a long-term follow-up of children in whom maternal hPL levels were determined during intra-uterine life, though clearly such studies would be of great interest and importance. Placental lactogen levels are often found to be decreased in association with severe *congenital abnormalities* of the fetus (Cadle and Gau, 1976). This presumably reflects the reduced weight of the placenta, which is a feature of such cases.

Specific disorders of pregnancy. Hypertension and pre-eclampsia are associated with reduced levels of hPL. Most workers agree that the levels are still further reduced when the fetus is at particular risk. For example, Spellacy and his colleagues (1971) defined a 'fetal danger zone' of values less than $4 \mu g/ml$ after the 30th week; subjects falling into this category had a fetal mortality of 24 per cent. Keller and his colleagues (1971) compared plasma hPL determinations with a number of other tests and concluded that hPL was the only one to give no false-negative results related to fetal complications, although because of the higher false-positive rate it was best combined with urinary oestriol determination. On presently available information, a patient with hypertension or pre-eclampsia and a low hPL level would be a candidate for intensive management and for planned early delivery.

Prolonged pregnancy. There is no specific published information on the value of maternal hPL levels in the management of prolonged pregnancy. Nevertheless, comparison with other complications would suggest that low or falling levels should be an indication for induction of labour.

Antepartum haemorrhage. In most cases maternal hPL levels are normal prior to the occurrence of the placental separation. Since they are of little or no predictive value, hPL estimation would not play more than an ancillary part in the management of this condition, and then only in the less severe cases.

Tobacco smoking. Maternal hPL levels are lower in those who smoke, but paradoxically the reduction is confined to light rather than heavy smokers (Moser et al, 1974). Whether the measurement has any practical contribution to make in the management of such patients is not known.

Diabetes. Placental lactogen levels associated with diabetes mellitus have been reviewed by Gillmer and Beard (1975). They are generally elevated in pregnancy, but in cases with evidence of placental dysfunction are relatively reduced. It should be emphasised that this reduction is only significant when compared with the range for 'normal' diabetics, rather than that for the normal non-diabetic population (Figures 19.11 and 19.12). Levels which are consistently below 5 μg/ml are an indication of increased risk for the fetus.

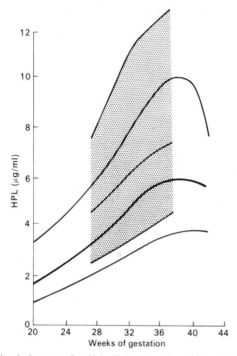

Figure 19.11. Plasma hPL levels (mean ± 2 s.d.) in diabetic women with uncomplicated pregnancies (shaded area) shown superimposed on the normal. Redrawn from Ursell, Brudenell and Chard (1973) with kind permission of the editor of *British Medical Journal*.

Rhesus isoimmunisation. Placental lactogen levels are elevated in this condition, presumably associated with the abnormally large placenta. The degree of elevation is related to the severity of the disease. Ward and his colleagues (1974) have shown that in mild and moderately affected cases maternal hPL levels are almost normal, while in severely affected cases they are raised above the normal range; a patient presenting before the 26th week with levels lying more than two standard deviations above the normal mean has a 90 per cent chance of delivering a severely affected child. Elevation of hPL levels in amniotic fluid has a similar significance (Niven, Ward and Chard, 1974). The estimation of hPL is therefore a useful adjunct to the management of this condition, particularly in the late second trimester when other tests, such as the antibody levels and liquor bilirubin, may give ambiguous results.

Multiple pregnancy. Placental lactogen levels are elevated in multiple pregnancy in proportion to the increased mass of the fetoplacental unit (Garoff and Seppala, 1973). Insufficient data are available to yield a normal range for this situation, and there is no information on the clinical significance in the management of these pregnancies.

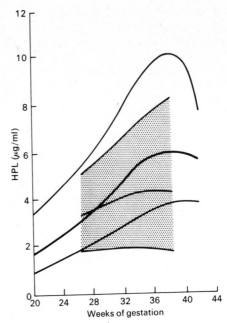

Figure 19.12. Plasma hPL levels (mean ± 2 s.d.) in diabetic pregnancies with complications (shaded area) shown superimposed on the normal. Redrawn from Ursell, Brudenell and Chard (1973) with kind permission of the editor of *British Medical Journal.*

Premature labour. Placental lactogen levels show no alteration in association with the onset of spontaneous labour at term (Gillard, Letchworth and Chard, 1973). Though no published evidence is available, there is little reason to suppose that they would be of any clinical value in the prediction of premature spontaneous labour.

Screening for the 'at risk' pregnancy. Spellacy, Buhi and Birk (1975) have found the incidence of low hPL values in clinically selected high-risk pregnancies to be about eight per cent. In a prospective study of such cases these authors found that when hPL values were low the incidence of intra-uterine fetal death was reduced by 75 per cent if prompt delivery was effected. However, half of all stillbirths, and the majority of those without hypertension, are not associated with low hPL values, so it remains to be seen what effect screening of all pregnant women with hPL measurements might have on overall perinatal mortality.

CONCLUSIONS

The available hormonal tests of fetal well-being are based on important physiological functions of the feto-placental unit and thus should provide a powerful method of diagnosis. However, their application has often fallen short of the optimistic predictions made by their originators, for a number of reasons:

1. The variety of pathophysiology of the disorders of pregnancy.
2. The overlap of values in normal and abnormal pregnancies.

3. Methodological deficiencies resulting from lack of biological and methodological specificity, and methodological error.
4. Limited clinical studies, which have often been retrospective, anecdotal and uncontrolled. Biochemical tests of this type are unlikely to indicate the exact risk to the fetus, merely that a risk exists, perhaps of greater or lesser degree. Only if the results of a test are interpreted in terms of risks rather than certainties will their full value—as an adjunct to other methods—be realised.

Of the presently available hormonal tests of fetal well-being, only two seem likely to withstand the test of time: measurement of oestrogens in maternal urine or blood, and measurement of hPL in maternal blood. Although in their application these materials are not necessarily intrinsically superior to others, they have the advantages that the technique of estimation is widely available, and that they are backed by a substantial literature on their clinical application. Clinical comparisons of determinations of various substances have been too limited to be conclusive; although urinary oestrogens have not been bettered, this can only be expected to apply mainly to disorders affecting fetal nutrition. There are insufficient clinical data yet to choose between oestrogens in urine and blood, but there are good biological reasons for preferring the unconjugated oestrogens, particularly E_3, in blood. In urine there are clear advantages in measuring conjugated total oestrogens rather than conjugated E_3.

For the future it is likely that the approach to placental function tests will be very different in the 1980s from that which obtains at the present time. First, the disadvantages of urine collection are such that it is bound to be replaced, and all tests are likely to be performed on blood samples. Second, unless this technique is replaced by a better one, all tests for hormone products will be performed by radioimmunoassay, for it offers immense advantages in terms of both precision and the ability to process large numbers. Third, objective interpretation of results will be considerably facilitated by means of computers. Fourth, every unit will have available a spectrum of tests: for instance, unconjugated E_3 as a test of fetus and placenta together and hPL as a test of the placenta alone. Finally, and most important, these tests may not be confined to those patients who have obvious clinical abnormalities, but will probably be extended to all pregnant women. The collection of a blood sample for biochemical determinations may become as routine a part of an antenatal visit as is the taking of blood pressure.

REFERENCES

Abraham, G. E. & Samojlik, E. (1974) Correlation between plasma unconjugated estriol and 16α-hydroxyprogesterone during human pregnancy. *Obstetrics and Gynecology,* **44,** 767–768.
Adlercreutz, H. & Luukkainen, T. (1970) Identification and determination of oestrogens in various biological materials in pregnancy. *Annals of Clinical Research,* **2,** 365–380.
Beischer, N. A. & Brown, J. B. (1972) Current status of estrogen assays in obstetrics and gynecology. *Obstetric and Gynecological Review,* **27,** 303–343.
Beling, C. G. (1974) Hormone biogenesis in the foeto-placental unit. In *Hormonal Investigations in Human Pregnancy* (Ed.) Scholler, R., pp. 3–16. Paris: Sepe.
Broditsky, R. S., Reyes, F. I., Winter, J. S. D. & Faiman, C. (1975) Serum human chorionic gonadotrophin and progesterone patterns in the last trimester of pregnancy: relationship to fetal sex. *American Journal of Obstetrics and Gynecology,* **121,** 238–241.
Brombacher, P. J., Gijzen, A. H. J. & Verheeson, P. E. (1968) Simple and rapid determination of total oestrogens in pregnancy urine. *Clinica Chimica Acta,* **20,** 360–361.

Buster, J. E., Abraham, G. E., Kyle, F. W. & Marshall, J. R. (1974) Serum steroid levels following a large intravenous dose of a steroid sulfate precursor during the second trimester of human pregnancy. I Dehydroepiandrosterone-sulfate. *Journal of Clinical Endocrinology and Metabolism*, **38**, 1031–1037.

Cadle, G. & Gau, G. (1976) Placental lactogen levels in association with congenital abnormalities of the fetus. *Obstetrics and Gynecology*, in press.

Christner, J. E. & Fetter, Marion C. (1974) Sephadex column radioimmunoassay of unconjugated estriol in pregnancy plasma. *Steroids*, **24**, 327–342.

Crystle, C. D., Dubin, N. H., Grannis, G. F., Stevens, V. C. & Townsley, J. D. (1973) Investigation of precursor availability in the regulation of estrogen synthesis in normal human pregnancy. *Obstetrics and Gynecology*, **42**, 718–724.

Csapo, A. I., Pohanka, O. & Kaihola, H. L. (1974) Progesterone deficiency and premature labour. *British Medical Journal*, **i**, 137–140.

Diczfalusy, E. & Mancuso, S. (1969) Oestrogen metabolism in pregnancy. In *Foetus and Placenta* (Ed.) Klopper, A. & Diczfalusy, E. pp. 191–248. Oxford: Blackwell.

England, P., Lorrimer, D., Ferguson, J. C., Moffatt, A. M. & Kelly, A. M. (1974) Human placental lactogen: the watchdog of fetal distress. *Lancet*, **i**, 5–7.

Fishman, J. (1973) Metabolism and measurement of 15α-hydroxyestriol in late pregnancy. In *Endocrinology. Excerpta Medica International Congress Series*, **273**, 1038–1044.

Fliegner, J. R. H., Schindler, Irene & Brown, J. B. (1972) Low urinary oestriol excretion during pregnancy associated with placental sulphatase deficiency or congenital adrenal hypoplasia. *Journal of Obstetrics and Gynaecology of the British Commonwealth*, **79**, 810–815.

Garoff, L. & Seppala, M. (1973) Alpha fetoprotein and human placental lactogen levels in maternal serum in multiple pregnancies. *Journal of Obstetrics and Gynaecology of the British Commonwealth*, **80**, 695–700.

Gillard, M., Letchworth, A. T. & Chard, T. (1973) Human placental lactogen levels in relation to the initiation and maintenance of labour. *Obstetrics and Gynecology*, **41**, 774–776.

Gillmer, M. D. G. & Beard, R. W. (1975) Fetal and placental function tests in diabetic pregnancy. In *Carbohydrate Metabolism in Pregnancy and the Newborn* (Ed.) Sutherland, H. W. & Stowers, J. M. pp. 168–194. Edinburgh: Churchill Livingstone.

Goebelsmann, U. & Jaffe, R. B. (1971) Oestriol metabolism in pregnant women. *Acta Endocrinologica*, **66**, 679–693.

Goebelsmann, U., Chen, L-C., Saga, M., Nakamura, R. M. & Jaffe, R. B. (1973) Plasma concentration and protein binding of oestriol and its conjugates in pregnancy. *Acta Endocrinologica*, **74**, 592–604.

Goldman, B. D. & Zarrow, M. X. (1973) The physiology of progestins. In *Handbook of Physiology*, Section 7, Vol. II, Part I (Ed.) Greep, R. O. pp. 547–572. Washington: American Physiological Society.

Greene, J. W., Beargie, R. A., Clark, B. A. & Smith, K. (1969) Correlation of estriol excretion patterns of pregnant women with subsequent development of their children. *American Journal of Obstetrics and Gynecology*, **105**, 730–747.

Heap, R. B. (1972) Role of hormones in pregnancy. In *Reproduction in Mammals 3. Hormones in Reproduction* (Ed.) Austin, C. R. & Short, R. V. pp. 73–105. Cambridge: Cambridge University Press.

Heikkila, J. & Luukkainen, T. (1971) Urinary excretion of estriol and 15α-hydroxyestriol in complicated pregnancies. *American Journal of Obstetrics and Gynecology*, **110**, 509–521.

Hull, M. G. R. (1975) The clinical application of plasma oestrogen assays in human late pregnancy. *Bibliography of Reproduction*, **26**, 1–6, 111–115.

Hull, M. G. R. & Monro, P. P. (1975) Automated radioimmunoassay of plasma oestriol: unexpected problems. *Clinical Science and Molecular Medicine*, **48**, 3P.

Hull, M. G. R., Braunsberg, H. & Irving, D. (1975) Urinary total oestrogen values determined by an automated method in normal and abnormal pregnancies. *Clinica Chimica Acta*, **58**, 71–76.

Jorgensen, P. I. & Trolle, D. (1972) Low urinary oestriol excretion during pregnancy in women giving birth to infants with Down's syndrome. *Lancet*, **ii**, 782–784.

Josimovitch, J. B., Reynolds, M. & Cobo, E. (1974) *Lactogenic Hormones, Fetal Nutrition and Lactation*. New York: Wiley.

Keller, P. J., Baertschi, U., Bader, P., Gerber, C., Schmid, J., Solterman, R. & Kopper, E. (1971) Biochemical detection of fetoplacental distress in risk pregnancies. *Lancet*, **ii**, 729–731.

Klopper, A. & Gardner, J. (1973) *Endocrine Factors in Labour*. Cambridge: Cambridge University Press.

Klopper, A., Masson, G., Campbell, Doris & Wilson, G. (1973). Estriol in plasma: a compartmental study. *American Journal of Obstetrics and Gynecology*, **117**, 21–26.

Laga, E. M., Driscoll, Shirley G. & Munro, H. N. (1974) Human placental structure: relationship to fetal nutrition. In *Lactogenic Hormones, Fetal Nutrition and Lactation* (Ed.) Josimovitch, J. B., Reynolds, Monica & Cobo, E. pp. 143–181. New York: Wiley.

Lauritzen, Ch. (1974) Dynamic tests of fetoplacental function and endocrine therapy. In *Hormone Investigation in Human Pregnancy* (Ed.) Scholler, R. pp. 399–418. Paris: Sepe.

Letchworth, A. T. & Chard, T. (1972) Placental lactogen levels as a screening test for fetal distress and neonatal asphyxia. *Lancet*, **i**, 704–706.

Letchworth, A. T., Boardman, R., Bristow, C., London, J. & Chard, T. (1971) A rapid semi-automated method for the measurement of human chorionic somatomammotrophin. The normal range in the third trimester and its relation to fetal weight. *Journal of Obstetrics and Gynaecology of the British Commonwealth*, **78**, 542–548.

Lindberg, B. S. & Nilsson, B. A. (1973) Human placental lactogen (HPL) levels in abnormal pregnancies. *Journal of Obstetrics and Gynaecology of the British Commonwealth*, **80**, 1046–1053.

Lindberg, B. S., Johansson, E. D. B. & Nilsson, B. A. (1974) Plasma levels of nonconjugated oestradiol-17β and oestriol in high risk pregnancies. *Acta Obstetrica et Gynecologica Scandinavica*, Supplement **32**, 37–51.

Lockwood, G. F. & Newman, R. L. (1974) Estriol determinations in random urine samples. *Obstetrics and Gynecology*, **43**, 343–346.

MacLeod, S. C., Mitton, D. M. & Avery, C. R. (1971) Relationship between elevated blood pressure and urinary estriols during pregnancy. *American Journal of Obstetrics and Gynecology*, **109**, 375–382.

Mathur, R. S., Leaming, A. B. & Williamson, H. O. (1973) Assessment of 'free' and conjugated estriol in uncomplicated and complicated pregnancy plasma. *American Journal of Obstetrics and Gynecology*, **117**, 316–320.

Michie, E. A. & Robertson, J. G. (1971) Amniotic and urinary oestriol assays in pregnancies complicated by rhesus isoimmunisation. *Journal of Obstetrics and Gynaecology of the British Commonwealth*, **78**, 34–40.

Moser, R. J., Hollingsworth, D. R., Carlson, J. W. & Lamotte, L. (1974) Human chorionic somatomammotrophin in normal adolescent primiparous pregnancy. I Effect of smoking. *American Journal of Obstetrics and Gynecology*, **120**, 1080–1086.

Niven, P. A. R., Ward, R. H. T. & Chard, T. (1974) Human placental lactogen levels in amniotic fluid in Rhesus isoimmunisation. *Journal of Obstetrics and Gynaecology of the British Commonwealth*, **81**, 988–990.

Oakey, R. E., Cawood, M. L. & Macdonald, R. R. (1974) Biochemical and clinical observations in a pregnancy with placental sulphatase and other enzyme deficiencies. *Clinical Endocrinology*, **3**, 131–148.

Pavlou, C., Chard, T., Landon, J. & Letchworth, A. T. (1973) Circulating levels of human placental lactogen in late pregnancy: the effect of glucose loading, smoking and exercise. *European Journal of Obstetrics, Gynaecology and Reproductive Biology*, **3**, 45–49.

Sciarra, J. J., Sherwood, L. M., Varma, A. A. & Lundberg, W. B. (1968) Human placental lactogen (HPL) and placental weight. *American Journal of Obstetrics and Gynecology*, **101**, 413–416.

Scommegna, A. (1973) Clinical uses of estriol assays. In *Obstetrics and Gynecology Annual*, Vol. 2 (Ed.) Wynn, R. M. pp. 455–79. New York: Appleton-Century-Crofts.

Scommegna, A. (1974) Concentrations of steroids and other hormones in amniotic fluid: changes in estrogen concentrations and their interpretation. In *Amniotic Fluid—Physiology, Biochemistry and Clinical Chemistry* (Ed.) Natelson, S., Scommegna, A. & Epstein, M. B. pp. 259–272. New York: Wiley.

Simmer, H. H., Tulchinsky, D., Gold, E. M., Frankland, Marjorie, Greipel, Margaret & Gold, Anita S. (1974) On the regulation of estrogen production by cortisol and ACTH in human pregnancy at term. *American Journal of Obstetrics and Gynecology*, **119**, 283–296.

Spellacy, W. N., Buhi, W. C. & Birk, S. A. (1975) The effectiveness of human placental lactogen measurements as an adjunct in decreasing perinatal deaths. *American Journal of Obstetrics and Gynecology*, **121**, 835–844.

Spellacy, W. N., Teoh, E. S., Buhi, W. C., Birk, S. A. & McCreary, S. A. (1971) Value of human chorionic somatomammotrophin in managing high risk pregnancies. *American Journal of Obstetrics and Gynecology*, **109**, 588–598.

Stringer, J., Anderson, M., Beard, R. W., Fairweather, D. V. I. & Steele, S. J. (1975) Very early termination of pregnancy (menstrual extraction). *British Medical Journal*, **iii**, 7–9.

Swapp, G. H., Masson, G. M. & Klopper, A. (1975) The renal clearance of oestriol in late human pregnancy. *British Journal of Obstetrics and Gynaecology*, **82**, 132–136.

Tamby Raja, R. L., Anderson, Anne B. M. & Turnbull, A. C. (1974) Endocrine changes in premature labour. *British Medical Journal*, **iv**, 67–71.

Targett, C. S., Gunesee, H., McBride, F. & Beischer, N. A. (1973) Evaluation of the effects of smoking on maternal oestriol excretion during pregnancy and on fetal outcome. *Journal of Obstetrics and Gynaecology of the British Commonwealth*, **80**, 815–821.

Townsley, J. D., Rubin, Elizabeth J. & Crystle, C. D. (1973) Evaluation of placental steroid 3-sulfatase and aromatase activities as regulators of estrogen production in human pregnancy. *American Journal of Obstetrics and Gynecology*, **117**, 345–50.

Tulchinsky, D. (1973) Placental secretion of unconjugated estrone, estradiol and estriol into the maternal and fetal circulation. *Journal of Clinical Endocrinology and Metabolism*, **36**, 1079–1087.

Tulchinsky, D. & Okada, D. M. (1975) Hormones in human pregnancy. IV Plasma progesterone. *American Journal of Obstetrics and Gynecology*, **121**, 293–299.

Tulchinsky, D., Frigoletto, F. D., Ryan, K. J. & Fishman, J. (1975) Plasma estetrol as an index of fetal well-being. *Journal of Clinical Endocrinology and Metabolism*, **40**, 560–567.

Tulchinsky, D., Hobel, C. J., Yeager, E. & Marshall, J. R. (1972) Plasma estradiol, estriol and progesterone in human pregnancy. II Clinical applications in Rh-isoimmunisation disease. *American Journal of Obstetrics and Gynecology,* **113,** 766–770.

Ursell, W., Brudenell, M. & Chard, T. (1973) Placental lactogen levels in diabetic pregnancy. *British Medical Journal,* **ii,** 80–82.

Wallace, Sheila J. & Michie, Eileen A. (1966) A follow-up study of infants born to mothers with low oestriol excretion during pregnancy. *Lancet,* **ii,** 560–563.

Ward, H., Rochman, H., Varnavides, L. A. & Whyley, G. A. (1973) Hormone and enzyme levels in normal and complicated pregnancies. *American Journal of Obstetrics and Gynecology,* **116,** 1105–1113.

Ward, R. H. T., Letchworth, A. T., Niven, P. A. R. & Chard, T. (1974) Placental lactogen levels in Rhesus isoimmunisation. *British Medical Journal,* **i,** 347–349.

Wilde, C. E. & Oakey, R. E. (1975) Biochemical tests for the assessment of fetoplacental function. *Annals of Clinical Biochemistry,* **12,** 83–118.

20

PLACENTAL FUNCTION (NON-HORMONAL ASPECTS)

Peter Baillie

The first human right is the right to be well born (Reid, 1970) and a major object of contemporary obstetrics is to ensure that this happens. At present the cornerstone of the medical practice designed to achieve this objective is accurate detection of a compromised fetus so that appropriate steps are taken to avoid further compromise. A bewildering profusion of tests for fetal condition has emerged in recent years. There is confusion in the minds of most clinicians about the value of these tests in clinical practice and careful evaluation is needed. Apart from the number of tests, the following factors contribute to this confusion and it is mandatory to keep these in mind when a particular test is being evaluated.

THE END-POINT AGAINST WHICH THE TEST IS EVALUATED

The traditional end-point is perinatal mortality but there is a growing realisation that this is too crude as subsequent neurological dysfunction in survivors is in many ways a greater disaster to both the community and the parents than is a perinatal death. Neurological condition is an ideal end-point but is unfortunately affected by many postnatal influences which make it difficult to relate the outcome to obstetric care and antenatal monitoring.

Three end-points that are being used increasingly as an index against which to compare tests of fetal well-being are a decreased fetal weight for gestational age (small for gestational age, dysmaturity), condition at birth and fetal distress in labour.

Neonatal weight for age is easy to measure and is widely used but has several disadvantages. Three different types of fetal growth retardation occur (Winick, Basel and Velasco, 1973), each with a different risk of subsequent neurological deficit. Ounsted and Ounsted (1973) have shown, furthermore, that up to 20 per cent of some subgroups may actually be advanced in infancy and childhood when compared with normally grown fetuses. In addition, appropriately grown fetuses may die in utero of a decreased placental margin of reserve (Gruenwald, 1970). Such deaths should be preventable by a test that gives adequate warning of the condition of the fetus.

Fetal condition at birth is an attractive end-point to the obstetrician as it relates immediately to the fetal condition, albeit intrapartum. It can be measured biologically or biochemically. The general relationship of both Apgar score (Drage et al, 1966) and the acid–base status at birth (Dawes, 1968; James, 1970) to subsequent neurological status is undoubted, and furthermore Apgar score and acid–base status are directly related (James et al, 1958; Crawford, 1965). Unfortunately, in clinical practice, these two measures often conflict and it is uncertain which is the better measure. When they are concordant, it has been suggested by Baillie (1974) that a one-minute Apgar score of 6 or less combined with a base excess gradient (maternal and fetal arterial) of more than 5 mEq/l is unacceptable in terms of the right to be well born. The critical question is whether minor degrees of disturbance of homeostasis which these values represent are likely to affect the infant in any way in its future development. Other measures have been used and it is possible that recent objective developments such as nerve conduction velocity, electroencephalogram and REM deep sleep ratios (Parmelee and Michaellis, 1971) will be more precise.

Fetal distress in labour has also been used as a measure of efficiency of antenatal tests (Letchworth and Chard, 1972) but, because of the many variables affecting especially the fetal heart rate, it bears an inadequate relationship to subsequent neurological outcome.

In summary therefore, the end-point against which the predictive value of antenatal tests must be measured is uncertain at present. It is likely that some measure of status at birth or soon thereafter is appropriate if the right to be well born is to be ensured.

FACTORS INTERFERING WITH EVALUATION OF ANTENATAL TESTS

Many conditions endanger the fetus, and some of them, such as the assessment of fetal condition by monitoring, will not assist in the management of, for example, accidental haemorrhage and prolapsed cord. Fetal compromise or death caused by such conditions should be excluded if the value of a test is to be assessed. Other variables interfere with the end-point, especially if the status at birth is considered. Such factors include prematurity, prolonged and difficult labour, sedation, operative delivery, cord compression, as well as technical errors in measurement of acid–base balance. Unpredictable events such as a sudden onset of severe pre-eclampsia may nullify the predictive value of an antenatal test performed a short time beforehand. It is apparent that if the predictive value of any measure is being tested, interfering or unpredictable factors should be excluded in the first instance. Unfortunately this is seldom apparent in the literature.

ATTITUDE OF CLINICIANS

The clinician must bear some responsibility for the present state of confusion. A clearcut answer is expected in most circumstances, and when in a few cases this is not forthcoming, the test is often discarded as useless (Dalley, 1961). A cursory application of fetal physiology is sufficient in order to conclude that many variables may affect the results of any test. It must be admitted that no evaluation of antenatal condition of the fetus is foolproof. Equally, however, clinicians should not expect too much of a test but should rather assess results obtained in the light of available physiological knowledge, with a clear understanding of what one is trying to achieve with the test. Excessive importance is often attached in a clinical situation to fetal size and age rather than to the actual condition of the fetus.

It is apparent from the above discussion that no ideal test of fetal well-being is available at present. The characteristics of an ideal test have been discussed by Baillie (1974). The most important are a sound physiological basis, precision and easy applicability to all patients attending an antenatal clinic. In general, these characteristics tend to be conflicting as the more precise tests are usually complicated. Antenatal monitoring is potentially more useful than intrapartum monitoring, as it will detect the fetus at risk of death prior to labour and hopefully those cases where labour should not be allowed, whereas even though intrapartum monitoring detects fetal distress during labour, appropriate delivery is not always immediately available and neurological damage continues. At the present time, however, intrapartum monitoring has played a highly significant role in reducing perinatal mortality in many institutions. The two methods are, of course, complementary.

METHODS OF MONITORING

Hormone assays, ultrasonic measurements and fetal breathing are discussed in Chapters 19, 15 and 16. The first two are the most widely utilised, although enzyme analysis, tests of transfer of substances and stress tests are of increasing interest.

Epidemiological associations

Although epidemiological risk factors are easily recognisable and have the advantage of broad application in conditions such as toxaemia and postmaturity, the amount of energy required to obtain an improvement in perinatal salvage is enormous. For example, the perinatal mortality of these conditions is raised by 50 per cent but is of a low order of magnitude, 17.6 and 17.9 per 1000 at 40 and 42 weeks respectively (Butler and Bonham,

1963). In addition, some of the fetuses that might be salvaged would be lost as a direct result of interference from conditions such as cord prolapse, infection and prematurity. In addition the majority of fetuses dying of a decreased placental reserve do not have a recognised epidemiological risk factor. It is unlikely that further studies of epidemiological associations will uncover risk factors of high probability as biological factors, beyond clinical control or measurement, are likely to be operative (Ounsted and Ounsted, 1973). Nevertheless Tipton and Lewis (1975) attributed a marked decrease in perinatal mortality to elective induction of labour near term. This was not found by Cole et al (1975) and has been challenged by Singer and Cooke (1975) as being consequent upon a liberalised abortion law rather than elective induction. There is therefore a strong argument for regarding epidemiological risk factors as warning indicators of the need to measure feto-placental reserve.

Maternal weight

Strand (1966) suggested that a failure of production of oestrogens by the feto-placental unit may result in maternal weight not increasing or even decreasing, because oestrogen production is largely responsible for water retention which accounts for about half of the increase of maternal weight in pregnancy.

Elder et al (1970) performed a three-phase study of maternal weight and girth changes (retrospective, prospective and changes in hypertension). Retrospectively in 703 patients they found a highly significant difference between the growth-retarded neonates and normal neonates when the average maternal weight gain from 34 weeks was considered (0.4 lbs/week among the growth-retarded group versus 0.68 lbs/week in normals, $P < 0.001$). In terms of weight change, 58.8 per cent of the growth-retarded group and 21.5 per cent of the normal controls had a static or falling weight after 34 weeks which was highly significant. Prospectively, 1128 patients were studied, of whom 431 were ultimately excluded because of insufficient data or interfering conditions. Again a highly significant relationship between static or falling maternal weight and growth retardation ($P < 0.001$) was found. However, only some 15 per cent of static or falling weight was associated with dysmaturity and five per cent of normal weight gain mothers delivered a growth-retarded fetus. No predictive value for fetal distress in labour was found. In essential hypertension, weight change was a clearer predictor of fetal weight for age. Of a total of nine perinatal deaths in the entire study, eight demonstrated static or falling maternal weight prior to fetal death.

Maternal weight and weight change is a crude measure and is subject to interference by dieting, anorexia, vomiting, diarrhoea and disease as well as being disguised by oedema. Eastman and Jackson (1968) have shown furthermore that weight gain is related to prepregnancy weight so it is probable that other more subtle influences are operative. Nevertheless, because of its simplicity and consequent wide applicability, weight change may result in a similar fetal salvage to more sophisticated measures which require preselection. Intelligent interpretation is necessary, however, and conditions in developing countries may be different to those in Western Europe.

Clinical examination

The detection of fetal growth retardation by clinical examination has been held back by a generation of clinicians more concerned with the mechanics of obstetrics than with the health of the intra-uterine patient. Beazley and Underhill (1970) have demonstrated that fundal height is an unsatisfactory guide to fetal age, particularly after 30 weeks gestation, because of the wide variation in maternal measurements and fetal size after this time. Many external measures have been made of uterine size and its changes during pregnancy (McSweeney, 1958; Insler et al, 1967; Niswander, Capraro and Van Coevering, 1970). Some include an allowance for the thickness of the abdominal wall (Poulos and Langstadt, 1953; Johnson, 1957). Furthermore, Loeffler (1967) has claimed that when attention is paid to these assessments some improvement in accuracy will result. Unfortunately these measurements were all attempts to calculate fetal size or gestational age and fetal outcome was not discussed. Elder et al (1970) attempted to relate girth measurement and fetal well-being. They found that girth measurement added nothing to the information gained by weighing patients. More recently, Baillie (1975) has found that change in 'uterine volume' as measured by girth and corrected fundal height is a more precise predictor of condition at birth than plasma oestriol and hPL. The reason for the discrepancy between these results and those of the Hammersmith group may be explained on several grounds. Firstly, differing end-points were utilised. Furthermore, mathematically the girth at its widest should be measured at right angles to the long axis of the uterus and not at right angles to the couch at the level of the umbilicus. Thirdly, changes in uterine volume are three-dimensional and not two-dimensional as measured by girth alone. Although observer differences are to be expected, and measurement must be exceptionally meticulous (Greene, Durhring and Smith, 1965), the rate of change in a normally growing fetus is greater than observer differences in most cases. It is probable that more precise measurement can be obtained with ultrasound.

In the acute situation a severely compromised fetus can be recognised clinically without recourse to the more desirable serial changes described above. An inappropriately decreased amount of liquor (Gadd, 1966) for the fetal and more especially uterine size is probably the best guide. Other clinical impressions such as inappropriate hardness of the fetal skull, abnormal uterine irritability and premature cervical ripening may suggest a compromised fetus (Greene, Durhring and Smith, 1965). This description conforms very closely to the description by Clifford (1954) of 'a uterus full of fetus' in postmaturity. It behoves clinicians to realise that adequate individual fetal survival depends far more precisely on fetal health than on fetal age and that the presence or absence of the 'preterm Clifford syndrome' should be evaluated at every antenatal examination.

Clinical suspicion at an antenatal clinic of the possibility of preterm labour supervening should be entertained in addition to an assessment of fetal health, as premature delivery and its sequelae account for a large proportion of perinatal mortality and morbidity. Inappropriate uterine activity with an apparently healthy fetus indicates either a risk of preterm delivery (which should be prevented) or normal labour at term in an individual with a fetus misdiagnosed as growth-retarded. Amniocentesis and assessment of amniotic fluid surfactant, which is discussed in Chapter 17 is helpful. In the present context of differentiation of the patient that requires suppression of uterine activity from the patient that requires delivery because of fetal growth retardation, difficulty in performing the procedure should alert the clinician to the latter possibility. Early appearance of surfactant activity (Gluck and Kulovich, 1973; Fairbrother, DuToit and Cheifitz, 1975) is significantly associated with growth retardation.

Enzyme analysis

More than 85 enzymes have been characterised in the placenta and evidence for the presence of many more is available (Hagerman, 1969). For use as a test, however, the presence of the enzyme in altered concentrations in maternal blood during pregnancy is essential. This characteristic is present in only a few placental enzymes.

Heat-stable alkaline phosphatase (HSAP)

The heat-stable isoenzyme has been clearly shown to originate in the cytotrophoblast and its function is related to and probably is a measure of mobilisation of calcium from maternal bone in order to provide material for skeletal calcification of the growing fetus (Weingold, 1968). The estimations present some difficulty in that not all authorities use an identical method, as is discussed by Weingold (1968). Sadovsky et al (1969) have utilised leucocyte alkaline phosphatase which has been shown to be related to urinary oestrogen excretion in pregnancy. The strongest protagonist of the usefulness of this enzyme is the Belfast School (Hunter, 1969; Hunter, Pinkerton and Johnson, 1970) although Curzen and Varna (1971) claim very limited usefulness. An abnormal result is usually regarded as one in which serial estimations are abnormally low or are rising rapidly above normal in the third trimester. Hunter has claimed excellent predictability for HSAP in pre-eclampsia, although most authorities claim that the wide range of normality limits clinical usefulness (Hagerman, 1969; Leroux and Perry, 1970). Quigley, Richards and Shier (1970) found no critical value denoting fetal death. Shane and Susuki (1974) found the test to be useless, and it suffers by comparison with other enzymes (Petrucco, Cellier and Fishtall, 1973; Ward et al, 1973).

Diamine oxidase (DAO)

Recently a sensitive, highly specific radioassay has been developed enabling the enzyme to be used as a screening procedure (Weingold, 1968). It is formed in the decidua but the fetus is necessary to induce enzyme production. Histamine, a major substrate, is important in the metabolism of all rapidly growing tissue with primary action in the microcirculation of damaged tissue (Kahlson, Rosengren and White, 1960). Fetal levels of histamine are far in excess of lethal concentrations to adults. Harrison, Peat and Heese (1974) have found urinary histamine excretion of value in assessing lung maturation in late pregnancy.

The level of DAO in maternal serum increases rapidly to 20 weeks, thereafter exceeding 500 mu/l of plasma and rising slowly to term. Weingold claims, therefore, a usefulness of this radioassay in early pregnancy and a good correlation between its use and fetal outcome in diabetics. The condition of a pregnant diabetic is one of hyperplacentation in which the antepartum condition of the fetus is often difficult to determine with the usual tests. Resnik and Levine (1969), however, found the estimation too variable for clinical use as did Ward et al (1972, 1973).

Cystine aminopeptidase (CAP)

The Commission of Enzymes of the International Union of Biochemistry (1964) decided to name enzymes according to the nature of the reaction they catalysed rather than according to substrates. The older name of 'oxytocinase' is therefore redundant. This enzyme acts on a number of substrates and is increased up to 100 times in pregnancy plasma. Leucine aminopeptidase does not increase in pregnancy (Hurry et al, 1972). There is no decline in levels at the end of pregnancy and therefore it is not related to the onset of labour (Titus, Reynolds and Glendenning Pace, 1960). Lower levels are found in pre-eclampsia, suggesting the possibility of vasopressin inactivation. Serial values show less fluctuation than is seen in the excretion of oestriol (Weingold, 1968). As it is produced in the placenta it is not useful in conditions where fetal jeopardy is due to fetal factors per se but serial determinations appear to be a valuable tool in predicting fetal death in certain pathologic pregnancies where placental dysfunction is the responsible factor (Babuna and Yenen, 1966). Hensleigh and Krantz (1970) showed that normal results did not exclude fetal compromise. Hurry et al (1972) showed that when the trend was downwards 4 out of 15 cases had a depressed fetus at birth, which is not significantly different from the incidence found in an unselected population.

Where enzyme tests have been compared with the more widely used ultrasonography or urinary oestriol excretion, they have generally suffered by comparison (Robinson et al, 1973; Ward et al, 1972, 1973). Combinations of values obtained with two or more enzyme tests give a high proportion of false-positive results, although a significant relationship between enzymes and other parameters is usually found (Weingold, 1968). In general CAP appears to correlate best with the condition of the fetus (Petrucco, Cellier and Fishtall, 1973; Pathak, Himaya and Mosher, 1974). Pathak, Himaya and Mosher (1974) have claimed that a low CAP and a high HSAP in combination reflect inadequate placental function.

In summary, enzyme estimations have found limited usefulness in general usage but several comments are worth bearing in mind:

1. None of the evaluation studies has been carried out under even relatively steady-state conditions, although one must accept that this may be unattainable in clinical practice.
2. The end-point to most studies is fetal death rather than fetal well-being. Weingold has pointed out that low levels of DAO may indicate a low reserve pregnancy with a poor infant prognosis.
3. It is apparent that a changing level (either up or down) of enzymatic activity may indicate a poor prognosis. This suggests that turnover or amount of substrate utilised may be a more appropriate measure of enzyme activity than simple random levels.

Tests of transfer of substances

Numerous tests of transfer of substances between mother and fetus have been proposed, but only two have had any degree of acceptance.

Atropine

The transfer and action of atropine were extensively studied by Hellman and Fillisti (1965). They found the end-point of transfer not clearly defined and required five points from the direct record, the analogue and a computer to ascertain it. The results were extremely variable and they considered the test to be of no clinical value. More recently Ionascu (1970) has reported that intravenous administration of atropine to the mother is 100 per cent successful in predicting the fetus that is in trouble. A physiological response is an increase in the fetal heart rate of 20 to 35 beats per minute. An abnormal response is either no change or a limited increase up to 10 beats per minute. John (1965a) administered a weight-graded dose intravenously in 51 cases. Ten cases, which showed no alteration of the fetal heart rate within 30 minutes, all showed evidence of 'reduced placental function', whereas only one of the responsive cases demonstrated this but was delivered three weeks after the test. Boyd, Chamberlain and Fergusson (1974) found the isoxsuprine transfer test to be of no value.

The atropine test has not found widespread popularity in obstetric practice in Britain, although most published reports attest to its value. Possibly standardisation will allow a clearer evaluation to be made. Whether by blocking the vagal reflex in an already asphyxiated fetus the use of atropine may be dangerous, is uncertain at present.

Selenomethionine

Garrow and Douglas (1968) and Lee and Garrow (1970) administered [75] Se selenomethionine intravenously to the mother. The count over the uterus (compared with that over the sternum) was taken for 20 minutes and repeated one to three days later. Excellent results are claimed, the apparatus being one-quarter the cost of ultrasonography, requiring 30 minutes training for the average house officer and providing an answer to high precision within 20 minutes. A total of 517 patients was studied altogether. The test can be repeated but requires 5 to 8 μCi the second time. All intra-uterine deaths were predicted and fetal growth retardation was significantly associated with a low uptake ratio. A specific advantage was that in two cases where the fetus was obviously clinically dysmature, but had a high uptake ratio, congenital abnormalities were found. The disadvantages of the test are that it can only be repeated twice, the source geometry is a problem and it is dependent upon gestational age. The final disadvantage is the uncertainty about the extent to which the selenomethionine uptake reflects ultimate fetal prognosis and well-being.

Stress tests

Davie (1969), in a follow-up study of the 1958 British Perinatal Mortality Survey, stated that 'certain perinatal events increase the likelihood of subsequent dysfunction but the extent or even the nature of this dysfunction is rather determined by the capacity of the fetus or baby to withstand the insult'. It would appear logical, therefore, to stress the fetus in a controlled measurable manner in order to predict the outcome of continued intra-uterine existence and/or labour for a particular fetus. The two natural stresses which have a direct relationship to fetal outcome are oxytocin-induced uterine activity and hypoxia.

Oxytocin stress tests

This is the most widely utilised of the two methods, but a surprising degree of variation exists in case selection, methodology, criteria for abnormality and end-point utilised (Table 20.1). It is therefore not surprising that opinions range from enthusiastic (Spurrett, 1971; Ray et al, 1972) to condemnatory (Baillie, 1974; Ewing, Farina and Otterson, 1974). The results obtained by these authors are summarised in Table 20.2.

It appears clear from Table 20.2 that, in the presence of a testing stimulus, oxytocin challenge could predict fetal status at birth. The most extreme challenge in the form of sufficient oxytocin to produce hyperstimulation was administered by Baillie (1974) and a positive response was obtained in all depressed neonates. He found the challenge to be potentially harmful and unquantifiable and therefore abandoned the test. Where the stress was less precise, a less clearly defined predictive value was obtained, extending even to Christie's findings (Christie and Cudmore, 1974) that the test was of no predictive value. Where the test was compared with urinary oestriols and ultrasonic cephalometry, it was found to be superior, both in predictive ability (Kubli, Kaeser and Hinselmann, 1969; Tchilinguirian, 1973) and in the time taken to obtain a result (Ray et al, 1972). Kubli, Kaeser and Hinselmann (1969) found, however, that amnioscopy was a better predictor of a low Apgar score.

In general, if an abnormal response is obtained with a mild stress, it can be stated with considerable confidence that the fetus is severely compromised. A normal response to a mild stress, however, does not exclude a compromised fetus, as it would be foolhardy to consider

Author	Method	Positive results	End-point
Kubli et al (1969)	Start at 2 mu. Increase until contractions occur and continued for 10 to 30 min. No oxytocin if spontaneous activity.	Late deceleration. Baseline tachycardia. Loss of beat-to-beat fluctuation.	Light for dates. IUD. Low Apgar score. Fetal distress in labour.
Spurrett (1971)	If doubtful FHR, oxytocin to produce contractions. If no abnormality then painful contractions for 10 min.	Late deceleration.	Not stated.
Ray et al (1972)	10 min baseline. Head of bed raised 30°. Start at 0.5 mu/min. Increased every 10 min until contractions every 3 to 4 min or late deceleration.	Uniform deceleration of FHR which reflects the waveform of uterine contractions with onset at or beyond acme of contraction or similar changes later.	Fetal distress in labour. Low Apgar scores. IUD.
Tchilinguirian (1973)	Oxytocin beginning at 0.5 mu/min. Doubled every 20 min (up to 4 mu) until 3 to 4 contractions every 10 min. Maintained for 30 min.	Late deceleration.	Not stated.
Boyd, Chamberlain and Fergusson (1974)	Contractions (painful or otherwise) 3 per 10 min lasting 30 sec with 90 sec in between, for 8 to 10 contractions.	Late deceleration.	Acidaemia during labour.
Christie and Cudmore (1974)	Baseline for 10 min. Head of bed raised 30 °. Slow increase until uncomfortable contractions with intervals 90 sec. Maintained for 10 min.	Late deceleration (lag > 15 sec, recovery > 15 sec, amplitude > 15 beats).	Urinary oestriols. Fetal distress in labour. Low Apgar score. High risk index. Gestational age.
Ewing et al (1974)	Baseline for 10 min. Start at 0.65 mu/min and increased every 10 min until uterine contractions every 3 to 4 min.	Uniform deceleration of FHR at or beyond peak of contraction or repetition during subsequent contractions.	Not stated.
Shifrin, Doctor and Lapidus (1974)	Infuse oxytocin if contractions < 150 Montevideo units.	Repeated late decelerations.	Not stated.
Baillie (1974)	Baseline for 10 min. Oxytocin to produce 8 painful uterine contractions. If no FHR changes, rate doubled to produce tetany for 3 to 7 min (augmented test).	Late deceleration during recovery from tetanic contraction.	Low Apgar scores.
Pose et al (1970)	A few uterine contractions (similar to normal labour) (intra-uterine pressure).	Late deceleration with intra-uterine pressure > 30 mm Hg.	Low Apgar scores.

Table 20.2. *Oxytocin stress tests—results.*

Author	Positive results		Negative results		Comment
	No.	Outcome	No.	Outcome	
Kubli et al (1969)	8	3 SFD 4 low Apgar 1 IUD	34	2 SFD 6 low Apgar	2 borderline responses. Missed 60% of low Apgar scores. Meconium a better prediction. Test time-consuming.
Spurrett (1971)	23	12 SFD 13 low Apgar 2 deaths	170	23 SFD 30 low Apgar	
Ray et al (1972)	15	9 low Apgar 3 IUD	43	3 low Apgar	5 suspicious, 13 technically unsatisfactory. Better than urinary oestriol and gives an earlier positive response. Time-consuming—90 minutes.
Tchilingiurian (1973)	9%	Not stated	81%	Not stated	
Boyd, Chamberlain and Fergusson (1974)	5	1 asphyxial NND 1 scalp pH < 7.25	30	1 IUD 1 asphyxial NND 4 scalp pH < 7.25	6 traces unsatisfactory. Should be used twice weekly. Not a good test.
Christie and Cudmore (1974)	9	4, with $\frac{1}{16}$ high risk score	35	3 low oestriol 1 fetal distress 5 low Apgar 2.4 high risk score	6 unsatisfactory. Value of negative test undisputed. Positive test not good—depends on stage of gestation and oxytocin.
Ewing et al (1974)	8	3 low Apgar 1 NND	47	Not stated other than normal	3 suspicious. 7 tests unsatisfactory. Mature fetus and positive OCT—deliver as soon as possible. Immature and positive OCT—other tests.
Schifrin, Doctor and Lapidus (1974)	5	3 IUD	45	All normal	Valuable test.
Baillie (1974)	5	5 low Apgar	53	Normal	Standard test useless. Augmented test good but dangerous.
Pose et al (1970)	8	6 low Apgar at 5 min	12	Vigorous at 5 min	Time-consuming.

that a few mild contractions could in any way be predictive of fetal condition after a full labour up to one week later, although no perinatal deaths have occurred where this has been found. Better standardisation of techniques and end-point would allow a better evaluation of this most promising avenue of antenatal investigation. At present, it appears best utilised where some other index of fetal compromise is present as it is time-consuming.

Hypoxic stress tests

Less attention has been paid to this than to oxytocin challenges. The reason is probably a fear of possible harm to the mother and fetus. Maternal welfare was not significantly altered by administration of 11.6 per cent oxygen (Fisher and Baillie, 1974) apart from a decreased Po_2 and mild hyperventilation. This is in accordance with Huckabee's findings (1958) that tissue oxygen debt as measured by excess lactate formation did not occur until the oxygen percentage was reduced to between 10 and 14 per cent. The effect on the fetus has been the subject of several studies (Hellman et al, 1961; John, 1965b; Copher and Huber, 1967; Baillie, 1974). Concentrations of oxygen ranging from 8 to 15 per cent were used for between and 20 minutes (Table 20.3). Wood et al (1971) utilised 10 per cent oxygen during early labour, for up to 20 minutes. This is not strictly comparable to the antenatal studies as the stress of contractions is superimposed. The test was considered to be harmful and was abandoned on ethical grounds. A striking discrepancy between the findings of Baillie and the other workers is apparent if predictive value is considered (Table 20.4). This was thought to be due to the lack of steady state conditions in the other studies, as the fetal heart rate is normally extremely labile, even when the mother is resting quietly (Hon, 1968).

In animal experiments, fetal tachycardia is thought to be an early response to mild asphyxia, whereas bradycardia is a late response (Mann, Prichard and Symmes, 1970). Bradycardia must therefore be considered dangerous when used as an end-point. Dawes (1974) has stated that, in chronic sheep preparations, the fetal heart changes are too variable to allow adequate interpretation, but he did not sedate the animals and used nine per cent oxygen in order to produce a similar maternal Po_2. The alarming and sometimes persistent bradycardia (associated with severe acidaemia) often encountered under these circumstances clearly points to profound tissue hypoxia. In a clinical application of this test Baillie achieved a reduction in the perinatal mortality rate as well as the incidence of depressed neonates, although the latter improvement was not statistically significant. No confirmation of these findings has been published and further evaluation must be awaited before definite conclusions about their value can be drawn.

Hyperoxic stress tests

Copher and Huber (1967) and Hellman et al (1961) administered 100 per cent oxygen and in a few cases showed bradycardia, i.e. possibly 'more normal'. Details of outcome are not available from the text and it would seem that this approach, which surmounts the danger of possible harm to the mother and fetus, is an avenue for future development.

Maternal exercise

Stembera and Hod (1968) described a three-minute two-step test in 15 healthy gravidas and 52 with pathological conditions (toxaemia, postmaturity, diabetes and previous repeated

Table 20.3. *Hypoxic stress tests.*

Author	Method	Positive results	End-point
Wood et al (1971)	10% oxygen with a face mask for 3 to 20 min.	Alteration in fetal heart rate or acidaemia.	Apgar scores at 2 minutes.
Hellman et al (1961)	12% oxygen for 10 min.	Fetal tachycardia.	Not assessed.
John (1965)	10% oxygen for 20 min. One-way valve.	Tachycardia followed by bradycardia.	Reduced placental function.
Copher and Huber (1967)	Randomised stimulation. 15% oxygen for a minimum of 7 min.	*Mild*: Post-stimulation tachycardia with loss of accommodation. *Gross*: Profound bradycardia with delayed recovery.	Fetal bradycardia (<110) in labour with return to normal > 30 sec.
Baillie (1974)	I.V. Pethidine 50 mg. When steady fetal heart rate, 12% oxygen for 15 min. with one-way valve.	Tachycardia with recovery delayed >4 min.	Apgar scores and feto-maternal pH and base excess gradients.

Table 20.4. *Hypoxic stress tests—results.*

Author	Positive results		Negative results		Comment
	No.	Outcome	No.	Outcome	
Wood et al (1971)	3	Not stated	11	Not stated	12 Apgar 7 to 10. Stress greater than labour. Abandoned because scalp Po_2 drop could not be predicted.
John (1965)	11	Normal	17	3 Abnormal	3 'delayed' responses abnormal.
Copher and Huber (1967)					Measures reduction of placental reserve capacity. 100% oxygen immediately afterwards resulted in augmentation of response in abnormals.
(a) Retrospective	43	13 Fetal distress	298	Not stated	
(b) Prospective	16	13 Fetal distress	116	0	
Baillie (1974)					The one abnormal negative response was performed 25 days before delivery. Explanations for other cases of abnormal response with good condition fetus (short labour, time interval and time to settle).
(a) Evaluation	10	6 Abnormal	56	1 Abnormal	

obstetric fetal deaths). The test was later modified to utilise a specially constructed bicycle. The fetal heart rate was recorded beforehand and for 10 minutes afterwards. They divided the fetal outcome into four groups:

  I. Normal pregnancy with normal neonate (N = 15). In this group there was no change in the fetal heart rate.
 II. Abnormal pregnancy with a normal neonate (N = 17). A shift towards tachycardia occurred in about one-quarter of the cases.
III. Variation in the fetal heart rate during labour, meconium staining of the liquor amnii but a vigorous neonate (N = 15). In this group, both tachycardia ($\pm$ 8 per cent) and bradycardia ($\pm$ 5 per cent) occurred after exercise.
 IV. Depressed neonates with a Wulf score of 6 or less (N = 20). A shift towards bradycardia occurred in $\pm$ 20 per cent of cases.

They noted that the shift may last a short time, but despite their suggestion of usefulness, this test has not found a place in present day obstetrics and their findings remain unconfirmed. The reasons for this are apparently a lack of standardised stress, no steady state conditions initially and difficulties in recording the fetal heart rate.

Fetal arousal

Goodlin and Schmidt (1972) utilised 2000 Hz pure-tone sound for 5 sec after a baseline fetal heart rate recording had been obtained. This was delivered through a 5-inch speaker fixed to the abdominal wall. The responses were divided into five categories (Table 20.5).

Table 20.5. *FHR variability and pattern of response to pure tone sound related to condition of babies at birth.*

Group	Baseline beat to beat variation	Response to sound
I	Reactive	Acceleration
II	Reactive	Deceleration
III	Reactive	No change
IV	Flat	No change
V	Flat	Deceleration

Adapted from Goodlin and Schmidt (1972).

Groups I and II comprised 411 women, all of whom gave birth to vigorous newborns, except for five difficult deliveries. Groups IV and V indicated that the fetus was asleep, medicated or asphyxiated. Group V comprised six fetuses out of 1700, all of whom were premortem or had neonatal seizures. He does state that the unresponsive pattern was not seen antenatally and that the same fetus responded with different patterns. It seems likely, therefore, that this test may well have a place intrapartum (subject to confirmation) but that it will be of limited use antepartum.

Fetal movements

Sadovsky, Yaffe and Polishuk (1974) recently summarised their extensive experience. They studied 80 normal and pathological pregnancies (diabetes, rhesus disease, polyhydramnios and postmaturity). The patients recorded fetal movements for 30 to 60 minutes three time

ng the day. A diurnal rate of movements for 12 hours was then calculated. If there were
than three movements per hour, then 6 to 12 hours were recorded. They noted a wide
e of movements (4 to 840) and confirmed that the patients recorded 87 per cent of the
ements (Sadovsky and Yaffe, 1973). Variables that appeared to affect the number of
ements were the character, occupation and cooperation of the mother, as well as the
e of pregnancy. A positive response was the cessation of fetal movements in the presence
pulsating fetal heart. Fifteen such cases resulted in one normal newborn and ten intra-
ine deaths (after one day in eight cases, two days in one patient and twelve days in one
ent). They state that five intra-uterine deaths could have been prevented if they had acted
heir findings. Sixty-five cases apparently resulted in a normal fetus, 17 showing 4 to 10
ements per 12 hours. Brotanek and Scheffs (1973) related increased movements and
ociated saltatory fetal heart rate patterns in maternal conditions that compromise the
s but give no results. Matthews (1972, 1973) reports similar encouraging results. He in-
ly reported nine stillbirths and two hypoxic neonatal deaths, and differentiated between
ll-for-dates and normally grown fetuses. In six small-for-dates fetuses, death was.
eded by decreased fetal movements for one to eight weeks. Low urinary oestriol excre-
was found in only one case. The remaining five fetuses were all normally grown (one,
ever, was below the 10th percentile) and retained vigorous movement up to the date of
death or delivery. His second publication reported 31 small-for-dates fetuses with no
births. He does not specify what he considers to be decreased fetal movement but in such
s 50 per cent (four out of eight) demonstrated 'fetal distress', whereas this was only
rded in one out of 22 with vigorous fetal movement. He noted that the decrease of fetal
vity was definite and gradual and persisted for at least one week, and stressed that the
ject of fetal movements should be raised casually in order to avoid maternal distress and
alarms.

David, Weaver and Pearson (1975) studied increases in fetal activity when a Doppler
em of recording the fetal heart rate was utilised for one hour, the movements being
rded for 24 hours. They noted that four fetuses associated with absent movements for at
12 hours before the fetal heart tones disappeared. In summary, fetal movement or its
onse to a stimulus such as the Doppler effect appears to be a simple and extremely
mising avenue of antenatal fetal monitoring, perhaps combined with fetal heart rate
itoring. The shortcomings (e.g. in normally grown fetuses) have not yet been fully
ified.

cellaneous

onium

ham (1973) found that when dark green or yellow meconium was observed by am-
copy prior to onset of labour in 17 cases, there were three perinatal deaths and five
ses had an Apgar score of less than six. He also noted that when liquor was decreased, a
per cent perinatal mortality had been obtained as well as a 10 per cent incidence of
ressed neonates and therefore considered amnioscopy to be an extremely useful clinical
. Mandelbaum (1973) suggests amniocentesis rather than amnioscopy. Beard (1968), in
trospective analysis of antepartum stillbirths, found that there was usually no indication
amnioscopy prior to death, and analysis of individual case histories revealed that
conium was present in only 40 per cent of the stillbirths. He did state, however, that an
ence of liquor amnii was an ominous sign that required further investigation including
nioscopy, which Henry (1969) subsequently confirmed. It appears therefore, that when

the cervix permits passage of an amnioscope, meconium is an indication for immediate delivery and that a decreased amount of liquor should put the clinician on his guard. Unfortunately the cervix is usually uneffaced until near term and a negative result does not exclude fetal compromise. The results of several larger studies do not appear to justify the considerable time required from medical personnel and patient discomfort in this investigation.

Alpha-fetoprotein (AFP)

This is discussed in Chapter 17. Seppala and Ruoslahti (1973) have found fetal distress in 59 per cent of cases where abnormal levels were found and in only 11 per cent of cases where normal levels were found. Garoff and Seppala (1973) found HPL and AFP to be complementary. Cohen, Graham and Lau (1973) found in seven cases that the maternal serum level was greater than 250 ng/ml. All were morbid or suffered a perinatal death. This test holds great promise in the future for reducing the incidence of congenital defects.

Physical measures

MacDonald (1972) found that persistent or recurrent ferning in early pregnancy related very well to subsequent dysmaturity, and this simple parameter has perhaps not been as widely used as it warrants. The value has not been confirmed. Organ et al (1974) in animal studies has used the pre-ejection period of the fetal heart which is shortened in asphyxia and lengthened in cord compression. It is far more suitable for intrapartum use and technical difficulties abound. Wheeler and Guerard (1974) have commented on the potential use of beat-to-beat variations antenatally, but no study is available.

CONCLUSIONS

No ideal antenatal test of fetal well-being is yet available. Tests may be grouped into those that can be applied to all cases in a population and those which specifically elucidate the intra-uterine status of a selected individual fetus. The former group tends to be simple but crude and imprecise, whereas the latter group tends to be complicated and requires preselection and an excellent physiological knowledge in order to interpret results, a quality lacking in many obstetrics departments.

Recent physiological knowledge about the intra-uterine patient and development of non-invasive measuring techniques has opened up many avenues of study, and it is highly likely that this 'second generation' of tests will outmode the first generation of urinary oestriols, serum enzymes and biparietal diameters, although at present most are in the preliminary stages of evaluation. It is worth noting that many measures have strong protagonists but few studies can be compared adequately because of imprecision of end-point and differences in case studies. Because many of the physiological variables of the intra-uterine patient are unknown or unmeasurable, it is likely that the future lies in dynamic tests such as fetal movement, breathing or heart recording with an initially imposed steady state. Finally, the end-point against which the results are to be evaluated must conform to the aim of modern obstetrics, that is, the right to be well born. This is of necessity more stringent than that widely used parameter perinatal death.

REFERENCES

Babuna, C. & Yenen, E. (1966) Enzymatic determination of placental function. *American Journal of Obstetrics and Gynecology*, **95**, 925.

Baillie, P. (1974) Nonhormonal methods of antenatal monitoring. *Clinics in Obstetrics and Gynaecology*, **1**, 103.

Baillie, P. (1975) *The State of the Fetus at Birth*. MD Thesis, University of Cape Town.

Barham, K. A. (1973) Amnioscopy . . . Is it worthwhile? *Australian and New Zealand Journal of Obstetrics and Gynaecology*, **11**, 209.

Beard, R. W. (1968) The effect of fetal blood sampling on Caesarean section for fetal distress. *Journal of Obstetrics and Gynaecology of the British Commonwealth*, **75**, 1291.

Beard, R. W. & Roberts, G. M. (1970) A prospective approach to the diagnosis of intrauterine growth retardation. *Proceedings of the Royal Society of Medicine*, **63**, 501.

Beazley, J. M. & Underhill, R. A. (1970) The fallacy of fundal height. *British Medical Journal*, **iv**, 404.

Boyd, I. E., Chamberlain, G. V. P. & Fergusson, I. L. C. (1974) The oxytocin stress test and isoxsuprine placental transfer test in the management of suspected placental insufficiency. *Journal of Obstetrics and Gynaecology of the British Commonwealth*, **81**, 120.

Brotanek, V. & Scheffs, J. (1973) The pathogenesis and significance of saltatory patterns of fetal heart rate. *International Journal of Gynaecology and Obstetrics*, **11**, 223.

Butler, N. R. & Bonham, D. G. (1963) *British Perinatal Mortality Survey 1958. First Report*. Edinburgh: Livingstone.

Christie, G. B. & Cudmore, D. W. (1974) The oxytocin challenge test. *American Journal of Obstetrics and Gynecology*, **118**, 327.

Clifford, C. H. (1954) Postmaturity—with placental dysfunction. *Journal of Pediatrics*, **44**, 1.

Cohen, H., Graham, H. & Lau, H. L. (1973) Fetoprotein in pregnancy. *American Journal of Obstetrics and Gynecology*, **115**, 881.

Cole, R. A., Howie, P. G. & MacNaughton, M. C. (1975) Elective induction of labour. *Lancet*, **i**, 767.

Copher, D. E. & Huber, C. P. (1967) Heart rate response of the human fetus to induced maternal hypoxia. *American Journal of Obstetrics and Gynecology*, **98**, 320.

Crawford, J. S. (1965) Maternal and cord blood at delivery. *Biologia Neonatorum*, **8**, 131.

Curzen, P. & Varna, R. (1971) A comparison of heat stable alkaline phosphatase and urinary estriol excretion in the mother as placental function tests. *Journal of Obstetrics and Gynaecology of the British Commonwealth*, **78**, 686.

Dalley, G. (1961) Experience with the vacuum extractor. *Proceedings of the Third World Congress of Obstetrics and Gynaecology, Vienna, 1961*. Vol. 3, p. 93.

David, H., Weaver, J. B. & Pearson, J. F. (1975) Doppler ultrasound and fetal activity. *British Medical Journal*, **i**, 62.

Davie, R. (1969) In *Perinatal Problems* (Ed.) Butler, N. R. & Alberman, E. D. Edinburgh: Livingstone.

Dawes, G. S. (1968) *Fetal and Neonatal Physiology*. Chicago: Year Book Publishers.

Dawes, G. S. (1974) Fetal circulation and breathing. *Clinics in Obstetrics and Gynaecology*, **1**, 139.

Drage, J. S., Kennedy, C. & Berendes, H. W. (1966) The 5 minute Apgar scores and 4 year psychological performance. *Developmental Medicine and Child Neurology*, 141.

Eastman, N. J. & Jackson, E. (1968) Weight relationships in pregnancy; the bearing of maternal weight gain and pre-pregnancy weight on birth weight in full term pregnancies. *Obstetrical and Gynecological Survey*, **23**, 1003.

Elder, M. G., Burton, E. R., Gordon, H., Hawkins, D. F. & McClure Browne, J. C. (1970) Maternal weight and girth changes in late pregnancy and diagnosis of placental insufficiency. *Journal of Obstetrics and Gynaecology of the British Commonwealth*, **77**, 481.

Ewing, D. E., Farina, J. R. & Otterson, W. N. (1974) Clinical application of the oxytocin challenge test. *Obstetrics and Gynecology*, **43**, 536.

Fairbrother, P. F., DuToit, I. L. & Cheifitz, R. L. (1975) The amniotic fluid foam test and fat cell count in malnourished and well-nourished fetuses. *British Journal of Obstetrics and Gynaecology*, **82**, 182.

Fisher, A. & Baillie, P. (1974) Nonhormonal methods of antenatal monitoring. *Clinics in Obstetrics and Gynaecology*, **1**, 114.

Gadd, R. L. (1966) The volume of the liquor amnii. *Proceedings of the Royal Society of Medicine*, **59**, 1131.

Garoff, L. & Seppala, M. (1973) α-Fetoprotein and human placental lactogen levels in maternal serum in multiple pregnancies. *Journal of Obstetrics and Gynaecology of the British Commonwealth*, **80**, 695.

Garrow, J. S. & Douglas, C. P. (1968) A rapid method for assessing intrauterine growth by radio-active selenomethionine uptake. *Journal of Obstetrics and Gynaecology of the British Commonwealth*, **75**, 1034.

Gluck, L. & Kulovich, M. V. (1973) Lecithin:sphingomyelin ratios in amniotic fluid in normal and abnormal pregnancies. *American Journal of Obstetrics and Gynecology*, **115**, 539.

Goodlin, R. C. & Schmidt, W. (1972) Human fetal arousal levels as indicated by heart rate recordings. *American Journal of Obstetrics and Gynecology,* **114,** 613.

Greene, J. W., Durhring, J. L. & Smith, K. (1965) Placental function tests. *American Journal of Obstetrics and Gynecology,* **92,** 1030.

Grunewald, P. (1970) Perinatal death of full sized and full term infants. *American Journal of Obstetrics and Gynecology,* **107,** 1022.

Hagerman, D. D. (1969) Enzymology of the placenta. In *Fetus and Placenta* (Ed.) Klopper, A. & Diczfalusky, E. p. 413.

Harrison, V. C., Peat, G. & Heese, H. deV. (1974) Fetal growth in relation to histamine concentration in urine. *Journal of Obstetrics and Gynaecology of the British Commonwealth,* **81,** 686.

Hellman, L. M. & Fillisti, L. P. (1965) Analysis of the atropine test for placental transfer in gravidas with toxaemia and diabetes. *American Journal of Obstetrics and Gynecology,* **91,** 797.

Hellman, L. M., Johnston, H. L., Tolks, W. E. & Jones, E. H. (1961) Some factors affecting the fetal heart rate. *American Journal of Obstetrics and Gynecology,* **82,** 1055.

Henry, G. R. (1969) The role of amnioscopy in the prevention of antepartum hypoxia of the fetus. *Journal of Obstetrics and Gynaecology of the British Commonwealth,* **76,** 790.

Hensleigh, P. H. & Krantz, K. E. (1970) Oxytocinase and placental function. *American Journal of Obstetrics and Gynecology,* **107,** 1233.

Hon, E. H. (1968) *An Atlas of Fetal Heart Rate Patterns.* New Haven: Harty.

Huckabee, W. E. (1958) Relationships of pyruvate and lactate during anaerobic metabolism. III. Effect of breathing low oxygen gases. *Journal of Clinical Investigation,* **37,** 264.

Hunter, R. J. (1969) Serum heat stable alkaline phosphatase: an index of placental function. *Journal of Obstetrics and Gynaecology of the British Commonwealth,* **76,** 1057.

Hunter, R. J., Pinkerton, J. H. & Johnston, H. (1970) Serum placental alkaline phosphatase in normal pregnancy and pre-eclampsia. *Obstetrics and Gynecology,* **36,** 536.

Hurry, D. J., Tovey, J. E., Robinson, D. A., Beynon, C. L. & Cooper, K. (1972) Lower abdominal pain in normal and complicated pregnancies. *Journal of Obstetrics and Gynaecology of the British Commonwealth,* **79,** 788.

Insler, V., Bernstein, D., Rikover, M. & Segal, T. (1967) Estimation of fetal weight in utero by simple external palpation. *American Journal of Obstetrics and Gynecology,* **98,** 292.

Ionascu, D. R. (1970) Screening for fetal distress before the onset of labour using the atropine test. *Obstetrics and Gynecology,* **70,** 465.

James, L. S. (1970) Experimental production of brain lesions in subhuman primates by asphyxia at birth. In *Fetal Growth and Development* (Ed.) Waisman, H. A. & Kerr, G. R. p. 253. New York: McGraw Hill.

James, L. S., Weisbrot, I. M., Prince, C. E., Holaday, D. A. & Apgar, V. (1958) The acid base status of human infants in relation to birth asphyxia and the onset of respiration. *Journal of Pediatrics,* **52,** 379.

John, A. H. (1965a) Placental transfer of atropine and the effect on the fetal heart rate. *British Journal of Anaesthesia,* **37,** 57.

John, A. H. (1965b) The effect of maternal hypoxia on the heart rate of the fetus in utero. *British Journal of Anaesthesia,* **36,** 515.

John, A. H. (1966) The accuracy of direct auscultation and the normal variation of the fetal heart rate. *Journal of Obstetrics and Gynaecology of the British Commonwealth,* **73,** 983.

Johnson, R. (1957) Calculations in estimating fetal weight. *American Journal of Obstetrics and Gynecology,* **74,** 929.

Kahlson, G., Rosengren, E. & White, T. (1960) Fetal histamine formation. *Journal of Physiology,* **151,** 131.

Kubli, F. W., Kaeser, O. & Hinselmann, M. (1969) In *The Feto-Placental Unit* (Ed.) Pecile, A. & Finzic, p. 323. Amsterdam: Excerpta Medica.

Lee, P. & Garrow, J. S. (1970) A clinical evaluation of the selenomethionine uptake test. *Journal of Obstetrics and Gynaecology of the British Commonwealth,* **77,** 982.

Leroux, M. & Perry, W. F. (1970) Serum heat stable alkaline phosphatase in pregnancy. *American Journal of Obstetrics and Gynecology,* **108,** 235.

Letchworth, A. T. & Chard, T. (1972) Placental lactogen levels as a screening test for fetal distress and neonatal asphyxia. *Lancet,* **i,** 704.

Loeffler, F. E. (1967) Clinical fetal weight prediction. *Journal of Obstetrics and Gynaecology of the British Commonwealth,* **74,** 675.

MacDonald, R. R. (1972) Ferning in early pregnancy. *Journal of Obstetrics and Gynaecology of the British Commonwealth,* **79,** 1087.

Mandelbaum, B. (1973) Gestational meconium in the high risk pregnancies. *British Journal of Obstetrics and Gynaecology,* **42,** 87.

Mann, L. I., Prichard, J. & Symmes, D. (1970) E.E.G., E.C.G. and acid base observations during acute fetal hypoxia. *American Journal of Obstetrics and Gynecology,* **106,** 39.

Matthews, D. D. (1972) Measuring placental function. *British Medical Journal,* **i,** 439.

Matthews, D. D. (1973) Fetal movements and fetal well being. *Lancet*, **i**, 1315.

McSweeney, D. (1958) Fetal weight estimation. *American Journal of Obstetrics and Gynecology*, **76**, 1279.

Niswander, K. R., Capraro, V. J. & Van Coevering, R. J. (1970) Estimation of birth weight by quantified external uterine measurements. *Obstetrics and Gynecology*, **36**, 294.

Organ, L. W., Bernstein, A., Smith, K. C. & Rowe, I. H. (1974) Pre-ejection period of the fetal heart. *American Journal of Obstetrics and Gynecology*, **120**, 49.

Ounsted, M. & Ounsted, C. (1973) *On Fetal Growth Rate; its Variations and their Consequences*. London: Heinemann.

Parmelee, A. H. & Michaellis, R. (1971) *Neurological Examination of the Newborn Exceptional Infant*, Vol. 2. New York: Bruner, Mazel.

Pathak, S., Himaya, A. & Mosher, R. (1974) Small for dates syndrome. Some biochemical considerations in prenatal diagnosis. *American Journal of Obstetrics and Gynecology*, **120**, 32.

Petrucco, O. M., Cellier, K. & Fishtall, A. (1973) Diagnosis of intrauterine fetal growth retardation by serial serum oxytocinase, urinary estrogen and serum heat stable alkaline phosphatase. *Journal of Obstetrics and Gynaecology of the British Commonwealth*, **80**, 499.

Pose, S. V., Castillo, J. B., Mora-Rojas, E. O., Soto-Yances, A. & Caldeyro-Barcia, R. (1970) Test of fetal tolerance to induced uterine contractions for the diagnosis of chronic fetal distress. *International Journal of Gynaecology and Obstetrics*, **8**, 142.

Poulos, P. & Langstadt, J. (1953) The volume of the uterus during labour and its correlation with birth weight. *American Journal of Obstetrics and Gynecology*, **65**, 233.

Quigley, G. J., Richards, R. T. & Shier, K. J. (1970) Heat stable alkaline phosphatase. *American Journal of Obstetrics and Gynecology*, **106**, 340.

Ray, M., Freeman, R., Pine, S. & Hesselgesser, R. (1972) Clinical experience with the oxytocin challenge test. *American Journal of Obstetrics and Gynecology*, **114**, 1.

Reid, D. E. (1970) The right and responsibility. *American Journal of Obstetrics and Gynecology*, **108**, 825.

Resnik, R. & Levine, R. J. (1969) Plasma diamine oxidase activity in pregnancy in re-appraisal. *American Journal of Obstetrics and Gynecology*, **104**, 1061.

Robinson, H. P., Chatfield, W. R., Logan, R. W., Tweedie, A. K. & Barnard, W. P. (1973) A scoring system for the assessment of multiple methods of monitoring. *Journal of Obstetrics and Gynaecology of the British Commonwealth*, **80**, 230.

Sadovsky, E. & Yaffe, H. (1973) Daily fetal movement recording and fetal prognosis. *Obstetrics and Gynecology*, **41**, 845.

Sadovsky, E., Yaffe, H. & Polishuk, W. K. (1974) Fetal movement monitoring in normal and pathological pregnancy. *International Journal of Gynaecology and Obstetrics*, **12**, 75.

Sadovsky, E., Diamant, Y. Z., Suckerman, H. & Polishuk, W. Z. (1969) Leucocyte alkaline phosphatase in pre-eclampsia. *Journal of Obstetrics and Gynaecology of the British Commonwealth*, **16**, 538–541.

Schifrin, B. S., Doctor, G. S. & Lapidus, M. (1974) Evaluation of the oxytocin challenge test. *Obstetrics and Gynecology*, **43**, 617.

Seppala, M. & Ruoslahti, E. (1973) α-Fetoprotein in maternal serum. A new marker for detection of fetal distress and intrauterine death. *American Journal of Obstetrics and Gynecology*, **115**, 48.

Shane, J. M. & Susuki, K. (1974) Placental alkaline phosphatase: A review and revaluation of its application in monitoring fetoplacental function. *Obstetrical and Gynecological Survey*, **29**, 97.

Singer, A. & Cooke, I. D. (1975) Induction of labour and perinatal mortality. *British Medical Journal*, **ii**, 35.

Spurrett, B. (1971) Stressed cardiotocography in late pregnancy. *Journal of Obstetrics and Gynaecology of the British Commonwealth*, **78**, 894–900.

Stembera, Z. K. & Hod, R. J. (1967) The 'exercise test' as an early diagnostic aid for fetal distress. In *Intrauterine Dangers to the Fetus* (Ed.) Horsky, J. & Stembera, Z. K. p. 349. Amsterdam: Excerpta Medica.

Strand, A. (1966) The function of the placenta and 'placental insufficiency' with special reference to the development of prolonged fetal distress. *Acta Obstetrica et Gynecologica Scandanavica*, **45**, Supplement 1, 125.

Tchilinguirian, N. G. O. (1973) Fetal monitoring in high risk pregnancy. *Clinical Obstetrics and Gynecology*, **16**, 329–346.

Tipton, R. H. & Lewis, B. V. (1975) Induction for labour and perinatal mortality. *British Medical Journal*, **i**, 391.

Titus, M. A., Reynolds, D. R. & Glendenning Pace, E. W. (1960) Plasma aminopeptidase activity (oxytocinase) in pregnancy and labour. *American Journal of Obstetrics and Gynecology*, **80**, 1124.

Ward, H., Whyley, G. A. & Millar, M. D. (1972) Serial serum diamine oxidase estimations in normal singleton and twin pregnancies and in abnormal pregnancies. *Journal of Obstetrics and Gynaecology of the British Commonwealth*, **79**, 216.

Ward, H., Whyley, G. A., Fricker, E. S. A. & Stoten, A. E. (1973) Serum heat stable alkaline phosphatase compared with urinary estriol in abnormal pregnancy. *Australian and New Zealand Journal of Obstetrics and Gynaecology*, **13**, 22.

Weingold, A. G. (1968) Enzymatic indices of fetal environment. *Clinical Obstetrics and Gynecology*, **11**, 1081.

Wheeler, T. & Guerard, P. (1974) Fetal heart rate during late pregnancy. *Journal of Obstetrics and Gynaecology of the British Commonwealth,* **81,** 348.

Winick, M., Basel, J. A. & Velasco, E. G. (1973) Effects of prenatal nutrition upon pregnancy risk. *Clinical Obstetrics and Gynecology,* **16,** 184–198.

Wood, C., Hammond, J., Lumley, J. & Newman, W. (1971) Effect of maternal inhalation of 10% oxygen upon the human fetus. *Australian and New Zealand Journal of Obstetrics and Gynaecology,* **11,** 85.

21

FACTORS INFLUENCING PERINATAL WASTAGE

Eva Alberman

Perinatal wastage comprises late fetal deaths and neonatal deaths occurring in the first week. In the United Kingdom late fetal deaths are stillbirths of 28 weeks gestation or more. Similar definitions are used by the World Health Organization for international comparisons, but many countries use different definitions and such variations are described individually in international publications. Comparisons which are carried out without taking account of the differences in definition can be very misleading (Chase, 1967). When expressed as a rate, perinatal mortality is usually calculated as the rate per thousand total live and stillbirths from which the deaths were derived. The combined rate is used because of the difficulty in defining signs of life after birth, and because many of the causes of stillbirth and very early neonatal death are the same.

Like other mortality rates in the maternal and child health field, the perinatal rate has fallen fairly consistently since 1931 when it was first recorded in this country (Figure 21.1). There is still little evidence that the rate is levelling out, even in countries with lower rates than our own.

Until comparatively recently the neonatal component of perinatal deaths was responsible for a relatively small proportion of first year (infant) deaths, and this is still true in the developing countries and very poor communities. Table 21.1 shows how first week (early

415

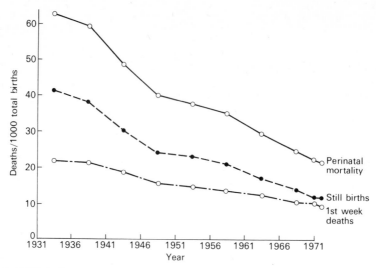

Figure 21.1. Stillbirth, first week death and perinatal mortality rate in England and Wales 1931–1971. Derived from *Statistical Review for the Year 1972* (Office of Population, Censuses and Surveys, 1974).

neonatal) deaths tend to make up an increasing proportion of infant mortality as the latter falls. This is because in communities with very high infant mortality rates the majority of these deaths are due to gastrointestinal or respiratory infections, mostly preventible by simple hygienic measures. It is the rapid reduction of these diseases that has focused attention on the more resistant neonatal and late fetal deaths.

The ratio of stillbirths to early neonatal deaths also varies in a systematic fashion, the stillbirth rate having fallen faster than the neonatal death rate in this country. During 1931 to 1935 in England and Wales stillbirths made up 66 per cent of the perinatal rate, while in 1972 this proportion had fallen to 55 per cent.

The present account outlines the causes of perinatal deaths, and their relative importance, the measures which have already effected improvements, and those which will be necessary to accelerate the rate of improvement.

Table 21.1. *Infant and early neonatal mortality rates—1972.*

	Infant mortality rate	Early neonatal mortality rate	$\dfrac{\text{Early neonatal mortality rate}}{\text{Infant mortality rate}} \times 100$
Sweden	10.8	7.5	69.4
Netherlands	11.7	7.4	63.2
Japan	11.7	6.1	52.1
England and Wales	17.2	9.8	57.0
Venezuela	51.7	16.7	32.3
Mauritius	63.8	24.9	39.0
Chile	71.1	19.2	27.0

Data from *World Health Statistics Annual for 1972* (Published 1975).

PERINATAL DEATHS BY CERTIFIED CAUSE

Meaningful data on causes of perinatal death are still surprisingly difficult to obtain. In the majority of such deaths the causes are multifactorial and it is misleading to try to give a single cause. However, this problem is compounded by the current International Classification of Diseases (1967) which is used in selecting and coding the causes as assigned on death certificates. In particular, unless the death of a premature infant is coded as 'immaturity unqualified', one has no indication of its maturity. Thus a death from pneumonia in a baby of 28 weeks maturity might be coded exactly as would such a death at 44 weeks, although the pathology may be quite different. In this country data on gestational age are not routinely collected. The only data on birthweight in livebirths are those on births weighing 2500 g or less and these stem from birth notifications, which cannot at present be related to birth or death certificates. The importance of such data can be gauged from Table 21.2, which shows that in 1972 60.7 per cent of all perinatal deaths (58.7 per cent of stillbirths and 63.3 per cent of first week deaths) weighed 2500 g or less.

Table 21.2. *Perinatal deaths by birthweight, England and Wales, 1972.*

Birthweight group (g)	Stillbirths		First week deaths		Perinatal deaths		Total births	
	No.	%	No.	%	No.	%	No.	%
Up to 2000	3878	44.1	3628	50.8	7506	47.1	17 245	2.3
2001–2500	1283	14.6	891	12.5	2174	13.6	35 871	4.9
over 2500	3638	41.3	2625	36.7	6263	39.3	681 123	92.8
Total	8799	100.0	7144	100.0	15 943	100.0	734 239	100.0

Data from Department of Health and Social Security (personal communication, 1972).

There is an International Classification of Diseases (ICD) coding specifically designed for perinatal deaths, the 'P' coding, and in Table 21.3 an attempt has been made to group this in a meaningful way in order to obtain a picture of the relative importance of different types of cause, including immaturity. These causes for 1972 in England and Wales (Office of Population, Censuses and Surveys, 1974) have been grouped as follows: congenital malformations; those ascribed by the author to intrapartum causes; those ascribed to antepartum causes; other specific causes and those considered to be associated with premature labour, 'immaturity'.

The congenital malformations group is self-explanatory. Intrapartum causes comprise those from birth trauma or asphyxia, that is, difficult labours, birth injury, cord complications, placenta praevia and premature placental separation. Most of these cause intrapartum or early neonatal deaths. Macerated stillbirths, placental infarction and 'other fetal causes' are those deaths assumed to have occurred before the onset of labour.

The causes considered to be associated primarily with immaturity comprise hyaline membrane disease, immaturity unqualified, cervical incompetence and multiple births. Certainly these do not comprise all deaths associated with immaturity, and probably they include some which are not. However, these are the causes which are known to be associated with very low birthweight, and it seems likely that this group overlaps largely with the first week deaths of babies weighing 2000 g or less (Table 21.2), after excluding congenital malformations.

The major groups of perinatal deaths are due to birth injury and asphyxia, to immaturity, and congenital malformations. If we consider only stillbirths, immaturity is not important; in

Table 21.3. *Registered causes of perinatal deaths in England and Wales (1972)—percentage distribution of different groups.*

International classification of causes of death; Abbreviated list 'P'	Registered causes grouped as in text	Still-births	First-week deaths	Stillbirths and first-week (perinatal) deaths
69–80	Congenital malformations	22.5	18.0	20.5
36–37; 40; 57; 61	'Immaturity'	2.8	40.6	19.7
21–35; 42–43; 47–52; 58–60; 62–66	'Intrapartum' difficult labour cord complications placenta praevia placental separation	28.6	29.2	28.9
67–68; 44–46	'Antepartum' maceration unknown cause placental infarction placental insufficiency	25.1	0.5	14.1
12–17	Maternal toxaemias	9.0	1.0	5.4
53–56	Haemolytic disease	3.1	1.7	2.5
1–11; 18–20; 38–39; 41	Maternal diseases and other complications	8.9	2.2	5.9
81–100	Fetal or neonatal infection, diseases or external injury	0.0	6.8	3.0
1–100	Total % No.	100.0 8799	100.0 7144	100.0 15 943

Data from *Statistical Review for the Year 1972* (Office of Population, Censuses and Surveys, 1974).

the case of neonatal deaths the immaturity group dwarfs all others. As classified by the ICD, maternal conditions, toxaemia and others, remain important causes of stillbirths though not of neonatal deaths, although toxaemia certainly plays a large part in deaths certified as due to other causes. Fetal and neonatal infections are relatively unimportant numerically as causes of death but like haemolytic disease are vitally important to diagnose because they may be easily treated.

UNDERLYING CAUSES OF MORTALITY

The causes underlying these groups of fetal deaths may usefully be described according to the time at which they appear to operate.

Congenital anomalies

The majority of the causes for these act either before, or very early in pregnancy, so that by the time their effects are suspected the damage is usually irreversible. The causes range from genetic to environmental, but probably the majority are multifactorial and are due to interactions between genetic disposition and environment, both external and intra-uterine. In general, predisposing factors are parental, particularly maternal, ageing, multiparity, low social class, irradiation before conception, viral infections and some drugs (Eriksson, Catz and Jaffe, 1973), including anaesthetics (American Society of Anesthesiologists, 1974). It will be seen later that many of the same adverse factors which contribute to the risk of congenital anomaly also contribute to other perinatal hazards in normally formed fetuses, and indeed may lead to different deleterious long-term effects in survivors.

Gestational immaturity

There is a second group of causes which acts somewhat later in pregnancy, and whose effects are manifested predominantly by expulsion of the fetus during the second, or early in the third trimester. Although not all are well understood, they lead to a very important group of wasted pregnancies, usually of apparently normal fetuses, whose extremely high mortality seems to be accounted for mainly by their premature expulsion. Important causes are pre-eclamptic toxaemia and premature separation of the placenta; their epidemiology will be discussed below.

One special subgroup is that of multiple births, where the premature onset of labour may be unrelated to any fetal factor. In this subgroup the mortality rate is actually lower than that of singletons of the same birthweight, possibly because they are relatively more mature gestationally than singletons of the same weight (Butler and Alberman, 1969a). Even so their perinatal mortality is considerably higher than that of all singletons, due to immaturity, growth retardation and to the hazards of labour.

Singletons born prematurely are often those of mothers who have had other shortened pregnancies or repeated late abortions. Surprisingly little is known about the causes of this clinical picture, which may indeed be responsible for a substantial proportion of total reproductive wastage. One accepted cause for this 'syndrome' is incompetence of the cervical os, and this has led to the practice of inserting a Shirodkar suture in early pregnancy in vulnerable women. There are very few published data showing either how often this condition accounts for premature labour or how successful the procedure is in preventing it. In the Collaborative Perinatal Study (Niswander and Gordon, 1972) the syndrome was reported in three per cent of all white mothers who gave birth to babies weighing 2500 g or less. It is probably considerably more common in gestationally premature labour. It may follow obstetric or surgical cervical injury or even dilatation (Naver, 1969). Possibly the dilatation of an unprepared cervical canal, resulting from early fetal expulsion, predisposes to permanent subsequent cervical incompetence and repeated early loss. Such a hypothesis is supported by the findings that second trimester abortion and premature labour are unduly common after both spontaneous and therapeutic abortion (Papaevangelou et al, 1973). Certainly this is a group which warrants more epidemiological research.

There are many other conditions which are known to predispose to this 'premature expulsion' syndrome. Abnormalities of the shape of the uterus, which may be congenitally or otherwise deformed by fibroids or other tumours, certainly increase the risk of late abortions and of premature labour. Moreover, there is an interesting suggestion that cervical incompetence may often be superimposed in the case of a congenitally malformed uterus (Craig, 1973).

Another probably very important but little understood subgroup is that in which anomalies of the normal hormonal cycle are found. Once again there are surprisingly few data on any relationship between abnormal menstruation, infertility, abortion and premature expulsion. One wonders what effect an abnormal hormonal profile, such as is found in the years before the menopause (Adamopoulos, Loraine and Dove, 1971), or in the years just after the menarche, has on conception and implantation. May not such anomalies have far-reaching implications that later, in pregnancy, lead to either premature expulsion or placental insufficiency? Klopper (1971) discussed the question of whether hormonal deficiency early in pregnancy can lead to abortion and concluded that this is still unproven. However, he went on to suggest that premature labour can only come about when certain combinations of events, leading to uterine contractions, cervical dilatation and possibly low implantation of the membranes, occur together. Hormonal anomalies need not be of purely maternal origin for undoubtedly the fetus plays an important part in maintaining pregnancy. One interesting recent finding has been that babies born after premature labour for no apparent cause had larger adrenals than those born prematurely after pre-eclamptic toxaemia or antepartum haemorrhage (Anderson et al, 1971).

Other causes of premature labour are immunological, including blood group incompatibility, toxic effects of drugs, for instance anaesthetic agents (*British Medical Journal*, 1972) and maternal ill health such as heart disease, or infection, both chronic and acute. Recently there has been a resurgence of interest in the effect of bacteriuria in pregnancy. In an early classic series of papers Baird (1935) described this as a complication of severe urinary infections of pregnancy. More recently it has been suggested that even subclinical urinary infections increase the risk of premature labour (Wren, 1970). Many of these factors are discussed in a series of review articles on prematurity by Abramowicz and Kass (1966).

In two recent articles Fedrick (1976) and Fedrick and Anderson (1976) have looked again at factors indicative of premature delivery, and have devised a scoring system to predict this dangerous complication. Unfortunately the best predictors are the outcomes of previous pregnancies, so that prediction is poor in primiparas, but promises to be very successful in multiparas.

Birth trauma and/or asphyxia during or before labour

The causes of these deaths overlap very considerably and almost certainly the time of death varies with the severity of the conditions. Although the basic causes may have been present throughout pregnancy, the occurrence of the damage is probably predominantly in the third trimester.

Acute fetal distress

The pregnancy apparently proceeds entirely normally until the onset of labour, and the damage is largely or entirely inflicted during labour and delivery. In these groups the fetal distress as described by Gruenwald (1963) is acute and not chronic. Examples are maternal–fetal disproportion and placenta praevia. This is a subgroup in which prompt and effective intervention should ensure an intact surviving baby if the fetal distress is detected quickly.

Chronic fetal distress

Often a complicated labour follows a pregnancy in which the fetus has already been threatened with other hazards, the most severe forms of which lead to antepartum death, and the less severe to a dangerously weakened fetus. Here one may be faced with the problem of acute superimposed upon chronic distress. These hazards have in common a tendency to interfere with fetal growth and development and usually manifest themselves in the light-for-dates baby which has come into such prominence in recent years, but sometimes the distress results from accelerated growth. Both these states, but particularly retarded development, render the fetus or baby abnormally vulnerable to death from asphyxia and/or trauma. The causes for these are numerous and may reside in the fetus, the placenta, or in both, and have recently been very fully discussed by Ounsted and Ounsted (1973).

Fetal causes for growth disorders are themselves manifold. One cause is a genetic abnormality such as Down's syndrome, which itself imposes some form of growth restraint. Fetal infections such as those due to rubella or cytomegalic virus have a similar effect (see Chapter 18). In other cases the growth restraint, or acceleration, seems itself to be genetically determined through the maternal line, so that siblings or other maternal relatives have similar birthweight patterns (Ounsted, 1965). Irradiation has been shown to cause retardation of the growth of the fetal head (Miller and Blot, 1972). A particularly important effect is that caused by maternal smoking. It has been postulated that much of the observed growth retardation is attributable to the action of carbon monoxide on the fetus itself, either directly or secondarily to hypoxia due to the affinity of carbon monoxide for fetal haemoglobin (Longo, 1972). The effect of smoking on the fetus was recently fully reviewed (*British Medical Journal*, 1973). Finally, a most important factor is sex, which affects fetal growth considerably, boys being on average 140 g heavier than girls (Butler and Alberman, 1969b).

Nutritional factors

In the last analysis the effect on the fetus results from the interaction between fetal and placental factors. Relative placental insufficiency can come about either when an enhanced growth potential of the fetus outstrips the resources of a normal placenta or when a placenta becomes structurally or functionally unable to support even normal growth. The latter situation may arise when a fetus outstays its normal time in the uterus and continues to grow, or attempts to grow, at a time when the placenta is beginning to involute. The resulting state of relative malnutrition is merely an exaggeration of the normal slowing down of growth near term, but may become lethal if it continues too long or is followed by a prolonged or difficult labour. It is this danger which threatens postmature pregnancies, and which may present the obstetrician with the well-known dilemma of deciding whether to induce labour, possibly prematurely, or to risk fetal death. It is in this situation that current methods of assessing fetal maturity and fetal well-being can, and do, contribute enormously to the reduction of perinatal mortality.

There are many other situations which mimic that met in postmaturity, but appear earlier in pregnancy and are therefore more dangerous. These occur in any condition in which the fetus is unable to obtain the nourishment it needs for its growth potential. In this country it is very rare for the nutritional state of the mother to be the reason for fetal growth retardation, but this is probably a common cause in the developing countries and has certainly been documented as occurring in wartime situations (Antonov, 1947; Smith, 1947). However, even in Western countries a positive relationship has been reported between weight gain in pregnancy and birthweight. Furthermore, women in poor socioeconomic circumstances who are poorly grown, often due to malnutrition in childhood, and are of low weight for their height, tend to produce light-for-dates babies, regardless of their nutritional state in pregnancy. Illegitimate babies seem to be at high risk of this complication. These are situations to be distinguished from those of genetically determined small stature, in which the babies may be small but show no signs of malnutrition.

Placental factors

More common causes for fetal growth retardation are abnormalities of the placenta. These may be caused by premature placental separation—either many small separations, as may occur in threatened abortion, or massive separation. This latter condition is one of the most important single antecedents of fetal death, and possibly in its less severe form, of fetal growth retardation. The causes are still not established. Folic acid deficiency has been incriminated (Hibbard and Hibbard, 1963) but this has been questioned (Pritchard, Whalley and Scott, 1969). It is known to be associated with toxaemia (Butler and Bonham, 1963a) and its frequency seems to rise with age rather than parity. The incidence of placenta praevia certainly rises with parity, but this is a rarer and less dangerous complication, provided that good obstetric care is available.

Maternal conditions

Pre-eclamptic toxaemia itself also threatens placental function. The precise causes of this complication are also still disputed. It is known to be most common in primiparas, and to become more frequent with rising age in both primiparas and multiparas, so that mothers

Table 21.4. *Incidence of severe pre-eclampsia by age and parity, excluding essential hypertension.*[a]

Parity	Age	Percentage incidence
Primiparas	under 25	8.2
	25–34	9.4
	over 34	15.5
Multiparas	under 25	3.4
	25–34	3.4
	over 34	5.7

[a]Based on *Perinatal Mortality Survey* (1958), and adapted from Butler and Alberman (1969).

having their first babies over the age of 34 are at highest risk (Table 21.4). Multiple pregnancy also increases the risk. It has also been suggested that the incidence of hypertension in pregnancy is raised in the presence of bacteriuria (McFadyen et al, 1973). Maternal smoking may protect the mother against the onset of pre-eclampsia (Duffus and MacGillivray, 1968), but, as previously mentioned, may independently adversely affect placental function as well as the fetus by affecting oxygen transport by fetal blood.

Maternal diseases cause a multitude of possible complications, most of which are reflected in fetal growth anomalies. The most important are infections, which are discussed in detail in Chapter 18. However, many other forms of maternal illness may threaten fetal health. One common complication is anaemia which may, when very severe, lead to fetal hypoxia. It has already been mentioned that folic acid deficiency, as well as leading to a maternal megaloblastic anaemia, may increase the risk of placental separation. Maternal diabetes is known to increase perinatal mortality unless it is very well controlled (see Chapter 8). This effect is due to a number of causes such as growth retardation, an increased incidence of congenital anomalies and neonatal complications, and possibly, an undetermined effect linked with the tendency to fetal macrosomia. Other maternal endocrine disorders may create problems during and shortly after pregnancy if untreated. Certainly as a general rule, any woman suffering from chronic ill health must be regarded as at high risk as far as the fetus is concerned.

RELATIVE IMPORTANCE OF DIFFERENT CAUSES OF PERINATAL MORTALITY

When the overall effect of fetal growth retardation is compared with that of a curtailed pregnancy, it is quite clear that the latter is by far the more lethal complication. Table 21.5

Table 21.5. *Mortality ratio by birthweight and gestational age.*[a]

	Birthweight 2500 g or less			All mothers of singletons in survey
	under 34 weeks	34–37 weeks	38+ weeks	
No. births	232	342	436	16 994
Mortality ratio[b]	1680	746	344	100

[a]Based on *Perinatal Mortality Survey* (1958).

[b] $\dfrac{deaths}{population} \times \dfrac{total\ population}{total\ deaths} \times 100.$

gives the mortality of babies weighing 2500 g or less at different gestational ages. Fortunately extremely preterm birth is very uncommon, labour before 34 weeks occurring in only two per cent of total births. The overall importance of the light-for-dates condition lies in the fact that it occurs much more often, if one takes into account the increased growth potentials of boys, babies of high birth rank and others. Indeed it can be seen from Table 21.5 that in the 1958 British Perinatal Mortality Survey, 43.2 per cent of babies of 2500 g or less were born at 38 weeks or later (Butler and Bonham, 1963b). The corresponding figure in the 1970 British Births Survey (Chamberlain et al, 1975) was 46.3 per cent.

It is important to distinguish between the epidemiology of these conditions themselves, and the effect they have on perinatal mortality in different groups of mothers. All the complications mentioned above are a greater threat to the survival of firstborn, and fourth or later-born, than to second-born babies. This is well illustrated in Table 21.6 which gives the incidence of a maternal diastolic pressure of 110 or more and perinatal mortality rate by parity. As in the case of postmaturity it is the babies who by virtue of their birth rank have a

Table 21.6. *Diastolic pressure of 110+ in singleton pregnancies—incidence and perinatal mortality.*

Diastolic pressure ≥ 110 mm Hg	Parity				
	0	1	2	3	4+
Percentage incidence in population	4.3	1.9	2.1	2.5	2.4
Mortality ratio	304	246	274	275	338

Based on *Perinatal Mortality Survey* (1958) and adapted from Butler and Bonham (1963).

growth rate which is either slower or faster than average who are most vulnerable to this complication. In the case of the firstborn, it may be that intrinsic growth rate is too slow to leave much margin of safety when adverse extrinsic influences impose further constraint. In a fourth or later-born fetus the initially accelerated growth rate may impose demands which a damaged placenta cannot meet. For similar reasons boys are more vulnerable to relative malnutrition than girls. The population effect of these factors is illustrated in Figure 21.2, showing the incidence of antepartum and intrapartum stillbirths, as grouped in Table 21.3, rising with increasing parity.

These then are the most important causes of death, but what of long-term effects in survivors?

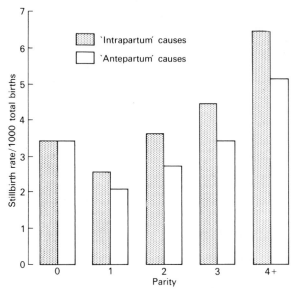

Figure 21.2. Intrapartum and antepartum causes (as in Table 21.3) for legitimate stillbirths in England and Wales, 1972. Derived from *Statistical Review for the Year 1972* (Office of Population, Censuses and Surveys, 1974).

HANDICAPS IN SURVIVING INFANTS

Perhaps the most important aspect of perinatal wastage is the fact that many of the causes leading to death are the same as those leading to chronic handicap in survivors. Although fears have been expressed that the consequences of saving fetal lives will be an increase in later deaths and handicaps, the little evidence that is available suggests that the opposite is true, and that measures which reduce mortality will also reduce later mortality and morbidity (Rawlings et al, 1971; Alberman, 1974).

The causes of perinatal death that have been described may lead to many different types of handicap, although the natural history of some is better understood than others. The causes leading to lethal congenital malformations are the same as those leading to less severe defects compatible with life. Only 'secondary' prevention can be carried out once an affected child is born, in order to prevent the worst consequences of the defect.

When it comes to the causes which lead to intrapartum death the long-term situation is far more complex, and not always well understood. It is in the subgroup of women in whom regnancy had proceeded normally up to the time of labour that swift preventive action, even fter the fetus had been temporarily affected, may avoid any long-term damage. Certainly at he present time in this country the clinical impression is that long-term damage following irth trauma has become very unusual and accounts for only a minute fraction of the total of nfants with handicap in later life.

On the other hand, the situation following prolonged or chronic fetal distress, especially vhen followed by a difficult labour, has a worse prognosis. Such a situation arises particular-y often in multiple pregnancy. It has now been shown repeatedly that in severe fetal growth etardation, brain development, and therefore intellectual development, may be permanently stunted or abnormal (Dobbing and Smart, 1974). It is not easy to estimate how important a :ause of handicap this may be, but in its most severe form it may account for a substantial proportion of all cases of cerebral palsy, or be followed by minor signs and symptoms of neurological damage. The risk of this has probably been reduced since developments in neonatal care have prevented such dangerous complications as neonatal hypoglycaemia.

Much more important than the rare occurrence of overt neurological damage is the possibility that intellectual performance may frequently be just slightly impaired in such babies. This is the more important because it may occur in whole social or racial strata and contribute considerably to existing divisive socioeconomic differences. It is highly probable hat the current policy of inducing labour early in pregnancies which show signs of fetal distress s lowering the incidence of such damage in survivors, but this is difficult to prove because of the paucity of good population data. The overall influence of intra-uterine nutrition on subsequent development has recently been reviewed by Osofsky (1975).

Without doubt, the most important risks of very early delivery are those of long-term damage in survivors. Up to recently the incidence of chronic neurological handicap in babies born before 33 weeks was of the order of 10 or more times that found in all births. An impor-ant finding by McDonald (1967) was that the incidence of neurological handicap was similar whatever the cause for the premature birth. This supported the hypothesis that the handicap followed birth rather than preceded it, and indeed it has been reported that with in-ensive neonatal care, the long-term adverse effects of prematurity can be considerably educed (Rawlings et al, 1971; Davies and Tizard, 1975). An important warning has however been given by Cross (1973) who pointed out that over-enthusiastic and uncritical acceptance of new ideas, such as the reduction of oxygen concentration to prevent retrolental ibroplasia, may indeed reverse the benefits gained. However, of all measures, prevention of premature labour, or the subsequent neonatal respiratory complications, would probably be he most important both in terms of perinatal death and later handicap.

PRESENT AND FUTURE MEASURES TO REDUCE PERINATAL WASTAGE

Comparison with other countries

One indicator of the success of present preventive measures is to compare our own mortality ates with those in other developed countries. Such comparisons must be made with caution because of the wide disparity between countries in ascertainment and definition of deaths. The annual statistics produced by the World Health Organization are standardised as far as

Table 21.7. *Causes of early neonatal death in England and Wales, Netherlands and Sweden, 1972.*

International classification		Groups of causes	Rate per 1000 livebirths		
A list	Equivalent on P list		England and Wales	Netherlands	Sweden
126–130	69–80	Congenital malformations	1.77	1.28	1.68
131	21–35, 50–51	Birth injury and difficult labour	1.05	1.37	1.27
132	42–49	Conditions of the placenta and cord	0.21	0.34	0.15
133	53–56	Haemolytic disease of the newborn	0.18	0.13	0.07
134	57–60[a]	Anoxic and hypoxic conditions not classified elsewhere	3.31	2.16	2.44
135	1–20, 52[b], 61–68	Maternal conditions; other conditions of fetus and newborn, including immaturity	2.65	1.78	1.68
Remainder	36–41	Other complications	0.67	0.36	0.23
All causes	P1–80	All early neonatal deaths	9.84	7.42	7.54

[a]Includes hyaline membrane disease and respiratory distress.
[b]Termination of pregnancy without mention of cause.

Data from *WHO Statistics Annual for 1972* (published in 1975).

possible, and Table 21.7 shows how the incidence of causes of neonatal death varies between ourselves and the two European countries that lead the league table of perinatal mortality. No similar comparison is available for stillbirths, and unfortunately the grouping of the ICD categories is somewhat different from that in Table 21.3. However, it can be seen that the excess of neonatal deaths in this country lies mainly in codes A134 and 135, which comprise the largest proportion of the 'immaturity' category in Table 21.3, and in the congenital malformations.

It is clear that our problems lie less in the areas of obstetrical complications, and more in the causes determined by the environment, genetics and social circumstances. This means that our obstetricians and paediatricians need to practice a more active management than their colleagues in Holland and Sweden, and underlines the importance of hospital delivery in this country. However, there has recently been an increased demand for home delivery from articulate mothers at low risk because of their socioeconomic status, and it is worth looking at the Netherlands experience. In 1965 70 per cent of all Dutch babies were born at home (although by 1973 this figure had fallen to 52 per cent; Van Alten, unpublished data, 1973) and yet their perinatal mortality is amongst the lowest in the world. However, in 1974 Haspels, referring to the small proportion of home-booked deliveries that had to be transferred to hospital, said, '. . . even with the most meticulous selection during pregnancy the necessity for hospitalization during labour cannot be avoided'. He warned that the Dutch system is not for export to countries with a low density of population and/or transport problems. It is very difficult to assess the safety of home delivery in any country since the reasons for this may vary from gross maternal negligence to extreme privilege. The scanty evidence available suggests that even the most privileged home confinement cannot equal the best that a well-staffed and well-equipped consultant hospital can offer in terms of perinatal safety. However, there is a real danger that the complex technology of delivery in such units may frighten mothers into preferring home delivery.

Measures to reduce the incidence of low birthweight

From the description given of the causes of low birthweight it is clear that the prevention of this dangerous condition will have to be tackled in many different ways. First, the continuous though slow improvement in the health and development of young girls in recent decades should express itself in a steady decline in prematurity rates. However, one would have expected this decline to be evident by now, and Figure 21.3 shows how little the proportion of

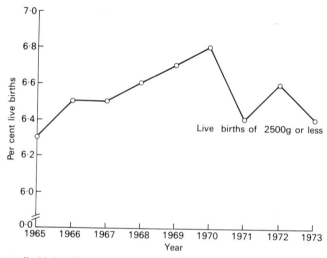

Figure 21.3. Per cent livebirths of 2500 g or less, England and Wales, 1965 to 1973. From Alberman (1974) and personal communication from DHSS.

premature births (2500 g or less) has fallen. The increase in the smoking habit of young girls may have militated against this hoped-for improvement, and certainly one urgent measure should be a massive increase of the campaign against smoking in pregnancy. It is also possible that since the introduction of legal termination, a certain proportion of premature labours have followed such interference. Recent advances in techniques of termination should reduce this complication. On the other hand, one should consider the possibility that the recent increasing tendency to induce labour may have contributed towards keeping up the low birthweight rate.

The persistence of this complication underlines the comments made earlier, namely that this has stimulated active measures both by obstetricians and paediatricians. Figure 21.4 shows clearly how improvements in neonatal care have reduced the mortality of low birthweight infants, but the cost of this improvement has been very great, and we are still not confident about the quality of the survivors. Moreover, even the most recent figures show that a baby of a weight of 2000 g or less still has a 29 per cent chance of dying in the neonatal period.

The last five years have, however, seen some very encouraging new obstetric developments, promising both measures to arrest premature labour (Thomlinson, 1974) and the ability to predict the onset of such a complication (Tamby Raja, Anderson and Turnbull,

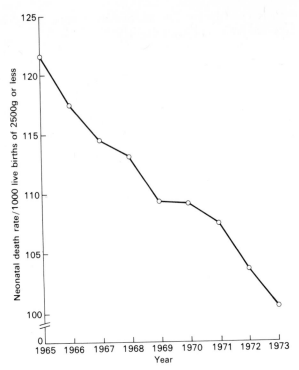

Figure 21.4. Neonatal mortality rate (up to 28 days) of babies of 2500 g or less, England and Wales, 1965 to 1973. From Alberman (1974) and personal communication from DHSS.

1974). The difficulty with the latter is that it would entail frequent monitoring, and the problem now is to delineate a group of high-risk mothers for monitoring. Fedrick (1976) has defined such a group, largely on previous obstetric history, and trials on such monitoring are likely to be carried out shortly. Whether successful preventive measures can follow the identification of a woman at risk remains to be proved. Another very promising development is the ability to predict lung maturity before induction of premature labour for maternal or fetal complications, thereby avoiding the planned delivery of an infant liable to the respiratory distress syndrome (Nelson, 1975).

Antepartum and intrapartum causes

It is in this field that preventive measures seem to have been most successful in recent years. Table 21.8 shows how the incidence of the groups of deaths as categorised in Table 21.3 has changed between 1968 and 1972, the earliest and most recent years in which comparable data are available.

The largest group in both years was that of deaths classed as due to intrapartum causes, and this has fallen by 17 per cent. Deaths due to antepartum causes have fallen by 14 per cent, the small group due to 'toxaemias of pregnancy' by 29 per cent, and haemolytic disease by 44 per cent. This is in contrast with a small rise in incidence of deaths from congenital malformations, and only a four per cent drop in deaths due to immaturity.

Almost certainly much of the fall in the ante- and intrapartum causes can be attributed to

Table 21.8. *Falls in the incidence per 1000 total births of the causes of perinatal deaths grouped as in Table 21.3 between 1968 and 1972.*

Groups	1972	1968	Percentage difference
Congenital malformations	4.4	4.3	+2
'Immaturity'	4.3	4.5	−4
'Intrapartum'	6.3	7.6	−17
'Antepartum'	3.1	3.6	−14
Maternal toxaemias	1.2	1.7	−29
Haemolytic disease	0.5	0.9	−44
Maternal diseases	1.3	1.4	−7
Fetal or neonatal infection	0.6	0.7	−14
All perinatal deaths	21.7	24.7	−12

Data from *Statistical Review for the Year 1972* (Office of Population, Censuses and Surveys, 1974).

aggressive obstetrics, with the policies of antenatal monitoring, induction upon signs of impending fetal distress, intrapartum monitoring and caesarian section as soon as necessary. Certainly part of the fall is also due to a demographic change, namely a drop in the proportion of very high-risk mothers, such as those of parity four or more. One can, however, calculate from annual statistics that the fall in stillbirths due to antepartum causes between 1968 and 1971 was 15 per cent over all, and seven per cent in mothers of parity of four or more, and in the intrapartum causes group the falls were 23.2 per cent and 38 per cent respectively (Office of Population, Censuses and Surveys, 1974). The improvement thus extends to the high-risk groups themselves.

There is every reason to believe that these improvements are continuing, and indeed from St Mary's Hospital there are indications that improved surveillance by monitoring the babies of all women in labour results not only in the elimination of intrapartum death but a reduction in neonatal mortality and morbidity (Edington, Sibanda and Beard, 1975).

Measures to prevent congenital malformations

As in the case of immaturity, no success has been achieved in reducing the incidence of perinatal deaths due to congenital malformations, and even the demographic changes in maternal age and parity seem to have had little effect on incidence over the last decade.

Again one is forced to active measures, and in this case they are confined to the termination of pregnancies known to be abnormal. The major advances in this field have been in the development of methods of prenatal diagnosis. Most important has been the development of prenatal diagnosis of neural tube defects, by the estimation of alpha-fetoprotein in the amniotic fluid. Such estimations involve amniocentesis and are at present limited to women who have previously delivered affected children. Recently it has been claimed that the screening of maternal blood together with the amniocentesis where the blood level is raised, may be sufficiently sensitive to enable the detection of more than half of all such affected pregnancies (Brock and Scrimgeour, 1975). Such a development, if validated, would indeed contribute to a fall in congenital malformations. Nevertheless the administration of such a two-stage screen could be extremely difficult and costly (Hagard, Carter and Milne, 1976).

Other abnormalities which can be diagnosed prenatally, but only by amniocentesis, include those due to numerical or structural chromosome aberrations, and certain biochemical defects. In addition, since fetal sex can be determined, pregnancies carrying fetuses at very high risk of sex-linked anomalies may be sexed and terminated if the fetus is of the vulnerable sex. The whole field of prenatal diagnosis is still changing very rapidly, but at present, however, it seems unlikely that we shall be able to diagnose more than 10 to 20 per cent of congenital malformations prenatally in the forseeable future, and that we will still be left with a substantial problem.

Role of medical care

The mothers at high risk of perinatal death are, above all, those with multiple hazards of social, biological and pathological nature. Figure 21.5 taken from the Second Report of the

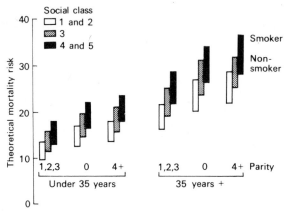

Figure 21.5. Theoretical cumulative perinatal mortality risk according to smoking habit, in mothers of different age, parity and social class groups. The top of each bar represents the high risk in smokers, and the bottom, the risk in non-smokers. Based on mothers 5 ft 2 in or more in height and without severe pre-eclampsia. Redrawn from Butler and Alberman (1969) with kind permission of the publishers (Edinburgh: Churchill Livingstone).

Perinatal Mortality Survey shows very clearly the cumulative risk of adverse maternal age, parity, social class and smoking habit. Maternal height and complications such as pre-eclamptic toxaemia have not been included in this figure, but the analysis carried out in the study (Goldstein, 1969) shows that their effects can be regarded as further cumulative risks in the vulnerable mother.

Inevitably built into the results of the survey was the demonstrable fact that mothers at particularly high cumulative risk were most often those receiving the poorest quality of medical care (Baird and Thomson, 1969). For example, the mothers of high parity and low social class are precisely those who are least likely to attend antenatal clinics early or often, or to deliberately seek the most skilled care. This is still one of the largest problems to be tackled for no amount of technical expertise can help a woman who cannot or will not accept it. The causes for this may be extremely mundane, such as mothers having been asked to attend clinics during working hours, or with no encouragement to bring their children with them. Furthermore, the high parity mother who is at increasing risk of perinatal death takes a casual attitude and remains unconvinced about the necessity for antenatal care, especially if previous pregnancies have gone well.

The full preventive effect of fetal monitoring and 'aggressive' obstetrics will not been seen until these particular high-risk mothers are persuaded to cooperate, and monitoring and relevant obstetric action is carried out for all the women who need it, rather than for those who demand it. However, it is already abundantly clear that we have in our power the ability to reduce perinatal mortality to a level very considerably below that which not long ago was considered to be an irreducible minimum. It is indicative of the present hopeful climate that this is a phrase which is no longer in current use.

REFERENCES

Abramowicz, M. & Kass, E. H. (1966) Pathogenesis and prognosis of prematurity. *New England Journal of Medicine,* **275,** 878, 938, 1001, 1053.
Adamopoulos, D. A., Loraine, J. A. & Dove, G. A. (1971) Endocrinological studies in women approaching the menopause. *Journal of Obstetrics and Gynaecology of the British Commonwealth,* **78,** 62–79.
Alberman, E. (1974) Stillbirths and neonatal mortality in England and Wales by birthweight, 1953–71. *Health Trends,* **6,** 14–17.
American Society of Anesthesiologists (1974) Occupational disease among operating room personnel. *Anesthesiology,* **41,** 321–339.
Anderson, A. B. M., Laurence, K. M., Davies, K., Campbell, H. & Turnbull, A. C. (1971) Fetal adrenal weight and the cause of premature delivery in human pregnancy. *Journal of Obstetrics and Gynaecology of the British Commonwealth,* **78,** 481–487.
Antonov, A. N. (1947) Children born during the siege of Leningrad in 1942. *Journal of Pediatrics,* **30,** 250–259.
Baird, D. (1935) Infection of the urinary tract during pregnancy. Pt. IV. *Journal of Obstetrics and Gynaecology of the British Empire,* **42,** 774–794.
Baird, D. & Thomson, A. (1969) In *Perinatal Problems* (Ed.) Butler, N. R. & Alberman, E. D. p. 236. Edinburgh, London: Livingstone.
British Medical Journal (1972) Leading article: Pollution in the operating theatre. *British Medical Journal,* **ii,** 123.
British Medical Journal (1973) Leading article: Smoking hazards to the fetus. *British Medical Journal,* **i,** 369–370.
Brock, D. J. H. & Scrimgeour, J. B. (1975) Screening for neural tube defects. *Lancet,* **i,** 745 (letter).
Butler, N. R. & Alberman, E. D. (1969) *Perinatal Problems* (a) p. 131, (b) p. 53, & (c) p. 38. Edinburgh, London: Livingstone.
Butler, N. R. & Bonham, D. G. (1963) *Perinatal Mortality* (a) p. 107, (b) p. 143, & (c) p. 91. Edinburgh, London: Livingstone.
Chamberlain, R., Chamberlain G., Howlett, B. & Claireaux, A. (1975) *British Births 1970,* p. 84. London: Heinemann.
Chase, H. C. (1967) *International Comparison of Perinatal and Infant Mortality: The United States and Six West European Countries. Vital and Health Statistics.* PHS Pub. No. 1000, Series 3, No. 6. Public Health Service. Washington: US Government Printing Office.
Craig, C. J. T. (1973) Congenital abnormalities of the uterus and foetal wastage. *South African Medical Journal,* **7,** 2000–2005.
Cross, K. W. (1973) Cost of preventing retrolental fibroplasia? *Lancet,* **ii,** 954–956.
Davies, P. A. & Tizard, J. P. M. (1975) Very low birthweight and subsequent neurological defect. *Developmental Medicine and Child Neurology,* **17,** 3–17.
Dobbing, J. & Smart, J. L. (1974) Vulnerability of developing brain and behaviour. *British Medical Bulletin,* **30,** 164–168.
Duffus, G. M. & MacGillivray, I. (1968) The incidence of pre-eclamptic toxaemia in smokers and non-smokers. *Lancet,* **i,** 994–995.
Edington, P. T., Sibanda, J. & Beard, R. (1975) The influence on clinical practice of routine intrapartum fetal monitoring. *British Medical Journal,* **iii,** 341–343.
Eriksson, M., Catz, C. S. & Jaffe, S. J. (1973) Drugs and pregnancy. *Clinical Obstetrics and Gynaecology,* **16,** 199–244.
Fedrick, J. (1976) Antenatal identification of women at high risk of spontaneous pre-term birth. *British Journal of Obstetrics and Gynaecology,* **83,** 351–354.
Fedrick, J. & Anderson, A. (1976) Factors associated with pre-term births. *British Journal of Obstetrics and Gynaecology,* **83,** 342–350.

Goldstein, H. (1969) In *Perinatal Problems* (Ed.) Butler, N. R. & Alberman, E. D. p. 45 Edinburgh, London: Livingstone.

Gruenwald, P. (1963) Chronic fetal distress and placental insufficiency. *Biologia Neonatorum*, **5**, 215–265.

Hagard, S., Carter, F. & Milne, R. (1976) Screening for spina bifida cystica: a cost–benefit analysis. *British Journal of Preventive and Social Medicine*, **30**, 40–53.

Haspels, A. A. (1974) Obstetric care in the Netherlands. *Public Health*, **88**, 183–188.

Hibbard, B. M. & Hibbard, E. D. (1963) Aetiological factors in abruptio placentae. *British Medical Journal*, **ii**, 1430–1436.

International Classification of Diseases, 1965 Revision (1967) Geneva: World Health Organization.

Klopper, A. (1971) Endocrine factors in abortion and premature labor. In *Endocrinology of Pregnancy* (Ed.) Fuchs, F. & Klopper, A. New York, Evanstone, London: Harper & Row.

Longo, L. D. (1972) Carbon monoxide in the pregnant mother and fetus and its exchange across the placenta. *Annals of the New York Academy of Sciences*, **174**, 312–341.

McDonald, A. D. (1967) *Children of Very Low Birthweight*. Spastics International Medical Publications, Monograph No. 1, p. 100. London: William Heinemann.

McFadyen, I. R., Eykyn, S. J., Gardener, N. H. N., Vanier, T. M., Bennett, A. E., Mayo, M. E. & Lloyd-Davies, R. W. (1973) Bacteriuria in pregnancy. *Journal of Obstetrics and Gynaecology of the British Commonwealth*, **80**, 385–405.

Miller, R. W. & Blot, W. J. (1972) Small head size after utero exposure to atomic radiation. *Lancet*, **ii**, 784–787.

Naver, E. (1969) The incompetent cervix and its treatment in habitual abortion and premature labour. *Obstetrical and Gynaecological Survey*, **24**, 1108–1109.

Nelson, G. H. (1975) Risk of respiratory distress syndrome as determined by amniotic fluid lecithin concentration. *American Journal of Obstetrics and Gynecology*, **121**, 753–755.

Niswander, K. R. & Gordon, M. (1972) *The Women and Their Pregnancies*, p. 395. Philadelphia, London, Toronto: W. B. Saunders.

Office of Population, Censuses and Surveys (1974) *Part I, Tables, Medical. The Registrar General's Statistical Review of England and Wales for the Year 1972*. London: Her Majesty's Stationery Office.

Osofsky, H. J. (1975) Relationships between nutrition during pregnancy and subsequent infant and child development. *Obstetrical and Gynaecological Survey*, **30**, 227–241.

Ounsted, M. K. (1965) Maternal constraint of foetal growth in man. *Developmental Medicine and Child Neurology*, **7**, 479–491.

Ounsted, M. & Ounsted, C. (1973) *Fetal Growth Rate*. Spastics International Medical Publications, London: William Heinemann. Philadelphia: Lippincott.

Papaevangelou, G., Vrettos, A. S., Papadatos, C. & Alexiou, D. (1973) The effect of spontaneous and induced abortion on prematurity and birthweight. *Journal of Obstetrics and Gynaecology of the British Commonwealth*, **80**, 418–422.

Pritchard, J. A., Whalley, P. J. & Scott, D. E. (1969) The influence of maternal folate and iron deficiencies on intrauterine life. *American Journal of Obstetrics and Gynaecology*, **104**, 388–395.

Rawlings, G., Reynolds, E. O. R., Stewart, A. & Strang, L. B. (1971) Changing prognosis for infants of very low birthweight. *Lancet*, **i**, 516–519.

Smith, C. A. (1947) Effects of maternal undernutrition upon newborn infants in Holland (1944–1945). *Journal of Pediatrics*, **30**, 229–243.

Tamby Raja, R. L., Anderson, A. B. M. & Turnbull, A. C. (1974) Endocrine changes in premature labour. *British Medical Journal*, **iii**, 67–71.

Thomlinson, J. (1974) In *Obstetric Therapeutics* (Ed.) Hawkins, D. F. pp. 321–327. London: Baillière Tindall.

World Health Statistics Annual (1974) *Vol. I. Vital Statistics and Causes of Death*. Geneva: World Health Organization.

Wren, B. G. (1970) Subclinical renal infection and prematurity. *Obstetrical and Gynaecological Survey*, **25**, 1045–1046.

22

PROBLEMS OF THE FETUS IN AFRICA

R. H. Philpott and P. F. Fairbrother

In Africa, fetal growth and development and the outcome of labour are so markedly influenced by environmental factors that they must be taken into consideration as doctors and midwives endeavour to improve the service that they are providing. The background circumstances of African obstetrics are often described as 'low socioeconomic status', but the components of that situation need more detailed analysis and description. Thus the doctor must be prepared to exert an influence beyond the labour ward, even into the area of government and the social life of the community. Though major improvements in fetal well-being in Africa are dependent on the economy of the people, it is rewarding to find that, while attending to these critical issues, much can also be accomplished within the strictures of the existing circumstances.

ENVIRONMENTAL FACTORS INFLUENCING FETAL OUTCOME

Facilities

In most parts of Africa maternity services are inadequate and poorly distributed. There are large population groups with no hospitals or maternity clinics within the range of available transport. This is particularly the case in the rural areas of the continent where 70 per cent of the population live. Health service patterns applicable to Europe and America have often been transferred to Africa without consideration of priorities and local circumstances, and enormous sums of money have been and are being spent on the construction and maintenance of a few large elaborate hospitals, with little awareness of the needs of the total population of the country. The hospitals and clinics that do exist are short of standard equipment and frequently find themselves without supplies of basic drugs. There is a comparable shortage of medical and nursing staff. In Rhodesia, for example, the proportion of doctors to population is 1 : 3000 in the urban areas and 1 : 80 000 in the rural areas. Even when hospitals are built in the rural areas, it is difficult to persuade doctors and midwives to staff them and, in the main, the maternity services on the continent depend on the maternity assistant with junior school education, one year of basic nursing and two years of midwifery training.

Availability of services

Large sectors of the population live in small scattered villages or in kraals dotted over the hills, far from the main centres and with very poor, or often no means of communication and transport. For this reason many patients are not booked for antenatal or intrapartum care; those that are booked often deliver before arrival at the maternity unit and there are many problems of neglected obstructed labour. At Harare Hospital in Salisbury, Rhodesia in 1974, 25.6 per cent of patients arrived with the cervix fully dilated or needing immediate delivery. The perinatal mortality rate for that group was 135 per 1000 live births compared with the overall rate for the unit of 44. With a large proportion of patients admitted late in the first stage of labour, it is not possible to give adequate attention to fetal condition during labour.

Nutrition

Malnutrition is common in Africa. It has, it is supposed, already limited the growth of the young mother and will, it is argued, limit the growth of her fetus in utero. The young mother has a very small pelvis by European standards. Her fetus may be growth-retarded because of a cell deficit in its growing tissues, and it is because the cell deficiency might involve the fetal brain that there is so much concern about malnutrition.

There is no doubt that severe malnutrition such as was seen in northwest Holland in 1944 to 1945, if experienced during the third trimester, will limit fetal growth (Smith, 1947). The question is whether the range of subnutrition found throughout Africa is enough to limit growth also, as suggested by Maletnlema and Bavu (1974). These authors demonstrated a good correlation between maternal protein intake and newborn weight. Their report must, however, be viewed with some caution because some of the newborn were not weighed at birth and it is not altogether clear that the authors took adequate account of gestational age.

Notwithstanding these objections, their report does suggest that the maternal diet in Africa is often so poor as to affect fetal growth.

The same problem was looked at in a different way by Naeye et al (1969) in the United States. They wished to examine the effect of poverty on fetal growth. They weighed, organ by organ, stillbirths from poor and non-poor mothers, having excluded any in which the pregnancy was complicated by factors known to affect fetal growth. The results showed that although the mean gestational ages of the stillbirths were similar, the weights of fetuses from the poor group were significantly less. In another study they showed that the difference between the poor and non-poor groups was due to differing maternal nutrition levels, as was expressed by the diet in pregnancy, the maternal gestational weight gain, and the maternal prepregnancy weight (Naeye, Blanc and Paul, 1973). It was further shown that the effect of nutrition was only significant after 33 weeks. It is fair to conclude that inadequate maternal nutrition limits fetal growth particularly in the third trimester, and that many African mothers are in the category at risk. The consequences for the fetus of this growth limitation are a matter for speculation. We must turn to the human infant and animal models for analogies. A full discussion of the consequences of human postnatal malnutrition on development is outside the scope of this chapter, but they have been well reviewed by Winick and Coombs (1972). Their conclusion was that malnutrition is often associated with retarded development, although it may not be its sole cause.

Animal experiments have given rise to two concepts. Most, but not all tissues have a time-limited cell division phase, during which the tissue is vulnerable to malnutrition. Malnutrition slows the rate of cell division and the full-grown tissue has a cell deficit. Dobbing and Smart (1973) have shown that the human brain has a second vulnerable period of growth which begins at about 30 weeks gestation and does not end until the second year of life. The onset of this vulnerable period coincides with the time at which fetal growth is beginning to be limited by maternal malnutrition. It is of added concern therefore that the second concept derived from animal work should be that there are two types of growth retardation, the brain spared and the symmetrical or brain involved. The brain-spared growth retardation is caused by interference with the placenta or its blood supply, whilst the symmetrical is caused by malnutrition (Winick, Brasel and Velasco, 1973). It is noteworthy that Naeye, Blanc and Paul (1973) described a symmetrical type of growth retardation amongst the stillbirths from under-nourished mothers, the brain weight being equivalently reduced with that of other organs.

There is good reason to suspect that if a fetus is small because of maternal malnutrition then its brain will also be small, and this in turn may be responsible for retarded development in the future. The question to be asked is 'does the range of subnutrition ordinarily seen in Africa affect the newborn body weight or—perhaps more to the point—brain weight, for gestational age, and if so is it associated with retarded development?' The claims that the ratio of urinary urea to total urinary nitrogen (Beydoun et al, 1972) and the maternal leucocyte enzyme profile (Yoshida et al, 1972) are good markers of maternal nutritional status need to be investigated. If these claims are justified then both the investigator and clinician will have access to important measurements which should be used to answer the stated question.

Parity

Although family planning is the national policy of a number of countries in Africa, it is not yet accepted as a way of life and high parity is the rule. In addition to the fact that the provision of suitable contraceptive methods is inadequate, there is limited incentive for those living in a subsistence economy with poor educational facilities to limit their family size. The woman with five or more children is a high risk patient for she is unable to give sufficient priority to her own health care during pregnancy when faced with her commitments to her other children. Fetal problems in the highly parous patient are related to the increased incidence of preterm labour, abruptio placentae, hypertensive disease and malpresentation in labour. In addition, the increased risk associated with induction of labour in the grand multipara makes obstetricians reluctant to perform an induction even when there is a definite indication to deliver the fetus.

Customs

Tribal customs relating to pregnancy and childbirth vary greatly from one part of the continent to another. In some areas the customs do not include any physical interference in the pregnancy or labour, whereas in others oxytocic preparations and manipulative procedures are used by village midwives and tribal doctors. However, traditional customs have not held back the acceptance of modern obstetric services where these have been introduced with efficiency.

Solving the environmental problems

The yardsticks of the efficiency of a perinatal service must be the maternal and perinatal mortality rates, and while these remain high, every effort must be made to deal with the causes. It is the doctor's responsibility to provide the government of the country with factual information relating to the quality of obstetric care being provided in the community and to alert the government to its responsibility to correct the environmental factors that have a deleterious effect on maternal and fetal well-being. Then, within the circumstances prevailing, there is much that can be done at fairly low cost to improve the existing standards of maternity care.

Foremost in the doctors' consideration will be the provision of adequate facilities for antenatal care and delivery, accepting that it is not possible in the immediate future to provide hospital beds for every delivery. Domiciliary deliveries have no place in the planning of maternity services, for they are dangerous and wasteful of staff time. The answer has been to establish satellite maternity and child welfare clinics, related to base hospitals, and strategically placed so that all women in the community have easy access to their nearest clinic. These clinics can be run efficiently by midwives and obstetric work done in the clinics should be limited to antenatal care and normal delivery. The base hospital is responsible for establishing criteria for referral in its satellite clinics and receives patients of high risk from the areas served by its clinics.

When family planning becomes part of maternal and child health care in these satellite clinics, then it becomes acceptable to the patient as part of a package deal health care programme. Part of the failure of family planning in the past has been due to major deficiencies in the provision of the actual clinic service as well as non-acceptance by the patients. In addition, contraceptive methods such as the pill need to be made freely available in every store and trading point for those who would prefer to separate their family planning from the clinic atmosphere.

One answer to the problem of great distance between patients' homes and the nearest maternity clinic or hospital is the establishment of villages for pregnant women near to delivery centres. Patients are accommodated at low cost during the last week of pregnancy, cook for themselves, and while waiting for delivery can be given instruction in various aspects of health care.

CURRENT CLINICAL PROBLEMS

The proportions in which the various clinical problems occur will probably vary from area to area. A study (Fairbrother and Connolly, 1975) has been carried out on the clinical statistics for the Harare Perinatal Service in Salisbury, Rhodesia, which comprised the integrated obstetric service of Harare Hospital and its seven satellite maternity clinics and covered a total of 15 259 deliveries in 1973. When these findings were submitted to workers in centres in East, North and West Africa, there was agreement that the figures were fairly typical for other areas. Table 22.1 shows the analysis of perinatal deaths by obstetric complication.

Table 22.1. *Perinatal deaths by obstetric complication. Harare Perinatal Service, Salisbury, Rhodesia, 1973.*

	Stillbirths	Neonatal deaths	Total
Asphyxia in labour	49	54	103
In consequence of preterm delivery	0	102	102
Minor antepartum haemorrhage	56	33	89
Unexplained intra-uterine death	81	0	81
Disproportion	53	28	81
Congenital defect	18	31	49
Cord prolapse	28	5	33
Hypertensive maternal disease	23	5	28
Placenta praevia	10	12	22
Accidental haemorrhage	15	0	15
Syphilis	9	3	12
Second twin	11	0	11
Miscellaneous (extra-uterine pregnancy, typhoid, rhesus disease, neonatal blood disorders, suffocation, sepsis, meconium aspiration)	3	18	21

Perinatal mortality rate per 1000 live births = 43.85.

From Fairbrother and Connolly (1975) with kind permission of the editor of *South African Medical Journal.*

Detailed consideration will be given to the five commonest obstetric complications causing perinatal death, which account for 71 per cent of the deaths, and comment will be made on the clinical areas in which progress is particularly needed.

It is important that each perinatal service conducts a quality control study at least annually, and reviews its own priority problems. In addition, there should be weekly perinatal mortality meetings attended by those working in the satellite clinics as well as by those in the base hospitals.

Asphyxia in labour

In the series studied by Fairbrother and Connolly (1975) two-thirds of the fetuses dying from asphyxia in labour weighed more than 2225 g and were therefore salvageable. These deaths occurred in spite of the fact that there were facilities for the intensive care of those patients who were regarded as being at highest risk. Patients were allocated to one of the three areas in the labour ward as determined by their priority rating. Those at greatest risk were monitored with the cardiotocograph and fetal blood sampling and they had a perinatal mortality rate of 16.6 per 1000 live births. There were a limited number of cardiotocographs and so the next priority group received continuous clinical supervision by the most experienced midwives. The perinatal mortality rate in this second group was 19.7 per 1000 live births. The rest of the patients, regarded as being of low risk, received standard half-hourly observations in the labour ward and their perinatal mortality rate was 55.5 per 1000 live births.

The results obtained in the first group were obtained in a busy unit where midwives did all the monitoring. It is recognised that the second group was at lesser risk than the first group, but the results were much better than in the general labour ward and do show what can be accomplished by skilled midwives who are providing intensive clinical supervision without the aid of monitors. The cause for real concern is the high mortality rate in the group regarded as being of low risk. There are two facets to this problem.

First, it is possible that current assumptions are not entirely correct as to which groups of patients form the high-risk category. Brown (1975) pursued this question by reviewing in the same obstetric department, the previously established grouping of high-risk factors. He prospectively studied 1080 patients admitted to the labour ward and determined which developed significant fetal heart rate (FHR) abnormalities in labour, regarding these to be truly at highest risk. On this basis he showed that, for the population being studied, the patients showing the greatest incidence of FHR abnormalities in labour were firstly those with meconium staining of the liquor, then patients with cephalo-pelvic disproportion and finally patients with a combination of two or more abnormal features. Thus, other conditions such as postmaturity, hypertension, antepartum haemorrhage and a poor past obstetric history, which were previously regarded as being high-risk factors, when seen alone were not associated with a high incidence of FHR abnormality. When two of these were present together or in association either with meconium staining of the liquor or cephalo-pelvic disproportion, then their risk was markedly increased. In this study it was noted that the small for gestational age fetus was seldom recognised before birth, probably because of late antenatal booking. Earlier recognition would have led to a high priority rating.

Second, there are the unpredictable cases of asphyxia that develop during labour in the otherwise healthy fetus. These are usually cord problems and cannot always be detected without continuous cardiotocographic monitoring of every labour. This is of course not feasible for economic reasons, but it is possible to improve the standard of FHR observations by midwife and doctor as shown in this series studied by Brown (1975) and also as shown by Steer and Beard (1970). This analysis served to establish priorities for the use of the limited intensive care monitoring facilities available in one particular department.

Premature labour

In the developed countries the immature newborn are usually managed with a minimum of mortality and residual damage, but the same cannot be said for most of Africa. The outlook is better in urban than rural areas, but not by as much as one would suppose. With a few shining exceptions child health services are not orientated towards the newborn, and the premature newborn is the first to suffer. In the developed countries premature birth is better avoided because of the increased risk of morbidity and occasional death. In Africa the situation is such that if premature labour is not prevented it is likely that the baby will die.

Beta-sympathomimetic drugs by themselves, or augmented by calcium ion antagonists (Neubuser, 1974) or practolol (Liggins and Vaughan, 1973), have the potential to arrest premature labour. These advances in technology are of little importance to the African woman in premature labour for she does not usually present until labour is too far advanced for treatment to have any significant effect. There are four common reasons for the late application of treatment. In the first place, the patient either fails to recognise or ignores the prodromal symptoms and signs of labour. These are inappropriate at eight months and their significance is not appreciated. Many African women feel that it is right to time one's entry into the delivery centre so as to spend as little time there as possible and the same applies to premature labour. Second, the patient who recognises the onset of labour may not be able to communicate with the ambulance service or transport may not be available to take her to the delivery centre. Third, the patients are often afraid to leave the house at night because in many areas assault is very common and police protection inadequate. Fourth, the diagnosis and significance of premature labour is often not appreciated by medical and nursing staff until it is too late.

This failure to provide appropriate care may be looked at in two ways. On the one hand it might be seen as an indication to educate patients and health care personnel to the dangers and prodromal features of premature labour, whilst at the same time to improve the patient's access to care. This is undoubtedly an immediate and a right approach, but it is not the ultimate. Beta-sympathomimetic drugs are not the answer to premature labour; they are only 'first aid'. An investigation of the cause and mechanism of term and premature labour is essential if the at-risk patient is to be identified and prophylaxis applied. It is only by prophylaxis that the patients in Africa will, in the long run, be really helped.

An understanding of the onset of labour is based on concepts derived from animal models and clinical associations, from which the clinician is left to make the best sense he can. It is not the place here to attempt to evaluate these, but there is one neglected association of premature labour which has practical significance. The mother of the small for gestational age (SGA) fetus, defined according to the 10th percentile on the standards of Lubchenco et al (1963), goes into spontaneous labour before that of the appropriately grown for gestational age (AGA) fetus. This association was shown amongst patients who delivered in the Cape Peninsula Maternity Service in 1973, when all spontaneous labours which occurred in patients in whom the gestational age of the fetus at birth was reliably known were analysed. The incidence of SGA relative to AGA infants was 7.5 per cent without hypertension and 11.1 per cent with hypertension. The incidence of SGA : AGA having a spontaneous onset of labour before 38 weeks was 13.9 per cent without hypertension and 33 per cent with hypertension. Therefore, the SGA fetus in both groups is associated with an early spontaneous onset of labour. This was particularly marked when hypertension complicated the pregnancy. It is essential for the clinician to be aware of the probability that the fetus of a particular premature labour is growth-retarded. The management is then not to arrest labour, but to allow it to proceed, whilst recognising that the fetus has a high risk of becoming hypoxic.

Minor antepartum haemorrhage

Antepartum haemorrhage excluding placenta praevia and clinical accidental haemorrhage was commonly found with perinatal deaths in the study of Fairbrother and Connolly (1975). The authors did not conduct a control study and could not ascribe an association between the two events. Their work points to an area which needs closer scrutiny.

Unexplained intra-uterine death

The unexplained intra-uterine death made up the major group amongst antepartum fetal deaths at Harare Hospital (see Table 22.1). History, examination and the special investigations at present available have not helped to define the reason for fetal death. Supposedly, autopsy would provide useful information, yet pathologists in general are extremely reluctant to examine the macerated stillbirth and its placenta. This attitude is surprising in view of the insight into disease given by the autopsy in other circumstances.

Detection of the small for gestational age fetus

It is a reasonable hypothesis that an intra-uterine death is caused by a severe degree of placental insufficiency, milder forms of which produce the SGA fetus. A system which aims to identify the SGA fetus antenatally should pari passu identify those at risk of dying unexpectedly with the result that there should be a decline in the number of babies dying in this group as appropriate management is introduced.

Table 22.2. *The discriminant score.*

Maternal weight in kg			WR		
Rate of weight gain kg/week			Single		
			Hypertension		

          Total A _____   Total B _____

Discriminant score is A − B

To calculate A

The earliest antenatal weight is recorded in kg. The rate of maternal weight gain over at least a three-week period between 30 and 36 weeks is added to the maternal weight according to the following transformation:

Weight gain	Negative to zero	Score 0
	0.01 to 0.19 kg/week	Score 3
	0.20 to 0.39 kg/week	Score 8
	0.40 to 0.59 kg/week	Score 14
	More than 0.60 kg/week	Score 20

To calculate B

If the WR is positive, score 25, to which 6 is added if the mother is single. The score derived from the blood pressure recordings between 30 and 36 weeks is then added. The score is calculated according to the following transformation:

No BP greater than 140/90	Score 0
BP greater than 140/90 but inconsistently	Score 10
BP consistently greater than 140/90 but diastolic never 110 or more ⌐ ᵒᵗ	Score 20
BP consistently greater than 140/90 and a diastolic 110 or more at sometime	Score 30

A further score of 10 is added when proteinuria occurred and persisted, except when the maximal score of 30 had already been achieved.

The final discriminant score is arrived at by subtracting the sum B from the sum A.

Any scheme which aims to identify the SGA fetus must take account of two facts which specially apply to the developing world. The antenatal clinics are large and impersonal and in the main run by midwives; furthermore, the facility of laboratory investigation is a luxury which is often lacking. Therefore, the scheme must be simple, quickly applied, based on objective and not subjective parameters and not require laboratory tests other than those that are simple enough for the clinician to do. It was with this specification in mind that a scheme was devised for Cape Coloured patients to identify the SGA fetus at about 36 weeks (Fairbrother, 1976). An SGA fetus was defined as one whose weight for gestational age fell below the 10th percentile on the standards reported by Lubchenco et al (1963).

Prior analysis of antenatal recordings by a step-wise discriminant function programme had shown that five parameters were outstandingly useful in distinguishing between an AGA and an SGA pregnancy: maternal weight, the rate of maternal weight gain, hypertension, the maternal Wassermann reaction and the maternal marital status. From the constants derived from this computer analysis, it was possible to establish a simple scoring system which weighed each of the parameters appropriately and allowed a score to be arrived at for each individual patient. The 'discriminant score' was established (Table 22.2). When the discriminant score was tested on 100 pregnancies at 36 weeks (50 AGA and 50 SGA) a significant but incomplete separation into their two groups was achieved (Table 22.3). The separation indicated its considerable value as a screening test, whilst overlap of

Table 22.3. *Application of the discriminant score to the study group of 50 SGA and 50 AGA pregnancies.*

	Score		
	≤49	50–59	60+
SGA	27	13	10
AGA	2	21	27

50 SGA and 50 AGA pregnancies were scored at 36 weeks by the scheme illustrated by Table 22.2. The numbers of each group which occurred in three discriminant score groups are shown. The separation of the group is clear: $Chi^2 = 31.24$, $P < 0.001$, but the overlap is considerable.

scores between the groups denied it any critical diagnostic role. It has, however, been shown that the liquor concentration of 'pulmonary surfactant' is higher if the fetus is SGA than if it is AGA in the gestational age range under study, namely around 36 weeks (Fairbrother, du Toit and Chiefitz, 1975). The possibility that this information might be used diagnostically together with the discriminant score was explored. The discriminant score was determined on 79 patients who came consecutively to amniocentesis for the usual clinical indications between 34 and 37 weeks of gestation (Table 22.4). Patients with multiple pregnancy, diabetes and hydramnios were excluded. The aim was to identify the SGA fetus. Ninety per cent (18 out of 20) of the SGA fetuses were associated with pregnancies scoring less than 60—so, however, were 45 per cent of the AGA fetuses. If the portion scoring less than 60 is further limited to those with a high liquor surfactant concentration however, 70 per cent of the SGA fetuses were included together with a bare eight per cent of the AGA fetuses. The actual composition of this group in this sample was 75 per cent SGA and 25 per cent AGA. The diagnostic implications are clear. Preliminary selection on the basis of a discriminant score followed by liquor analysis for some allowed a group to be selected which was composed of 75 per cent SGA and 25 per cent AGA fetuses and included 70 per cent of all the SGA fetuses. This is a considerable achievement, despite its apparent numerical shortcomings.

Table 22.4. *The diagnosis of an SGA fetus at about 36 weeks gestation by the combined use of discriminant score and liquor analysis.*

	49 Surfactant concentration			50–59 Surfactant concentration			60+ Surfactant concentration			
	High	Low	Absent	High	Low	Absent	High	Low	Absent	
Number of patients SGA	8	3	0	6	1	0	2	0	0	
Total		11			7			2		20
Number of patients AGA	1	5	5	4	3	9	5	11	16	
Total		11			16			32		59

The sample is composed of 79 consecutive patients, 20 SGA and 59 AGA, coming to amniocentesis between 34 and 37 weeks gestation inclusive. The discriminant score and liquor surfactant concentrations are shown for each group. Surfactant was measured by the modified foam test (Fairbrother, du Toit and Chiefitz, 1975). High concentration means a foam score of three or four, low a foam score of one or two, and absent a foam score of 0. It is clear that the SGA fetus has both a lower discriminant score, and a higher surfactant concentration than the AGA fetus.

Application of this scheme in practice demands antenatal attendance, a shrewd idea of gestational age and selected amniocentesis. It is to be expected that the accuracy of diagnosis of the SGA and AGA fetuses would be better than the figures above would suggest, because no account has so far been taken of the features of the pregnancy only appreciated by abdominal palpation or even more sophisticated laboratory investigations, both of which are known to be helpful in distinguishing between an AGA and SGA pregnancy.

The aim in presenting these data is to show what might be achieved with resources at present available in Africa, and it is suggested that these resources have not been fully used either in Africa or in places where more sophisticated tests are more freely available.

Cephalo-pelvic disproportion

Cephalo-pelvic disproportion is a common problem throughout Africa and will continue to present a major hazard to fetal well-being for many decades. Its effect on the fetus during labour may be direct or indirect, as a consequence of its influence on the management of other clinical conditions. The geographical variation in pelvic size is reflected in the following figures for mean pelvic brim area from different parts of the world. Nicholson (1938) in a series of British women gives a mean brim area of 121 cm²; Bernard (1952) quotes 106.8 cm² for Scottish women under 5 ft in height and 137.6 cm² for those over 5 ft. Heyns (1946) reports a mean area of 101.23 cm² for South African Bantu women in the Transvaal and Stewart and Philpott (1975) report a mean brim area of 102.2 cm² for a selected group of apparently normal Rhodesian African women who had delivered spontaneously.

The most important factor found to correlate with disproportion was that perinatal death from this cause is 32.5 times more common in unbooked than in booked patients (Fairbrother and Connolly, 1975). In booked patients the intrapartum mortality rate from disproportion was kept to the low figure of 10 per thousand births by the use of a regime of active trial of labour based on graphic recordings of the features of the first stage of labour as described by Philpott (1973).

Fetal response to increasing disproportion has been studied by Philpott and Stewart (1974) in an endeavour to alert the clinician to the early evidence of fetal jeopardy. The FHR responds by early decelerations typical of head compression, and then as the compression becomes excessive these decelerations become more and more prolonged into the phase of uterine relaxation. The FHR pattern is thus compounded of features of both early and late decelerations. Added to this there will be an increasing baseline tachycardia. These changes would of course be more easily picked up with the use of the cardiotocograph, but such equipment is seldom available, and it is possible to train the observer to detect these changes with an educated ear and hand.

Meconium which appears for the first time or increases during the labour is evidence of increasing fetal anoxia. Increasing head moulding without head descent is the other parameter of fetal distress in a mechanical trial of labour, and to be of value this sign needs to be gauged qualitatively and quantitatively. Philpott and Stewart (1974) have shown that moulding first appears and progresses more quickly at the occipito-parietal and fronto-parietal sutures and only later with increasing compression does it appear and progress at the suture between the two parietal bones. Further, it is possible to grade the degree of moulding. Thus it is recorded as negative if the bones are separate; 1, if they are touching; 2, if they overlap but reduce on digital pressure, and 3, if they overlap and do not reduce on digital pressure. This method of assessing the type and degree of head moulding enables the observer to recognise whether there is an increase in the degree of head compression.

The problem of cephalo-pelvic disproportion becomes an issue in a number of clinical circumstances and these warrant more detailed discussion.

In primigravidas

It would be ideal for fetal well-being, if it were possible to determine antepartum which patients have absolute cephalo-pelvic disproportion warranting caesarean section. This can probably be done in a community where there is very little underlying contraction of the pelvis, because if one erred on the side of fetal safety the caesarean section rate would still not be very high. However, where disproportion is prevalent, then the limitations of our predictive accuracy would result in an already high caesarean section rate becoming unacceptably so. Clinical assessment of disproportion based on patient height and bimanual pelvic examination in the antenatal period is of help, but is by no means accurate enough to determine whether a patient should have an elective caesarean section or a vaginal delivery. X-ray pelvimetry is only available to a minority of patients in Africa, and even when available it produces both false-negative and false-positive predictions. For these reasons a functional active trial of labour is indicated for all primigravidas unless there is another obstetric factor, e.g. malpresentation, cardiac disease or severe pre-eclamptic toxaemia.

To conduct an active trial of labour in a population group where there is so much underlying pelvic contraction, it is a prerequisite that there should be early detection of dysfunctional labour and then high quality clinical observation of the problem labour. To achieve these ends, the composite labour graph (Philpott, 1972) has been introduced into clinical practice at both satellite clinic level and in the intensive care area of the labour ward in the base hospital. As shown in Figure 22.1, the graph portrays the three main determinants in a trial of labour: fetal condition, progress of labour and maternal condition.

The early detection of dysfunctional labour is based on a simple analysis of the rate of progress in cervical dilatation in the first stage of labour and is based on the fact that when

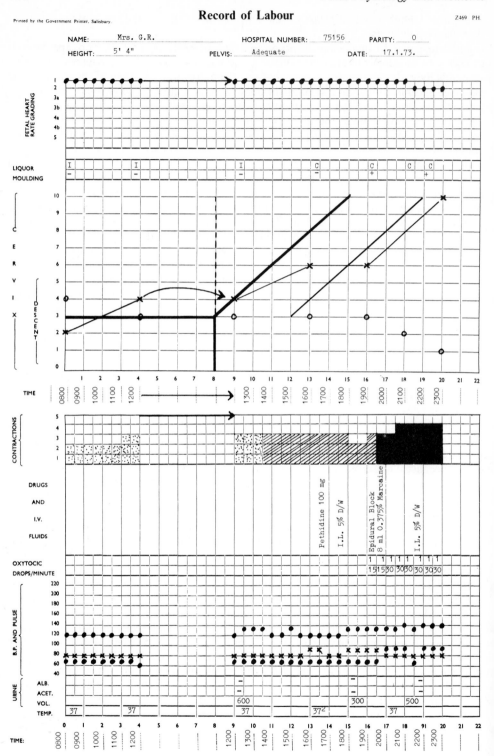

Figure 22.1. Example of a composite labour graph.

lisproportion is present in the primigravida there will be, with very few exceptions, delay in cervicographic progress. Philpott and Castle (1972) have shown that the problems of disproportion in the primigravida will be seen among those patients where the latent phase of labour (i.e. prior to 3 cm dilatation) lasts longer than eight hours from the time of admission to hospital, or the rate of cervical dilatation in the active phase (i.e. after 3 cm dilatation) is less than 1 cm/hour. These guides can be superimposed on the cervicograph portion of the composite labour graph as shown in Figure 22.2. Thus if there is prolongation of the latent

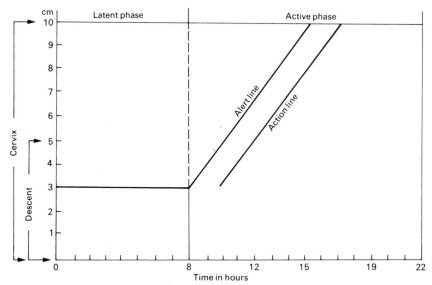

Figure 22.2. Cervicograph portion of the composite labour graph.

phase beyond the eight hour mark, or if progress in the active phase crosses the alert line (i.e. 1 cm/hour), then the patient is referred to a doctor. Dysfunctional labour at this stage will be due to disproportion, malpresentation or primary uterine inertia. If clinical examination at this juncture reveals a malpresentation, gross disproportion as evidenced by a high head and moulding, or significant fetal distress, then a caesarean section is indicated. All other patients warrant a carefully observed period of augmented uterine action and this should commence at or before the time when the rate of cervical dilatation reaches the action line on the cervicograph, which is a line two hours parallel and to the right of the alert line.

In hospitals in Africa where outlying clinics are at some distance, the action line can be placed four hours to the right of the alert line, as in the example in Figure 22.1. A few more patients will deliver spontaneously during this two-hour extension of time. The burden of supervision of oxytocic infusions in the busy labour ward is thereby reduced, but at the expense of delay in picking up cases of disproportion. This delay increasingly becomes a fetal hazard, and experience has shown that if active intervention is postponed beyond a four-hour action line, perinatal mortality and morbidity increase. During the period of augmented uterine action, significant disproportion will become clinically evident in sufficient time to avoid fetal damage, and patients without disproportion will deliver vaginally, either spontaneously or with assistance. Uterine action is augmented at the time when the rate of cervical dilatation reaches the action line by attending to the patients' fluid and nutritional needs by the intravenous infusion of dextrose solution, provision of adequate analgesia—preferably in the form of a lumbar epidural block, and by oxytocic infusion.

Intensive clinical monitoring of fetal condition and labour progress is now imperative, otherwise fetal condition may be seriously jeopardised. The evidence of disproportion becomes apparent within six hours of commencing oxytocic augmentation, and very often shortly after commencing infusion. This evidence will be either indirect, in the form of early fetal distress or failure of progress in cervical dilatation, or direct, as seen by the head that remains high with increasing moulding.

In multigravidas

The response of the uterus in the primigravida to cephalo-pelvic disproportion is predictable, whereas the multigravida may show a varying response which makes the detection and management of disproportion much more difficult. In the first place, although disproportion may be accompanied by delay in the rate of cervical dilatation in the active phase of the first stage of labour, it is not uncommon for the progress to be in excess of 1 cm/hour. The disproportion is then only recognised by the failure of the head to descend in the presence of increasing moulding or by delay of more than 20 minutes in completion of the second stage of labour. Where there is delay in the rate of cervical dilatation in the first stage of labour in the multigravida, oxytocin should only be employed for augmentation of the labour after very careful consideration. In the presence of disproportion the multigravid uterus may respond to even small doses of oxytocin with uninhibited action and the risk of early uterine rupture. Therefore, if there is any likelihood of disproportion underlying inefficient uterine action in the multigravida, oxytocin should not be used, and failure to progress should be treated by caesarean section. In the multigravida oxytocin should only be used to augment uterine action which is inefficient if the head is deep in the pelvis and there is negligible moulding, and then only if the labour is very strictly supervised.

Breech presentation

Delivery in breech presentation carries greater fetal hazards than in cephalic presentation, not only for immediate survival but also for infant and childhood development. For this reason, there is a trend towards delivering the patient with a breech presentation by caesarean section unless circumstances are optimal. In a population group where disproportion is known to be prevalent, the circumstances for vaginal breech delivery are very seldom optimal, regardless of parity of the mother or size of the baby. In most units in Africa, fetal outcome in breech presentation is very poor. To improve these results change is needed at three points: antenatal care needs to become the rule, so that the proportion of unbooked patients is reduced; a programme for halting premature labour is needed; and for the persistent breech there must be greater recourse to caesarean section.

Twins

In the case of twin delivery there will be a similar concern as stated for the singleton breech delivery, since malpresentation is so common. It is difficult to estimate the size of twin fetuses, and also it is necessary to have two cardiotocographs if the condition of each individual fetus is to be monitored during the first and second stage of labour. It is therefore important to assess pelvic size prior to the onset of labour with the same degree of accuracy and concern as in the singleton breech presentation. If there is any doubt about pelvic size, it is better to do a caesarean section than take the chance of a damaging manipulative procedure in the second stage of labour.

Induction of labour

Induction of labour plays an important role in the management of patients in whom placental insufficiency is suspected. Some obstetricians go so far as to induce labour routinely at or before term because it is assumed, on an epidemiological basis, that placental function fails thereafter. Recognising that in the African patient there are underlying mechanical problems that could increase the difficulties and hazards of induction of labour, Wilson (1975) has studied the particular problems of induction in the Rhodesian African patient. He made a prospective study of 175 consecutive inductions done for strict obstetric indications and showed that the risks of induction were greater than for comparable indications in a Caucasian racial group.

The caesarean section rate in his series was 21 per cent or approximately 2.5 times the overall hospital rate of eight per cent, and a study of the indications for these sections reflects the particular problems of induction in the African patient. An important indication was for failed induction, and this occurred in 5.7 per cent of all inductions, in spite of meticulous attention to the titration of the dose of oxytocin after rupturing the membranes. This contrasts with the series reported by Anderson, Turnbull and Baird (1968), who went so far as to say that failed induction had disappeared as an entity. In comparing the 'failed induction' group in Wilson's series with the successes, it was shown that the percentage of highly parous women (higher than para 4) was double in the former group, the head was higher at the time of amniotomy and the cervix was longer and less dilated.

The other large group that required caesarean section and which represented 7.4 per cent of all inductions, comprised those who showed evidence of disproportion as their labour progressed. This group would have been larger if it were not that patients with gross disproportion were excluded from the series and had elective caesarean sections. When working in a population group where there is a considerable amount of borderline disproportion present and delivery becomes indicated for reasons of placental insufficiency, it is common to meet the situation where the fetal head is above the pelvic brim, the angle of inclination at the brim is high, the pelvic capacity is suspect and the cervix is unfavourable. Then one either does an elective caesarean section, or awaits the onset of labour with the risk of intra-uterine death, or conducts a carefully controlled induction of labour. The latter is only possible where there are monitoring facilities or adequate experienced staff available to watch the labour closely. Without such facilities the approach to induction of labour has to be very conservative, induction only being carried out for definite obstetric indications.

Previous caesarean section

Where the previous caesarean section was done for cephalo-pelvic disproportion following a well-conducted trial of labour, the indication for a repeat caesarean section is obvious. However, when the previous section was done for some other cause, it is tempting to be conservative and to try for a vaginal delivery in the next pregnancy. This tendency can lead to major problems for fetus and mother where there is a background of disproportion, and particular attention has to be paid to the assessment of pelvic and fetal size. This will probably lead to an increase in the caesarean section rate, but this might be necessary in order to ensure fetal well-being.

Umbilical cord prolapse

A review of perinatal deaths in Harare Maternity Hospital, Salisbury, showed that there were very few deaths when the cord prolapsed before full cervical dilatation, but if it occurred with the cervix at full dilatation the mortality rate was high. The reason was that, in the group seen before full cervical dilatation, an immediate caesarean section was carried out, whereas in those seen at full dilatation attempts were nearly always made to deliver the baby vaginally, and at a late stage unrecognised disproportion often became apparent. This review led to a change in policy whereby a caesarean section was carried out regardless of the stage of labour unless the presenting part was low down and the cervix fully dilated, with a result that the perinatal mortality improved immediately.

Second stage of labour

Detailed observations in the first stage of labour have led to an awareness of a need for similar discipline in the second stage of labour. This is particularly true in the presence of possible cephalo-pelvic disproportion, as major fetal damage can occur even in a spontaneous vaginal delivery if the disproportion is not recognised early in the second stage. Past teaching that expected the multigravida to take up to one hour and the primigravida up to two hours in the second stage is certainly not true of the normal African patient and Wood et al

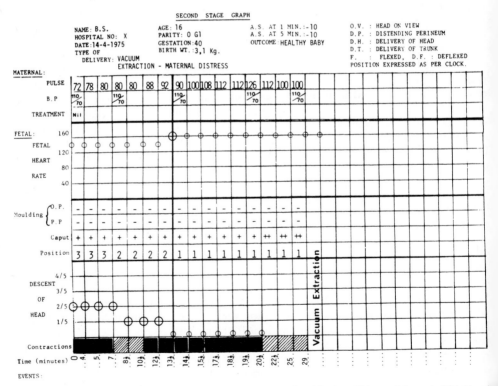

Figure 22.3. Portion of composite labour graph showing maternal and fetal condition and descent of fetal head through the pelvis.

(1973) have shown the improvement in fetal condition when the second stage was hastened by simple measures.

The recording of the features of maternal condition, fetal condition and labour progress on a graph in the second stage of labour, as shown in Figure 22.3, enables the midwife conducting the labour to recognise the indications for intervention as soon as they occur. Each feature is recorded in the same way as in the first-stage graph and in addition major events such as when the head is on view, when it is distending the perineum, the delivery of the head and the delivery of the trunk are marked on the time scale. Guide criteria are at present being established in order to ensure fetal safety in the second stage of labour.

Method of delivery

The provision and acceptance of modern obstetric care are in a stage of transition in Africa and this has a bearing on the selection of delivery method. Past experience has determined that, because many patients were unlikely to return for antenatal and intrapartum care in subsequent pregnancies, after having had a caesarean section, it was best to aim at a vaginal delivery wherever possible, often at the expense of the fetus. It is important to point out that in some parts of Africa these circumstances are changing, and with proper explanation to the patient and the provision of adequate maternity services an increasing number of patients are returning in subsequent pregnancies for whatever treatment is recommended. For these reasons it is necessary to assess the background of each individual patient before finally determining the most appropriate method of delivery.

Delay in progress in the second stage of labour in the African patient is almost always due to a degree of cephalo-pelvic disproportion, and it is impossible to emphasise too strongly just how critical it is to assess the situation accurately before selecting the method of delivery. For example, after 30 minutes of strong bearing down it is not uncommon to find that the head is impacted into a contracted pelvis, causing a remarkable degree of caput and moulding. In this case, due to the shallowness of the pelvis, the head might be visible at the introitus while still three-fifths above the pelvic brim. This picture of early impaction is a result of strong bearing-down effort, marked contraction of the pelvis and malrotation of the fetal head, all of which are present in the African patient to a degree rarely seen in the Caucasian. Fetal safety depends on an awareness of the severity of this problem and strict adherence to the principles relating to the use of each of the operative methods in the armamentarium of the doctor working in Africa.

When there is evidence of moderate disproportion the suitability of symphysiotomy should be considered. This operation is associated with a slightly greater incidence of side-effects than is caesarean section, and these include pain, instability of gait (both likely to recur in subsequent pregnancies) and urinary stress incontinence. However, the incidence of these side-effects is not sufficient to obviate the use of symphysiotomy in certain environmental circumstances and, indeed, where the operator is skilled, the side-effects become negligible. Thus, where there is concern that a particular patient might not return for hospital care in a subsequent pregnancy and where there is a desire for a large family, symphysiotomy is preferable to caesarean section in the management of selected patients with moderate disproportion. Because the decision to do a symphysiotomy is only made at the end of a trial of labour, suitability for the procedure needs to be considered in advance. The purpose of the operation is to avoid the difficult vacuum extraction and therefore to prevent fetal damage in the second stage of labour. Thus, if the head is two-fifths above the brim of the pelvis with marked moulding, it is in the fetal interests to relieve the disproportion before applying the vacuum extractor. Here the alternatives are symphysiotomy and caesarean section. If the head is higher with marked moulding, then even a symphysiotomy will not ensure an intact fetus and a caesarean section has to be done.

Even in centres where symphysiotomy is performed whenever there is an obstetric indication, caesarean section is still required for the majority of patients with moderate to severe disproportion, and a liberal approach to symphysiotomy does not bring about a marked reduction in the caesarean section rate. On the other hand, an obstetrician working in Africa has to accept a three-fold, or greater increase in caesarean section rate if, in the face of so much disproportion, he intends to take no chances on fetal outcome in such situations as breech presentation, multiple pregnancy and second-stage delay with a cephalic presentation. Liberal use of caesarean section is only appropriate where the medical services are adequate and accepted by the community. A very careful consideration of the social consequences of caesarean section is called for in the many places where this still does not apply.

When there is an indication to assist a vaginal delivery the vacuum extractor is used in preference to the forceps. The application of forceps is easy and suitable for a 'lift-out' procedure at the outlet, but it becomes extremely difficult and can cause soft tissue trauma if the head is any higher, due to the marked reduction in the subpubic angle and the forward projection of the sacral promontory. Not only is there limited space for the forceps but also it is very difficult to apply and rotate them. The vacuum extractor on the other hand is simple and does not cause maternal trauma, but herein lies a potential danger. In the well-selected and well-managed operation the results are excellent, but if there is more disproportion than is suspected, the application will still be simple, but the excessive traction that is necessary to deliver the baby can cause major intracranial damage.

Judgement of the most appropriate delivery method will depend on the level of the fetal head in relation to the pelvic brim, the degree of moulding and the condition of the fetus. Rigid instructions cannot be given, but the information provided in Table 22.5 can be used as a guide.

Table 22.5. *Suggested clinical guide to selection of final delivery method.*

Head level (in fifths above the pelvic brim)	Moulding (+ = moderate ++ = severe)	Fetal distress (− = absent + = present)	Method of delivery
$\frac{1}{5}$	+	−	VE
$\frac{1}{5}$	++	−	S or CS
$\frac{1}{5}$	+	+	S or CS
$\frac{2}{5}$	−	−	VE
$\frac{2}{5}$	+	−	Trial VE—probably S or CS
$\frac{2}{5}$	+	+	S or CS
$\frac{3}{5}$	+	−	CS

VE = Vacuum extraction. S = Symphysiotomy. CS = Caesarean section.

Inherent in this clinical guide is the principle that strong traction should not be applied when fetal distress is present, and also that no operative delivery should involve excessive traction. As a guide, the first sustained pull with the vacuum extractor must dislodge the fetal head, the second pull must bring it down to the pelvic floor and the third pull must accomplish delivery or imminent delivery. If any of these pulls fails to attain its stated purpose, then at that point the procedure must be halted and a symphysiotomy or caesarean section carried out.

Other causes of perinatal death

Most of the other causes of perinatal death here listed are conditions that occur elsewhere in the world, but with greater frequency and severity in Africa, and against a background of inadequate medical services. Little has been written on these subjects indicating that there is a real need for more research in this area.

Medical disorders in pregnancy

The incidence of maternal anaemia varies considerably depending on the local prevalence of malaria, sickle-cell disease, hookworm infestation and protein–calory malnutrition. Harrison and Ibeziako (1973) have reported from Ibadan that, when other factors known to reduce fetal birthweight were excluded, maternal anaemia was itself associated with intra-uterine fetal growth retardation. This was only true when the maternal anaemia had not been corrected by the end of pregnancy, and then a two per cent drop in the maternal haematocrit was associated with a fetal birthweight reduction of about 100 g. Malaria can lead to a haemolytic anaemia and thereby cause fetal growth retardation, but in addition, as shown by Cannon (1958), there is a reduction in fetal weight in proportion to the parasite count in the placenta, quite apart from the maternal anaemia. The various haemoglobinopathies have been studied by Hendrickse et al (1972) and they have shown that homozygous sickle cell anaemia (SS) alone is associated with intra-uterine growth retardation and an increased perinatal mortality rate. This is probably due to the long-standing chronic ill health of the mothers. Acute hypertension in the form of pre-eclamptic toxaemia has a geographic distribution in Africa in that it is most prevalent in coastal areas and relatively uncommon in the inland areas. Mild to moderate essential hypertension which usually runs a benign course during pregnancy is common, and mild proteinuria due to bilharziasis with no other complicating features is frequently seen.

Infections

In many parts of Africa syphilis is a major cause of perinatal loss with a high incidence of macerated stillbirths and neonatal disease. This is in part due to a way of life whereby husbands may work in industry and mining in the cities and then return to their families in the rural areas for short infrequent periods of the year. Premature labour due to early rupture of the membranes followed by established intra-uterine infection is particularly prevalent and warrants more detailed study. Poor vaginal hygiene has been implicated in other forms of pelvic sepsis and could be an underlying factor in this condition.

Multiple pregnancy

In many of the tribal groups in Africa the incidence of multiple pregnancy is twice that seen in Caucasian races. The problems of multiple pregnancy in the context of contracted pelvis and prematurity are discussed earlier in this chapter. The question of antenatal management of multiple pregnancy has been considered in Salisbury, where the high twinning rate in the Rhodesian African makes it difficult to provide hospital bed rest for lengthy periods of time for mothers with multiple pregnancy. A controlled trial was conducted to assess the benefits to the fetus of prolonged hospital bed rest from the 32nd week of pregnancy. It was found that, in comparison with continuous hospital admission from the 32nd week, it was possible to obtain as good results for the fetus by weekly observation in the antenatal clinic and selective admission up to the 38th week, with admission of all patients from the 38th week. Fetal results in this study were measured by birthweight, incidence of premature delivery, incidence of toxaemia and perinatal mortality. In the antenatal clinic, vaginal examinations were done at every visit, and if the cervix shortened or became dilated ahead of time, the patient was admitted. Any evidence of toxaemia or poor fetal growth was accepted as indication for admission. Hospitalisation prior to the onset of labour was important in avoiding many of the mechanical problems to the fetus that occurred in the rather rapid labour of the multiparous patient who delayed coming to hospital.

High parity

High parity is very common in many parts of Africa and so becomes a major associated factor in many perinatal deaths. It is associated with maternal anaemia, intra-uterine growth retardation, hypertensive disease and obstructed labour due to malpresentation and cephalopelvic disproportion. The background medical and socioeconomic reasons for the prevalence of very high parity are discussed earlier in this chapter. The solution can only come with attention to all these factors.

REFERENCES

Anderson, A. B., Turnbull, A. C. & Baird, D. (1968) The influence of induction of labour on Caesarean section rate, duration of labour and perinatal mortality in Aberdeen primigravidae between 1938 and 1966. *Journal of Obstetrics and Gynaecology of the British Commonwealth*, **75**, 800–811.
Bernard, R. M. (1952) The shape and size of the female pelvis. *Edinburgh Medical Journal*, **52**, 1–16.
Beydoun, S. N., Guenca, V. G., Evans, L. P. & Aubry, R. H. (1972) (1) Maternal nutrition. The urinary urea nitrogen/total nitrogen ratio as an index of protein nutrition. *American Journal of Obstetrics and Gynecology*, **114**, 198–203.
Brown, I. McL. (1975) A critical assessment of the criteria for selection of patients for an obstetric intensive care unit. *South African Medical Journal*, **49**, 2004–2006.
Cannon, D. S. H. (1958) Malaria and prematurity in the Western region of Nigeria. *British Medical Journal*, **ii**, 877–878.
Dobbing, J. & Smart, J. L. (1973) Early undernutrition, brain development and behaviour. In *Ethology and Development, Clinics in Developmental Medicine* (Ed.) Barnett, S. A. Vol. 47, Ch. 2 London: Heinemann.
Fairbrother, P. F. (1976) *Diagnosis of Intrauterine Growth Retardation*. To be submitted as DM thesis, University of Oxford.
Fairbrother, P. F. & Connolly, M. D. (1975) The quality of perinatal care received by patients in the Greater Harare Area during 1973. *South African Medical Journal*, **49**, 158–162.
Fairbrother, P. F., duToit, I. & Chiefitz, R. L. (1975) The amniotic fluid foam test and fat cell count in malnourished and well nourished fetuses. *British Journal of Obstetrics and Gynaecology*, **82**, 182–186.
Harrison, K. A. & Ibeziako, P. A. (1973) Maternal anaemia and fetal birthweight. *Journal of Obstetrics and Gynaecology of the British Commonwealth*, **80**, 798–804.
Hendrickse, J. P. deV., Watson-Williams, E. J., Luzzatto, L. & Ajabor, L. N. (1972) Pregnancy in homozygous sickle-cell anaemia. *Journal of Obstetrics and Gynaecology of the British Commonwealth*, **79**, 396–409.
Heyns, O. S. (1946) Classification of human pelvis. *Journal of Obstetrics and Gynaecology of the British Empire*, **53**, 242–250.
Liggins, G. C. & Vaughan, G. S. (1973) Intravenous infusion of salbutamol in management of premature labour. *Journal of Obstetrics and Gynaecology of the British Commonwealth*, **80**, 29–33.
Lubchenco, L. O., Hansman, C., Dressler, M. & Boyd, E. (1963) Intrauterine growth as estimated from liveborn birthweight data at 24 to 42 weeks of gestation. *Pediatrics*, **32**, 793–798.

Maletnlema, T. N. & Bavu, J. L. (1974) Nutrition studies in pregnancy. *East African Medical Journal,* **51,** 515–528.

Naeye, R. L., Blanc, W. A. & Paul, C. (1973) Effects of maternal nutrition on the human fetus. *Pediatrics,* **52,** 494–512.

Naeye, R. L., Diener, M. M., Dellinger, W. A. & Blanc, W. A. (1969) Urban poverty; effects of prenatal nutrition. *Science,* **106,** 1026.

Neubuser, D. (1974) Uber die Wirkung der Kalzium inhibitore Verapamil (Isoptin) und D 688 auf die neben Wirkungen der klinishen Tokolyse mit dem Beta-Stimulator Th 1165a (Partusisten). *Geburtshilfe und Frauenheilkunde,* **34,** 782–787.

Nicholson, C. (1938) Interpretation of radiological pelvimetry. *Journal of Obstetrics and Gynaecology of the British Empire,* **45,** 950–984.

Philpott, R. H. (1972) Graphic records in labour. *British Medical Journal,* **iv,** 163–165.

Philpott, R. H. (1973) Fetal quality preserved in cephalo-pelvic disproportion in the primigravida. *South African Medical Journal,* **47,** 2021–2025.

Philpott, R. H. & Castle, W. M. (1972) Cervicographs in the management of labour in primigravidae. I, The alert line for detecting abnormal labour. II, The action line and treatment of abnormal labour. *Journal of Obstetrics and Gynaecology of the British Commonwealth,* **79,** 592–602.

Philpott, R. H. & Stewart, K. S. (1974) Intensive care of the high-risk fetus in Africa. *Clinics in Obstetrics and Gynaecology,* **1,** 241–262.

Smith, C. A. (1947) Effects of maternal undernutrition upon the newborn infant in Holland (1944–1945). *Journal of Paediatrics,* **30,** 229–243.

Steer, P. J. & Beard, R. W. (1970) A continuous record of fetal heart rate obtained by serial counts. *Journal of Obstetrics and Gynaecology of the British Empire,* **45,** 950–984.

Stewart, K. S. & Philpott, R. H. (1975) A radiological study of the primigravid African pelvis in cephalo-pelvic disproportion. *South African Medical Journal,* in press.

Wilson, P. D. (1975) Induction of labour in African patients. *South African Medical Journal,* in press.

Wilson, P. D. & Philpott, R. H. (1976). Induction of labour in black patients. *South African Medical Journal,* **50,** 498–502.

Winick, M. & Coombs, J. (1972) Nutrition environment and behavioural development. *Annual Review of Medicine,* **23,** 149–160.

Winick, M., Brasel, J. R. & Velasco, E. G. (1973) Effects of prenatal nutrition upon pregnancy risk. In *Clinical Obstetrics and Gynaecology* (Ed.) Osofsky, H. J. Vol. 16, No. 1, Ch. 10. New York: Harper & Row.

Wood, C., Ng, K. H., Hounslow, D. & Bennings, H. (1973) Time—an important variable in normal delivery. *Journal of Obstetrics and Gynaecology of the British Commonwealth,* **80,** 295–300.

Yoshida, T., Metcoff, J., Morales, M., Rosada, A., Sasa, A., Yoshida, P., Urrusti, J., Freck, S. & Velasco, L. (1972) Human fetal growth retardation. II. Energy metabolism in leucocytes. *Pediatrics,* **50,** 559–567.

23

FETAL HEART RATE MONITORING

C. Wood and P. Renou

INNERVATION OF FETAL HEART

Field stimulation of adult cardiac muscle has been shown to be an effective way of exciting the intramural nerves of the isolated heart (Blinks, 1966; Bolton, 1967). The results of studies of the myocardium of the fetus of more than 14 weeks gestation are qualitatively identical to these, and are consistent with the view that field stimulation causes the release of neurotransmitters from the autonomic nerve plexus (Blinks, 1966). The abolition of both the excitatory and inhibitory responses by tetrodotoxin indicates that excitatory and inhibitory substances are released from nerves within the fetal myocardium.

The inhibitory response can be enhanced by the inactivation of acetyl-cholinesterase by neostigmine, and can also be blocked by atropine, which indicates that it is caused by the release of acetyl choline. The excitatory response is augmented by drugs which block the neural uptake of noradrenaline from the tissue space, and are blocked by the beta-receptor blocking agent propranolol. These observations suggest the neural release of noradrenaline.

Low doses of nicotine have no appreciable inhibitory effect on the fetal myocardium, indicating that there is an absence of active ganglionic (nicotinic) receptor sites in the developing heart. Parasympathetic ganglia and nerve fibres have been visualised histochemically in the heart of the early human fetus (Navaratnam, 1965; Smith, 1971), and this study has shown that acetyl choline can be released from a neural store by field stimulation. Hence it is possible that the vagal ganglia are functionally immature.

Although field stimulation of fetal atria beyond 14 weeks has shown that the heart contains a store of releasable autonomic transmitters, other evidence suggests that autonomic nerve transmission does not normally occur at this stage. For example, cardiac ganglia do not respond to nicotine. Histochemical studies of the developing adrenergic nerve fibre in a number of laboratory species show that noradrenaline first appears in the preterminal, non-varicose region of the neurone (Furness, McLean and Burnstock, 1970; Eranko, 1972), and it is considered that this is not likely to be associated with normal neuromuscular transmission (Furness, McLean and Burnstock, 1970).

Autonomic blocking or stimulating drugs given to the mother as uterine suppressants, hypotensives, antidepressives, anaesthetic and premedicating agents may also act upon the fetal cardiac autonomic system.

FACTORS INFLUENCING HUMAN FETAL HEART RATE

Gestational age

Several recent studies have shown that the fetal heart rate (FHR) falls throughout pregnancy from as early as the ninth week. This has been explained as being the result of an increase of parasympathetic nervous tone, which increases throughout gestation and restrains the activity of the sino-atrial node (SAN) by way of the vagus nerve. However, in vitro observations show that activity in the fetal pacemaker slows down during fetal development. An inverse relationship between the spontaneous rate of atrial systole and the fetal crown–rump length is not an in vitro artefact, since neither variations in the tension at which the tissue is mounted, nor variations in the degree of oxygenation of tissues of differing size appear to influence the activity of the pacemaker.

The significance of the in vitro findings is that it is possible to explain the dramatic fall in the FHR which occurs in vivo before 20 weeks of gestation (Wladimiroff and Seelen, 1972; Resch, Herczeg and Papp, 1973). The isolated human fetal heart does not respond to ganglion-stimulating drugs at this time, which makes it unlikely that vagal transmission takes place in ordinary physiological circumstances, and hence it is unlikely that the fetal heart is subject to tonic vagal control (Hon and Yeh, 1969; Schifferli and Caldeyro-Barcia, 1973) early in gestation. Beat-to-beat variation, which is considered to be a good indicator of parasympathetic tone (Hon and Yeh, 1969) probably develops some time after 20 weeks of gestation (Wladimiroff and Seelen, 1972).

Growth processes within the heart, along with electrophysiological changes, may lead to a natural decrease in the frequency of discharge from the fetal sino-auricular node, this being independent of the parasympathetic nervous system. Since the period when the basal FHR is decreasing fastest is also the time when the heart is growing at its greatest rate (Hislop and Reid, 1972), the coincidence suggests that the two phenomena are functionally related. That non-neurogenic mechanisms are important is suggested by the observation that the inherent pacemaker rate continues to fall after birth and throughout early childhood (Cumming and Mir, 1970). It may be that there is an interplay of nervous and non-nervous factors at any given time, with the autonomic nervous system assuming a more direct role in the final stages of pregnancy, while growth and maturational changes within the myocardium have the greatest significance in early gestation.

One can speculate that in those instances where neural development is either delayed or imperfect, the fall in FHR during gestation will differ from the normal case; similarly in those instances where growth is retarded or otherwise disturbed, the descent of the basal heart rate during pregnancy may also deviate from normal. Consequently, there is some importance to be attached to extending our knowledge with further in vivo and in vitro studies of the developing heart.

Autonomic control

By using the sympathetic blocking drug propranolol and the parasympathetic blocking drug atropine, the role of sympathetic and parasympathetic nerves in the control of the mature human fetal heart rate has been elucidated.

It has been shown that a dose of 0.04 mg atropine/kg body weight is adequate to block as effectively as possible parasympathetic control of the sino-atrial node in fit young people (Chamberlain, Turner and Sneddon, 1967). A comparable dose for a fetus of average weight 3200 g would be 0.13 mg, so that the fetal scalp injection of 0.1 to 0.6 mg atropine should block the parasympathetic control of fetal heart rate. The effects of atropine upon the heart rate are known to vary with age (Nalefski and Brown, 1950). The largest increase in heart rate in response to subcutaneous atropine (30 beats/min) is seen in the first decade of life, this being identical to the mean increase in the fetus of 31 beats/min. If the degree of vagal tone can be measured by the changes in heart rate after administration of atropine, then these results indicate that the degree of vagal tone is greatest in late fetal life and childhood.

Renou, Newman and Wood (1969) administered atropine to the fetus in doses varying from 0.1 to 0.6 mg, this being injected into the subcutaneous tissue of the scalp under direct vision through an endoscope. Atropine was administered intravenously to the mother 15 to 45 min after the fetal injection of atropine, the dose being 0.6 mg. Five min after the maternal injection of atropine, 10 mg propranolol was given intravenously over a period of 10 min. Atropine was administered before propranolol in order to prevent the possible ill effects of unopposed vagal tone, and ensured maintenance of atropinisation of the fetus during the period of action of propranolol. Within 10 min of the i.v. injection of 10 mg of propranolol to the mother, the fetal heart rate slowed 10 beats/min ($P = 0.002$). This fall of fetal heart rate was not due to the effects of the prior injection of atropine wearing off, as its action on fetal heart rate is maintained for at least 45 min. It was not possible to inject propranolol directly into a normal fetus, as tissue necrosis following its subcutaneous injection has been reported. However, 0.3 mg propranolol was injected directly into an anencephalic fetus and this resulted in slowing of the fetal heart rate by 30 beats/min. Thus, the fall in fetal heart rate after propranolol in the present study may be explained by the hypothesis that the human fetus normally has some sympathetic stimulation of its sino-atrial node.

Abdominal compression

External compression over the fetal head, neck or trunk frequently alters FHR by at least 15 beats/min or more (Walker, Grimwade and Wood, 1973). Slowing is more common with compression of the head or neck, whilst acceleration occurs more frequently during compression of the thorax or trunk.

There is general agreement that the bradycardia is a vagal response, since it is modified by atropine (Bradfield, 1961). There is little agreement, however, on the nature of the input that provokes this discharge, and the following mechanisms have been proposed: (1) increase of intracranial pressure per se (Mocsary et al, 1970); (2) neural hypoxia resulting from decreased cranial perfusion (Paul, Quilligan and MacLachlan, 1964), and (3) carotid body stimulation due to the increased arterial pressure resulting from cord compression (Bradfield, 1961).

Other mechanisms could conceivably play a part—such as volume receptors at the vena cava atrial junction, pressure receptors in the pulmonary artery, and the effects of pressure on the diaphragm and trachea (Rushmer, 1961)—although these have not yet been shown to have any function in fetal life. Tachycardia in the fetus is known to occur in response to sound and mechanical stimulation (Grimwade, Walker and Wood, 1971a) and as a response to brief hypoxaemia (Dawes, 1968). Conceivably, a tachycardia could also result from decreased venous return due to partial cord compression, causing a fall in cardiac output and carotid pressure; tachycardia would then be due to vagal withdrawal. Of relevance is the observation in dogs that pressure applied over the thoracic spinal cord evokes a sympathetic discharge (Kaminsky, Meyer and Winter, 1970). Pressure would thus produce a tachycardia by increased sympathetic drive.

Insufficient evidence makes a decision between all the above possibilities difficult. However, the very short latency of onset of both the rises and falls in heart rate argues against hormonal and blood gas changes as the responsible agent in initiating the response and implicates a neural mechanism. Rapid recovery of all tachycardias and some bradycardias may be explained likewise; the slow recovery of some bradycardias produced by pressure over the head and neck suggests anoxia or ischaemia. It is difficult to believe that pressing on the fetus always compresses such a mobile structure as the umbilical cord. Since pressure on the spinal cord and cranium can produce both sympathetic and vagal discharge, one is attracted toward the hypothesis that pressure per se on these structures can initiate a change in fetal heart rate and when complicated by local neural ischaemia, is associated with delayed recovery.

The foregoing is presented at the risk of making the subject more complex. It is evident, however, that abdominal pressure produces a wider range of heart rate changes in the fetus than is usually acknowledged. Such changes sometimes exceed 60 beats/min (BPM) and may result in a mistaken diagnosis of fetal distress. The change in FHR may be produced by compression of the abdomen during palpation or auscultation. Rarely, slowing of the FHR associated with abdominal pressure may indicate there is an abnormality. In one case the FHR decreased by more than 100 beats/min on two occasions when abdominal pressure was exerted. Subsequent caesarean section, during labour, revealed a firm true knot in the umbilical cord. One can tentatively conclude that a profound fall in FHR on abdominal compression is likely to be associated with fetal asphyxia.

Hypoxaemia

Acute maternal hypoxaemia, resulting from the administration of 10 per cent oxygen in nitrogen, produced slowing of the FHR at the end of uterine contractions in two of 11 patients. The slowing of FHR occurred after 6 and 11 min of inhalation of the mixtures, maternal Po_2 fell by 61 and 51 mm Hg and fetal scalp blood Po_2 by 19 and 6 mm Hg. However, the occurrence of slowing could not be predicted by either the degree of fall or the absolute level of the maternal and fetal Po_2, and one must conclude that the FHR does not precisely mirror acute change in fetal blood Po_2 (Wood et al, 1971). Slowing of the FHR at the end of contractions has also been found in monkeys subject to experimental hypoxaemia (James et al, 1972).

Administration of 15 per cent oxygen in nitrogen has also been studied. Again no consistent change in FHR was seen in four patients, and in particular there was no slowing during or at the end of contractions. It may be considered that the degree of restriction of oxygen uptake by the mother is insufficient to affect fetal oxygen levels but this is not so. Using a fetal scalp tissue Po_2 electrode, the mean fetal tissue Po_2 was found to fall by 30 per cent when the mother breathed 15 per cent oxygen in nitrogen. This means that FHR is insensitive to a fall of tissue Po_2 of this degree. What is important to understand is that lesser degrees of hypoxaemia (e.g., under anaesthesia, shock) are not detectable by observation of FHR (Walker et al, 1971). The clinical significance of this observation has not been properly investigated as yet. A number of clinical situations cause hypoxaemia and if this is severe enough then FHR change, particularly slowing at the end of a contraction, may follow. While the conditions causing hypoxaemia may also act in other ways to change FHR, it is convenient to categorise them in two groups as follows:

Maternal factors (many reversible)

1. Hypoxaemia as a result of poor induction of anaesthesia or respiratory depression from excessive drug administration, e.g., of pethidine or morphine.
2. Hypotension associated with drugs, the supine position, anaesthesia or haemorrhage.
3. Uterine hypoperfusion in the absence of systemic hypotension or hypovolaemia. This occurs when the patient is supine in labour and is thought to be due to aortic and/or vena caval compression (Poseiro effect).
4. Uterine hypersystole which may be spontaneous or drug-induced.

Fetal and/or placental factors (many irreversible)

1. Obstruction to oxygen interchange such as occurs in pre-eclampsia, severe hypertension, placental separation, placenta praevia, abruptio placentae, placental infarction and severe cord complications. There may be a physiopathological explanation of the FHR abnormality in these situations.

    Aladjem et al (1971) have been able to relate fetal placental capillary area to the occurrence of fetal heart rate abnormalities. They measured the capillary area of the placenta by planimetric study using a projected microphotograph of fresh placental tissue and expressed the fetal capillary area as a percentage of the total area. In a high-risk group of patients a reduction of capillary area below 50 per cent was associated with late deceleration patterns.
2. Fetal cardiac failure, either congenital or acquired, as in myocardial depression from local anaesthetic agents.

Acidosis

Both maternal and fetal metabolic acidosis have been seen in the clinical and experimental situation without change in FHR so that one can conclude that in the absence of asphyxia, acidosis does not influence FHR. However, in the presence of asphyxia, scalp blood pH levels can be related to the frequency and severity of FHR changes. Fetal scalp pH in the following groups of patients is as follows: normal FHR, 7.32; slowing of FHR in the early or mid-phase of contractions, 7.27 (12 patients); slowing of FHR at the end of contractions, 7.14 (19 patients) (Wood et al, 1969). Therefore, the relation between total acidosis and FHR is not a direct one and is dependent upon another coincident variable, asphyxia.

The effect of alterations in CO_2 and H^+ upon FHR has not been properly studied. Lowering fetal P_{CO_2} significantly by voluntary hyperventilation does not consistently alter FHR nor does increasing base by means of maternal alkali infusions.

Head compression

Schwarcz et al (1968) studied the effect of uterine contractions on the human fetal head during labour. In some patients transient drops in the FHR occurred synchronously with the uterine contractions ('a mirror image' of the contraction). This was called a type 1 dip, and it was concluded that they were due to the rise in intracephalic pressure which caused a temporary increase in vagal tone. This explanation is not necessarily correct. A general increase in pressure in the skull at the time of uterine contractions, if the intracranial contents behave as a pascalian system, would not provide a stimulus for receptors influencing vagal tone. However, vagal stimulation during contractions may result from uneven changes of intracranial pressure affecting venous distensibility and blood pooling. This is analogous to the slowing of pulse rate which occurs in the presence of raised intracranial pressure resulting from a cerebral tumour or subdural haemorrhage.

When head compression exceeds trunk compression, or when head compression is uneven, venous obstruction may occur. This may be more important when the head is large and the pelvis small, when excessive deformation of the skull (and brain) occur. Whilst FHR slowing may be related to pressure between the head and uterus, it is difficult to be certain that this is the actual cause of the bradycardia because other mechanisms may be operating (see section on abdominal compression above).

Apart from uterine contractions, head compression may also occur when the head is tightly wedged in the pelvic cavity, during the application of forceps or in the occurrence of an intracranial haemorrhage.

Sound and vibration

A number of studies have shown that the human fetus responds to stimulation by *sound* or *vibration*. Grimwade, Walker and Wood (1970) demonstrated a significant increase in FHR and movement during *intra-uterine* stimulation by sound or vibration, the stimulus–response time being less than five sec. Under these circumstances a considerable attenuation in the sound audible through the abdominal and uterine wall was noted. This suggests that the only negative study reported in this field may have been due to an inadequate external stimulus.

Under normal environmental conditions external sound or vibrational stimuli rarely penetrate to the fetus. Only in unusual circumstances, such as proximity to aircraft engines, would external sounds reach the fetal ear. Nevertheless, environmental stimuli may influence FHR indirectly through their effect on the mother. Studies have shown that when mothers listen to pleasant music, the FHR increases within 90 sec and continues for a time after its cessation.

Sexual intercourse

Slowing of the FHR has been described during orgasm in a patient near term (Goodlin, Schmidt and Creevy, 1972). The slowing was ascribed by these authors to fetal distress or hypoxia, but when, as in the case Goodlin describes, the FHR slowing is short and not profound, there is probably no deleterious effect on the fetus. Moreover, Goodlin's explanation of the FHR slowing during orgasm may not be correct. Pressure on the fetus may cause slowing of the FHR (Walker, Grimwade and Wood, 1973), and abdominal pressure may be increased during coitus by the husband or by contracting of muscles during orgasm.

Transient bradycardia also has been seen when mothers defaecate, urinate or vomit in late pregnancy or labour.

Emotional change

FHR has changed after mothers have become anxious or frightened. Although no control study has been carried out, it appears that FHR is sometimes affected by maternal emotion (Hellman et al, 1961; Welford and Sontag, 1969). In assessing the cause of FHR change, it is necessary to consider the possibility of excessive anxiety influencing baseline FHR. Unfortunately neither the frequency of this occurrence nor the mechanism by which this occurs is understood. As causes of anxiety are known, a pragmatic approach to this problem is possible. Reassurance concerning specific anxieties and sedation may resolve this FHR change.

Temperature change

During the four hours prior to delivery a positive correlation has been found between fetal scalp temperature and heart rate (Walker, Walker and Wood, 1969). Scalp temperature was found to vary in different fetuses by as much as 3°C, a fact which may account for a normal variation of 30 beats/min in baseline FHR. A case has been described in which hypothermia to 30°C during cardiac surgery resulted in progressive slowing of both maternal and fetal heart rate. The FHR of 80 beats/min was maintained for eight hours, the slow rate possibly being a feature of reduced tissue O_2 consumption. Maternal blood pressure, P_{O_2} and P_{CO_2} were normal.

In two of the patients in Walker's study maternal and fetal temperature rose simultaneously, and in both the fetal heart rate increased by more than 30 beats/min. This increase in heart rate may have been due to the temperature rise itself, or to toxins produced as a result of infection.

The largest increase in fetal temperature (0.6°C) occurred independent both of change in maternal temperature and evidence of intra-uterine infection. The rise of fetal temperature was associated with a rise of baseline FHR and slowing of the FHR at the end of contractions (type 2 dips). In this instance the high fetal heart rate and temperature may be due to the release of increased amounts of noradrenaline in response to the stress of asphyxia.

Uterine contractions

The influence of uterine contractions is considered in more detail later, as pathological patterns of FHR change in relation to contractions can be related to fetal prognosis.

The influence of uterine contractions upon FHR depends upon the stage of labour and the strength of contractions. The change may be either an increase or decrease, or a combination of these (Renou et al, 1968). Early in labour FHR is usually unaffected, while late in labour FHR frequently changes. Bradycardia occurs during birth.

Uterine contractions may change FHR by several different mechanisms. During a contraction uterine blood flow and intervillous space oxygen may decrease, fetal placental blood flow may slow as a result of external pressure (sluice effect), or cord or head compression may occur. It is also possible that sensory stimulation of the face or torsion of the neck may occur during a contraction and alter FHR.

Drugs

A variety of drugs may affect FHR, either by directly affecting the feto-placental circulation or indirectly by altering maternal cardiovascular or respiratory status.

Injection of atropine sulphate into the mother increases the baseline FHR by up to 30 beats/min (Renou, Newman and Wood, 1969), while atropine methylbromide has no effect (Padua and Gravenstine, 1969). The electrical charge of this last drug is thought to limit its transfer across the placenta. Adrenaline, administered to the mother, increases FHR, possibly by a direct effect on the fetus (Beard, 1962; Sandler, Ruthven and Wood, 1964), although in species other than the human there is no evidence that adrenaline crosses the placenta.

Cloeren, Lippert and Fridrich (1974) studied the influence of smoking on the fetal heart rate in pregnant women. The most common change was a tachycardia or alternatively a decrease in the baseline fluctuation in heart rate. They also measured the maternal placental and cardiac blood pools by the use of radioactive indium. No constant change in the blood pool was found—in a few patients there was increase in the uteroplacental blood pool and in a small number there was a decrease.

Propranolol (Renou, Newman and Wood, 1969), digoxin and the local anaesthetic agents decrease FHR (Rosefsky and Pertersiel, 1968; Rogers, 1969).

Mepivacaine hydrochloride (Carbocaine) is thought to depress the fetal myocardium as the effect is dose-dependent and ECG changes occur. Two fetal deaths have been recorded after paracervical block with mepivacaine hydrochloride. Fetal bradycardia was present for 5 and 80 min respectively before death. Local anaesthetic agent is found in significant amounts in the fetus after epidural anaesthesia is induced in the mother. The maternal injection of 0.2 mg/kg of morphine is also followed by a significant fall in FHR (Hon and Yeh, 1969; Grimwade, Walker and Wood, 1971b), the average fall in FHR being 17 beats/min, the range being 12 to 20. Morphine also lowers fetal scalp pH, the average fall being 0.03 pH unit, although the exact mechanism of the effect is not known. Diazepam (Valium), morphine and atropine (Hon and Yeh, 1969; Grimwade, Walker and Wood, 1970) reduce the normal beat-to-beat variation of FHR (Scher, Hailey and Beard, 1972). Valium has no effect on fetal pH.

It is important for the obstetrician to recognise drug-induced FHR change, otherwise unnecessary caesarean section may be performed. The time relationship between the administration of the drug and the FHR change will help in determining whether the drug has changed the FHR.

Cardiac arrhythmias

Cardiac arrhythmias, such as paroxysmal supraventricular tachycardia, atrial flutter an fetal trigeminy from multiple extrasystoles may cause an increase in FHR, while heart bloc may slow FHR.

Tuxen, Kaplan and Ueland (1971) reported a case of paroxysmal atrial tachycardia an suggested that abrupt alterations between tachycardia and normal rhythm suggest th diagnosis. In their case the cause was not found, the fetus was healthy and the arrhythmi disappeared at birth. Usually this type of arrythmia persists after birth and requires therapy resolution occurring weeks or months after birth.

Teteris, Chisholm and Ullery (1968) have described a number of cases of intra-uterin heart block which are often associated with fetal cardiac defects and have sometimes led t death in the early neonatal period. In other cases complete heart block has been compatibl with normal growth and development.

Hon (1968) states that the detection of an intra-uterine fetal arrhythmia is an indicator o fetal distress. Generally speaking, however, most infants with congenital supraventricula arrhythmias appear to do well (Klapholz, Schifrin and Rivo, 1974). In their experienc arrhythmias occur in three to five per cent of all births during labour. The majority are shor lived, benign and usually disappear shortly after birth.

CLASSIFICATION OF FETAL HEART RATE CHANGES

The definition of FHR normality depends upon the population sample, the conditions fo study of the sample and the criteria used for distinguishing abnormality. Failure to recognis the need to standardise experimental conditions probably accounts for some of the con tradictions in the current literature. Undefined variables which may affect FHR have bee described and clearly it is often impossible to be sure that the fetal environment from one cas to the next is identical. Contemporary studies have attempted to define abnormality by cor relating FHR changes with two phenomena: fetal scalp blood measurements of pH, $P\text{co}$ and $P\text{o}_2$, and the condition of the fetus at birth as judged by the Apgar score, but both ap proaches have limitations.

Scalp blood measurements (see Chapter 25) may not always reflect fetal conditio because of inherent errors (Lumley et al, 1971). Circulatory disturbances which ar associated with changes in FHR frequently do not correlate with the biochemical composi tion of fetal blood. Apgar scoring, on the other hand, has the disadvantage that it may be in fluenced by neonatal respiratory depression from drugs or events which occur only at birth such as shoulder dystocia.

A disadvantage of the Apgar score is that it is a measure of the condition of the baby at th end of the second stage whereas, in practice, the obstetrician is most interested in th prognostic value of FHR change in the first stage. The second stage is a time of considerabl stress that may have no relationship to events occurring in the first stage. Even so, it is unlike ly that FHR patterns will ever predict fetal condition with a high degree of reliability although it has proved possible by standardising the sample, the conditions of study, th monitoring equipment and the method for records analysis, to improve predictive reliability

The correlation between FHR abnormalities and Apgar scores has largely concentrate on heart-rate patterns in which slowing occurred in relation to uterine contractions. Ou classification is based upon the two most simple observations that can be made from a heart ate record: the degree of slowing or deceleration and the timing of this slowing in relation to contraction. In general, early decelerations are synonymous with Caldeyro-Barcia's type 1 dips and late decelerations with type 2 dips (Caldeyro-Barcia, 1969). The degree of slowing is classified as 30 to 60 or more than 60 beats/min for early–mid decelerations and more than 5 beats/min for late decelerations. Late decelerations of such a minor degree are included since, in our experience they may precede fetal death. Hon's predictive classification requires the assessment of 13 separate criteria and is, therefore, difficult to use in practice (Hon, 1967).

The same FHR pattern has a different prognostic significance for the healthy as compared with the malnourished fetus. The latter, if severely depleted of glycogen stores, may rapidly succumb to mild hypoxaemia resulting, for example, from cord compression in labour. Until shortly before death the FHR changes of the malnourished fetus may be quite indistinguishable from those of the healthy fetus.

Because of these limitations and variations in present methods of study, what constitutes an abnormal FHR trace is more difficult to define. Nevertheless, there is agreement between most investigators that the following patterns are significant:

. Slowing of the FHR in relation to the contraction cycle.

A baseline FHR of less than 100 beats/min which is falling (based on individual case reports) and a FHR of more than 170 beats/min. Views differ on the significance of FHR between 100 and 120 and between 160 and 170.

Loss of the normal beat-to-beat variation of FHR.

ETAL PROGNOSIS IN RELATION TO FETAL HEART RATE

Changes in the FHR trace have been analysed in association with the Apgar score at delivery in 132 cases from the authors' department. The most severe FHR change during the 60 min preceding delivery, providing this change was present for at least 20 of the 60 min, was correlated with the fetal blood gas and acid–base status and the Apgar score. Both late decelerations of more than 5 beats/min and early–mid decelerations of more than 60 beats/min, when the baseline FHR was more than 160 beats/min, were associated with significant depression of Apgar scores (Renou and Wood, 1974).

What is the degree of confidence that the obstetrician can place in FHR changes? This may be determined by considering the range of Apgar scores determined by the 95 per cent confidence limits. A marked range of Apgar scores occurs within each abnormal FHR group. For example, late decelerations are associated with a mean Apgar score of about five, but the range, expressed as 95 per cent confidence limits, is two to seven (Renou and Wood, 1974). In other published data the mean Apgar score has been expressed without a range or expressed as one standard deviation or standard error, giving a false favourable impression of the confidence which can be placed in FHR patterns.

In a previous study, different classifications of FHR patterns were compared (Wood et al, 1969). Statistically, none was proved superior to the others. All showed that late decelerations or their equivalents, type 2 dips or late dips, are associated with lower Apgar scores. Tipton and Finch (Shelley and Tipton, 1971; Tipton, 1972; Tipton and Finch, 1972) consider that the temporal relationship of fetal bradycardia to uterine contractions is not important and prefer to measure the dip area. They believe the greater significance is attached to late decelerations merely because they are usually larger than early to mid decelerations.

Dip area does correlate well with Apgar score when tracings are analysed up to birth, but the correlation with first stage FHR data is not so good.

Detailed analysis of late decelerations with a lag time of more than 18 sec in a small sample showed that the amplitude and duration of each dip were unimportant, but the frequency with which they appeared over a period of time was important (Wood et al, 1969). This result differs from Hon (1967), who regards the degree of slowing in 'late deceleration' (type 2 dips) as being important in prognosis. In 21 patients Kubli et al (1969) found a weak relationship between the degree of the late deceleration and the extent of the fall of fetal scalp pH. No such correlation in 13 patients with late decelerations was demonstrated in the study of Wood et al (1969).

The difficulty of classifying the variability of fetal heart rate and the lag time between the deceleration and the contraction have been studied statistically by Chik, Rosen and Hirsch (1974). Their study compared three methods of lag time measurement and they established the definition of variability. However, given a sufficiently large number of patterns, arbitrary division between early and late deceleration patterns enables a reasonable distinction between infants who will be in good and poor condition to be made.

In the above studies prognosis was assessed by analysis of FHR changes which occurred immediately prior to the time of delivery. In clinical practice, however, there is always a delay between making a decision to deliver the baby and its accomplishment, whether the delivery is by caesarean section, forceps or spontaneous vaginal expulsion. During the delay the FHR abnormality may worsen, improve or remain the same. A method for testing the prognostic value of FHR changes when there is a period of delay was devised in a further study.

FHR changes present up to the end of the first stage were checked in 38 infants who were born vaginally in poor condition (Apgar score 0 to 3). The average duration of the second stage was 35 min which is approximately the time taken to accomplish delivery by forceps or caesarean section in this hospital. Employing our classification, a low Apgar score between and 6 would have been predicted in 28 of the 38 cases. In six the abnormal FHR pattern appeared for the first time in the second stage of labour and in the remaining four FHR remained normal up until the time of birth. Depression at birth in the latter four may have resulted from the use of analgesics, shoulder dystocia or breech delivery. In contrast to Goodlin (1972) beat-to-beat variation was not found to be more helpful than slowing in predicting the baby in poor condition. This may be because drugs used in labour, which often reduce beat-to-beat variation, diminish the diagnostic value of this sign for detecting fetal asphyxia. However, the presence of normal beat-to-beat variation is a more reliable sign that the condition of the baby is satisfactory.

FETAL SCALP BLOOD AND FETAL HEART RATE

Beard et al (1971) studied the relationship between fetal heart rate and pH of fetal blood in 279 high-risk patients. The incidence of fetal acidosis was low when the fetal heart rate showed good beat-to-beat variation and no slowing during contractions. Decelerations of fetal heart rate accompanied by a baseline tachycardia and/or loss of beat-to-beat variation were the changes most commonly associated with fetal acidosis and hence, by inference, with fetal asphyxia.

FHR changes have been analysed and related to the pH of scalp blood collected during the first stage of labour by Renou and Wood (1974). The correlation was made from the FHR immediately preceding the blood collection. The mean fetal scalp pH for both late decelerations and early–mid decelerations were statistically significantly different from normal. The percentage of cases with a pH less than 7.24 is shown and indicates how often particular FHR patterns are associated with fetal acidosis. The imprecision of the association between pH and FHR abnormalities is best understood by considering the range of pH found in 95 of every 100 patients with a particular FHR change (Renou and Wood, 1974). For example, late decelerations are associated with fetal scalp pH varying from 6.95 to 7.45. Kubli et al (1969) have also correlated pH and FHR changes. Late deceleration (similar to type 2 dips or late slowing) and severe variable deceleration (slowing to 70 beats/min for more than 60 sec, either type 1 or 2 dips) were found to be associated with fetal acidosis.

It is important to know whether the FHR or fetal blood pH more accurately predicts fetal condition. Insufficient data are available to answer this question with certainty, but the following is relevant. The severity of fetal acidosis and the Apgar score are positively correlated (Wood et al, 1969; Lumley and Wood, 1969, 1973). When the pH is less than 7.10, 80 per cent of fetuses are born with an Apgar score between 0 and 3, and when pH is between 7.10 and 7.25, one in three is born in similar condition. In addition, more precise diagnosis may be achieved by determining the nature of the acidosis, i.e. whether this is metabolic, respiratory or mixed. FHR abnormalities can be quantitated, but not as precisely as pH values.

It is also necessary to determine whether FHR or pH changes provide the earliest evidence of fetal asphyxia. In a study of this relationship it was concluded that abnormal FHR changes usually precede significant changes in fetal pH (Wood et al, 1969). In 14 of 15 cases FHR abnormalities were present before the pH fell below normal. This observation is relevant clinically because circulatory disturbance may continue for some time before fetal acidosis occurs. FHR monitoring does have the advantage over pH measurement in that it provides a record that immediately reflects changes in the condition of the fetus. Unexpected complications, such as cord compression, can be more quickly detected than is possible with the intermittent technique of fetal blood sampling.

In practice, fetal monitoring is most useful when FHR and fetal pH are used in a complementary fashion. Individually each parameter is better than clinical criteria for assessing fetal prognosis, although both are subject to errors of different types. In situations in which the two tests agree, confidence in diagnosis is increased whether they are both normal or abnormal. When they disagree, e.g., FHR is abnormal and pH is normal, the pH measurement should be repeated at intervals. When pH is abnormal and FHR is normal, the pH measurement is repeated. Before or during early labour, pH may be low with a normal FHR. Although this is rare, two patients in this category have been delivered of severely depressed infants after caesarean section, asphyxia being confirmed from cord blood measurements.

Beard (1974) is of the opinion that the role of continuous fetal heart rate monitoring is an indicator that the fetus is in good condition if the trace is normal. He considers that it is rarely possible to determine the significance of an abnormal trace with confidence without the aid of fetal pH. In one study there were 138 continuous fetal heart rate traces with some abnormality, but in only 32 of these was the pH less than 7.25 (Beard et al, 1971).

SPECIAL CLINICAL TOPICS

Abdominal decompression

Fetal monitoring has been used to test the efficacy of fetal therapy. Koubenec (1970) has studied the effect of abdominal decompression, according to the method of Heyns, upon fetal heart rate. Normal fetal heart rates were unaffected by decompression. In one patient a fetal respiratory acidosis (pH 7.20) in association with fetal tachycardia was improved by decompression treatment for 35 min. While the author thought that decompression may improve the blood supply to the placenta, he also considered that decompression was too complicated a method. Other studies have shown that abdominal decompression has no effect on normal acid–base or oxygen levels when given during labour (Newman and Wood, 1967).

Fetal monitoring may be helpful in checking the effects of therapy on the fetus, but it has two limitations: FHR changes lack specific pathophysiological interpretation, so one does not know exactly what one is treating, and FHR changes may disappear spontaneously, so that case reports describing resolution of FHR changes may be a chance phenomenon. Monitoring would be a useful tool in therapeutic trials if used in a standard scientific manner with appropriate controls. So far, monitoring has not been used in this way to test the efficacy of decompression.

Artificial rupture of the membranes

The possibility that artificial rupture of the membranes may harm the fetus has often been expressed. Sudden reduction of uterine volume leading to disturbance of placental function, and cord compression, are mechanisms whereby membrane rupture may affect the fetus adversely.

The effect of artificial rupture of the membranes has been studied by Gabert and Stenchever (1972) in 749 patients. Rupture of the membranes was artificial in 303 and spontaneous in 446. In 21 cases abnormal fetal heart rate patterns, delayed or variable decelerations developed at the time of rupture. All of them had some abnormality such as breech presentation, cephalo-pelvic disproportion or cord complications. The author concluded that there did not appear to be any greater risk in artificial than in spontaneous rupture of the membranes as the incidence of fetal heart rate abnormality in the two groups was not different.

On theoretical grounds it would seem possible that artificial rupture of the membranes would be more hazardous to the fetus than spontaneous rupture as the presenting part is higher and cord complications may occur more often. However, in the absence of evidence, it would seem reasonable to accept the findings of Gabert and Stenchever.

Auscultation

While auscultation is not satisfactory for accurate monitoring of fetal heart rate, it is still used more often than electronic equipment. Therefore, knowledge of its limitations and how best to use the method is important.

Auscultation of fetal heart rate has been shown to be subject to three types of error: a random error, an error biased towards normality when the heart is fast or slow, and an error based on the inability to count the heart rate during contractions (Day, Maddern and Wood, 1968). The overall error of auscultation of the hospital staff was considerable, 20 per cent of observations being inaccurate by more than ± 15 beats/min. The error of the hospital staff showed that it had two components: when the fetal heart rate was 130 to 150 beats/min the error was random, but when the fetal heart rate was more than 150 or fewer than 130 beats/min, the error was biased, so that measurements would tend to lie between 130 and 150 beats/min. Fetal heart rate changes in relation to a contraction, which is important in determining fetal prognosis, were not detected by auscultation. In contrast, the auscultation error of two medical students, trained by using an electronic monitor, was much smaller, one per cent of observations being inaccurate by more than $\pm$ 15 beats/min. Thus, when obstetric personnel are properly motivated and trained, auscultation between contractions can be reasonably accurate.

The method of counting the fetal heart rate introduced by Caldeyro-Barcia et al (1966) has merit. The counting is begun during or immediately before a contraction, and is continued until two min after the contraction, the count being taken over 15-sec periods with 5-sec intervals. This technique might involve the observer in making as many as ten separate counts, and a more realistic schedule in our own hospital would be six counts each of 15 sec, two taken during the contraction and four spaced over the two min after the contraction. In this manner change in the fetal heart rate may be detected both during and immediately after the contraction. Steer and Beard (1970) found that the nearest approximation to the continuous FHR trace resulted when serial 10-sec counts of the FHR were made.

Some value in auscultation of fetal heart rate has been confirmed from the findings of the Collaborative Project (Benson et al, 1968). This involved the evaluation of fetal heart rate recordings from 24 863 labours which resulted in single births—either a live birth or a fresh stillbirth. Observers were trained especially for this study. The most valuable recordings were those utilising:

1. A standard deviation of the fetal heart rate.
2. A maximum drop from the average fetal heart rate.

The lowest fetal heart rate recorded also correlated to some extent with prenatal morbidity and mortality.

Breech delivery

Fetal heart rate has been monitored throughout breech deliveries by Teteris et al (1970) and their changes compared to those occurring during delivery of cephalic presentations. Characteristically in a breech delivery bradycardia of less than 100 beats/min occurs almost immediately the buttocks are delivered and persists until some time after completion of the delivery. The average fetal heart rate during birth is 60 to 80 beats/min.

Fetal bradycardia occurred during all breech deliveries and was comparable to that previously found during delivery in cephalic presentations. However, after breech delivery, recovery to normal levels of heart rate occurred more slowly and Apgar scores were lower. The delivery time was longer for breech than for cephalic presentations, and it was thought that this factor might be responsible for the delay in recovery of the heart rate when the fetus was delivered as a breech. The importance of time during a breech delivery would also be consistent with the investigations of Wood et al (1973) who have shown that time is an important variable determining fetal pH in a cephalic delivery.

Because of the extra hazards of breech delivery, it would be advisable to monitor all such cases. Extra care has to be taken to obtain satisfactory records during delivery. However, the obstetrician would be able to gauge the length of time that bradycardia has been present and modify his delivery technique accordingly. In skilled hands hastening a breech delivery does not pose an extra hazard of cerebral trauma. However, if an obstetrician cannot speed delivery without also adding the risk of fetal brain trauma, then monitoring has no positive benefit, except as a record of events which may relate to neonatal condition.

Oxytocin

When oxytocin is properly used by continuous intravenous infusion, i.e. the frequency, duration and basal tone remain within normal limits, the fetus is not usually affected. In a number of studies fetal heart rate, umbilical cord pH and Apgar scores have been compared in oxytocin and normal labours and found to be the same. One exception is the study reported by Bartschi, Huter and Romer (1972). They compared the effects of oxytocin, methyl-oxytocin and desamino-oxytocin on fetal heart rate and fetal scalp pH during labour. Oxytocin was administered at 1 to 10 mu/min. All three substances had no action on the fetal heart rate but oxytocin significantly reduced pH, whereas methyl and desamino-oxytocin did not. The reason for the difference may be that oxytocin increased the basal tone of the human uterus, an effect not found with methyl-oxytocin.

Stress tests using oxytocin before the onset of labour have been used as an index of fetal condition (Spurrett, 1971; Christie and Cudmore, 1974; Ewing, Farina and Otterson, 1974). While the correlation between a positive test and the occurrence of fetal distress or low Apgar scores is not close, there is general agreement that a negative test indicates the fetus is in good condition, whereas a positive test is too difficult to interpret to be of practical value. Thus a negative test in a high-risk pregnancy may be a guide in allowing the pregnancy to continue.

The criteria for using the test vary, the general indication being a high-risk pregnancy. Most investigators carry out the test by gradually increasing the oxytocin infusion until regular uterine contractions occur every three to four minutes. Deceleration of the fetal heart rate in relation to uterine contractions is considered a positive response, some investigators regard other fetal heart rate changes as significant, e.g. both loss of baseline fetal heart irregularity and marked baseline bradycardia (Spurrett, 1971).

It is uncertain how effective oxytocin tests are in testing fetal condition, both in comparison to clinical criteria and other antenatal diagnostic tests. A controlled trial would be illuminating. In the absence of this type of evidence our view is that the test may be beneficial in high-risk cases, providing the infusion is carefully given, uterine pressure is measured, and only significant FHR changes are accepted as indications of a positive response.

Paracervical block

Paracervical block may adversely affect the fetus by accidental injection of local anaesthetic into the fetal brain, by the myocardial depressant effect of the local anaesthetic agent passing from maternal to fetal circulation or by disturbance of uterine blood flow as a direct result of the physical trauma of the injection or vasoactive drugs used in the injection, such as adrenaline. Paracervical block has been shown to be associated with fetal heart rate change. Gabert and Stenchever (1973) studied 326 patients. Thirty-six per cent had a bradycardiac episode immediately after the paracervical block. However, low Apgar scores appeared to be related to factors other than the paracervical block.

The incidence of fetal bradycardia has been halved following the use of prilocaine compared to lidocaine or mepivacaine when administering a paracervical block (Schnider and Gildea, 1973), suggesting that it is the anaesthetic agent of choice.

Paracervical blocks are less popular in obstetrics because of the risks and observed FHR change following their use. However, where pain relief is required and other methods are not available or have failed, then using prilocaine, a small injection volume and no adrenaline, paracervical block may still have a place in obstetrics.

Pre-eclamptic toxaemia

Wood et al (1968) have shown that FHR abnormalities are more common in patients with hypertension and pre-eclampsia than normal. The incidence of abnormality was much commoner in the presence of proteinuria and hypertension, rather than hypertension alone.

Weingold et al (1970) have compared the fetal heart rate response to pre-eclamptic hypertensive patients during spontaneous and oxytocin-stimulated labour. Each patient was used as her own control, bouts of normal labour being alternated with oxytocin-stimulated labour. The oxytocin dosage was 5 to 6 mu/min and the control and oxytocin periods were each one hour. The incidence of late decelerations in the active phase of labour was three times higher during the oxytocin periods. The sample was small and there was no evidence that the oxytocin produced a serious effect on the infant when examined clinically at birth. However, the authors raised the question as to whether the use of oxytocin when the fetus is already compromised may sometimes be harmful. Normally there is some variation in uterine contractions while progress in labour is satisfactory. They suggest that a local control mechanism may be operative and be of benefit to the fetus which is in a precarious state of oxygen perfusion. Fetal monitoring is indicated in this condition, particularly in the presence of proteinuria. The use of a wide variety of drugs in this disease, some of which may decrease beat-to-beat variation of the FHR, should be taken into account when interpreting the FHR record. In addition, if morphine is used in pre-eclampsia, its depressive effect on FHR average decrease 17 beats/min) should be remembered.

Respiratory distress syndrome

Hobel, Hyvarinen and Oh (1972) have carried out an interesting study where they showed that respiratory distress syndrome was higher among infants with abnormal heart rate patterns. Abnormal patterns were observed in 15 low birthweight (650 to 2500 g) fetuses by continuous monitoring during labour. Fetal scalp blood and umbilical cord blood pH and gases were also measured. The clinical condition of the infant was evaluated during the first week of life and the results compared with those from 10 low birthweight infants with normal heart rate patterns. Infants with abnormal heart rate patterns had significant metabolic and respiratory acidosis during the intrapartum and immediate postnatal period, lower Apgar scores, and 10 of the 15 required resuscitation. The incidence of respiratory distress syndrome was higher among infants with the abnormal heart rate patterns (10 out of 15 compared to 1 out of 10).

This finding may be related to the aetiology of the respiratory distress syndrome and also may be used to warn the paediatrician of the possibility of neonatal depression and respiratory distress occurring in small fetuses exhibiting FHR abnormality.

Sympathomimetic drugs

The effect of orciprenaline, buphenine hydrochloride and tyramine (an indirect sympathomimetic) upon FHR has been tested by Dücker, Fischer and Thomsen (1972). There is an increase of maternal heart rate with orciprenaline and buphenine hydrochloride and a decrease using tyramine. The order of these changes varied from 16 to 45 per cent. However, none of the three agents altered FHR indicating that either the compounds do not permeate the placental barrier to any great extent, that the fetus is less sensitive to them or that metabolic breakdown of these substances in the feto-placental unit is very rapid.

These data are of importance as sympathomimetic agents are now used commonly in the treatment of premature labour and fetal distress. Ritodrine, another sympathomimetic drug also has no effect on FHR. Ritodrine has been shown in controlled trials to be effective in the treatment of premature labour, although its use in the management of fetal acidosis in the first and second stages of labour is still disputed.

Table 23.1. *Comparability of some obstetric variables in control and trial groups.*

	Control group	Trial group	Statistical test	
Mean maternal age	25.3 years	24.9 years	$t = 0.56$	NS
Parity 0	76	78		
1	38	31	$\chi^2 = 5.63$	NS
2	14	26		
3+	22	15		
Mean gestation	274 days	277 days	$t = 1.76$	NS
Mean birthweight	3300 g	3257 g	$t = 0.67$	NS

NS = not significant.

Table 23.2. *Comparability of intrapartum variables in control and trial groups.*

	Control group	Trial group	Statistical test	
Mean length labour	9.0 hours	9.5 hours	$t = 0.67$	NS
Mean induction delivery interval	9.8 hours	10.4 hours	$t = 0.47$	NS
Oxytocin				
Incidence	94	90	$\chi^2 = 0.86$	NS
Mean length	6.9 hours	7.1 hours	$t = 0.28$	NS
Mean maximum dose	18.0 mu/min	14.5 mu/min	$t = 1.69$	NS
I.V. fluids				
Incidence	104	114	$\chi^2 = 1.36$	NS
Time administration	7.4 hours	7.5 hours	$t = 0.07$	NS
Mean total volume	950 ml	850 ml	$t = 0.64$	NS
Epidural				
Incidence	37	46	$\chi^2 = 1.07$	NS
Mean length	1.3 hours	1.5 hours	$t = 0.02$	NS
Ketosis—incidence	29	32	$\chi^2 = 0.26$	NS
Assisted delivery—incidence	60	62	$\chi^2 = 0.01$	NS
Difficult delivery—incidence	8	4	$\chi^2 = 0.60$	NS
Caesarean section—incidence	20	30	$\chi^2 = 1.94$	NS
Infection incidence				
Intrapartum obstetric	6	3	$\chi^2 = 0.62$	NS
non-obstetric	3	5		
Puerperal obstetric	43	45	$\chi^2 = 2.62$	NS
non-obstetric	5	11		
Analgesic dose 0	13	18		
1	82	71		
2	45	40	$\chi^2 = 6.02$	NS
3	8	15		
4+	2	6		

NS = not significant.

FETAL INTENSIVE CARE—RESULTS OF CONTROL TRIAL

1. The Queen Victoria Memorial Hospital has a Fetal Intensive Care Unit which consists of a medical director, a medical technologist who carries out fetal blood analysis and equipment maintenance, and midwives who are trained in the use and interpretation of fetal heart rate (FHR) monitors. Prior to the commencement of the trial the Unit had been running for two years. The medical staff found the service attractive and monitoring was rarely omitted in high-risk cases. The senior medical staff came to rely on these techniques, the results of monitoring being used in determining the management of patients.
2. The unit was organised in the following manner. The FHR was monitored if there was a poor obstetric history, a medical or obstetric complication occurred or an abnormal FHR was detected by auscultation, or meconium was present in the liquor (Renou and Wood, 1974). If a monitored FHR was abnormal, then fetal scalp blood pH was measured.

Table 23.3. *Comparability of fetal variables in control and trial groups.*

	Control group	Trial group	Statistical test	
Apgar score—mean	8.0	8.0	$F = 1.12$	NS
grouped 0 to 3	5	3		
4 to 6	14	22	$\chi^2 = 2.42$	NS
7 to 10	131	125		
Resuscitation—*immediate*				
nil	5	6		
routine suction and oxygen	102	114	$\chi^2 = 3.07$	NS
i.v. therapy, intubation	43	30		
—*late* No	125	141	$\chi^2 = 8.49$	c
Yes	25	9		
Neurological symptoms/signs	11	0	$\chi^2 = 13.59$	c
Isolette care				
incidence	64	73	$\chi^2 = 0.86$	NS
mean time	2.7 days	2.3 days	$t = 1.21$	NS
Nursery care				
incidence	92	108	$\chi^2 = 3.58$	NS
mean time	3.8 days	3.0 days	$t = 2.25$	a
Gavaging				
incidence	27	18	$\chi^2 = 2.61$	NS
mean time	3.2 days	3.4 days	$t = 0.44$	NS
Neonatal infection	6	3	$\chi^2 = 1.03$	NS
Delivery blood gases				
Umbilical vein—pH	7.313	7.345	$t = 2.03$	a
—Po_2	24.4	30.4	$t = 3.26$	c
—Pco_2	43.5	38.0	$t = 2.68$	a
Umbilical artery—pH	7.266	7.293	$t = 1.54$	NS
—Po_2	13.4	18.7	$t = 3.28$	b
—Pco_2	54.2	47.2	$t = 2.81$	c

NS = not significant.
[a] $P = {<}0.05$
[b] $P = {<}0.01$
[c] $P = {<}0.001$

Clinical management was determined by the combined assessment of the clinical history and the prognosis known to be associated with FHR and fetal scalp pH findings (Renou and Wood, 1974). Because the value of fetal monitoring has been debated without evidence being available from a controlled trial, its value was tested by a controlled trial involving 300 consecutive patients whose fetuses were at increased risk of fetal death.

3. The patients were allocated to the control or trial group by the use of randomised cards in sealed consecutively numbered envelopes. There was one breach of protocol and we were obliged to remove all the patients of one of the eight doctors submitting patients to the trial. In order to test comparability of the control and trial groups, the mothers' age and parity, the gestations at delivery and the infants' birthweights were compared and were found not to differ significantly (Table 23.1).

4. Intrapartum and postpartum events were also examined in the control and trial groups (Table 23.2). No differences were found. This suggests not only that the groups were comparable, but also that monitoring does not alter usual obstetric procedures. In particular, the use of oxytocin, analgesia and the mode of delivery were similar in the two groups.

5. During the trial there was one stillbirth and one neonatal death. The stillbirth was asphyxial, was in the control group and was thought to be avoidable. The neonatal death was in the trial group, was due to pulmonary haemorrhage a week after birth and was thought to be unavoidable. From Table 23.3 it can be seen that monitoring had no significant influence on the 2-min Apgar score; need for resuscitation, special nursery care and incubator care; gavage feeding and the neonatal infection rate.

There were two major differences between the control and dual group. Eleven infants in the control group and only one in the trial group showed minor neurological symptoms and signs such as irritability and 'jitteriness'. This difference was highly significant ($P < 0.001$). A

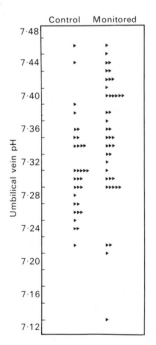

Figure 23.1. Distribution of umbilical vein pH in control and monitored groups. $t = 2.03$, $P < 0.05$.

paediatrician not associated with the trial considered perinatal hypoxia the most likely cause of the neurological findings.

The analysis of umbilical cord blood at delivery for pH, Po_2 and Pco_2 also showed significantly better results in the trial group as compared with the control group (Table 23.3, Figure 23.1).

It is apparent that fetal monitoring improves the biochemical status of the fetus at birth and the neurological status of the newborn at the Queen Victoria Hospital.

Using statistical methods (factorial analysis), it was also shown that fetal monitoring had more influence than any clinical factor in determining the biochemical acid–base and gaseous status of the fetus at birth. The details of this trial will be reported.

REFERENCES

Aladjem, S., Kahn, K., Dingfelder, J., Holzheimer, R., Cummings, R. & Michailov, D. (1971) Placental aspects of fetal heart rate patterns. *Obstetrics and Gynecology,* **38,** 671.

Bartschi, R., Huter, J. & Romer, V. M. (1972) Der Einfluss von Intravenosem Oxytocin, Methyoxytocin und Desamino Oxytocin auf die Wehentatigkeit, die fetale Herzfrequenz und das fetale aktuelle pH. *Gerburtshilfe und Frauenheilkunde,* **32,** 826.

Beard, R. W. (1962) Response of human fetal heart and maternal circulation to adrenaline and noradrenaline. *British Medical Journal,* **i,** 443.

Beard, R. W. (1974) The detection of fetal asphyxia in labour. *Pediatrics,* **53,** 157.

Beard, R. W., Filshie, G. M., Knight, C. A. & Roberts, G. M. (1971) The significance of the changes in the continuous fetal heart rate in the first stage of labour. *Journal of Obstetrics and Gynaecology of the British Commonwealth,* **78,** 865.

Benson, R. C., Shubeck, F., Deutschberger, J., Weiss, W. & Berendies, H. (1968) Fetal heart rate as a predictor of fetal distress. *Obstetrics and Gynecology,* **32,** 259.

Blinks, J. (1966) Field stimulation as a means of effecting graded release of autonomic transmitters in isolated muscle. *Journal of Pharmacology and Experimental Therapeutics,* **151,** 221.

Bolton, T. (1967) Intramural nerves in the ventricular myocardium of the domestic fowl and other animals. *British Journal of Pharmacology,* **31,** 253.

Bradfield, A. (1961) The vagal factor in fetal heart rate change: I. The effect of abdominal pressure. *Australian and New Zealand Journal of Obstetrics and Gynaecology,* **11,** 106.

Caldeyro-Barcia, R. (1969) Papers contributed by staff members of the Servico de Fisiologia Obstetrica Hospital de Clinicas, Montevideo, Uruguay, to the *Proceedings of the Special Session on Perinatal Factors Affecting Human Development held during the VIIIth Meeting of the P. A. H. O. Advisory Committee on Medical Research, Washington, D.C.*

Caldeyro-Barcia, R., Mendéz-Bauer, C., Poseiro, J., Escareena, L. A., Pose, S. V., Bierniarz, J., Arnt, I., Gulin, L. & Althabe, O. (1966) In *The Heart and Circulation in the Newborn and Infant* (Ed.) Cassels, D. E. New York: Grune & Stratton.

Chamberlain, D. A., Turner, P. & Sneddon, J. M. (1967) Effects of atropine on heart rate in healthy man. *Lancet,* **ii,** 12.

Chik, L., Rosen, M. G. & Hirsch, V. J. (1974) An analysis of lag time and variability of fetal heart rate measurements. *American Journal of Obstetrics and Gynecology,* **118,** 237.

Christie, G. B. & Cudmore, D. W. (1974) The oxytocin challenge test. *American Journal of Obstetrics and Gynecology,* **118,** 327.

Cloeren, S. E., Lippert, T. H. & Fridrich, R. (1974) The influence of cigarette smoking on fetal heart rate and uteroplacental blood volume. *Archiv für Gynäkologie,* **216,** 15.

Cumming, G. & Mir, G. (1970) Heart rate and hemodynamics after autonomic blockade in infants and children. *British Heart Journal,* **32,** 766.

Dawes, G. (1968) *Fetal and Neonatal Physiology.* p. 120. Chicago: Year Book Medical Publishers.

Day, E., Maddern, L. & Wood, C. (1968) Auscultation of foetal heart rate—an assessment of its error and significance. *British Medical Journal,* **iv,** 422.

Dücker, R., Fischer, W. M. & Thomsen, K. (1972) Das Verhalten von maternaler und fetaler Herzfrequenz nach Applikation direkter und indirekter Sympathicomimetica. *Archiv für Gynäkologie,* **213,** 127.

Eranko, L. (1972) Postnatal development of histochemically demonstrable catecholamines in the superior cervical ganglion of the rat. *Histochemical Journal,* **4,** 225.

Ewing, D. E., Farina, J. R. & Otterson, W. N. (1974) Clinical application of the oxytocin challenge test. *Obstetrics and Gynecology*, **43**, 563.

Furness, J., McLean, J. & Burnstock, G. (1970) Distribution of adrenergic nerves and changes in neuromuscular transmission in the mouse vas deferens during postnatal development. *Developmental Biology*, **21**, 491.

Gabert, H. A. & Stenchever, M. A. (1972) Effect of ruptured membranes on fetal heart rate patterns. *Obstetrics and Gynecology*, **41**, 279.

Gabert, H. A. & Stenchever, M. A. (1973) Electronic fetal monitoring in association with paracervical blocks. *American Journal of Obstetrics and Gynecology*, **116**, 1143.

Goodlin, R. (1972) Fetal heart rate patterns. *Journal of the American Medical Association*, **220**, 1015.

Goodlin, R., Schmidt, W. & Creevy, D. (1972) Uterine tension and fetal heart rate during maternal orgasm. *Obstetrics and Gynecology*, **39**, 125.

Grimwade, J., Walker, D. & Wood, C. (1970) Response of the human fetus to sensory stimulation. *Australian and New Zealand Journal of Obstetrics and Gynaecology*, **10**, 222.

Grimwade, J., Walker, D. & Wood, C. (1971a) Human fetal heart rate change and movement in response to sound and vibration. *American Journal of Obstetrics and Gynecology*, **109**, 86.

Grimwade, J., Walker, D. & Wood, C. (1971b) Letter. Morphine and fetal heart rate. *British Medical Journal*, **iii**, 373.

Hellman, L. M., Johnson, H. L., Tolles, W. E. & Jones, E. H. (1961) Some factors affecting the fetal heart rate. *American Journal of Obstetrics and Gynecology*, **82**, 1055.

Hislop, A. & Reid, L. (1972) Weight of the left and right ventricles of the heart during fetal life. *Journal of Clinical Pathology*, **25**, 534.

Hobel, C. J., Hyvarinen, M. A. & Oh, W. (1972) Abnormal fetal heart rate patterns and fetal acid base balance in low birth weight infants in relation to respiratory distress syndrome. *Obstetrics and Gynaecology*, **39**, 83.

Hon, E. H. (1967) Detection of fetal distress. In *Vth World Congress of Gynaecology and Obstetrics, Sydney* (Ed.) Wood, C. & Walters, W. A. W. p. 58. London: Butterworth.

Hon, E. H. (1968) *An Atlas of Fetal Heart Rate Patterns*. New Haven, Connecticut: Harty Press.

Hon, E. H. & Yeh, S-Y. (1969) Electronic evaluation of fetal heart rate, X. The fetal arrhythmia index. *Medical Research Engineering*, **8**, 14.

James, D., Morishima, O., Daniel, D., Bowe, T., Cohen, H. & Niemann, W. (1972) Mechanism of late deceleration of the fetal heart rate. *American Journal of Obstetrics and Gynecology*, **113**, 578.

Kaminsky, R., Meyer, G. & Winter, D. (1970) Sympathetic unit activity associated with Mayer waves in the spinal dog. *American Journal of Physiology*, **219**, 1768.

Klapholz, H., Schifrin, S. & Rivo, E. (1974) Paroxysmal supraventricular tachycardia in the fetus. *Obstetrics and Gynecology*, **43**, 718.

Koubenec, H. J. (1970) Fetale Herzfrequenz und intrauteriner druck bei Anwendung der abdominalen dekompression unter der Geburt. *Geburtshilfe und Frauenheilkunde*, **30**, 781.

Kubli, F. W., Hon, E. H., Khazin, A. F. & Takemura, H. (1969) Observations on heart rate and pH in the human fetus during labour. *American Journal of Obstetrics and Gynecology*, **104**, 1190.

Lumley, J. & Wood, C. (1969) Fetal acidosis. *Australian and New Zealand Journal of Obstetrics and Gynaecology*, **9**, 145.

Lumley, J. & Wood, C. (1973) The effect of changes in maternal oxygen and carbon dioxide tensions on the fetus. In *Clinical Anaesthesia* (Ed.) Marx, G. F. Oxford: Blackwell.

Lumley, J., Potter, M., Newman, W., Talbot, J., Wakefield, E. & Wood, C. (1971) The unreliability of a single estimation of fetal scalp blood pH. *Journal of Laboratory and Clinical Medicine*, **77**, 535.

Mocsary, P., Gaal, J., Komaromy, B., Mihaly, G., Pohanka, O. & Suranyi, S. (1970) Relationship between fetal intracranial pressure and fetal heart rate during labour. *American Journal of Obstetrics and Gynecology*, **106**, 407.

Nalefski, L. A. & Brown, C. F. G. (1950) Action of atropine on the cardiovascular system in normal persons. *Archives of Internal Medicine*, **86**, 898.

Navaratnam, V. (1965) The ontogenesis of cholinesterase activity within the heart and cardiac ganglia in man, rat, rabbit and guinea pig. *Journal of Anatomy*, **99**, 459.

Newman, J. & Wood, C. (1967) Abdominal decompression and foetal blood gases. *British Medical Journal*, **iii**, 368.

Padua, D. C. B. & Gravenstine, J. S. (1969) Atropine sulfate vs. atropine methyl bromide. *Journal of the American Medical Association*, **208**, 1022.

Paul, W., Quilligan, E. & MacLachlan, T. (1964) Cardiovascular phenomenon associated with fetal head compression. *American Journal of Obstetrics and Gynecology*, **90**, 824.

Renou, P. & Wood, C. (1974) Interpretation of the continuous fetal heart rate record. *Clinics in Obstetrics and Gynaecology*, **1**, 191.

Renou, P., Newman, W. & Wood, C. (1969) Autonomic control of fetal heart rate. *American Journal of Obstetrics and Gynecology*, **105**, 949.

Renou, P., Newman, W., Lumley, J. & Wood, C. (1968) Fetal scalp blood changes in relation to uterine contractions. *Journal of Obstetrics and Gynaecology of the British Commonwealth,* **75,** 629.

Resch, B., Herczeg, J. & Papp, J. (1973) On the fetal heart rate in early pregnancy. *American Journal of Obstetrics and Gynecology,* **116,** 293.

Rogers, R. E. (1969) Fetal bradycardia associated with para-cervical block anesthesia in labour. *American Journal of Obstetrics and Gynecology,* **106,** 913.

Rosefsky, J. B. & Pertersiel, M. E. (1968) Perinatal deaths associated with mepivacaine paracervical block anesthesia in labour. *New England Journal of Medicine,* **289,** 530.

Rushmer, R. (1961) *Cardiovascular Dynamics.* p. 57. Philadelphia: W. B. Saunders.

Sandler, M., Ruthven, C. K. J. & Wood, C. (1964) Metabolism of C^{14}-norepinephrine and C^{14}-epinephrine and their transmission across the human placenta. *International Journal of Neuropharmacology,* **3,** 123.

Scher, J., Hailey, D. M. & Beard, R. W. (1972) The effects of diazepam on the fetus. *Journal of Obstetrics and Gynaecology of the British Commonwealth,* **79,** 635.

Schifferli, P-Y. & Caldeyro-Barcia, R. (1973) Effects of atropine and β-adrenergic drugs on the heart rate of the human fetus. In *Boreus Fetal Pharmacology.* New York: Raven Press.

Schwarcz, R., Strada Saenz, G., Althabe, O., Fernandex-Funes, J., Alvarez, L. & Caldeyro-Barcia, R. (1968) Compression received by the head of the human fetus during labor. In *Physical Trauma as an Etiological Agent in Mental Retardation* (Ed.) Angle, Carol. Fourth Multidisciplinary Conference on the Etiology of Mental Retardation.

Shelley, T. & Tipton, R. (1971) Dip area. A quantitative measure of fetal heart rate patterns. *Journal of Obstetrics and Gynaecology of the British Commonwealth,* **78,** 694.

Shnider, S. M. & Gildea, J. (1973) Paracervical block anaesthesia in obstetrics III. Choice of drug: fetal bradycardia following administration of lidocaine, mepivacaine and prilocaine. *American Journal of Obstetrics and Gynecology,* **116,** 320.

Smith, R. (1971) Intrinsic innervation of the human heart in fetuses between 70 mm. and 420 mm. crown–rump length. *Acta Anatomica,* **78,** 200.

Spurrett, B. (1971) Stressed cardiotocography in late pregnancy. *Journal of Obstetrics and Gynaecology of the British Commonwealth,* **78,** 894.

Steer, P. & Beard, R. W. (1970) A continuous record of fetal heart rate obtained by serial counts. *Journal of Obstetrics and Gynaecology of the British Commonwealth,* **77,** 908–914.

Teteris, N. J., Chisholm, J. N. & Ullery, J. C. (1968) Antenatal diagnosis of congenital heart block. *Obstetrics and Gynecology,* **32,** 851.

Teteris, N. J., Botschner, A. W., Ullery, J. C. & Essig, G. F. (1970) Fetal heart rate during breech delivery. *American Journal of Obstetrics and Gynecology,* **107,** 762.

Tipton, R. H. (1972) Continuous fetal heart rate. *British Medical Journal,* **i,** 439.

Tipton, R. H. & Finch, A. (1972) The measurement and significance of transient fetal bradycardia during labour. *Journal of Obstetrics and Gynaecology of the British Commonwealth,* **79,** 133.

Tuxen, P., Kaplan, E. L. & Ueland, K. (1971) Intrauterine paroxysmal atrial tachycardia. *American Journal of Obstetrics and Gynecology,* **109,** 958.

Walker, A., Maddern, L., Day, E., Renou, P., Talbot, J. & Wood, C. (1971) Fetal scalp tissue oxygen tension measurements in relation to maternal dermal oxygen tension and fetal heart rate. *Journal of Obstetrics and Gynaecology of the British Commonwealth,* **78,** 1.

Walker, D., Grimwade, J. & Wood, C. (1973) The effects of pressure on fetal heart rate. *Obstetrics and Gynecology,* **41,** 351.

Walker, D., Walker, A. & Wood, C. (1969) Temperature of the human fetus. *Journal of Obstetrics and Gynaecology of the British Commonwealth,* **76,** 503.

Weingold, A. B., Feit, A., O'Sullivan, M. J. & Stone, M. L. (1970) Fetal heart rate response in the pre-eclamptic hypertensive patient during spontaneous and oxytocin stimulated labor. *Journal of Reproductive Medicine,* **5,** 35.

Welford, N. T. & Sontag, L. W. (1969) Recording fetal heart as a behavioural message. *American Journal of Psychology,* **24,** 276.

Wladimiroff, J. & Seelen, J. (1972) Fetal heart action in early pregnancy. Development of fetal vagal function. *European Journal of Obstetrics and Gynaecology,* **2,** 55.

Wood, C., Hammond, J., Lumley, J. & Newman, W. (1971) Effects of maternal inhalation of 10% oxygen upon the human fetus. *Australian and New Zealand Journal of Obstetrics and Gynaecology,* **11,** 85–90.

Wood, C., Lumley, J., Hammond, J. & Newman, W. (1968) The assessment of the foetus during labour in patients with hypertension. *Medical Journal of Australia,* **2,** 707.

Wood, C., Newman, W., Lumley, J., & Hammond, J. (1969) Classification of fetal heart rate in relation to fetal scalp blood measurements and apgar score. *American Journal of Obstetrics and Gynecology,* **105,** 942.

Wood, C., Ng, K. H., Hounslow, D. & Benning, H. (1973) Time—an important variable in normal delivery. *Journal of Obstetrics and Gynaecology of the British Commonwealth,* **80,** 295.

24

FETAL ELECTROENCEPHALOGRAPHY

Robert J. Sokol, Mortimer G. Rosen and Lawrence Chik

The direction of modern obstetric thinking has been not only to eliminate fetal and neonatal death, but also to ensure that infants are born in optimal condition with full potential for normal development. It is reasonable to suspect that some of those who experience severe fetal distress at any time prior to birth may survive with neurological damage that reduces their potential as future citizens. The fetus born from an abnormal intra-uterine environment, such as the dysmature infant or the infant of the toxaemic or diabetic mother, is known to have behavioural defects in later life which are not found in individuals who started life with nine months in an appropriate intra-uterine environment.

Other chapters in this volume discuss progress in identification of the many causes of fetal distress during the antepartum period. The intrapartum period undoubtedly may present significant stress for the fetus with increased risks of both trauma and asphyxia. Fetal response to these stresses during labour is amenable to study. Considerable experience has been gathered from monitoring intra-uterine pressure (IUP), fetal electrocardiogram (FECG), fetal heart rate (FHR) and fetal scalp microblood analysis.

Electroencephalography has been used for a long time by neurologists for assessing the central nervous system, but until recently the technique had rarely been used to study the fetus. As a result of the introduction of improved recording techniques, a relatively new application of this laboratory test has been developed. This method for studying the fetus during labour is termed fetal electroencephalography. At the beginning of our fetal monitoring programme, it was hypothesised that the fetal electroencephalogram (FEEG) might serve as a time marker for acute stressful events during labour, as they are reflected in alterations of the electrical energy of the fetal brain. The ability to study the brain more closely might be helpful in separating antepartum from intrapartum and postpartum events and make possible earlier identification of infant neurological morbidity.

In this chapter, the historical background of fetal electroencephalography and the development of the methodology for obtaining and analysing FEEG will be reviewed. Normal FEEG will be described as an introduction to studies of fetal environmental changes as they alter the FEEG. FEEG events associated with changes in other fetal monitoring parameters will be described. In addition, FEEG changes associated with abnormal neurological development will be discussed.

HISTORICAL BACKGROUND

Caton (1875) first documented the electrical energy of the brain from studies on rabbits. Berger (1929) successfully demonstrated the human brain wave. Jasper, Bridgman and Carmichael (1937) reported early studies in fetal electroencephalography by recording the developing potentials of the externalised fetal guinea-pig. These authors noted the earliest signs of electrical activity as well as FEEG changes with increasing fetal weight and maturity. Since then, FEEG has been studied by many investigators in several species, including the guinea-pig, sheep and man. Electrical activity of the human brain has been demonstrated as early as eight weeks after conception when studied in abortuses (see Rosen and Satran, 1965; Rosen, 1969).

Lindsley (1942) attempted to record both fetal heart and brain potentials with electrodes applied to the abdomen of his pregnant wife, and Bernstine, Borkowski and Price (1955) reported their attempts to use both abdominal and vaginal electrodes for recording electroencephalograms (EEG) of the human fetus. The latter technique, although the first to obtain FEEG directly from the fetal scalp, did not allow for continuous recording, since the electrodes were held in place for only short periods of time.

Investigators in the authors' laboratory reported the recording of FEEG using metal scalp clip electrodes which remained in place throughout labour. No abrupt changes in EEG were noted at the time of umbilical cord clamping or at the time of the infant's first breath (Rosen and Satran, 1965). Nonetheless, FEEG recording at that time was quite limited, since only a small portion of the recording was free of electrical artifact. It was apparent that a more adequate recording device would be needed.

PRINCIPLES OF RECORDING TECHNIQUE

The problem of obtaining FEEG of a technical quality equal to that obtained after birth centred around the development of an appropriate electrode. An electrode which may be used successfully to record FEEG must fulfil several criteria. It should be easily applied to the fetal scalp at a time early enough in labour to provide useful information, and be free of harmful effect. The recording point must be isolated from the highly conductive amniotic fluid, in addition to environmental electrical sources, such as the fetal heart. Without isolation, low scalp potentials of the FEEG are overshadowed by the higher potentials of the FECG. Finally, artifacts produced by uterine contractions, maternal body movements, pulse and respirations, and possibly by fetal movement, must be minimised if the information is to be useful.

The electrode

The electrode, as developed in the authors' laboratory (Rosen et al, 1973), has recently been modified. As shown in Figure 24.1, the electrode measures 2.5 cm in diameter. The outer surface is covered with silicone rubber which is inert to the environment and facilitates insertion. The recording point is a tapered platinum pin which does not easily penetrate the fetal scalp. The pin is embedded in the centre of a plastic disc which provides a stable recording base for the electrode. The recording wire cable assembly is shielded and is enclosed in a silicone sheath together with a suction tube. A platinum wire wrapped about the handle and back of

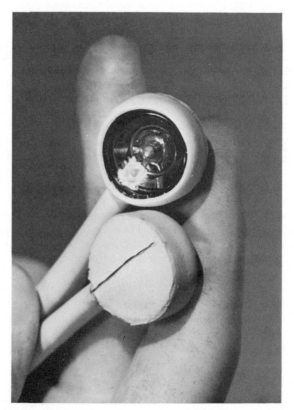

Figure 24.1. The suction electrode. Two electrodes are shown. The fetal surface contains the recording pin. The wire on the maternal surface acts as a patient reference. Two electrodes are required for recording bipolar FEEG. A single electrode can be used if only FECG is required.

the electrode acts as the patient reference. Continuous suction, provided by a connector assembly, draws the skin up to the recording pin, the grooved sides of the disc preventing the skin from occluding the suction. The use of suction helps to provide both isolation of the recording pin (eliminating conductive amniotic fluid) and mechanical stability. Utilisation of a platinum recording pin provides electrical stability, because of the non-polarisable property of the material. Electrode pairs are carefully matched for impedance and meticulously cleaned to eliminate polarisable contaminants.

Application of the electrode

Once the cervix is 2 to 3 cm dilated, the amniotic sac is ruptured and two electrodes are sequentially passed through the cervix and placed against the fetal scalp. About 250 to 400 mm Hg of negative pressure is exerted to keep the electrode in place. When properly applied, the electrodes remain in place for the duration of labour and delivery. Superficial fetal scalp abrasions may be seen following the use of these electrodes, but skin infections, lacerations or haematomata have not occurred.

The FEEG recorded in this manner is bipolar. Because of different rates of maturation of areas of the fetal brain, the central brain regions (parietal areas) show more electrical activity than the low occipital or temporal regions. To achieve the most reliable tracing, it is desirable to have at least one electrode in a parietal location.

Inter-electrode distance is also important. If this is less than 4 cm, an artifactual low voltage pattern is created, which may not reflect the true electrical state of the brain.

Recording methods

The morphology of the FEEG recorded depends upon the electrical characteristics of the electrode and amplifier systems. The signals from the electrodes are processed through differential amplifiers, which may be balanced to eliminate ECG artifact. The resulting voltages represent FEEG and are recorded on a high input impedance polygraph. Band pass filters are used to admit frequencies between 0.5 and 30 cycles/sec (Hz), at a paper speed of 25 mm/sec. Amplification of 50 μV/cm allows adequate visual discrimination of the wave forms.

Simultaneous FECG is also recorded from the electrodes and is processed through a cardiotachometer to yield FHR. IUP is obtained with the use of an open-ended catheter and strain gauge in the usual manner. FHR and IUP are displayed on a trend recorder with a paper speed of 30 mm/min. Determinations on fetal scalp blood samples include pH and base excess.

Data collection

Paper tracings of FEEG are interpreted visually in the light of clinical information, such as high-risk factors, labour progress, drugs and FHR/IUP findings. To aid in this integrated assessment, the authors' laboratory is developing a number of computer programmes for the analysis of patient information, labour progress (Sokol et al, 1973a, 1973b, 1974a, 1974b), intra-uterine pressure (Chik, Rosen and Hirsch, 1974; Chik et al, 1975) and FHR (Chik, Rosen and Hirsch, 1974; Chik et al, 1974a). A programme for FEEG pattern recognition (Chik et al, 1975) generates outcomes of each 10-sec epoch in a standard terminology, adapted from neonatal EEG interpretation (Anders, Emde and Parmelee, 1971).

FETAL ELECTROENCEPHALOGRAPH PATTERNS

The observations presented here are a summary of results obtained since 1969. When used on a general labour floor, about half the time a clean recording of FEEG, as defined by at least 20 min of useful tracing, is obtained. Many recordings are taken continuously throughout labour and may occasionally last 12 hours or more. With increasing experience and persistence in application of the electrodes, successful recording of FEEG is possible in almost every vertex presentation. The low success rate noted earlier is in part due to the training programme, in which all new physicians on the service as well as some nurses apply the monitoring devices.

During labour, the FEEG seen in the unmedicated mother can be compared with EEG in the neonate. In addition, there are two major categories of FEEG change which the authors believe represent other than normal electrical events recorded from the brain. The first category is a series of events, transient in time and associated with a specific clinical event occurring at that moment, e.g. certain FHR decelerations. These electrical changes do not persist after the termination of that event and are labelled as *transient*. The second general category of FEEG change is described as *non-transient*. These changes in wave form or voltage are persistent in time and, at least on visual interpretation, are less influenced by the acute events which occur during labour. They are present at the start of recording or may develop during the monitoring study; they may persist throughout major portions of the recording.

Normal FEEG patterns

FEEG patterns resemble patterns found in the neonate of the same gestational age or maturity. For more complete descriptions of the neonatal EEG patterns, the reader is referred to the

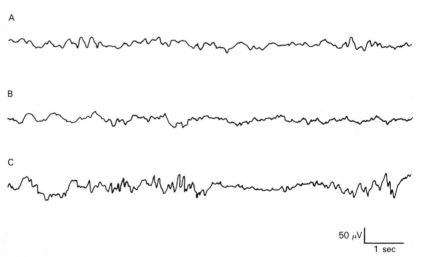

Figure 24.2. (A) Normal FEEG. Mixed activity recorded from a mature fetus with amplitude to 50 μV and wave frequencies between 1.5 and 7 Hz. (B) Neonatal EEG. Recorded from the same infant while alert, immediately after birth. Note similarity to FEEG. (C) Normal FEEG. Burst suppression (trace alternant) pattern in same unmedicated fetus. From Rosen, Scibetta and Hochberg (1970) with kind permission of the editor of *Obstetrics and Gynecology.*

neonatal studies of Dreyfus-Brisac (1964) and Anders, Emde and Parmelee (1971). In the mature fetus, as shown in Figure 24.2, wave frequency varies between 0.5 and 25 Hz with the predominant frequency in the 2.5 to 5 Hz range (theta waves). Delta waves (0.5 to 2.5 Hz) also occur. Voltage varies from approximately 10 to 100 μV. Low voltage irregular (LVI), mixed (MIX), high voltage slow (HVS) and trace alternant (T/A) patterns can be identified in the FEEG. Brain electrical activity does not change abruptly with birth, being the same as that seen in the FEEG immediately prior to birth. This has been confirmed in a computer analysis of FEEG patterns seen during labour (more than 14 000 ten-sec epochs from 11 subjects) and compared with records from the same neonate.

The FEEG of the premature infant may show discontinuous activity which increases with immaturity on an isoelectric (flat) baseline. The appearance is similar to that of the neonatal EEG of an infant at the same gestational age, as described by others.

Transient changes

The transient FEEG changes described below occur in association with acute events of labour. However, it is not certain that these electrical events are necessarily associated only with these events of labour.

Effect of medication

Examination of the FEEG obtained during labour and delivery documents the rapid transplacental passage of drugs from the mother to the fetus. These changes may be abrupt (Figure 24.3). For example, approximately 90 sec after intravenous injection of pethidine, a

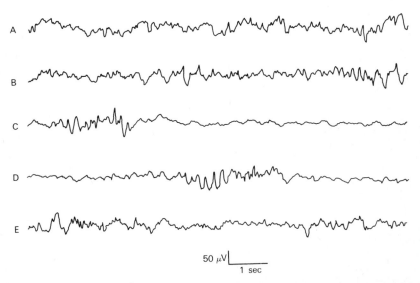

50 μV | _____
                1 sec

Figure 24.3. (A) FEEG prior to administration of pethidine 50 mg i.v. to the mother. (B) One min after administration of pethidine. (C) and (D) 20 min after drug administration. Note trace alternant activity. (E) 60 min after drug administration. Note appearance of faster activity. From Steinbrecher (1970) with kind permission of the author and the editor of *American Journal of EEG Technology*.

transient increase in theta wave frequencies (2.5 to 5 Hz) of about 50 μV in amplitude occurs. This is followed by a trace alternant-like pattern of burst suppression activity within five
min. This pattern may persist for as long as two hours, differentiating it from the trace
alternant-like pattern seen in non-medicated fetuses, which is considerably less persistent and
has less fast activity seen in the 'bursts'. Gradually, as the time after injection lengthens,
faster (15 to 25 Hz) and lower voltage (5 to 10 μV) wave forms in the beta range become
more obvious. Thus, with respect to pethidine, visual inspection reveals both changes in
amplitudes and frequencies, as well as changes in incidence of patterns usually seen.

Several more preliminary observations have also been made following the use of local
anaesthetics in paracervical blocks. The appearance of higher voltage activated EEG
patterns after the use of mepivacaine (Carbocaine) has been noted (Rosen, Scibetta and
Hochberg, 1970).

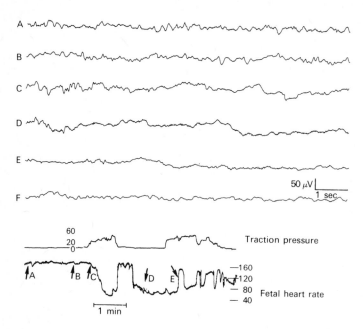

Figure 24.4. EEG and obstetric forceps. (A) FEEG prior to forceps application. (B) Forceps blades in place. (C)
FEEG shows 'flattening' starting in this case at 25 mm Hg of traction pressure as measured at the forceps handle.
(D) Despite relaxation of forceps traction, FHR remains depressed. FEEG is isoelectric. (E) FHR elevated tran-
siently but FEEG remains isoelectric. (F) Neonatal EEG immediately after birth. Note similarity to FEEG prior
to forceps application. From Rosen et al (1973) with kind permission of the editor of *American Journal of
Obstetrics and Gynecology*.

Effect of forceps

FEEG has been recorded prior to, during and following forceps rotation and traction (Figure
24.4). Transient EEG changes occur with a loss of faster frequency waves and decreasing
voltage to isoelectricity. The EEG appears to revert to the pre-forceps pattern after delivery
or when the forceps are unlocked and pressure is released prior to birth, although this did not
occur in the case shown in Figure 25.4. These changes may occur independently of FHR

decelerations and are not seen during normal spontaneous delivery, despite maternal 'pushing' pressure on the fetal head (Rosen, Scibetta and Hochberg, 1973).

Fetal heart rate decelerations

FHR decelerations have been described by Hon (1968) as 'early', associated with pressure on the fetal head; 'late', associated with 'utero-placental insufficiency'; and 'variable', associated with compression of the umbilical cord. Association of change or lack of change in the FEEG with these FHR deceleration patterns has been made difficult by the fact that the FEEG paper trace is recorded at 50 times the speed of the FHR/IUP paper trace. Thus, the recordings can be extremely long, making it impractical to compare all the data visually with the slower speed FHR/IUP tracing, but by means of a computer it will be possible to develop cross correlative evaluations.

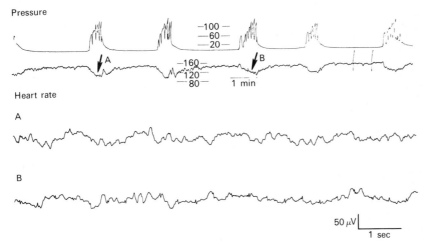

Figure 24.5. Early FHR decelerations. FEEG at times A and B (arrows at low points of decelerations) shows no significant voltage suppression. Note different calibration scales for FHR, IUP, and FEEG. From Rosen et al (1973) with kind permission of the editor of *American Journal of Obstetrics and Gynecology*.

FHR decelerations meeting with the criteria for early decelerations do not appear to be associated with changes in voltage or frequency of the FEEG. As shown in Figure 24.5, the EEG pattern seen prior to the deceleration, in this case, of mixed activity, tends to persist through the time of the early cardiac deceleration. Late and variable FHR decelerations are often associated with FEEG change (Figures 24.6 and 24.7). These changes progress in a very characteristic pattern. From a pre-existing pattern, present prior to the onset of the FHR deceleration, the FEEG first appears to lose the faster rhythms, followed by more apparent slowing. This trend persists to the development of isoelectric or almost flat periods with rare irregularly interspersed bursts of FEEG which disappear, giving rise to a totally isoelectric interval. This isoelectric interval is clearly distinct from the suppressed FEEG activity seen during spontaneous trace alternant activity or following maternal medication, inasmuch as it lasts for longer than 10 sec. As the FHR returns to its baseline value, the FEEG changes, as described above, occur in reverse progression from isoelectricity to occasional bursts of EEG activity, to more persistent electrical activity, finally returning to the previously visualised tracing. This entire sequence may last thirty sec or longer than one min.

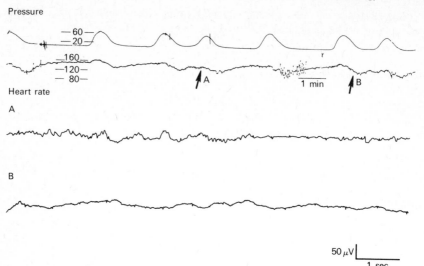

Figure 24.6. Late FHR decelerations. FEEG at time A, initially low voltage irregular, begins to become isoelectric (arrow A at onset of a late deceleration). Later in a late deceleration (arrow B, line B). FEEG shows isoelectric interval. Note calibration scales. From Rosen et al (1973) with kind permission of the editor of *American Journal of Obstetrics and Gynecology.*

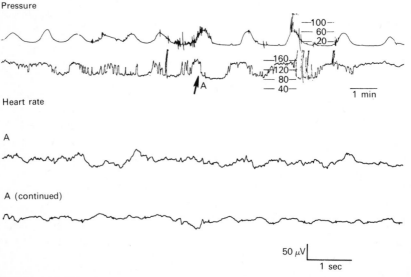

Figure 24.7. Variable FHR decelerations. At time A, the onset of a variable deceleration, FEEG changes to almost isoelectric recording. Note calibration scales. From Rosen et al (1973) with kind permission of the editor of *American Journal of Obstetrics and Gynecology.*

Fetal tachycardia

Fetal tachycardia is sometimes observed in association with other signs of fetal distress, such as FHR decelerations and meconium; it also tends to be present when the mother is febrile. FEEG patterns have been noted to show voltage suppression, i.e. lower wave amplitudes, and sometimes isoelectricity in association with tachycardia.

Non-transient changes

Our initial approach to the identification of significant non-transient changes in the FEEG was through retrospective studies. The FEEGs of infants known to be neurologically abnormal on follow-up examinations were carefully examined for electrical findings. On this basis, three varieties of FEEG were identified.

Sharp waves

These can be defined as repetitive waves in the same polarity (during that recording) which are generally higher in amplitude than the surrounding EEG and of short duration. Most often they are present at the onset of the recording and continue throughout labour. They generally occur during periods of relative EEG silence and are clearly distinguished from bursts of theta waves seen during trace alternant activity.

This finding has been identified in FEEGs of infants with neurological and developmental

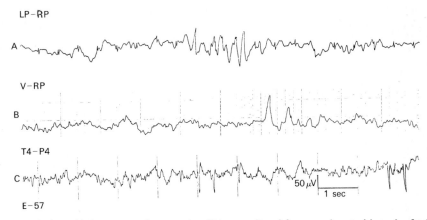

Figure 24.8. Mother with intrapartum hypertension. Fetus monitored for meconium and irregular fetal heart tones. (A) FEEG shows presence of high voltage sharp waves. (B) EEG at age three days. Note presence of sharp waves. Infant had been jittery but did not develop clinical myoclonic seizures until age eight days. Seizures responded to diphenylhydantoin and phenobarbitol therapy. (C) EEG at three years of age shows prominent spike discharges. Child, on diphenylhydantoin, showed retarded behavioural development and eye blinking and rolling without clinical seizure activity.

Table 24.1. *Relationship of FEEG to neurological examination at one year.*

FEEG		Neurological examination at 1 year [a]	
Normal (absence of sharp waves)	73	Normal	61
		Abnormal	12
Abnormal (presence of sharp waves)	23	Normal	10
		Abnormal	13

Adapted from Borgstedt et al (1975).

[a] The relationship of FEEG findings to the results of the neurological examinations at one year is significant ($\chi^2 = 12.58$ $P < 0.001$)

abnormalities at one year of age (Rosen et al, 1973). Moreover, sharp waves, both isolated and in runs, have been seen in patients who later developed neonatal seizures (Sokol et al, 1974c). In these cases, the sharp waves seen in the FEEG and neonatal EEGs were very similar in frequency, amplitude, and wave form. Figure 24.8 shows examples of tracings from one such case. More recently, data have been published for 96 children studied prospectively with FEEG and followed for one year in a neurological evaluation study (Borgstedt et al, 1975). As shown in Table 24.1, the presence of sharp waves in the FEEG was significantly related to neurological abnormality at one year of age.

Prolonged voltage suppression

This FEEG finding may be defined as the persistence of all recorded voltages below 20 μV with intervals of isoelectricity. Distinguishing this persistent finding from the rapidly changing tracing associated with FHR decelerations is not difficult but to delineate pathological prolonged voltage suppression, present from beginning to end of a tracing, from low voltage associated with poor electrode placement can be more difficult. However, as pointed out earlier in this chapter, if at least one of the electrodes is in a parietal location and the inter-electrode distance is more than 4 cm, a diagnosis of abnormal low voltage is made with more certainty. Indeed, persistent low voltage has been identified in neonatal EEGs in hydrocephalic and acutely ill infants. This finding may indicate an already stressed infant prior to the onset of monitoring and perhaps prior to the onset of labour.

A more easily distinguished pattern of prolonged voltage suppression which seems to be associated with neonatal depression is seen in the FEEG record which begins with normal amplitude and pattern of recording, but which, during the course of labour, progresses to persistent low voltage with prolonged periods of isoelectricity (Figure 24.9). Clinically, this

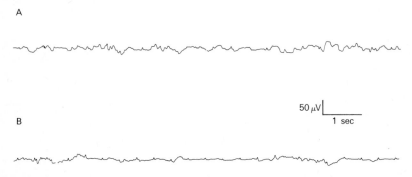

Figure 24.9. (A) EEG early in monitoring study of term fetus. Note continuous activity. (B) FEEG later in same patient showed development of prolonged voltage suppression which persisted through birth. Apgar score was normal, but the infant reverted to a lethargic state when not stimulated. From Rosen et al (1973) with kind permission of the editor of *American Journal of Obstetrics and Gynecology*.

pattern may be seen in premature infants whose mothers have received analgesic medication before delivery. It would appear that less mature infants are more sensitive to medication, as reflected by EEG events, than mature infants. Moreover, the persistence of low voltage without the recovery to a pre-existing normal EEG pattern, described in association with FHR decelerations, may suggest a more severely stressed infant with greater compromise of cerebral function. Prolonged voltage suppression has been associated clinically with neonatal depression and a complicated postnatal course (e.g. apnoeic episodes).

In a prospective study of Apgar scores of infants monitored with FEEG during labour, the presence of prolonged voltage suppression has been found to be significantly associated with decreased one and five-min Apgar scores and with the need for resuscitation in the delivery room (Borgstedt et al, 1976). In addition, preliminary findings based on programmed analysis of FEEG from 20 subjects appear to confirm the association of low voltage with decreased Apgar score at one min.

Periodic trace

In the neonate, periodic trace, also referred to as paroxysmal trace, is believed to be an abnormality of grave prognostic significance (Rose and Lombroso, 1970; Monod, Pajot and Guidasci, 1972). It may be defined as the presence of bursts of irregular sharp and spike wave activity of relatively high voltage compared to the very low voltage background activity. In the fetus, this sequence is characterised by abnormal patterns of higher amplitude than that usually recorded in the FEEG. It is remarkable for its repetitive similarities and is not to be confused with the burst suppression or trace alternant patterns seen in the neonate during deep sleep and also seen in the FEEG. Periodic trace is quite uncommon in the FEEG; the authors have identified it only once with absolute certainty (Sokol et al, 1974c). Figure 24.10 shows a sample of FEEG from a patient who developed infantile spasms and a hypsarrhythmic EEG at age four months.

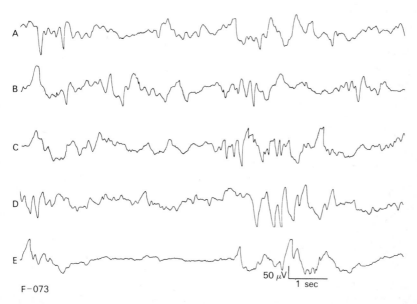

Figure 24.10. FEEG showing periodic trace. Mother with chronic hypertension. Fetus monitored because of meconium and abnormal labour. Pattern of repetitive bursts of high amplitude sharp waves and slow waves, as shown in this continuous example, was present from the beginning of monitoring study, suggesting cerebral damage prior to labour. Infant developed infantile spasms with a hypsarrhythmic EEG at age four and a half months.

CLINICAL ASSOCIATIONS

Intrapartum fetal distress and brain damage

Factors of importance in the aetiology of perinatal brain damage fall into general categories, two of which are trauma and asphyxia. In recent years, with the decrease of traumatic and difficult midforceps operations and the increasing utilisation of caesarean section in cases of relative cephalo-pelvic disproportion and prolonged labour, the importance of overt trauma in the aetiology of antenatally incurred brain damage may have declined (Burnard, 1962). On the other hand, the possible significance of intra-uterine hypoxia continues to be of interest.

Intrapartum hypoxia may produce brain damage. Windle (1968) compared monkey fetuses who had been asphyxiated totally with non-asphyxiated control monkeys for up to 10 years. Asphyxiation for more than seven min produced both transient neurological signs and permanent brain damage. In humans, an increased risk of neurological abnormality at age one year has been identified in infants, particularly prematures, who were the product of pregnancies complicated by abruptio placentae and placenta praevia, which both carry a risk to the fetus of hypoxia (Niswander et al, 1966a, b).

Intrapartum monitoring

FHR and MBE are parameters which are utilised as indirect indicators of the adequacy of fetal oxygenation; cardiovascular and biochemical changes may act as markers for in-adequate oxygenation of the fetal brain. Walker et al (1971) using a membrane-covered tissue O_2 electrode applied to the fetal scalp, were able to correlate a fall in fetal scalp Po_2 with FHR decelerations and accelerations. Myers, Mueller-Heubach and Adamsons (1973) using the monkey as an analogue to the human fetus, induced asphyxia by lowering maternal blood pressure in the distal maternal aorta. Components of late deceleration accurately reflected the state of fetal oxygenation. Myers (1972), also in the monkey, described fetal stress associated with hypotension and pathophysiological metabolic changes resulting in a small number of surviving monkeys who exhibited permanent brain damage. Finally, elsewhere in this book, Wood and Renou have clearly shown that the earlier detection and delivery that result from monitoring eliminate neurological abnormalities from neonates.

FEEG as an intrapartum monitor

Inasmuch as the central concern of intrapartum monitoring (apart from avoiding perinatal mortality) is the avoidance of brain damage, a parameter more directly reflecting brain func-tion is desirable. The authors believe FEEG to be such a monitor.

As pointed out earlier, early investigators without appropriate recording techniques could not consistently obtain useful FEEG. Since 1969, with the development of an adequate elec-trode, continuous recording of fetal brain wave during labour has been practical. Application of the electrodes to the fetal scalp is easily mastered; the obstetrician is not hindered in the normal conduct of labour, and acceptance by patients of the technique has been high. Once the electrodes have been set in place, the patient is no more aware of their presence than with ordinary FHR and IUP monitoring devices. Further improvements in electrode design are contemplated.

Wave forms and voltages recorded as EEG reflect the electrical activity of the superficial areas of the brain underlying the electrode locations. However, the electrical activity perceived in those superficial areas may also reflect signals from underlying and deeper areas of the brain. In fetal electroencephalography, electrical abnormalities may suggest areas of pathology or tissue injury. However, since only two electrodes are used, rather than montages of many electrodes, this technique does not allow one to locate the sites of possible damage.

Evidence that FEEG reflects the effects of asphyxia on the fetal brain as it does in the more mature brain has been demonstrated (Rosen, 1967). Asphyxia in pregnant guinea-pigs was induced by maternal tracheal clamping. This produced progressive diminution in voltage and slowing of wave frequencies (i.e. flattening) to isoelectricity in the FEEG, as well as in the maternal EEG, and was associated with FHR decreases. With release of the tracheal clamp, FEEG returned to the previously recorded patterns. The changes are similar to those already described in the asphyxiated human fetus. While such episodes are unlikely to be associated with neurological damage if an adequate cerebral circulation exists or if the duration of stress is brief, it is possible that persistent voltage suppression during labour developing from a pre-existing normal FEEG pattern is associated with cerebral damage.

Antepartum brain damage

Histological documentation has shown that fetal brain damage can be incurred prior to the onset of labour. Towbin (1970), studying serial sections of whole brain histologically, has postulated two general patterns of hypoxic damage, the appearance of which depend on fetal maturity at the time of the insult. Both patterns are consequences of hypoxic circulatory failure with venous stasis/thrombosis producing local infarctional damage. Moreover, both focal lesions and a diffuse depletion of neurons have been associated with significant neurological disability throughout the life of the individual. The authors' work with FEEG suggests that this situation may be reflected in FEEG tracings with non-transient changes of low voltage, sharp waves and periodic trace, present from the beginning to the end of the tracings. These FEEG patterns appear to be associated with developmental abnormality and are still being studied by visual and computer analysis.

Continuing fetal electroencephalograph research

A massive volume of FEEG data generated during intrapartum monitoring has accumulated. Programmed FEEG analysis eliminates subjective visual sampling problems and will facilitate specific correlative studies quantitating transient and non-transient FEEG changes and their relationships to prepartum and intrapartum events. For example, the characteristics of FEEG related to pethidine administration to the mother are being studied using programmed pattern recognition techniques. Clinical data from a computerised patient information file is being linked with programmed analysis of FEEG. In addition, on-line real time, computerised FEEG, FHR/IUP and labour analysis are being tested.

CONCLUSIONS

At this time, the FEEG is a research technique for although characterisation of the wave forms is well documented, clinical correlations need further study. It would seem that the

FEEG can reflect events which may occur prior to labour as well as electrical events seen to occur during monitoring. If abnormalities in the FEEG predict the later appearance of developmental neurological abnormality, the FEEG could become a valuable tool, not only for aetiological study and identification, but also for the prevention and treatment of brain damage.

ACKNOWLEDGEMENT

Work reported in this chapter was supported in part by USPHS grant HD-05566-01A1, the Grant Foundation, USPHS grant 5M01-RR00210-11, and the John A. Hartford Foundation.

REFERENCES

Anders, T., Emde, R. & Parmelee, A. (Editors) (1971) *A Manual of Standardized Terminology, Techniques and Criteria for Scoring of States of Sleep and Wakefulness in Newborn Infants.* Los Angeles: ULCA Brain Information Service/BRI Publications Office, NINDS Neurological Information Network.

Berger, H. (1929) Über das Electroenkephalogramm des Menschen. *Archiv für Psychiatrie und Nerven Krankheiten,* **87,** 527–570.

Bernstine, R. L., Borkowski, W. J. & Price, A. H. (1955) Prenatal fetal electroencephalography. *American Journal of Obstetrics and Gynecology,* **70,** 623–630.

Borgstedt, A. D., Heriot, J. T., Rosen, M. G., Lawrence, R. A. & Sokol, R. J. (1976) Fetal electroencephalography and one-minute and five-minute Apgar scores. Submitted for publication.

Borgstedt, A. D., Rosen, M. G., Chik, L., Sokol, R. J., Bachelder, L. & Leo, P. (1975) Fetal electroencephalography: Relationship to neonatal and one-year developmental neurological examinations in high risk infants. *American Journal of Diseases of Children,* **129,** 35–38.

Burnard, E. (1962) The relative dangers of asphyxia and mechanical trauma at birth. *Medical Journal of Australia,* **2,** 487–492.

Caton, R. (1875) The electric currents of the brain. *British Medical Journal,* **ii,** 278.

Chik, L., Rosen, M. G. & Hirsch, V. J. (1974) An analysis of lag time and variability of fetal heart rate measurements. *American Journal of Obstetrics and Gynecology,* **118,** 237–242.

Chik, L., Rosen, M. G. & Sokol, R. J. (1975) An interactive computer program for studying fetal electroencephalograms. *Journal of Reproductive Medicine,* **14,** 154–158.

Chik, L., Rosen, M. G., Hirsch, V. J. & Sokol, R. J. (1974a) Programmed identification of fetal heart rate deceleration patterns. *American Journal of Obstetrics and Gynecology,* **119,** 816–820.

Chik, L., Hirsch, V. J., Sokol, R. J. & Rosen, M. G. (1974b) Temporal characterization of intrauterine pressure data. *American Journal of Obstetrics and Gynecology,* **120,** 496–501.

Chik, L., Hirsch, V. J., Sokol, R. J. & Rosen, M. G. (1975) An optimized algorithm for the detection of uterine contractions in intrauterine pressure recordings. *Computers and Biomedical Research,* **8,** 294–301.

Dreyfus-Brisac, C. (1964) The electroencephalogram of the premature infant and the full term newborn. In *Neurological and EEG Correlative Studies in Infancy.* New York: Grune & Stratton.

Hon, E. H. (1968) *An Atlas of Fetal Heart Rate Patterns.* New Haven: Harty Press.

Jasper, H. H., Bridgman, C. S. & Carmichael, L. (1937) An ontogenetic study of cerebral electrical potentials in the guinea pig. *Journal of Experimental Psychology,* **21,** 63–71.

Lindsley, D. B. (1942) Heart and brain potentials of human fetuses in utero. *American Journal of Psychology,* **55,** 412–416.

Monod, N., Pajot, N. & Guidasci, S. (1972) The neonatal EEG: statistical studies and prognostic value in full-term and pre-term babies. *Electroencephalography and Clinical Neurophysiology,* **32,** 529–544.

Myers, R. E. (1972) Two patterns of perinatal brain damage and their conditions of occurrence. *American Journal of Obstetrics and Gynecology,* **112,** 246–276.

Myers, R. E., Mueller-Heubach, E. & Adamsons, K. (1973) Predictability of the state of fetal oxygenation from a quantitative analysis of the components of late deceleration. *American Journal of Obstetrics and Gynecology,* **115,** 1083–1094.

Niswander, K. R., Friedman, E. A., Hoover, D. B., Pietrowski, H. & Westphal, M. C. (1966a) Fetal morbidity following potentially anoxigenic obstetric conditions. I. Abruptio placentae. *American Journal of Obstetrics and Gynecology,* **95,** 838–845.

Niswander, K. R., Friedman, E. A., Hoover, D. B., Pietrowski, H. & Westphal, M. C. (1966b) Fetal morbidity following potentially anoxigenic obstetric conditions. II. Placenta previa. *American Journal of Obstetrics and Gynecology*, **95**, 846–852.

Rose, A. L. & Lombroso, C. T. (1970) Neonatal seizure states. A study of clinical, pathological, and electroencephalographic features in 137 full-term babies with a long-term follow-up. *Pediatrics*, **45**, 404–425.

Rosen, M. G. (1967) Effects of asphyxia on the fetal brain. *Obstetrics and Gynecology*, **29**, 687–693.

Rosen, M. G. (1969) Studies of brain damage in the fetus and the newborn. *Hospital Topics*, **47**, 91–93.

Rosen, M. G. & Satran, R. (1965) Fetal electroencephalography during birth. *Obstetrics and Gynecology*, **26**, 740–745.

Rosen, M. G., Scibetta, J. J. & Hochberg, C. J. (1970) Human fetal electroencephalogram. III. Pattern changes in presence of fetal heart rate alterations and after use of maternal medications. *Obstetrics and Gynecology*, **36**, 132–140.

Rosen, M. G., Scibetta, J. J. & Hochberg, C. J. (1973) Fetal electroencephalography. IV. The FEEG during spontaneous and forceps births. *Obstetrics and Gynecology* **42**, 283–289.

Rosen, M. G., Scibetta, J. J., Chik, L. & Borgstedt, A. D. (1973) An approach to the study of brain damage. *American Journal of Obstetrics and Gynecology*, **115**, 37–47.

Sokol, R. J., Nussbaum, R. S., Chik, L. & Rosen, M. G. (1973a) Computer diagnosis of labour progression. I. Development of an on-line interactive digital computer program for the diagnosis of normal and abnormal cervical dilatation patterns. *Journal of Reproductive Medicine*, **11**, 149–153.

Sokol, R. J., Nussbaum, R. S., Chik, L. & Rosen, M. G. (1973b) Computer diagnosis of labour progression. II. Application of an on-line interactive program in 45 high-risk labors. *Journal of Reproductive Medicine*, **11**, 154–158.

Sokol, R. J., Nussbaum, R. S., Chik, L. & Rosen, M. G. (1974a) Computer diagnosis of labor progression. IV. An on-line interactive digital computer subroutine for evaluating descent of the fetal presenting part during labor. *Journal of Reproductive Medicine*, **13**, 177–182.

Sokol, R. J., Nussbaum, R. S., Chik, L. & Rosen, M. G. (1974b) Computer diagnosis of labor progression. V. Reliability of a subroutine for evaluating station and descent of the fetal presenting part. *Journal of Reproductive Medicine*, **13**, 183–186.

Sokol, R. J., Rosen, M. G., Borgstedt, A. D., Lawrence, R. A. & Steinbrecher, M. (1974c) Abnormal electrical activity of the fetal brain and seizures in the infant. *American Journal of Diseases of Children*, **127**, 477–483.

Steinbrecher, M. (1970) Human fetal EEG monitoring during labor and delivery. *American Journal of EEG Technology*, **10**, 7–11.

Towbin, A. (1970) Central nervous system damage in the human fetus and newborn infant: mechanical and hypoxic injury incurred in the fetal-neonatal period. *American Journal of Diseases of Children*, **119**, 529–542.

Walker, A., Maddern, L., Day, E., Renou, P., Talbot, J. & Wood, C. (1971) Fetal scalp tissue oxygen tension measurements in relation to maternal dermal oxygen tension and fetal heart rate. *Journal of Obstetrics and Gynaecology of the British Commonwealth*, **78**, 1–12.

Windle, W. F. (1968) Brain damage at birth: functional and structural modifications with time. *Journal of the American Medical Association*, **206**, 1967–1972.

25

MATERNAL AND FETAL ACID–BASE BALANCE

James F. Pearson

UNITS OF ACID–BASE MEASUREMENT

A consideration of the units of acid–base measurement forms a good starting point for discussion of fetal and maternal acid–base physiology and pathology.

492

Whole blood pH

Hydrogen ion concentration is expressed in nanomols (1 nanomol $= 10^{-9}$ mol/l) or, more commonly, as the pH. The latter is the logarithm of the reciprocal of the hydrogen ion concentration; thus a unit change in pH is, in absolute terms, a tenfold change in hydrogen ion concentration.

The pH of a solution containing a single buffer can be calculated if the pK value of the buffer and the ratio between the concentrations of acid and base are known, from the Henderson–Hasselbalch equation, thus:

$$pH = pK + \log_{10} \frac{[base]}{[acid]}$$

(The pK of a buffer is the pH value at which the buffer is 50 per cent dissociated.) The pK of blood is more difficult to quantitate because it contains several buffers each with a different pK value and each present in different quantities.

The pH of the blood is influenced mainly by two groups of factors, *respiratory* and *metabolic*.

The respiratory component of acid–base balance

The respiratory component of acid–base balance is dependent on the carbon dioxide content of blood. The partial pressure of carbon dioxide is measured as $P\text{co}_2$ and is expressed in mm Hg.

The metabolic component of acid–base balance

Buffer base

This is defined as the sum of the bicarbonate, phosphate, plasma protein and haemoglobin ions in whole blood. The relative contributions of these elements to the buffering power of whole blood are detailed below.

Table 25.1. *The proportions in which the main buffers of whole blood contribute to its buffering capacity.*

Buffer acid $\rightleftharpoons$ H$^+$ + Buffer base	Approximate percentage contribution
$H_2CO_3 \rightleftharpoons H^+ + HCO_3^-$	64
$H_2PO_4^- \rightleftharpoons H^+ + HPO_4^{2-}$	1
H Proteinate $\rightleftharpoons$ H$^+$ + Proteinate$^-$	6
H Hb $\rightleftharpoons$ H$^+$ + Hb$^-$	29
	100

At any given pH all the buffer systems are in equilibrium. The total buffer base is conventionally measured at a standard $P\text{co}_2$ of 40 mm Hg, and is therefore independent of the actual $P\text{co}_2$ of the sample. When hydrogen ions are added to the system there is an overall reduction of buffer base. Buffer base measurements vary according to the haemoglobin and plasma protein concentrations of the blood sample. For this reason, direct comparisons between mother and fetus cannot be made.

Standard bicarbonate

This is a measurement of the bicarbonate ion in fully oxygenated whole blood which has been equilibrated to a P_{CO_2} of 40 mm Hg at 37°C. Thus it is independent of the actual P_{CO_2} of the blood sample. As standard bicarbonate constitutes only a proportion of the total buffer base it cannot be used to calculate the amount of acid or base required to correct an acid–base disturbance.

Base excess

The great advantage of this measurement is that the acid–base status of blood samples with differing concentrations of haemoglobin and plasma protein can be directly compared. Base excess is the amount of acid or base needed to titrate blood to a pH of 7.40 at a P_{CO_2} of 40 mm Hg and a temperature of 37°C. It is expressed in mEq/l. A negative base excess sometimes termed a base deficit, indicates a metabolic acidosis and a positive value of base excess indicates a metabolic alkalosis.

Base excess is useful in the calculation of the number of milliequivalents of bicarbonate required to correct a metabolic acidosis. A commonly used formula is:

$\frac{1}{3}$ of body weight (kg) × base deficit (mEq/l) equals approximately the number of milliequivalents of bicarbonate required to correct a metabolic acidosis.

Base excess can be expressed either as base excess 'fully oxygen saturated', or base excess at the actual oxygen saturation of the sample.

THE MOTHER

Maternal acid–base adaptations in pregnancy

Hasselbalch and Lundsgaard (1912) showed that blood P_{CO_2} values of women in late pregnancy are lower than normal. In 1915, Hasselbalch and Gammeltoft related the low P_{CO_2} to maternal metabolic acidosis, which they detected as early as the second month of pregnancy. It has since become apparent that over-breathing during pregnancy causes increased loss of carbon dioxide. Estimates by Bouterline-Young and Bouterline-Young (1956) and Lyons and Antonio (1959) suggested that the mean blood P_{CO_2} falls from about 38 mm Hg in non-pregnant women down to about 31 mm Hg during pregnancy. The increased maternal ventilation is out of proportion, being in excess of maternal oxygen requirements by a factor of two (Cugell et al, 1953). At high altitude, the fall in P_{CO_2} due to pregnancy is superimposed upon the altitude effect.

Pregnancy hyperventilation is attributed to hormonal influences. Ever since 1915 it has been known that a similar type of hyperventilation occurs during the luteal phase of the menstrual cycle (Hasselbalch and Gammeltoft, 1915), and Tyler (1960) showed that intramuscular injections of progesterone produced the same effect in patients with emphysema and hypercarbia. Progesterone itself has a pronounced effect in causing hyperventilation but synthetic analogues tend to be ineffective. In 1959, Wilbrand et al showed that progesterone lowers the threshold of the respiratory centre to P_{CO_2}, and oestrogen increases the sensitivity of the centre. Normal subjects increase their ventilation by about 1.5 l/min for each rise of

1 mm Hg in Pco_2. In pregnancy the equivalent in ventilation is about 6 l/min (Prowse and Gaensler, 1965). However, as progesterone does not readily cross the blood–brain barrier (Lurie and Weiss, 1967), the exact mechanism whereby hyperventilation is stimulated by progesterone has not been determined. The unified concept of Mitchell (1966), which hinges upon the active regulation of CSF hydrogen ion concentration, explains the general train of events. The fall in arterial Pco_2 brings about a respiratory alkalosis which is reflected initially in a higher than normal pH both in blood and cerebrospinal fluid. Within a few days, both CSF and blood pH values are restored to normal levels by means of compensatory renal excretion of bicarbonate. By means of active transport mechanisms across the blood–brain barrier the concentration of bicarbonate within the CSF is lowered. The superficial chemoreceptors in the medulla are then gradually 'reset' in such a way that they are able to discharge normally under conditions of lower than normal blood and CSF Pco_2 (Novy and Edwards, 1967). Thus pregnant patients, despite a lower than normal Pco_2, are able to adjust their ventilatory response to exercise in much the same way as do non-pregnant patients (Dahlström and Ihrman, 1960). The excretion by the kidney of bicarbonate ion results in a loss of base and this is reflected as a metabolic acidosis and base excess levels are reduced by 1 to 3 mEq/l (Sjostedt, 1962; Macrae and Palavradji, 1967). With the excretion of bicarbonate, sodium is also excreted. This has the effect of reducing the mother's plasma osmolality by about 10 mosmol (Robertson, 1968). The effect of reducing plasma osmolality by this amount would be that a diuresis would normally occur. However, the pregnant woman secondarily adapts her osmoreceptors to accept and preserve this new low level of osmolality in much the same way that her respiratory centre accepts and preserves a new low level of Pco_2. The fall in maternal Pco_2 in pregnancy makes good teleological sense in that the fetus can develop in a Pco_2 environment in keeping with an extra-uterine existence.

Much of the acid–base work on maternal blood has been performed using nomograms derived from the Henderson–Hasselbalch equation. These nomograms have been validated by Fadl and Utting (1969a).

Maternal acid–base changes in labour

The first stage of labour

Respiratory component. Normal labour is characterised by intermittent episodes of acute hyperventilation which recur in response to the pain of uterine contractions. These episodes recur with ever increasing frequency as labour progresses. As a result, arterial Pco_2 falls early in labour and continues to fall until full cervical dilatation, by which time Pco_2 values between 20 and 25 mm Hg are often obtained. The provision of pain-free conditions prevents this hyperventilation and maternal Pco_2 is maintained at its normal pregnancy value (Pearson and Davies, 1973a).

Metabolic component. The first stage of labour is associated with a metabolic acidosis which develops mainly during the active phase of labour and is exacerbated in prolonged and difficult labour. The main metabolite responsible for the acidosis is lactic acid, the levels of which correlate well with standard bicarbonate values. Ketonuria, which is a feature of the accelerated starvation of pregnancy, is a fairly common finding in labour and, although it is popularly considered to be an indicator of acidosis, there is no obligatory association between ketonuria and metabolic acidosis (Paterson et al, 1967). Other organic acids such as glutamic acid and alpha oxoglutaric acid are present in small concentrations in maternal blood. The plasma pyruvate concentration is very small by comparison with plasma lactate and the lactate: pyruvate ratio is mainly determined by the concentration of lactate. As pain-free labour causes minimal maternal metabolic acidosis (Pearson and Davies, 1973a), the probability is that a large proportion of the metabolic acidosis is due to loss of bicarbonate by the kidney to compensate for the respiratory alkalosis. This is supported by the fact that in response to acute hyperventilation for about 20 minutes, there is a prompt renal bicarbonate excretion which is reflected by a rapid fall of plasma bicarbonate. Active hyperventilation, such as is recommended by some proponents of psychoprophylaxis, results in the production of more lactate than occurs in women who do not consciously hyperventilate.

Skeletal muscular activity in response to pain may increase lactate production to a variable extent. Fear and apprehension, with consequent adrenaline production, may also be incriminated. In man, the administration of adrenaline leads to a significant rise in plasma lactate and pyruvate. At one time, it was thought that the muscular activity of the contracting uterus was a major factor in the production of maternal metabolic acidosis, but in the light of current knowledge this seems unlikely. It has been suggested that pain may induce changes in peripheral blood flow leading to inadequate tissue perfusion and that the metabolic acidosis seen in normal labour may in part reflect chronic tissue hypoxia.

The second stage of labour

Respiratory component. The expulsive efforts made by the mother during the second stage of labour can be regarded, from a respiratory standpoint, to consist of a series of Valsalva manoeuvres performed during uterine contractions, interspersed with periods of hyperventilation in order to eliminate accumulated CO_2. The effect upon maternal P_{CO_2} is reflected in a transient rise during contractions with a transient fall between contractions. The overall tendency during the second stage of labour is for CO_2 values to remain constant within the limits imposed by the transitory changes just described (Pearson and Davies, 1973b), or to increase slightly (Fadl and Utting, 1969b).

Metabolic component. The normal second stage is usually associated with a marked metabolic acidosis in the mother due mainly to lactate accumulation. It has been suggested that the duration of the second stage of labour determines the degree of metabolic acidosis and Jacobson (1970) showed that in multiparas the second stage was associated with less maternal metabolic acidosis than in nulliparas. The degree of maternal metabolic acidosis and lactic acidaemia has since been shown to depend on the duration of the second stage and not on parity (Pearson and Davies, 1973b). They also showed that, when, by use of epidural analgesia, maternal 'supplementary' expulsive efforts in the second stage of labour were abolished, no maternal metabolic acidosis occurred. Thus the progressive maternal metabolic acidosis of the second stage of labour is probably the result of expulsive and ventilatory efforts made by the mother.

The effect on maternal pH. The pH of the mother falls rapidly and, like base excess, is time-dependent. A mother bearing down during the second stage of labour will have a fall of blood pH at a rate of about 0.025 units per 15 min (Pearson and Davies, 1973b).

Placental gas exchange

Anatomical considerations

Recent advances in the understanding of the functional anatomy of the placenta require a re-evaluation of the mechanics of transplacental exchange. The placental cotyledon is subdivided into 60 to 100 lobules. Each lobule is supplied by a single end artery derived from the umbilical artery. The lobule is shaped rather like a brandy glass and the lobular branch of the umbilical artery, entering via the stem, subdivides into numerous capillary loops. Each loop, covered by trophoblast, constitutes a villus. The villi are packed closely together facing inwards, towards the cavity of the lobule. On the maternal side, each lobule is served by a single maternal spiral artery which spurts blood towards the apex of the bowl; the blood then spreads downwards towards its rim. This anatomical arrangement implies that the composition of intervillous space blood is far from uniform. It has been suggested that the maternal spiral arteries operate on a fully open or totally closed principle and seem to function intermittently, although recent studies using the electron microscope show that the internal elastic lamina is absent from the spiral arteries in the pregnant uterus (Sheppard and Bonnar, 1974). This finding suggests that the flow through the arteries may not be pulsatile and it is possible that they may not function intermittently.

Oxygen transfer

The factors which influence the transplacental diffusion gradient for oxygen are here considered separately.

Maternal and fetal Po_2 relationships. The maximum Po_2 issuing from the spiral artery is about 100 mm Hg; the maximum Po_2 gradient between the maternal blood and the fetal blood (Po_2 approximately 17 mm Hg) is at the apex of the lobule and diminishes towards the rim of the bowl where maternal Po_2 is about 33 mm Hg and fetal Po_2 about 28mm Hg.

Maternal and fetal oxygen dissociation curves. This subject has been reviewed in great detail by Metcalf, Bartels and Moll (1967). Fetal haemoglobin has a greater affinity for oxygen than does adult haemoglobin. Oxygen affinity is defined as the percentage oxygen saturation at a given Po_2, pH and temperature and is reflected in the oxygen dissociation curve. Examination of the oxygen dissociation curves of maternal and fetal blood shows that the fetal curve lies to the left of the maternal curve. This means that, for any given Po_2, fetal blood contains a larger quantity of oxygen per gram of haemoglobin than does maternal blood.

Maternal and fetal haemoglobin concentrations. The oxygen carrying capacity of both fetal and adult haemoglobin is 1.24 ml/g. Assuming a fetal haemoglobin concentration of approximately 17 g/100 ml and that of the mother about 11 g/100 ml, at full saturation 100 ml of fetal blood would contain 23 ml of oxygen and maternal arterial blood 14.7 ml of oxygen. So, in addition to the increased oxygen affinity of fetal haemoglobin, fetal blood has an inherently greater oxygen binding capacity.

The Bohr effect (see Figure 25.1). Maternal blood releases oxygen to the fetal blood and at the same time accepts fetal metabolites which cause a fall in maternal pH. This causes a shift to the right of the maternal oxygen dissociation curve (the Bohr effect) which of itself increases the mass transfer of oxygen from mother to fetus. As the fetal blood sheds its metabolites, the fetal blood pH rises, shifting the fetal oxygen dissociation curve to the left. This increases the oxygen affinity of fetal haemoglobin enabling it to accept more oxygen. The transplacental movement of hydrogen ions from fetus to mother effectively shifts both oxygen dissociation curves further away from each other. The greater the degree of separation of the respective dissociation curves of mother and fetus, the more rapid is the transfer of oxygen. This effect is called the 'double Bohr effect' and is unique to the placenta.

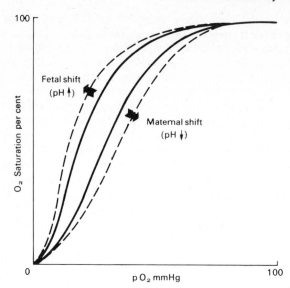

Figure 25.1. Diagram of the oxygen dissociation curves of fetal and maternal blood showing how the transfer of hydrogen ions from fetus to mother across the villus further separates the two curves, thus increasing the oxygen tension gradient between fetal and maternal circulations (the double Bohr effect).

Carbon dioxide transfer

As CO_2 enters the maternal blood from the fetus, some of it, under the influence of carbonic anhydrase, combines with water within the erythrocyte to form H_2CO_3 which then dissociates into HCO_3^- and H^+. The H^+ is buffered by haemoglobin and only a small fall in maternal blood pH results. The HCO_3^- moves out of the red cell in exchange for Cl^-, thus promoting the processing of more CO_2. Some CO_2 in the erythrocyte reacts with an amino group of haemoglobin to form carbaminohaemoglobin. At equilibrium about 8 per cent of CO_2 is in solution, 30 per cent is present as carbaminohaemoglobin and about 62 per cent passes out of the cell as HCO_3^-. As fetal blood traverses the villus the reverse reaction occurs and CO_2 is released which then diffuses into the maternal blood.

The Haldane effect. The CO_2-combining power of blood depends largely on the amount of haemoglobin within the erythrocyte which is not bound to oxygen and is thus free to buffer the H^+ formed by the dissociation of carbonic acid. Therefore, as maternal blood releases its oxygen it can accept an increased amount of CO_2 at the same level of carbon dioxide tension. This is known as the Haldane effect. As the fetal blood accepts oxygen, CO_2 is released from the fetal erythrocyte without alteration in environmental P_{CO_2}. This is known as 'the double Haldane effect' which like the 'double Bohr effect' is a unique characteristic of the placenta. It has been estimated that the double Haldane effect, under physiological conditions, is responsible for nearly half the total amount of transplacental carbon dioxide exchange.

Metabolic acidosis and the Haldane effect. Hydrogen ions from fixed acids, i.e. acids other than carbonic acid, diffuse across the placenta and are buffered by maternal haemoglobin. This reduces the amount of haemoglobin available to buffer the hydrogen ions derived from carbonic acid. Thus, by diminishing the Haldane effect, a metabolic acidosis either in the mother or fetus may adversely affect the transplacental transfer of carbon dioxide. However, the magnitude of this effect is generally regarded as being small.

THE FETUS

The investigation of fetal acid–base balance was pioneered by Ylppö (1916) who reported that by adult standards the cord blood of the fetus was acidotic. For the 40 years following this observation cord blood analysis remained the only method of investigation by which the acid–base status of the fetus could be determined. The introduction of fetal blood scalp sampling has enabled us to examine changes taking place in the fetus during parturition.

Fetal scalp blood sampling

Fetal scalp blood sampling (FBS) was introduced by Saling (1963). When properly performed, the sample conforms to the criteria set for arterialised capillary blood by the Report of the Ad Hoc Committee on Acid–Base Terminology (1966) and therefore is reflective of the acid–base status of the fetus as a whole.

Validity of fetal scalp blood sampling

On the basis of the evidence detailed below, it seems reasonable to accept that the acid–base values obtained from fetal scalp blood are reflective of the changes taking place within the fetus.

1. Samples of scalp blood taken just before delivery, compared to blood taken from the umbilical vessels at the time of delivery and before the first cry, have shown significant degrees of correlation with respect to the parameters of acid–base balance (Saling, 1963, 1966; Beard and Morris, 1965; Kubli, 1968).
2. Chronic catheters implanted in the blood vessels of rhesus monkey fetuses provided positive correlation between the acid–base and blood–gas characteristics of scalp and arterial blood (Adamsons et al, 1968).
3. Using exteriorised fetal lamb preparations, Gare, Whetham and Henry (1967) showed that blood taken from fetal hyperaemic scalp closely approximated the fetal arterial blood values of pH, Po_2 and Pco_2.
4. Good correlation exists between fetal scalp blood pH, glucose, lactate and pyruvate, and values found in cord blood, both at vaginal delivery and caesarean section (Yoshioka and Roux, 1970).

Technique of fetal blood sampling

The parturient patient is placed in the lithotomy position. In order to minimise the effects of aorto-caval occlusion a pillow or rubber wedge is placed under one or other buttock so that she tilts at least 15° from the dorsal position. Alternatively, especially during the second stage, samples can be easily obtained by utilising the full Sim's position.

The usual aseptic precautions are taken and, following a vaginal examination to check cervical dilatation, an endoscope of suitable size is introduced and digitally guided through the cervix to rest evenly against the fetal scalp. As a matter of personal preference this technique is modified as follows. The endoscope and obturator are introduced into the posterior fornix blindly. The obturator is removed; the fibreoptic light is attached and the endoscope is manoeuvred onto the fetal scalp under direct vision. This modification in technique causes much less discomfort to the patient and is particularly useful when the cervix is only minimally dilated. In order to place the endoscope tip evenly against the scalp, it is important to angle the endoscope correctly; otherwise leakage of amniotic fluid is likely to occur around the edges of the endoscope, thus contaminating the field. Therefore, as a general rule, it is advised that the higher the fetal head the lower should be the operator. Many operators in fact kneel on a small cushion placed on the floor or alternatively a low stool can be provided. The angle of the endoscope within the pelvic axis should be the same as that which would be subtended by the shanks of Kielland's forceps were they to be applied at that level.

If the membranes are intact, they are ruptured with swab-holding forceps, and if the head is not engaged, it is important that it be steadied by an assistant. If this practice is not followed, the fetus, being stimulated into activity by the procedure, will move about during the operation and spoil the field.

It must be remembered that the aim is to obtain arterialised capillary blood. Therefore, after the scalp has been carefully dried with a dental swab on a holder, it is sprayed with ethyl chloride. This is best done under direct vision by the operator. It is of the greatest importance that a hyperaemic flush develops on the scalp. Should the initial ethyl chloride spray fail to result in the development of hyperaemia the scalp is rubbed, perhaps several times, with the dental swab until a good hyperaemic flush develops in the operating field. Silicone grease is then smoothed *thinly* over the area. It is good practice at this point, if the scalp is hairy, to make a parting in the hair with the butt end of the scalp blade holder, otherwise the capillary action of the hair will cause the blood to run along the hairs and not along the collecting tube.

Two stab incisions in the scalp are made at about 12 o'clock with a plastic mounted knife. It is important that the knife is sharp and that the knife is used for one operation only and then discarded. This practice prevents unnecessary trauma to the fetal scalp. The incisions are best made just before the onset of a uterine contraction and the globule of blood which forms (Figure 25.2) is collected into preheparinised tubes—the straight pattern, which is extremely useful when the cervix is only one or two centimetres dilated, or the angled pattern

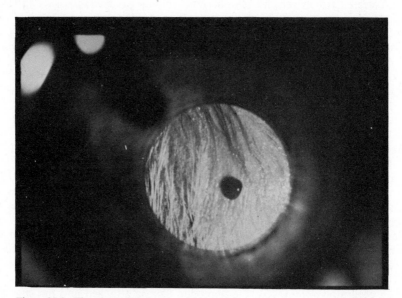

Figure 25.2. View through endoscope showing globule of blood formed after incision.

with tapered tips, which is probably easier to use. It is useful to fix a 6 to 8-inch piece of flexible polythene tubing to the end of the tube, which can be put in the operator's mouth and capillary action can be aided by gentle suction. The flow from the fetal scalp is always maximal during uterine contractions and should sufficient blood not be obtained with the first contraction, it is well worthwhile rubbing the scalp with a mounted dental roll and awaiting the onset of the next contraction before obtaining further blood. Under ideal conditions the aim is to obtain one full tube of blood for pH investigations and these require to be done, if possible, in triplicate. It is important that at least two estimations of pH agree with each other with an accuracy of ± 0.02 pH. If this modest level of agreement is not achieved, there is usually some methodological error and it is best not to accept the result. For research purposes two full tubes are required. It is best to avoid air bubbles in the tube but if the pH is tested immediately no great error will result.

Bleeding from the scalp is, in the author's experience, always controlled by swab pressure, but very occasionally, severe bleeding has been reported in severely asphyxiated infants because of an associated consumptive coagulopathy (Hull, 1972).

Acid–base measurement

The specimen is mixed with the heparin by use of a magnet which runs a short steel rod up and down the lumen of the tube. The blood samples are analysed by means of micro blood sample pH equipment which should be readily accessible to the obstetrician and be accurately calibrated with precision buffer before obtaining the sample. It is the practice of the author's department to ensure that all resident medical staff are fully conversant with the apparatus and are trained in the calibration of the equipment and are also responsible for its day-to-day maintenance. The pH values should be measured immediately. Measurements of fetal P_{CO_2} and base excess in the past were more difficult as they involved equilibration of the fetal blood with two CO_2/oxygen mixtures (containing four and eight per cent CO_2 respectively). However, of recent years more expensive automated equipment has become available which is capable of giving a readout of the absolute values of the different components of acid–base balance without preliminary gas equilibration.

Accuracy of measurement can only be achieved by attention to detail and a comment of Seligman (1968) is well worth remembering: 'In order to obtain meaningful results, it is essential that estimations are made on an apparatus in constant use by a constant user. The blood gas analysis apparatus which is left switched off in the labour ward for use once or twice a month by whichever resident happens to be on duty will give unreliable results which would probably be bettered by the use of litmus paper'.

Fetal acid–base balance

The normal acid–base range of fetal scalp blood

There has been considerable disagreement about what constitutes the normal range of scalp blood acid–base values. This problem was highlighted by Lumley, McKinnon and Wood (1971), who compared corrected values obtained by 14 different workers. Their conclusions were as follows.

The differences in acid–base values (Table 25.2) could not be explained by the method of selection of the study group, viz. clinically normal, normal by continuous fetal heart rate tracing or normal in terms of the delivery of a healthy infant. Nor could the differences be explained by the choice of analytical apparatus.

Table 25.2. *The range from lower to upper limits of normal ranges (mean ±
2 sd) given for fetal scalp blood–gas and acid–base parameters in a review of
the published work of 14 authors.*

	Lower limits	Upper limits
pH	7.15 to 7.30	7.33 to 7.47
P_{CO_2} mm Hg	22 to 34	50 to 67
P_{O_2} mm Hg	7 to 17	23 to 36
Base-excess (fully saturated) mEq/l	−14.1 to −5.3	−4.3 to +3.0

Adapted from Lumley, McKinnon and Wood (1971).

They attributed the differences to inaccuracies of measurement and variations of the composition of scalp blood over short periods of time. They pointed out that an associated factor might be the relative degree of acquaintance with fetal scalp sampling, which the writer feels is probably the factor of greatest relevance. As Table 25.2 illustrates, the range of published values is wide. In order to arrive at the likely normal range Lumley, McKinnon and Wood (1971) analysed acid–base values derived from 600 mainly abnormal patients and calculated a lower limit for pH at 7.25, base excess—8 mEq/l (fully oxygen saturated) and an upper limit for P_{CO_2} of 60 mm Hg. These values agree with those illustrated in Figures 25.3, 25.4 and

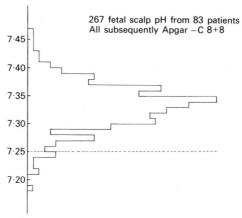

Figure 25.3. Histogram showing the distribution of 267 fetal scalp blood pH values obtained from 85 patients delivering of infants scoring Apgar (minus colour) 8 at one and five min. The lower limit of the normal range described by Lumley, McKinnon and Wood (1971) is indicated by the dotted line.

25.5. These histograms refer to values of pH, base excess (fully oxygen saturated) and P_{CO_2} in fetal scalp blood. All the mothers were subsequently delivered of infants in good clinical condition with an Apgar (minus colour) score of eight at one and five min respectively. Methodology was standardised. All scalp samples were taken during a contraction to improve sample comparability. Appropriate corrections were made for ambient barometric pressure and percentage oxygen desaturation. All samples were taken and all acid–base measurements were made by the writer.

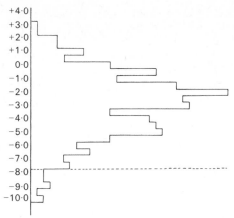

Figure 25.4. Histogram showing the distribution of 267 fetal scalp blood values of base-excess (fully oxygen saturated) in mEq/l obtained from 83 patients delivering of infants scoring Apgar (minus colour) 8 at one and five min. The lower limit of the normal range described by Lumley, McKinnon and Wood (1971) is indicated by the dotted line.

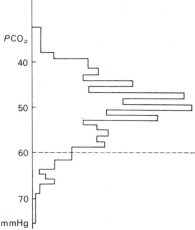

Figure 25.5. Histogram showing the distribution of 267 fetal scalp blood values of Pco_2 obtained from 83 patients delivering of infants scoring Apgar (minus colour) 8 at one and five min. The lower limit of normal range described by Lumley, McKinnon and Wood (1971) is indicated by the dotted line.

The lower limits of normal suggested by Lumley, which are strongly supported by the author's own observations, do not presuppose that values below these 'limits' are inevitably associated with fetal depression. The concept of 'pre-acidosis' (pH 7.20 to 7.25) and 'acidosis' (pH less than 7.20) proposed by Saling (1966) has some value for the clinician but is potentially dangerous for it presupposes that a fetus with a pH of more than 7.20 is not truly asphyxiated.

Fetal asphyxia

Total anoxia in the experimental animal results in a fall in oxygen content of the blood to zero in 2.5 min; the Pco_2 rises at a rate of about 10 mm Hg/min and the pH falls at a rate of 0.1

pH unit/min. These values reveal how sensitive pH is to oxygen lack, but have little relevance to the clinical situation, for, with the possible exception of major separation of the placenta (abruptio) the oxygen supply to the human fetus is rarely cut off so abruptly or so completely. Asphyxia in the human fetus is usually the result of partial oxygen deprivation, which in the fetus causes the following sequence of events to occur.

Glycolysis

Hepatitic glycogen is mobilised and broken down anaerobically along the glycolytic pathway (Embden–Meyerhof pathway), releasing energy and producing pyruvate. Normally, pyruvate is fed into the Kreb's tricarboxylic acid cycle where it is further metabolised aerobically. Under conditions of oxygen deprivation pyruvate production increases and, in order to maintain a rapid rate of glycolysis, is removed almost as fast as it is formed by conversion to lactate which then accumulates in the fetal tissues causing a metabolic acidosis and a fall in blood pH.

Hypercarbia

During hypoxia the fetal Pco_2 rises, increasing the level of H_2CO_3 in the fetal blood and giving rise to a respiratory acidosis and a fall in blood pH. The combination of hypoxia, metabolic acidosis and hypercarbia constitutes asphyxia. At any given level of oxygen deprivation, the survival time of the hypoxic fetus will depend primarily on its glycogen reserve, i.e. a well-nourished fetus can be expected to withstand a hypoxic insult better than for example, a growth-retarded fetus.

As the fetus is unable to compensate for acute metabolic acidosis by increasing pulmonary CO_2 excretion, the acidosis is combated mainly by utilising buffer systems. Of paramount importance in this respect is haemoglobin. If a pure metabolic acidosis is produced in fetal blood, the oxygen dissociation curve shifts to the right (Bohr effect) causing a change in oxygen affinity such that for a given Po_2 the oxygen saturation falls. This has the dual beneficial effect of increasing the quantity of reduced haemoglobin which is then utilised as buffer, and releasing oxygen from red cells, which then becomes available to the tissues. The buffering ability of the normal fetus is considerable because of its high concentration of haemoglobin. It also follows that the fetus with erythroblastosis is at a great disadvantage in this respect. The maintenance of blood pH is of vital importance in the maintenance of efficient glycolysis, for as pH falls, the rate of glycolysis is progressively inhibited and ceases altogether at pH 6.900, and it seems likely that when the buffer systems have become saturated with hydrogen ions the pH then falls abruptly to levels incompatible with life.

In 1963, the British Perinatal Mortality survey revealed that asphyxia was responsible for about 30 per cent of intrapartum deaths. Mortality statistics do not take into account fetal morbidity which may result from asphyxia. Brown et al (1974) reviewed 14 200 liveborn infants in Edinburgh and found an incidence of cerebral palsy directly attributable to asphyxia of 1.2 per 1000 live births and that if all grades of handicap were considered there were 34 such infants in this population (2.4 per 1000 livebirths).

The maintenance of an oxygen supply to the brain is of paramount importance. The oxygen consumption of the brain is 55 per cent higher in children than in adults (Richter, 1967) amounting to over one-fifth of the child's total oxygen consumption. Himwich et al (1955) have shown that the brain stem in the human neonate is selectively more vulnerable to anoxia than the cerebral cortex. Anoxic damage to the brain stem is likely to produce disorders of muscle tone and reflexes, disordered respiration, cranial nerve palsies and disturbances of temperature regulation. Hypoxia and carbon dioxide retention can cause cerebral vasodilatation and congestive brain swelling. The resultant cerebral oedema may further impair cerebral circulation with secondary cerebral ischaemia (Brock, 1971). Myocardial depression and systemic hypotension secondary to asphyxia may diminish cerebral perfusion. Furthermore, consumption coagulopathy caused both by the release of thromboplastin from ischaemic tissues and the consumption of coagulation factors in infarcted organs may result in an increased bleeding tendency.

All these factors serve to exacerbate the effects of cerebral birth trauma and the Edinburgh Study showed that of 94 severely asphyxiated infants with abnormal behaviour patterns in the neonatal period, one-third of them had been subject to traumatic delivery usually associated with unrecognised disproportion. It is therefore of the greatest importance that the mode of delivery of a severely asphyxiated infant is carefully considered. Davidson et al (1975) have shown that the duration of the deceleration phase of labour as determined by the time taken for the cervix to dilate from 7 to 10 cm is of considerable predictive value in separating those instrumental deliveries which are likely to be uncomplicated from those which are likely to be difficult. It is the present practice in the University Hospital of Wales to treat severe asphyxia at full dilatation of the cervix by caesarean section when a difficult forceps delivery has been thus predicted in order to minimise cerebral birth trauma amongst this vulnerable group of infants.

Fetal scalp blood sampling in clinical practice

In spite of considerable advances in continuous fetal heart rate monitoring, as Wood and Renou have also pointed out in Chapter 23, fetal scalp sampling remains the most reliable index of fetal asphyxia during labour. It is becoming generally accepted that scalp sampling is an essential step in confirming or refuting evidence of fetal asphyxia derived from other sources. Fetal scalp pH values of < 7.25 represent the beginning of fetal deterioration or 'preacidosis' and values of < 7.20 indicate fetal asphyxia or 'acidosis'. There are, however, several problems in the interpretation of the scalp pH and these are briefly discussed.

The false negative pH

Occasionally the situation arises when a scalp pH value within the normal range has been recorded before delivery and unexpectedly the fetus is born in a depressed condition. This is the 'false-negative' result, the frequency of which has been estimated by Beard (1970) to be of the order of ten per cent of all scalp samples taken for clinical indications. Although this figure may be regarded as rather high, there is no doubt that it does occur and that it may result from the interaction of several factors:

1. The pH value of the scalp sample can only be regarded as being reflective of the state of the infant at the time of sampling—a fact which limits its predictive value. Most samples are taken to assess the state of the fetus during the first stage of labour where a decision as to the most appropriate route of delivery may need to be made. During the second stage clinical evidence of fetal deterioration is usually taken at face value and as the infant is readily accessible, delivery is usually expedited with forceps or ventouse. It must also be remembered that fetal asphyxia occurs more commonly in the second stage of labour. Therefore, unless delivery is imminent, poor overall correlation between the clinical state of the infant at birth and a scalp blood pH performed during the first stage can be expected.

2. Cord entanglement, especially around the fetal neck, occurs in about 30 per cent of cephalic deliveries and causes fetal asphyxia in a haphazard manner.

3. The one-minute Apgar score can be dramatically depressed by vigorous and over-enthusiastic use of the mucus extractor. This device, impinging upon the larynx, may provoke laryngeal spasm and fetal apnoea.

4. Centrally acting drugs given to the mother cross the placenta and may result in the depression of a non-acidotic fetus. Most of these drugs are given for the purposes of pain relief or anaesthesia. A good rule of thumb guide for the obstetrician is that all drugs which act directly upon the central nervous system are likely to have the facility of passing from mother to fetus and the rate of onset of action of the drug upon the mother is probably reflective of the rapidity with which transplacental transfer occurs (Crawford, 1972). The only drugs that fail to obey this rule are those drugs which are destroyed by placental enzymes, the most notable examples being procaine and the catecholamines. Pethidine promptly crosses the placental barrier and causes respiratory depression in the newborn and is associated with carbon dioxide retention by the neonate. This may persist for up to five hours after delivery in infants whose mothers have received only one 100-mg dose of pethidine. The peak incidence of narcotic-induced depression occurs amongst those infants whose mothers receive pethidine three to three and a half hours before delivery (Roberts et al, 1957); morphine has a similar effect. The whole subject of drug transfer to the fetus and the effects of the drug upon the fetus is outside the scope of this discussion but is well reviewed by Crawford (1972).

The false-positive pH (infusion acidosis)

As the term implies, acid–base changes in the mother are reflected by the fetus. Significant correlations have been established between acid–base values obtained from scalp blood and maternal blood (Jacobson, 1970). It has furthermore been shown that it is possible to influence acid–base values in the fetus by inducing changes in the mother. Maternal lactic acidaemia induced by a hypertonic fructose (laevulose) infusion in the mother was shown to cause a metabolic acidosis in the fetus by Pearson and Shuttleworth (1971) and Otey et al (1964) established a direct relationship with respect to lactate and pyruvate between maternal and fetal blood. The consensus at present supports the contention that acid metabolites freely pass to and fro across the placenta, probably in response to simple diffusion gradients.

Maternal–fetal acid–base gradients

In an effort to discriminate between fetal acidosis of asphyxial origin and that caused by maternal–fetal infusion, many workers have sought to compare maternal and fetal acid–base values. These studies are sometimes difficult to compare because the values given for the maternal acid–base component have been derived from different sources. For instance, Beard and Morris (1965) and Beard (1968) used the concept of the Δ base deficit (the difference between the base deficit uncorrected for oxygen content in maternal peripheral venous blood and that of fetal scalp capillary blood). They found that the fetal base deficit was commonly lower than that of the mother and suggested that the extent of the difference might be a better index of fetal well-being than fetal values taken alone. Jacobson (1970), using maternal capillary blood, showed that at the beginning of labour the mean base deficit difference was near zero and the values remain close during labour, a finding confirmed by Pearson (1973), using maternal arterial blood. If the base deficit difference is near normal the fetal acidosis is more likely to be an infusion acidosis but the possibility still remains that an episode of hypoxia could coincide with maternal metabolic acidosis and thus give false reassurance to the clinician. In practice this occurrence is rare. The main requirement for use of the Δ base deficit is that good laboratory technique is essential and, if measured by someone not practised in acid–base measurement, could constitute a major source of error. A more practical method of discriminating between fetal asphyxia and materno-fetal infusion was presented by Rooth, McBride and Ivy (1973) who showed that the difference between maternal venous blood pH and fetal scalp pH tended to hold constant at about 0.10 pH units. They suggested that if fetal 'pre-acidosis' was redefined as a fetal pH of 0.15 to 0.19 pH units below that of the maternal pH and that fetal 'acidosis' was present when the fetal pH was more than 0.20 units below that of maternal venous blood, errors of pH interpretation caused by infusion acidosis would be minimised. Measurement of pH is relatively simple and therefore more useful in the clinical context than the Δ base deficit.

REFERENCES

Adamsons, K., Beard, R. W., Cosmi, E. V. & Myers, R. E. (1968) The validity of capillary blood in the assessment of the acid–base state of the fetus. In *Diagnosis and Treatment of Fetal Disorders* (Ed.) Adamsons, K. p. 175. New York: Springer-Verlag.

Beard, R. W. (1968) The results of foetal blood sampling. *Proceedings of the Royal Society of Medicine*, **61**, 488–489.

Beard, R. W. (1970) Fetal blood sampling. *British Journal of Hospital Medicine*, **3**, 523–534.

Beard, R. W. & Morris, E. D. (1965) Foetal and maternal acid–base balance during normal labour. *Journal of Obstetrics and Gynaecology of the British Commonwealth*, **72**, 496–506.

Bouterline-Young, H. & Bouterline-Young, E. (1956) Alveolar carbon dioxide levels in pregnant, parturient and lactating subjects. *Journal of Obstetrics and Gynaecology of the British Empire*, **63**, 509–528.

British Perinatal Mortality Survey (1963) *Perinatal Mortality. The First Report of the 1958 British Perinatal Mortality Survey* (Ed.) Butler, U. R. & Bonham, D. G. Edinburgh: E. & S. Livingstone.

Brock, M. (1971) Cerebral blood flow and intracranial pressure changes associated with brain hypoxia. In *Brain Hypoxia. Clinics in Developmental Medicine, No. 39/40*. (Ed.) Brierley, J. B. & Meldrum, B. S. London: S. I. P. with Heinemann Medical.

Brown, J. K., Purvis, R. J., Forfar, J. O. & Cockburn, F. (1974) Neurological aspects of perinatal asphyxia. *Developmental Medicine and Child Neurology*, **16**, 567.

Crawford, J. S. (1972) *Principles and Practice of Obstetric Anaesthesia*, 3rd edition, p. 16. London: Blackwell Scientific Publications.

Cugell, D. W., Frank, N. R., Gaenslar, E. A. & Badger, T. L. (1953) Pulmonary function in pregnancy—serial observations in normal women. *American Review of Tuberculosis and Pulmonary Diseases*, **67**, 568–597.

Dahlström, H. & Ihrman, K. (1960) A clinical and physiological study of pregnancy in a material from Northern Sweden. V. The results of work tests during and after pregnancy. *Acta Societatis Medicorum Upsaliensis*, **65**, 305–314.

Davidson, A., Weaver, J. B., Davies, P. & Pearson, J. F. (1976) The relation between ease of forceps delivery and speed of cervical dilatation. *British Journal of Obstetrics and Gynaecology*, **83**, 279–283.

Fadl, E. T. & Utting, J. E. (1969a) A study of plasma pK in women in labour. *British Journal of Anaesthesia*, **41**, 468–474.

Fadl, E. T. & Utting, J. E. (1969b) A study of maternal acid–base state during labour. *British Journal of Anaesthesia*, **41**, 327–337.

Gare, D. J., Whetham, J. C. G. & Henry, J. D. (1967) The validity of scalp sampling. *American Journal of Obstetrics and Gynecology*, **99**, 722–724.

Greene, N. M. (1961) Effect of epinephrine on lactate pyruvate and excess lactate in normal human subjects. *Journal of Laboratory and Clinical Medicine*, **58**, 682–686.

Hasselbalch, K. A. & Gammeltoft, S. A. (1915) Die Ventralitats—regulation des graviden Organismus. *Biochemische Zeitschrifte*, **68**, 206–264.

Hasselbalch, K. A. & Lundsgaard (1912) Blutreaktion und Lungenventilation. *Scandinavian Archives of Physiology*, **27**, 13–32.

Himwich, W. A., Sullivan, W. T., Kelley, B., Benaron, M. B. W. & Tucker, B. E. (1955) Chemical constituents of human brain. *Journal of Nervous and Mental Disease,* **122,** 441.

Hull, M. G. R. (1972) Perinatal coagulopathies complicating fetal blood sampling. *British Medical Journal,* **iv,** 319–321.

Jacobson, L. (1970) *Studies on Acid–Base and Electrolyte Components of Human Foetal and Maternal Blood during Labour.* Thesis, Studentlitteratur, Lund.

Khazin, A. F., Hon, E. H. & Quilligan, E. J. (1969) Biochemical studies of the fetus. III. Fetal base and Apgar scores. *Obstetrics and Gynecology,* **34,** 592–609.

Kubli, F. (1968) Influence of labor on fetal acid–base balance. *Clinical Obstetrics and Gynaecology,* **11,** 168–191.

Lumley, J., McKinnon, L. & Wood, C. (1971) Lack of agreement and normal values for fetal scalp blood. *Journal of Obstetrics and Gynaecology of the British Commonwealth,* **78,** 13–21.

Lurie, A. & Weiss, J. B. (1967) Progesterone in cerebrospinal fluid during human pregnancy. *Nature,* **215,** 1178.

Lyons, H. A. & Antonio, R. (1959) The sensitivity of the respiratory centre in pregnancy and after the administration of progesterone. *Transactions of the Association of American Physicians,* **72,** 173.

Macrae, D. J. & Palavradji, D. (1967) Maternal acid–base changes in pregnancy. *Journal of Obstetrics and Gynaecology of the British Commonwealth,* **74,** 11–16.

Metcalf, J., Bartels, H. & Moll, W. (1967) Gas exchange in the pregnant uterus. *Physiological Reviews,* **47,** 782.

Mitchell, R. A. (1966) In *Advances in Respiratory Physiology* (Ed.) Caro, C. G. p. 1. Baltimore: Williams & Wilkins.

Novy, M. J. & Edwards, M. J. (1967) Respiratory problems in pregnancy. *American Journal of Obstetrics and Gynecology,* **99,** 1024–1045.

Otey, E., Stenger, V., Eitzman, D., Gessner, I. & Prystowsky, H. (1964) Movements of lactate and pyruvate in the pregnant uterus of the human. *American Journal of Obstetrics and Gynecology,* **90,** 747–752.

Paterson, P., Sheath, J., Taft, P. & Wood, C. (1967) Maternal and fetal ketone concentration in plasma and urine. *Lancet,* **i,** 862–865.

Pearson, J. F. (1973) *The Effect of Epidural Analgesia on Maternal and Foetal Acid–Base Balance during Labour.* MD Thesis, University of London.

Pearson, J. F. & Davies, P. (1973a) The effect of continuous lumbar epidural analgesia on the acid–base status of maternal arterial blood during the first stage of labour. *Journal of Obstetrics and Gynaecology of the British Commonwealth,* **80,** 218–224.

Pearson, J. F. & Davies, P. (1973b) The effect of continuous lumbar epidural analgesia on maternal acid–base balance and arterial lactate concentration during the second stage of labour. *Journal of Obstetrics and Gynaecology of the British Commonwealth,* **80,** 225–229.

Pearson, J. F. & Shuttleworth, R. (1971) The metabolic effects of a hypertonic fructose infusion on the mother and fetus during labor. *American Journal of Obstetrics and Gynecology,* **111,** 259–265.

Prowse, C. M. & Gaensler, E. A. (1965) Respiratory and acid–base changes during pregnancy. *Anesthesiology,* **26,** 381.

Report of the Ad Hoc Committee on Acid–Base Terminology (1966) *Annals of the New York Academy of Sciences,* **133,** 251.

Richter, D. (1967) Biochemical changes in hypoxia. In *Brain Damage in the Fetus and Newborn from Hypoxia or Asphyxia. Report of 57th Ross Conference on Pediatric Research.* Columbus: Ross Laboratories.

Roberts, H., Caine, K. N., Percival, N., Snow, P. & Please, N. W. (1957) Effects of some analgesic drugs used in childbirth. *Lancet,* **i,** 128–132.

Robertson, E. G. (1968) Increased erythrocyte fragility in association with osmotic changes in pregnancy serum. *Journal of Reproduction and Fertility,* **16,** 323.

Rooth, G., McBride, R. & Ivy, B. J. (1973) Fetal and maternal pH measurements, a basis for common normal values. *Acta Obstetrica et Gynecologica Scandinavica,* **52,** 47–50.

Saling, E. (1963) Die Blutgasverhältnisse und der Saüre-Basen-Hanshalt des Feten bei ungestörtem Geburtsablaurt. *Zeitschrifte für Geburtshilfe und Gynäkologie,* **161,** 262.

Saling, E. (1966) Amnioscopy and fetal blood sampling: observations on foetal acidosis. *Archives of Disease in Childhood,* **41,** 472–476.

Seligman, S. A. (1968) Accuracy of blood pH determination. *Proceedings of the Royal Society of Medicine,* **61,** 491–492.

Sheppard, B. L. & Bonnar, J. (1974) The ultrastructure of the arterial supply of the human placenta in early and late pregnancy. *Journal of Obstetrics and Gynaecology of the British Commonwealth,* **81,** 497–511.

Sjostedt, S. (1962) Acid–base balance of arterial blood during pregnancy, at delivery and in the puerperium. *American Journal of Obstetrics and Gynecology,* **84,** 775–799.

Tyler, J. M. (1960) The effect of progesterone on the respiration of patients with emphysema and hypercapnia. *Journal of Clinical Investigation,* **39,** 34–41.

Wilbrand, U., Porath, Ch., Matthaes, P. & Jaster, R. (1959) Der Einfluss der Ovarialsteroide auf die Funktion des Atemzentrums. (Effect of ovarian steroids on the function of the respiratory centre.) *Archiv für Gynäkologie,* **191,** 507.

Ylppö, X. (1916) Neugeborenen, Hunger und Intoxikation-sacidosis in ihren Beziehungen Zueinander. *Zeitschrift für Kinderheilkunde,* **14,** 268.

Yoshioka, T. & Roux, J. F. (1970) Correlation of foetal scalp blood pH, glucose lactate and pyruvate concentrations with cord blood determinations at the time of delivery and caesarean section. *Journal of Reproductive Medicine,* **5,** 63.

26

METHODS FOR RECORDING FETAL HEART RATE AND UTERINE CONTRACTIONS

D. M. Serr

INTENSIVE CARE OF THE FETUS

Fetal monitoring and intensive care units have come of age and are now accepted as providing indispensable and reliable clinical information for pregnancy and labour. Changing trends and increasing availability and variety of instrumentation appear to be favouring an 'all-risk' approach to monitoring in place of the 'high-risk' approach. Although more staff and intensive care are required for the high-risk pregnancy and labour patient, it is recognised that during labour all fetuses are at some risk that cannot be detected other than by monitoring all deliveries. Whilst this is not possible in every centre, and although there will always be the fringe groups comprising precipitate labours and patients arriving late in labour, it does seem that the increasing simplicity and reliability of the fetal monitoring systems to be described favour a positive attitude to all-patient monitoring in the labour ward.

Extensive clinical experience of monitoring unselected labours shows that the fetal heart rate (FHR) record provides early evidence of fetal anoxia (Shenker, 1973). However, it has been shown that monitoring of the fetal heart does not provide an infallible parameter and

510

used on its own, without checking another parameter such as fetal pH, should be regarded more as a warning sign, since false signs of fetal asphyxia are not uncommon (Beard et al, 1971). Quilligan (1972) observed a slightly lower perinatal mortality amongst monitored high-risk patients than in unmonitored normal patients.

It must be realised that although equipment is available, trained personnel are going to be needed increasingly to apply the equipment and provide the intensive care prescribed; this must be taken into account when planning an obstetric monitoring system. Teamwork by monitoring-minded groups has proved that even in small obstetric units both doctors and midwives easily adapt to instrumental monitoring. The concept of the nurse–technician is rapidly becoming meaningful and is to be encouraged.

The challenge of adding an important parameter to the assessment of the fetal state before labour, by interpretation of fetal heart recordings, inspired the development firstly of indirect fetal electrocardiography and phonocardiography and later of ultrasonic rate-metering systems. The most important clinical application of electronic methods, which supplement, assist and, in fact, supersede the physical ability to evaluate the state of labour at a given time, has been in the combined systems for continuous recording of the FHR and of uterine contractions during active labour. Direct and indirect methods, invasive and non-invasive techniques need to be classified, so that any obstetric unit may adapt its needs, after weighing the advantages to patient and staff, to the many modular systems now available.

PATIENT SAFETY

Electronic instrumentation of any kind used in the care of patients must be designed with regard to patient safety. Although the fetus is relatively well insulated, the mother is more liable to possible accidents should the equipment not be up to the required standards, or should it be faulty. Complete isolation of the patient from the main power supply, isolated or floating input circuitry, avoidance of the combination of several types of instrument, all combine to make electronic monitoring safe. Some progress has been made in telemetric signal recordings, one of the few advantages of which is isolation of the patient from main-line equipment. Unger and Goodwin (1972) have reported on the use of a combined telemetric system for both fetal electrocardiography and intra-uterine pressure recordings. Strict enforcement of legislation for standards of safety in medical electronic equipment is necessary, and all members of the medical and paramedical staff should be trained to be aware of the possible dangers.

HOW A MONITOR WORKS AND WHAT IS BEING MEASURED

Monitoring systems are based on the cardiotocograph, measuring the basic parameters of FHR and uterine contractions.

Fetal heart rate

The FHR recorded electronically is measured by a rate-meter, which expresses the instantaneous heart rate in beats per min. This is the rate determined from a measurement of the

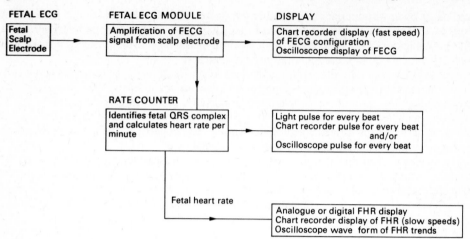

Figure 26.1. Scheme of direct fetal electrocardiogram recording system.

time interval between two similar events of two successive beats, such as the interval between the peaks of two successive R waves in the QRS complex of the fetal electrocardiogram. For the fetal electrocardiogram recording, the electronics involved make use of an input signal of approximately 10 mV peak-to-peak, which is amplified between 2000 and 10 000 times depending on the gain. In such apparatus everything above a 1 V output can be used for rate-metering (Figure 26.1). In ultrasonic systems, the input sensitivity will detect and process signals above 2 μV. For a 10 mV input pulse, the output voltage will be of the order of 6 V peak-to-peak in the circuit described as in Figure 26.2. Some rate meters record the heart rate as an average over a number of beats and these instruments do not record short-term fluctuations or 'beat-to-beat variations'. Table 26.1 is an assessment of systems in use at present.

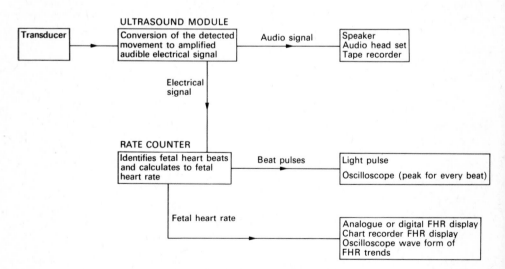

Figure 26.2. Scheme of ultrasound recording system.

Table 26.1. *Fetal heart and uterine activity recording systems.*

Parameter recorded	Direct/indirect (internal/external) (invasive/non-invasive)	Patient contact	Pregnancy/ labour	Reliability	Clinical value	Remarks
Fetal heart						
FECG	Indirect	Abdominal electrodes	Pregnancy and labour	Limited	Restricted	May soon be improved for clinical use
FECG	Direct	Fetal scalp electrodes	Labour only	Highly reliable	Excellent both for FHR and ECG complex	Widely accepted
FPCG	Indirect	Abdominal microphones	Pregnancy and labour	Good to fair	Good, but restricted during active labour	Largely being replaced by ultrasound
FHR (fetal heart-rate)	Indirect	Abdominal ultrasonic transducers + coupling medium	Pregnancy and labour	Good	Excellent	Instantaneous rate metering to be perfected
PEP (pre-ejection period)	Direct + indirect	FECG scalp electrode + abdominal Doppler transducer	Labour		Experimental	Appears promising
Uterine activity						
Uterine contractility	Indirect	Abdominal pressure transducer (tocodynamometer)	Pregnancy and labour	Fair	Good	Widely accepted
Intra-uterine pressure	Direct	Intra-uterine catheter (open end or balloon) and pressure transducer	Labour only	Good (if calibrated and checked)	Excellent	Allows mobility and acceptability increasing
EMG (electromyogram)	Direct/indirect	Abdominal or intra-uterine bipolar electrodes		Limited		

Display of data

Beat-to-beat variations are essential for true evaluation of FHR recordings. In instantaneous rate-metering an interval between two beats of half a second will be shown as 120 beats/min, whereas an interval of one second between two consecutive heart beats would record as 60 beats/min. Hon has shown how auscultation averaging techniques miss data on beat-to-beat variations when compared to electronic monitoring records (Hon, 1968) (Figure 26.3). The

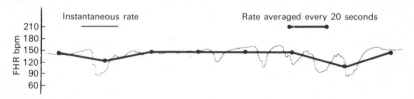

Figure 26.3. Comparison of electronic monitoring of instantaneous heart rate with classical auscultation every 20 sec. From Hon (1968) with kind permission of the author and the publisher (New Haven, Connecticut: Harty Press).

rate can be displayed in a number of ways such as strip chart recording, oscillographic display (non-fade or memory screens) and audiosignals, flashing lights and digital display units. For effective data recall a written record is necessary, and then the paper speed of the recording instrument becomes an important factor. Differing speeds on various types of equipment alter the forms of heart-rate patterns. Thus, for instance, a three-speed chart recorder allows a selection of two slow speeds for FHR and uterine contraction monitoring and one fast speed for direct writing of the fetal electrocardiogram signal and even of the Doppler ultrasonic wave form. The significance of these technical innovations will be referred to again later. In practical terms, however, it may be noted that a 1 cm/min speed is preferred in Europe, whereas a 3 cm/min speed is preferred in the United States. 1 cm/min offers an economy of paper and somewhat easier perusal of a lengthy period of recording, but this is at the expense of FHR detail. Pattern recognition is affected by the choice of a slow speed. For electrocardiogram (ECG) configuration and interpretation of the QRS complex a speed of 25 mm/sec is required. A committee of experts met to recommend accepted standards, and a summary of some of these recommendations is included at the end of this chapter (see Appendix).

Uterine contractility

It is important to read monitored fetal heart patterns in a combined system with a tocometer which simultaneously records the activity of the uterus. The tocometer on the instrument and trace both show in time the pattern of the contracting uterus and allow a comparison with the state of the fetal heart between, during and after contractions. However, not all tocometers measure the intra-uterine pressure, which measures more precisely the amplitude and duration of the contractions. External and internal tocometers, therefore, whilst differing in their precision and ease of application, provide a record from which the relationship of the uterine contraction to the changes in heart rate can be seen, but they do not necessarily measure true intra-uterine pressure. Further details of uterine activity records are discussed later.

In summary, the direct methods are more quantitative and the external methods are more qualitative. The direct method is limited to the period of time before delivery after the membranes are broken. The external method can be used at any time and is especially valuable for the oxytocin challenge test.

METHODS FOR LABOUR MONITORING

Indirect recording of fetal ECG (FECG) from abdominal leads

This is one of the earliest methods used for recording the fetal heart beat. Abdominal leads, however placed, pick up the FECG complex in an uncertain manner. The recording is always accompanied by the maternal ECG complex, which is of much greater amplitude than the fetal complex. Attempts have been made to retrieve a purely fetal recording by erasing the

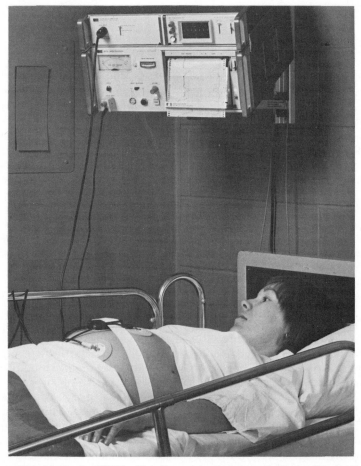

Figure 26.4. Monitoring FECG with indirect abdominal electrode display (Hewlett-Packard).

maternal complex. This can be done in a variety of ways, mainly based on electronic nega-
tion of the maternal QRS by an additional reversed maternal complex (Sureau, Chavinie and
Cannon, 1967). The filtered signal, until recently, has not been of sufficient strength to trigger
a rate-meter, or distinct enough from the maternal signal to be reliable, although data-
processing techniques are being applied for further development in this field. The main advantage of this technique lies in the innocuous application of abdominal electrodes, during
both pregnancy and labour. The more reliable interpretation of FECG complexes and rate-
metering during the various stages of high-risk pregnancies could add invaluable information
to the pathophysiology and clinical evaluation of such cases (Serr et al, 1968b). However, accurate instantaneous heart rate (beat-to-beat frequency) measurement by this method is
beset with difficulties, although finer interpretation of the ECG complex may be possible
(Pardi et al, 1971). The indirect FECG has a place in perinatal medicine, particularly in high-
risk pregnancies, and further attempts to improve its applicability could prove fruitful. There
are recent reports that manufacturers have overcome the technical problems involved in indirect FHR metering from abdominal electrodes, and a reliable electronic method has also
been described by Thieme and Eichmeier (1971). This approach will only be acceptable to
obstetricians as a practical clinical technique of fetal heart monitoring if it proves to be
efficient and reliable, free of noise disturbance and simple to apply (Figure 26.4).

Direct FECG

Direct recording of the FECG has become one of the most accepted methods and is certainly
the most reliable means of monitoring the fetal heart. The advantages are many. A reliable
beat-to-beat frequency is assured with a minimum of noise and a high signal-to-noise ratio.
Both rate-metering and visualisation by oscillograph or recording chart of the FECG complex are possible. The obvious main limitation of this method is its applicability only during
labour and then only when the membranes are ruptured. Much of the early reluctance to at-
tach electrodes to the fetal scalp has disappeared, with the increasing ease of application
of new types of electrodes (Figure 26.5a, b, c), and the low incidence of complications
reported.

Opinions differ as to the practicability of direct methods of monitoring which are dependent on whether staff are available for introducing electrodes and transducers. Paul and Hon
(1970) and Paul (1973) suggest that in teaching hospitals direct techniques are applied in 25
to 60 per cent of patients being monitored, whereas in private or community hospitals only 5
to 15 per cent of patients are so monitored. It must be remembered that these figures relate to
a period of expansion in the use of FHR monitoring and that with the acceptance of the 'all-
risks' concept, monitoring practice will change. Edington, Sibanda and Beard (1975) have
reported that in one year 92 per cent of patients coming to their obstetric unit were monitored
in labour, 82 per cent by direct methods for FHR. With the increasing ease of application of
new types of electrodes, it would seem reasonable to assume that smaller obstetric units will
tend to increase direct techniques both for heart-rate monitoring and pressure recording. It is
not long since obstetricians were using Drew–Smythe catheters for high rupture of the membranes to induce labour, and the use of scalp electrodes and Teflon pressure catheters is, after
all, no more of an intervention than this was, probably less because of the softer plastic
materials used. Some centres, encountering unwillingness to use intra-uterine pressure
records for displaying uterine contractility, now combine a system of cardiotocography
using a scalp electrode for direct FECG and an abdominal pressure transducer for uterine
activity (Edington, Sibanda and Beard, 1975). Equipment manufacturers are now offering
the possibility of various combinations, and it seems that this is among the most popular.

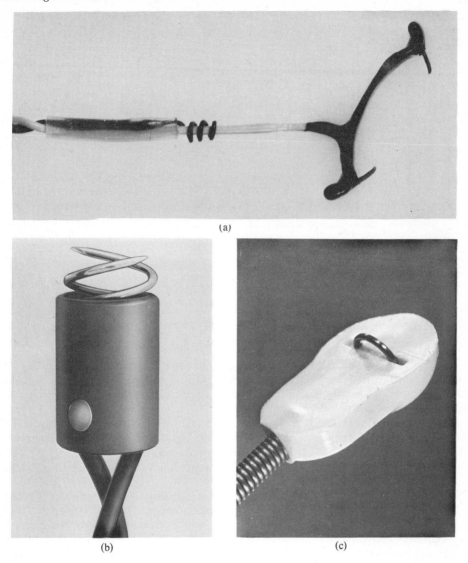

(a)

(b)   (c)

Figure 26.5. Fetal scalp electrodes and introducers.

Instruments allowing the use of either direct or indirect combination techniques are to be preferred (Figure 26.6).

The scalp electrode can be applied quite early in labour through a fairly narrow amnioscope. When in place, it does not interfere with microblood analyses often used for combined evaluation of the fetal state (Beard et al, 1971; Saling and Dudenhausen, 1973). Care is taken not to detach the electrode during vaginal examinations, but these can be carried out repeatedly. The FECG recording continues with delivery of the infant, and can even remain attached during resuscitation. It is easily removed when recording is no longer necessary. During labour, or before caesarean section, the electrode is easily disconnected.

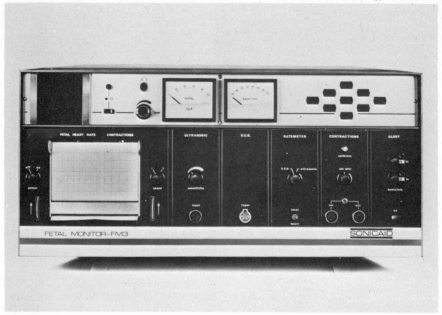

Figure 26.6. Example of modular type monitoring apparatus. Assembled monitor (Sonicaid FM 3).

The quality of the FECG tracing obtained with these direct techniques is far better than can be obtained from the abdominal wall. The FECG signal-to-noise ratio is much higher, permitting meaningful study of the FECG complex and a clean artifact-free record of FHR throughout labour and delivery.

A possible pitfall is that stillborn fetuses have been shown to conduct the ECG signal from the mother through a scalp electrode; thus care must be taken in interpretation (Schneiderman, Waxman and Goodman, 1972). Confirmation of fetal heart beats by another method should be made to avoid this possible error; when there is doubt a maternal electrocardiogram should be displayed simultaneously.

At the moment direct fetal electrocardiography is probably the most precise and reliable method for measuring beat-to-beat variations. Furthermore, it allows a far finer analysis of the FECG configuration than has been obtained by abdominal electrodes. Analysing the time constants and complexes obtained from scalp electrodes in relation to maternal and fetal acid–base status and plasma electrolytes in high risk cases, Symonds (1971) showed a relationship between fetal acidosis and prolongation of electric systole (Q–T) and T-wave inversion. The increasing information being gathered on the FECG configuration makes the direct fetal electrode modality even more important, and also gives added significance to the inclusion of display systems for FECG configuration in modern rate-metering equipment (Figure 26.7).

Fetal phonocardiogram (FPCG)

The FPCG is obtained indirectly by placing a microphone on the maternal abdomen, over the site of maximum intensity of fetal heart sounds. Developments in phonocardiographic techniques have been considerable, enabling continuous monitoring, recorded rate-metering

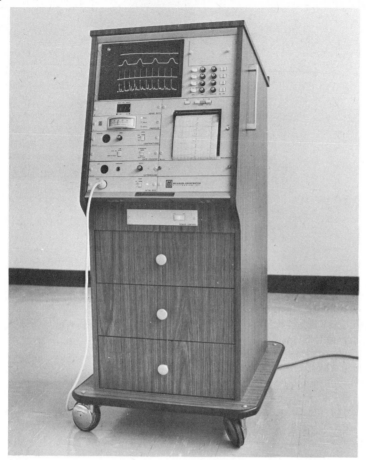

Figure 26.7. Fetal monitor with non-fade oscillograph display: (a) top channel—FHR trend, (b) uterine contractions, (c) ultrasound heart beat peak signal, (d) bottom channel—fetal electrocardiogram.

and even an approach to a qualitative analysis based on interpretation of the analogue phonocardiographic signals. In spite of the character of the fetal heart sounds and the introduction of more sophisticated transducers for fetal phonocardiography, there remain intrinsic disadvantages and pitfalls in the use of such systems. The use of signals within the acoustic range will be complicated by extraneous sounds from either the patient or her surroundings. Such interference may disturb the recording being picked up by the microphone. Instruments designed to take account of this have a mechanism which stops the stylus recording when the noise is interpreted as an artifact. Whilst preventing spurious patterns, this shows up as non-recorded areas thus reducing the continuity of the recording. Furthermore, the movements and progression of the fetal station sometimes make positioning in labour a factor requiring more personal attention than the instrument is meant to involve. Obesity also limits the applicability of abdominal microphones, and strong contractions usually interfere with the recording. However, a high quality microphone designed for phonocardiography allows the recording of a true beat-to-beat rate, and the built-in logic systems of some instruments give them the necessary reliability during pregnancy or quiescent periods of labour.

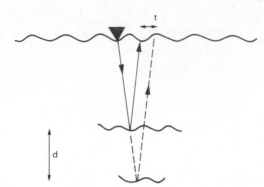

Figure 26.8. Doppler shift principle. Note the returning signal is delayed by time t, after passing distance d, thus altering frequency of the returning ultrasonic wave. Apparent frequency difference is processed as a signal (see also Figure 26.2). Redrawn from Donald (1972) with kind permission of author and the editor of *Obstetrics and Gynecology*.

The actual phonocardiographic signal can be displayed on an oscilloscope or paper record; thus both heart sounds of the beat can be viewed. Some observers have attributed significance to the form of the signal, but such factors as the type of filtration used and the position of the microphone considerably alter the tracing and the wave form.

The instrumentation available varies, and account should be taken of the size and comfort of the abdominally placed microphone. Older models combined in one head both microphone and pressure transducers. Most manufacturers are now producing separate transducers for phonocardiograph and contraction recordings. The combined head is somewhat heavy, and when locating the optimum acoustic heart sound, a separate microphone head is an advantage.

The popularity, simplicity and reliability of the external phonocardiograph makes it highly acceptable in units managing relatively uncomplicated pregnancies. Its application to the abdomen can be carried out by either medical or nursing staff, and the technique of readjustment as labour proceeds is easily mastered (Hammacher, 1969; Serr et al, 1969).

Ultrasound in fetal heart monitoring

Fetal heart rate recording

The use of the Doppler shift principle for demonstrating the FHR is now widely known and accepted, although it is a recent development in fetal heart monitoring techniques (Bishop, 1966). The principle is somewhat different to the B-scan or two-dimensional ultrasonic system, being designed to detect movement. Instead of the pulsed echo system used in A and B-scan ultrasonic units for measuring biparietal diameters by echo, the Doppler unit makes use of a continuous beam of ultrasound propagated by one transducer crystal, the echoes reflected from the structure under review being received by a second transducer placed alongside. Since the movement of the structure under review increases or decreases the length of time taken by each successive wave to return, the apparent alteration of frequency produced by such movement, which is known as the Doppler effect, is used as an electric signal. When the structure under the beam of sound is the heart, the rate can be recorded either from the movements of the myocardium or of the blood in the heart (Figure 26.8). The FHR can be recorded from the to-and-fro movement of blood in major vessels such as the umbilical cord. It is obvious therefore that whilst picking up the heart rate, as in a simple Doppler system applied even from the eleventh week of pregnancy, the signal obtained may be far more complex electronically than the phonocardiogram or electrocardiogram signals, since the structures moving and reflecting sound comprise the heart as an organ, the blood flow in the chambers and vessels and the main aortic and mitral valve openings and closures.

In practice an ultrasound beam of low energy intensity is directed through the abdominal wall to the fetal heart. The frequency of the beam is changed when it strikes a structure moving perpendicularly to its direction. Part of the transmitted beam, altered in frequency, is reflected back to the source to be picked up by a receiver, usually housed in the same head as the transmitting crystal. The signal is then processed. Whereas there are two fairly distinct components in the phonocardiograph—the first and second heart sounds—the Doppler effect signal as mentioned above reflects movements of valves and blood flow reverberations and when displayed on a tracing can be shown to have multiple components (Figure 26.9).

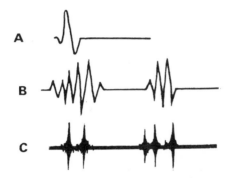

Figure 26.9. Comparison between signals of a single fetal heart beat. (a) QRS configuration from fetal electrocardiogram; (b) first and second heart sounds from fetal phonocardiogram; (c) multiple signals from a fetal heart beat recorded by an ultrasonic (Doppler shift) system.

Since these fetal heart movements are quite complex, considerable electronic damping is required, thus making it difficult to achieve a true beat-to-beat heart rate. The problem is further complicated by the necessity of having a wide-angle multiple crystal transducer in order to prevent the necessity for frequent readjustment as the fetus moves. One instrument available commercially uses a system that gives an averaged rate over 3 beats which the manufacturers (Roche, Paris) claim gives a reliable representation of true beat-to-beat variation. An alternative is the use of a double system possessing two interchangeable heads. One example of this is a narrow-beam transducer consisting of one pair of piezo-crystals and giving good beat-to-beat rate-metering, but only for short periods, since it requires frequent readjustment (Figure 26.10). A second type consists of a wide-angle transducer, having a convex crystal in the centre and surrounded by an array of receivers. This is easier to use and requires less frequent readjustment, but the result must be weighed in the light of requirements in the particular case. Combined models, which are adequate in most cases, and where less exact recording is not critical, are being put on the market. The ultrasound technique has its place in most labour room monitoring systems, and its usefulness is increasing. The advantage over phonocardiography is that it is relatively free of extraneous noise produced by sounds in the acoustic range and is quite comfortable for the patient. The transducer requires a coupling medium such as olive oil to obtain good contact with the skin, but the patient may lie on her side, and it can be applied by nurses and midwives with ease.

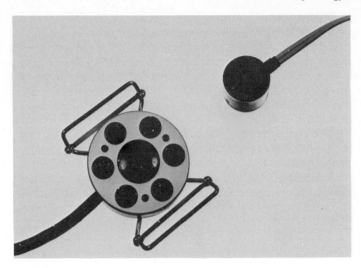

Figure 26.10. Narrow beam and multiple crystal head (Sonicaid Ltd).

A further and more refined development in the application of filtered Doppler ultrasound and FECG technique has been suggested by Organ et al (1973a) as a method of determining the 'pre-ejection period' (PEP) of the fetal cardiac cycle during labour. These observations are based on the use of ultrasonic echo cardiography showing the velocity of the aortic valve to be faster than that of the mitral valve. In the fetus this is immaterial, since the right and left ventricles work in parallel because of the ductus arteriosus, but the timing of the movement of the aortic valve is the parameter necessary for evaluating the PEP. Thus Organ et al (1973a) showed that by simultaneously recording the FECG and the filtered Doppler ultrasound, the evaluation of the aortic valve opening by ultrasound is reliable.

The possible importance of PEP lies in the relationship to myocardial contractility. The duration of the PEP decreases as myocardial contractility increases, and the availability of this parameter during labour relative to the FECG may offer a further means of assessing the fetal state. We may therefore be witnessing a refinement in the monitoring systems of the fetal heart by ultrasound to provide more information than just heart-rate patterns. Supporting evidence that the PEP may reflect changes in myometrial activity resulting from hypoxia, in contrast to FHR patterns which were variable in reaction during a similar period, has been reported by Organ et al (1973b) in experimental studies on lambs. Systems displaying comparative FECG complexes and ultrasonic timing devices are being developed (compare oscillographic tracings in Figure 26.7) and may bring about a practical application of this modality.

Safety of ultrasonics

The problem of safety in the prolonged use of ultrasonic irradiation has been examined carefully (Hellman et al, 1970; Serr, 1970; Serr et al, 1971). Although high intensity ultrasonic waves (over 3 W/cm²) are used in therapy and may be damaging to human tissues, instruments used for diagnostic purposes have an energy emission well below this level. The intensities of Doppler method equipment are in the order of 30 mW/cm² and this has been found to be innocuous in most human and animal experiments. Differences in interpretation of what is regarded as an aberrant chromosomal breakage frequency have in the past led to suspicion that ultrasound may have some effect on the developing embryo. Most later reports, however, agree that compared to controls or x-irradiated fetuses, ultrasound at present diagnostic levels is perfectly safe to mother and child (Mannor et al, 1972).

UTERINE ACTIVITY MEASUREMENTS

Studies on women with uncomplicated labours in which oxytocin is being used to stimulate the uterus have shown that the FHR is unchanged with uterine contractions occurring at the rate of three to four/10 min, being of 40 to 60 seconds duration and with peak amniotic pressures of 60 to 70 mm Hg and a tonus of 8 to 10 mm Hg (Hess and Hon, 1960). However, with an increase in frequency, fetal bradycardia may develop, although this effect is very variable. In cases where the patient has some complication of pregnancy such as pre-eclamptic toxaemia, even mild contractions may cause fetal bradycardia. Thus the stress of labour activity on the FHR is the basis of combining systems for measuring the FHR and contractility upon which monitoring is based.

The characteristics of myometrial contraction include a level of intercontraction tension (tonus), contraction intensity (peak minus tonus), frequency of contractions and their duration. These four parameters have a combined importance in their effect on labour and on the fetus through the relationship to uterine blood flow. The most frequently used method for measuring uterine activity is the amniotic fluid pressure test. This reflects the summated activity of all areas, provides little information on myometrial tension, but is a necessary and acceptable clinical index when interpreted together with the FHR. Mendez-Bauer, Fielitz and Caldeyro-Barcia (1961) have shown by using latex microballoons introduced into the myometrium that a contraction spreads slowly through the uterus, taking about 50 to 60 sec to reach the lower segment. Although there are observations (Borell et al, 1965) to support the concept that focal areas of contraction and relaxation occur during all phases of the uterine contraction cycle, placental blood flow must nevertheless be affected if amniotic fluid pressure exceeds the arterial blood pressure. Hypoxic fetal bradycardia would result, related in time to the increased intra-uterine pressure.

Smyth (1973), working with consecutive ultrasonic B-scans across the maternal abdomen in mid labour, has studied the biomechanics of uterine action with intact and with ruptured membranes. These studies show that following rupture or when the amount of amniotic fluid is reduced, it may not be correct to regard the pressure in the amniotic fluid as the pertinent parameter of force on the fetus or on the placental circulation. Pressure applied locally at the placental site may well exceed intra-uterine pressure.

Methods for recording myometrial activity vary from external pressure transducers to internal catheters and attempts to measure changes in impedance on the abdominal wall or recording from electrodes of fast action potentials arising from the spread of the contraction wave (electrohysterogram) (Serr, 1970; Wolfs et al, 1971). Recording of action potentials as a parameter of uterine muscle activity has been demonstrated by means of cervical electrodes from the tenth week of pregnancy. These potentials are irregular in amplitude and frequency (Serr et al, 1968a) (Figure 26.11). Wolfs et al (1971), measuring the electrical activity of the uterus by means of internal bipolar electrodes, compared their results with simultaneously recorded intra-uterine pressures by open-ended catheters. As labour

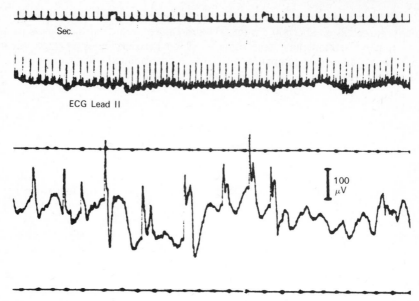

Figure 26.11. Irregular type action potentials recorded from the human cervix during pregnancy (20 weeks). Paper speed 2.5 mm/sec, time constant 0.03′, frequency 70 c.p.s. From Serr et al (1968) with kind permission of the editor of *Israel Journal of Medical Science*.

progressed electrical activity and overall pressure became more synchronised and electrical activity increased. The claim of a one-to-one relationship at full dilatation is only partially supported by later observations by Freundlich and Wingate (1973). These observers, using conveniently placed abdominal electrodes, concluded that although an electromyographic (EMG) system for recording uterine contractions constitutes a theoretically elegant means of monitoring this vital function during labour, they were unable to recommend it as a reliable system as yet.

The two most practical methods in use today, therefore, are the indirect (non-invasive) abdominal pressure transducer and the direct (invasive) intra-uterine catheter.

External tocometry (indirect)

All instruments in clinical use for external tocometry detect the hardening of the uterine wall and forward displacement of the uterus during a contraction. This activity pushes the end of a plunger in the centre of the abdominally placed transducer back into the body of the transducer. This small displacement is measured by a strain gauge and differential transformer. The transducer should be strapped firmly in place in the midline just below the fundus and re-positioned if necessary in order to obtain accurate recordings. The tracing produced by such recordings shows the duration and frequency of the contractions. The record contraction waveform is not a reliable indicator of intra-uterine pressure and should never be interpreted as such. External monitoring of uterine activity has found widespread acceptance, is easy to carry out and supplies useful information, particularly as regards the timing of the contraction, at no risk. It is, therefore, regarded as a necessary part of monitoring equipment in use in most labour units.

Internal intra-uterine pressure (direct)

The direct techniques for measurement of uterine activity use open-end catheters of polyethylene or Teflon, or catheters with water-filled or air-filled balloons. The intra-uterine catheter is connected by tubing to a pressure transducer working on the Statham strain-gauge principle (Figure 26.12). By flushing the open-ended catheter with fluid, air bubbles are

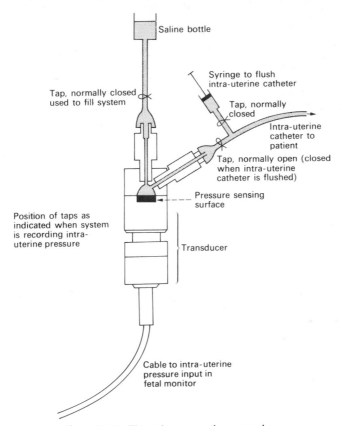

Figure 26.12. The catheter–transducer complex.

excluded and a continuity of the fluid column with the amniotic cavity is ensured. The changes in intra-uterine pressure are transferred via the catheter to the pressure transducer, which is attached to an amplifier and strip chart recorder enabling simultaneous reading with the heart rate-meter. Introduced transcervically, into the uterine cavity, this approach gives qualitative (tonus and intensity) as well as quantitative (duration and frequency) measurements of uterine contractions, thus providing a sounder basis for evaluating uterine activity during labour.

In comparing the direct technique with the external indirect approach, this latter point is stressed, since apart from qualitative assessment of labour activity, the indirect tocodynamometer records other parameters of uterine contractility just as well.

The direct method requires more care and experience in introducing the catheter. This is usually undertaken when the membranes are ruptured, but catheters can be introduced into the extra-ovular space with the membranes intact. Calibration of the instrument for zero pressure is necessary and care has to be taken that the transducer is at the correct level for the measurement required. Reports on pneumatic tocometry (Rodrigues-Lima and Montenegro, 1972) claim that air-filled balloons in a closed system eliminate the need for levelling in relation to the uterus, as is necessary in open-fluid systems. This means that recalibration is not required if the patient turns over or moves about. In the hydraulic systems every centimetre of elevation (such as getting on and off a bedpan) corresponds to $\pm$ 1 cm of water in the hydrostatic pressure.

Few complications have been reported. Haverkamp and Bowes (1971) have reported perforation of the uterus, but state that newer and softer Teflon-type cannulae are safer. The method has the advantage that when combined with a fetal scalp electrode, the maternal abdomen is quite free of cumbersome instrumentation, and the patient can then move freely in her bed from side to side. Some instrument manufacturers and obstetric centres prefer this freedom from abdominal straps, and this together with the superior precision of uterine activity measurement by intra-uterine presure recording justifies the extra care and effort needed in using this system.

COMBINED MONITORING SYSTEMS

The choice of fetal heart monitor and uterine activity recording system depends very much on the staff available. In centres where technical assistance is limited, only equipment which has to be turned on or off and having easily applied transducers should be recommended. Direct methods, although simple, are usually performed by doctors, but logically midwives should be capable of applying them, thus providing the continuity so necessary for monitoring. Indirect techniques can usually be applied by the nursing staff, and midwives should be incorporated in the teamwork engaged in fetal monitoring. Here it should be stressed that although the midwife has usually been trained to judge the fetal state by using a wooden monaural stethoscope, it is surprising how easily she adjusts to the new concept of fetal monitoring. In fact, most welcome the progress this offers, and the added information available induces more motivation in following the course of labour and delivery.

Another point for consideration when purchasing a monitor is the country of origin of the manufacturers and the availability of immediate service facilities. It is not an uncommon sight when visiting labour units to see 'out of order' monitoring trolleys adorning the walls. In this connection, those about to acquire equipment should ask around to find out which instruments are known to be the least frequently out of order and which agents offer a high standard of servicing.

For regular work on the labour ward, instruments with polygraph records using ink or requiring adjustment, should be avoided. The length of obstetric monitoring recordings may be expensive and the type of paper used should be as plain as possible. A module containing a cathode-ray oscillograph, particularly with non-fade display, is often a useful addition. FECG configurations can then be studied without reams of paper mounting up, since paper speed for ECG recordings must of necessity be far quicker than for rate-metering. Whereas for FECG–QRS complex recording, the paper speed needs to be in the order of 2.5 cm/sec, the paper speed for rate-meters ranges between 1.0 cm/min to 4 to 5 cm/min. Continuous rate-metering at the slowest speed will therefore result in a tracing 3 to 6 m long for a six-hour continuous recording.

Pressure recording equipment should have quick and easy calibration designs and attention should be paid to zero stability over a reasonable period of time.

Ultrasonic sensors and abdominal microphones are delicate and should have guard covers when not in use. Both nursing and medical staff must be instructed in handling the equipment and warned against unnecessary knocking or dropping of the transducer. If cared for, however, they are mostly trouble-free. In this connection, account must be taken of replacement parts, which at the moment in the case of ultrasonic transducer components are expensive. One abdominal heart sound sensor, at least, has a warning clearly labelled on its surface.

Alarm systems for which maximum and minimum rates can be set are available. The alarm systems available seem to be triggered off too easily, and experience shows that the staff in many units acquiring alarm systems have the alarm off and watch the records themselves for careful assessment. Evaluation over a period of time is more useful in fetal monitoring than an alarm of one particular episode of FHR abnormality.

Some instrument makers offer a modular cart in addition to the monitor, for which one can order optional extras such as oscilloscopes of varying sizes and on which central display systems can be arranged. The final choice depends on whether a central station is being planned and whether routine clinical monitoring is required. In this case the standard cardiotocometer provided with manufacturer's advice as to central stations is satisfactory. If, however, research is planned and a fetal intensive care unit is being equipped, it is wiser to make sure that the equipment will be sufficiently versatile and have adequate outlets for attachment to both central stations and research installations. The increased interest in data processing and promising work in computer analysis require connections to magnetic tape recorders, particularly of the frequency modulated type. Telemetric systems using wireless capsules are being offered and can often be used with the same basic equipment as in wired systems.

For smaller obstetric units or for the use of the younger physician wishing to consult his senior, a useful innovation by Xerox copying machines has been described by Boehn and Goss (1973). Using a Xerox 400 Telecopier (Xerox Corporation, Rochester, New York) 8-min strips from a fetal monitoring chart can be transmitted, two such sections usually sufficing for an expert opinion on interpretation of the pattern of the recording. Other dataphone systems relay directly to a distant centre signals by telephone lines which give an instantaneous read-out. Although analysis of the parameters of fetal distress should really be basic knowledge for all practitioners of perinatal medicine, a consultation system such as described, could, in certain units, be of definite value. It seems a worthwhile development in the field, even if not universally applicable. Minimum requirements for all labour rooms today, however, should include easily applied cardiotocometers as standard equipment.

APPENDIX

Following a symposium on fetal heart monitoring in Newark, U.S.A. in 1971 (*International Journal of Obstetrics and Gynaecology,* 1972) a committee was set up chaired by the editor, Dr H. Kaminetzky. The aim of the committee, which met in March 1972, was to suggest standards for classification of the terminology in use in fetal heart monitoring, and the standardisation of instrumentation. A summary of the suggestions regarding monitoring equipment follows.

Instrumentation

A fetal monitor should:

1. Be a single integrated unit which is easily movable, reliable, simple to operate and free of external interconnecting wires which may become disconnected or broken.

2. Be usable with both direct and indirect techniques for fetal heart rate (FHR) and uterine pressure (UP) monitoring.

3. Be safe from electrical hazards and meet or conform to minimum national specifications required of the Underwriters' Laboratories Inc., USA (UL) and/or the Verband Deutscher Electrotechniker of West Germany (VDE); the British Standards Institution (BSI); the International Electrotechnical Commission of Geneva, Switzerland (IEG).

4. Provide a continuous permanent written record (paper) of FHR and UP which conforms with the display standards set forth by this Committee. The recorder must have a full scale response of 500 msec or less and the complete recorder system must have a combined accuracy of $\pm$ 3 per cent full scale in the vertical axis (FHR–UP) and $\pm$ 0.5 per cent of the values indicated in the horizontal axis (time scale).

5. Have an instantaneous cardiotachometer which provides a linear presentation of FHR over a minimum range of 50–210 BPM with an accuracy of $\pm$ 1 per cent. (At 210 BPM this implies an accuracy of $\pm$ 2.8 msec.) For analogue systems, the time constant chosen should be such that the accuracy specified is maintained. This cardiotachometer accuracy is specified because of the desirable feature described in Section B, paragraph 3. In addition, signals with a signal to noise ratio (SNR) > 10 must be accepted by the monitor.

(For our purposes SNR is defined as $\dfrac{\text{peak value of signal}}{\text{peak value of noise}}$.)

6. Have a direct uterine pressure monitoring system which covers the range 0 to 100 mm Hg with an accuracy of $\pm$ 1 per cent full scale. Sensitivity of the direct pressure transducers must be such that the minimum range 0 to 300 mm Hg can be covered; the frequency response for catheter/transducer system should be in the range 0 to 3 Hz and the volume coefficient should be as small as necessary to maintain specifications.

7. Provide an accurate method of calibration of both FHR and UP recording apparatus.

8. Have some means of displaying the FHR signal source. This may be accomplished with an oscilloscope or the source may be displayed on the recording paper.

9. Have an audio signal (with adjustable volume) to present the raw signal output (ECG, phonocardiogram or ultrasonogram) and a flashing light which could represent the output of the counting logic. The purpose here, especially when indirect monitoring is used, is to be able to hear the raw signal which would tend to persist even if the counting logic display was inaccurate or temporarily unavoidable.

10. Have numbered Z-folded recording paper for convenient handling and storage.

11. Have ECG pre-amplifier with the following minimum characteristics:

1. Minimum input range — 10 µV to 1 mV r.m.s.
2. Common mode rejection — > 80 dB from d.c. to 200 Hz
3. Linearity — better than 1 per cent
4. Frequency response — 0.15 to 150 Hz   within 3 dB for EKG
   1.5 to 60 Hz   within 3 dB for FHR trigger
5. Input impedance — Dependent upon cable type or length but larger than 2.5 MΩ
6. Noise — > 1 µV r.m.s. or 1.414 µV peak-to-peak at input with input connected to a 2 KΩ resistance.

NOTE. The effect of a given level of ultrasonic energy is unknown; therefore the total input power of an ultrasonic system should be limited to the minimal amount compatible with reasonable function.

Additional desirable features

1. A meter or digital display of FHR for comparison with the strip chart display.
2. An inkless recording system such as carbon, or hot stylus.
3. A design which permits integration into a larger systems approach, with signal available from the rear panel in an IRIG format for recording.
4. A pen lift option activated by switch.
5. A 0 to 200 mm Hg recording option for UP also activated by switch.
6. A means of representing negative catheter pressure due to pressure from fetal parts. Electrical zero offset is not enough.
7. A real time encoder for the strip chart recorder.

REFERENCES

Beard, R. W., Filshie, G. M., Knight, C. A. & Roberts, G. M. (1971) The significance of the changes in the continuous fetal heart rate in the first stage of labour. *Journal of Obstetrics and Gynaecology of the British Commonwealth,* **78,** 865–881.

Bishop, E. H. (1966) Obstetric uses of the ultrasonic motion sensor. *American Journal of Obstetrics and Gynecology,* **96,** 863–867.

Boehn, F. H. & Goss, D. A. (1973) The Xerox 400 telecopier and the fetal monitor. *Obstetrics and Gynecology,* **42,** 475–478.

Borell, U., Fernstrom, I., Ohlson, L. & Wigvist, N. (1965) Influence of uterine contractions of the uteroplacental blood flow at term. *American Journal of Obstetrics and Gynecology,* **93,** 44–57.

Donald, (1972) In *Obstetrics and Gynaecology Annual* (Ed.) Wynn, R. M. p. 248. ACC Meredith Corporation, New York.

Edington, P. T., Sibanda, J. & Beard, R. W. (1975) Influence of clinical practice of routine intra-partum fetal monitoring. *British Medical Journal,* **iii,** 341–343.

Freundlich, J. J. & Wingate, M. B. (1973) An evaluation of an external electromyographic system for recording uterine contractions during labour. *American Journal of Obstetrics and Gynecology,* **116,** 822–826.

Hammacher, K. (1969) The clinical significance of cardiotocography. In *Proceedings of the 1st Congress of Perinatal Medicine* (Ed.) Huntingford, P. J., Hüter & Saling, pp. 80–93. Stuttgart: Georg Thieme.

Haverkamp, A. & Bowes, W. A. (1971) Uterine perforation; a complication of continuous fetal monitoring. *American Journal of Obstetrics and Gynecology,* **110,** 667–669.

Hellman, K. M., Duffus, G. M., Donald, I. & Sunden, B. (1970) Safety of diagnostic ultrasound in obstetrics. *Lancet,* **i,** 1133–1137.

Hess, O. W. & Hon, E. H. (1960) The electronic evaluation of fetal heart rate. III. The effect of an oxytocic agent for induction of labour. *American Journal of Obstetrics and Gynecology,* **80,** 558–568.

Hon, E. H. (1968) *Atlas of Fetal Heart Rate Patterns.* New Haven, Connecticut: Harty Press.

Mannor, S. M., Serr, D. M., Tamari, I., Meshorer, A. & Frei, E. H. (1972) The safety of ultrasound in fetal monitoring. *American Journal of Obstetrics and Gynecology,* **113,** 653–666.

Mendez-Bauer, V., Fielitz, C. & Caldeyro-Barcia, R. (1961) Recording of intramuscular pressure in the human myometrium. *Journal of Applied Physiology,* **16,** 573–575.

Organ, L. W., Bernstein, A., Rowe, I. H. & Smith, K. C. (1973a) The pre-ejection period of the fetal heart: detection during labour with Doppler ultrasound. *American Journal of Obstetrics and Gynecology,* **115,** 369–376.

Organ, L. W., Milligan, J. E., Goodwin, J. W. & Bain, M. J. C. (1973b) The pre-ejection period of the fetal heart: response to stress in the term fetal lamb. *American Journal of Obstetrics and Gynecology,* **115,** 377–386.

Pardi, G., Bramizati, B., Dubini, S., Luchetti, D., Polvani, F. & Candiani, G. B. (1971) Analysis of the fetal ECG by the group averaging technique. In *Proceedings of the 2nd European Congress of Perinatal Medicine, London, 1970* (Ed.) Huntingford, P. J., Beard, R. W., Hytten, F. E. & Scopes, J. W. pp. 76–84, Basel: Karger.

Paul, R. H. (1973) Intrapartum fetal monitoring: current status and the future. *Obstetrical and Gynecological Survey*, Supplement, **28**, 453–459.

Paul, R. H. & Hon, E. H. (1970) A clinical fetal monitor (1). *Obstetrics and Gynecology*, **35**, 161–169.

Quilligan, E. J. (1972) The obstetrical intensive care unit. *Hospital Practice*, **7**, 61–69.

Rodrigues-Lima, J. & Montenegro, C. A. B. (1972) Tocometry in obstetric practice; The development of a pneumatic system. *American Journal of Obstetrics and Gynecology*, **112**, 304–307.

Saling, E. Z. & Dudenhausen, J. W. (1973) The present situation of clinical monitoring of the fetus during labour. *Journal of Perinatal Medicine*, **1**, 75–103.

Schneiderman, C. I., Waxman, B. & Goodman, C. J. (1972) Maternal–fetal ECG conduction with intrapartum fetal death. *American Journal of Obstetrics and Gynecology*, **113**, 1130–1133.

Serr, D. M. (1970) The uterus and cervix. In *Scientific Foundations of Obstetrics and Gynecology* (Ed.) Philipp, E., Barnes, J. & Newton, M. Section II, Ch. 2, pp. 65–80. London: Heinemann.

Serr, D. M. (1972) Methods and problems of fetal heart monitoring. *International Journal of Gynaecology and Obstetrics*, **10**, 186–190.

Serr, D. M., Porath-Furedi, A., Rabau, E., Zakut, H. & Mannor, S. M. (1968a) Recording of electrical activity from the human cervix. *Journal of Obstetrics and Gynaecology of the British Commonwealth*, **75**, 369–363.

Serr, D. M., Zakut, H., Rabau, E. & Mannor, S. M. (1968b) Observations of the fetal electrocardiogram in postmaturity. *Israel Journal of Medical Sciences*, **4**, 949–952.

Serr, D. M., Mannor, S. M., Ron, A., Rabau, E., Zakut, H. & Schaudinishky, L. (1969) Phonocardiography in fetal heart monitoring. In *Proceedings of the 1st Congress of Perinatal Medicine* (Ed.) Huntingford, Huter & Saling, pp. 99–107. Stuttgart: Georg Thieme.

Serr, D. M., Padeh, B., Zakut, H., Shaki, R., Mannor, S. M. & Kallner, B. (1971) Studies on the effects of ultrasonic waves on the fetus. In *Proceedings of the 2nd European Congress of Perinatal Medicine, London, 1970* (Ed.) Huntingford, P. J., Beard, R. W. & Scopes, J. P. pp. 302–307. Basel: Karger.

Shenker, L. (1973) Clinical experiences with fetal heart rate monitoring of one thousand patients in labor. *American Journal of Obstetrics and Gynecology*, **115**, 1111–1116.

Smyth, C. N. (1973) Biomechanics of uterine action. *Lancet*, **i**, 208–209.

Sureau, C., Chavinie, J. & Cannon, M. (1967) Some technical aspects of fetal electrocardiography. *Proceedings of the 7th International Conference of Medical Biology and Engineering, Stockholm*, p. 146.

Symonds, E. M. (1971) Configuration of the fetal ECG in relation to fetal acid–base balance and plasma electrolytes. *Journal of Obstetrics and Gynaecology of the British Commonwealth*, **78**, 957–970.

Thieme, Y. & Eichmeier, J. (1971) Ein Verfahren zur Registrierung der fetalen Herzschlagfrequenz aus dem abdominalen Elektrokardiogramm. *Biomedizinische Technik*, **16**, 173–175.

Unger, F. W. & Goodwin, J. W. (1972) Instrumentation for fetal electrocardiography and intrauterine pressure. A new scalp electrode and radiotelemetry system. *American Journal of Obstetrics and Gynecology*, **112**, 351–357.

Wolfs, G., Van Leeuwen, M., Rottinghuis, H. & Boeles, J. Th. F. (1971) An electromyographic study of the human uterus during labour. *Obstetrics and Gynecology*, **37**, 241–246.

Index